HEALTH SYSTEM MANAGEMENT
and LEADERSHIP
for PHYSICAL
and OCCUPATIONAL THERAPISTS

HEALTH SYSTEM MANAGEMENT and LEADERSHIP

for PHYSICAL and OCCUPATIONAL THERAPISTS

EDITED BY

William R. VanWye, PT, DPT, PhD
Associate Professor
School of Physical Therapy
Florida Southern College
Lakeland, Florida
United States

Dianna Lunsford, OTD, MEd, OTR/L, CHT
Program Director, Professor
Occupational Therapy Doctorate
Gannon University
Ruskin, Florida
United States

ELSEVIER

Elsevier
3251 Riverport Lane
St. Louis, Missouri 63043

Notice

Practitioners and researchers must always rely on their own experience and knowledge in evaluating and
using any information, methods, compounds or experiments described herein. Because of rapid advances
in the medical sciences, in particular, independent verification of diagnoses and drug dosages should be
made. To the fullest extent of the law, no responsibility is assumed by Elsevier, authors, editors or
contributors for any injury and/or damage to persons or property as a matter of products liability,
negligence or otherwise, or from any use or operation of any methods, products, instructions, or ideas
contained in the material herein.

Content Strategist: Lauren Willis
Content Development Specialist: Priyadarshini Pandey
Publishing Services Manager: Deepthi Unni
Senior Project Manager: Manchu Mohan
Design Direction: Margaret M. Reid

Printed in India.

Last digit is the print number: 9   8   7   6   5   4   3   2   1

Working together
to grow libraries in
developing countries

www.elsevier.com • www.bookaid.org

To the future generations of physical and occupational therapy students: we hope you embrace your role as a healthcare provider and team member, as you will one day lead our profession.

Contributors

David L. Bell, PT, DPT, PhD, OCS, MTC, Cert DN
Assistant Professor
Physical Therapy
Western Kentucky University
Bowling Green, Kentucky

Jessica Bender, PT, EdD, PCS
Assistant Clinical Professor
Physical Therapy and Athletic Training
Northern Arizona University
Flagstaff, Arizona

Stephanie L. Bonk, OTD, OTR/L
Doctoral Capstone Coordinator/Assistant Professor
Occupational Therapy
Concordia University Wisconsin
Mequon, Wisconsin

Tammy Bruegger, OTD, MSED, OTR/L, ATP
Assistant Professor
Occupational Therapy
Rockhurst University;
Assistive Technology Practitioner
Occupational Therapy
The Children's Center for the Visually Impaired
Kansas City, Missouri

Kimberly Angel Bryant, OTD, OTR/L
Adjunct Instructor
Division of Occupational Therapy
Medical University of South Carolina
Charleston, South Carolina

Amy L. Brzuz, OTD, OTR/L
Occupational Therapy
Gannon University
Erie, Pennsylvania

Deborah Elgin Budash, PhD, OTR/L
Assistant Professor
Occupational Therapy
The University of Scranton
Scranton, Pennsylvania

Meredith Burd, OTR/L, MOT, MBA, CBIS
Director
Rehabilitation Services Center of Expertise
OSF HealthCare
Peoria, Illinois

Blair Carsone, PhD, MOT, OTR/L
Assistant Professor
Occupational Therapy
Gannon University
Ruskin, Florida

Jennifer Castelli, OTD, OTR/L, CHT
Academic Fieldwork Coordinator
Assistant Professor Occupational Therapy Doctorate Program
Gannon University
Ruskin, Florida

Sarah Corcoran, OTD, OTR/L
Assistant Professor
Occupational Therapy
Saint Joseph's University
Philadelphia, Pennsylvania

Carl DeRosa PT, DPT, PhD, FAPTA
Clinical Professor and Program Director
DPT Hybrid Program
Northern Arizona University
Flagstaff, Arizona

Karen Dishman, OTD, OTR, ATP
Assistant Professor
Occupational Therapy
Gannon University
Ruskin, Florida

Sarah Doerrer, PhD, OTR/L, CHT, CLT
Assistant Professor
School of Medicine and Health Sciences
George Washington University
Washington, District of Columbia

Steven D. Eberth, OTD, OTR/L, CDP, CFPS
Associate Professor
Occupational Therapy
Bradley University
Peoria, Illinois

Jennifer Edwards, MSPT
Chief Therapy Officer
Therapy
Reunion Rehabilitation Hospital–Denver
Denver, Colorado

Michele Favolise, PT, DPT, CFE
Associate Professor
Division of Physical Therapy
American International College
Springfield, Massachusetts

Carla Floyd-Slabaugh, DOT, OTR/L, CBIS
Assistant Professor
Occupational Science and Therapy
Grand Valley State University
Grand Rapids, Michigan

Matthew B. Garber, PT, DSc, OCS, FAAOMPT
Associate Professor and Assistant Director of Clinical Education
Department of Health, Human Function, and Rehabilitation
The George Washington University
Washington, District of Columbia

Melissa Goodman, PT, DPT, NCS
Assistant Teaching Professor
Physical Therapy
Gannon University
Ruskin, Florida

Aileen Gorman, MOT, OTR/L
Occupational Therapist, Clinical Coordinator of Inpatient
　Occupational Therapy
Occupational Therapy
Froedtert Pleasant Prairie Hospital
Pleasant Prairie, Wisconsin

Janice Hanshaw, MOT, OTR/L
Quality and Education Coordinator
Rehabilitation Services Center of Expertise
OSF HealthCare
Peoria, Illinois

Jeff Hartman, DPT, MPH
Assistant Professor, Doctor of Physical Therapy (DPT) Program
Department of Family Medicine and Community Health
University of Wisconsin School of Medicine and Public
　Health
Madison, Wisconsin

Julia Hawkins-Pokabla, OTD, OTR/L
Assistant Professor
Department of Occupational Therapy
Gannon University
Erie, Pennsylvania

Brandon Koehler, PT, DPT, PhD, MBA
Assistant Professor
Physical Therapy
The University of Findlay
Findlay, Ohio

Renée Lach-Sharon, PT, GCS, CEEAA, MSCS, CPHQ
Manager of Therapy Clinical and Quality Services
Home Office
Rehab Without Walls
Louisville, Kentucky

Patricia Laverdure, OTD, OTR/L, BCP, FAOTA
Assistant Professor, Program Director
Occupational Therapy
Old Dominion University
Norfolk, Virginia

Bridgette LeCompte, MS, OTR/L
Assistant Professor
Division of Occupational Science and Occupational Therapy
UNC Chapel Hill
Chapel Hill, North Carolina;
Consultant for Occupational Therapy
Department of Public Instruction
Raleigh, North Carolina

Dianna Lunsford, OTD, MEd, OTR/L, CHT
Program Director, Professor
Occupational Therapy Doctorate
Gannon University
Ruskin, Florida

Rose L. McAndrew, OTD, OTR/L, CHT
Assistant Professor Occupational Therapy Assistant Program
Saint Louis Community College
Saint Louis, Missouri

Patricia A. Meyers, OTD, OTR/L
Director and Associate Professor
Division of Occupational Therapy
American International College
Springfield, Massachusetts

Amy Estes Miller, PT, DPT
Physical Therapist
Special Education
Williamsburg–James City County Public Schools
Williamsburg, Virginia

Daniel Miller, MSPT, MBA
Director of Quality and Operational Policy
LHC Group, LLC
Newnan, Georgia

Mica Mitchell, PT, DPT
Assistant Professor
Physical Therapy
College of Saint Mary
Omaha, Nebraska

Karen Mueller, PT, DPT, PhD, NBC-HWC
Clinical Professor and Professor Emerita
Physical Therapy and Athletic Training
Northern Arizona University
Flagstaff, Arizona

Sarah Nechvatal, PT, DPT
Physical Therapist
Physical Therapy Department
UW Health University Hospital
Madison, Wisconsin

Tracey E. Recigno, OTD, OTR/L
Program Director and Assistant Professor
Occupational Therapy Program – Honolulu
Hawaii Pacific University
Honolulu, Hawaii

Theresa Rhett-Davis, EdD, OTR/L
Assistant Professor/Vice Chair
Occupational Therapy
Saint Joseph's University
Philadelphia, Pennsylvania

Amber Richardson, OTR/L, CHES, OMS
Community Relations Manager
Therapy Services
Pate Rehabilitation
Dallas, Texas;
Occupational Therapist
Therapy Services
Medical City
Fort Worth, Texas

Eileen Scanlon, OTD, MBA, OTR/L, CHT
Assistant Professor and Program Director
Occupational Therapy
Shenandoah University
Winchester, Virginia

Amanda Scott, OTD, OTR, BCG, CADDCT-CDP, CLT
Department Chair/Assistant Professor
Occupational Therapy
Bradley University
Peoria, Illinois

Cristina Reyes Smith, OTD, OTR/L, FAOTA
Assistant Professor and Admissions Director
Department of Rehabilitation Sciences Division of
    Occupational Therapy
Medical University of South Carolina College of Health
    Professions
Charleston, South Carolina

Rachael Frakes Spann, MOT, OTR/L, CDIS
Corporate Director of Patient Outcomes
Operations
Nobis Rehabilitation Partners
Allen, Texas

Melissa K. Travelsted, DNP, APRN, FNP-C, PTA, AANP
Associate Professor
School of Nursing and Allied Health
Western Kentucky University
Bowling Green, Kentucky

Scott Truskowski, PhD, OTR/L, ACUE
Associate Professor and Chair
Occupational Science and Therapy Department
Grand Valley State University
Grand Rapids, Michigan

Jonathan Ulrich, PT, DPT, OCS
Assistant Teaching Professor
Doctor of Physical Therapy Program
Gannon University
Erie, Pennsylvania

William R. VanWye, PT, DPT, PhD
Associate Professor
School of Physical Therapy
Florida Southern College
Lakeland, Florida

Jamie S. Way, PhD, DPT
Assistant Professor
Physical Therapy
Bradley University
Peoria, Illinois

Lauren Wengerd, PhD, MS, OTR/L
Assistant Professor
College of Medicine, Division of Neurological Surgery
The Ohio State University
Columbus, Ohio

Brett Windsor, PT, MPA, PhD
Clinical Professor
Physical Therapy
Northern Arizona University
Flagstaff, Arizona

Preface

This textbook delivers entry-level information from an outstanding group of experienced clinicians and educators, lending us their experience in health system management and leadership. This book was inspired by the need to provide physical and occupational therapy educators and students with a comprehensive text on health system management and leadership. The book has 21 chapters, divided into four parts: (I) Healthcare Systems and Policy, (II) Professional Conduct (III) Healthcare Management and Entrepreneurship, and (IV) Healthcare Settings.

Part I includes Chapters 1–4. Chapter 1, US Healthcare Service Systems, provides the historical origins of the US healthcare system and explains how complex and diverse conditions led to today's trillion-dollar healthcare industry. Chapter 2, Health Legislation, Laws, Policy, and Advocacy, details key US healthcare legislation, laws, and policies, as well as how advocacy can impact healthcare legislation, regulations, and procedures for the betterment of society. Chapter 3, Proposal and Grant Writing, outlines methods for writing proposals and applying for grants to finance and implement systematic improvement. Finally, Chapter 4, Current Issues in Healthcare: Barriers & Strategies, examines contemporary issues and trends and provides strategies for generating change and group development.

Part II includes Chapters 5–10. Chapter 5, Core Values and Ethical Implications, explores ethics and core values as a guide for personal and professional behaviors, organizations' mission and vision statements, and decision-making. Chapter 6, Professionalism, Professional Development, and Mentorship, details the importance of physical and occupational therapists as professionals, including professional development, reflective practice, and mentorship. Chapter 7, Interprofessionalism, describes how professionals from different disciplines collaborate as a team, working toward optimal outcomes.

Chapter 8, Diversity, Equity, and Inclusion, emphasizes that diversity, equity, and inclusion (DEI) operate at the macro-, meso-, and micro-system levels and offers a lens to understand the negative and positive impacts of social capital and DEI. Chapter 9, Communication With Clients and Providers, examines how therapists can successfully build rapport, interview clients, educate caregivers, collaborate with other healthcare providers, protect private health information, improve health literacy, and support those with various primary languages. Finally, Chapter 10, Leadership, presents physical and occupational therapy students with an understanding of leadership as the ethical, mindful application of a person's identity, strengths, and values.

Part III includes Chapters 11–14. Chapter 11, Healthcare Management and Administration, delves into the skills expected of healthcare managers to meet organizational goals and therapy staff needs. Chapter 12, Quality Assurance Performance Improvement, provides a means to assess the quality of a healthcare system regarding the structures and processes that affect outcomes. Chapter 13, Fundamentals of Insurance and Billing, explores various third-party payers and their documentation requirements and procedures to receive payment. Finally, Chapter 14, Starting a Business and Entrepreneurship, highlights points to consider when deciding to go into business for oneself and discover common qualities in entrepreneurs.

Part IV includes Chapters 15–21. This section describes the most common settings where physical and occupational therapists work. Each healthcare setting has unique accreditation standards, regulations, patient population, services, and setting characteristics. Although managers and administrators have similar responsibilities, each setting requires specific skills due to differences in reimbursement models, documentation, and quality improvement efforts. In addition, this section discusses discharge planning, care coordination, and case management, which are critical to reducing care fragmentation, inefficiencies, and costs.

William R. VanWye, PT, DPT, PhD
Dianna Lunsford, OTD, MEd, OTR/L, CHT

Acknowledgments

We want to thank the authors who made valuable contributions to this textbook. Your time and effort invested reflect your passion and commitment to future generations of physical and occupational therapists.

Contents

7 Interprofessionalism, 113
Patricia A. Meyers, OTD, OTR/L;
and Michele Favolise, PT, DPT, CFE

8 Diversity, Equity, and Inclusion, 125
Theresa Rhett-Davis, EdD, OTR/L;
and Sarah Corcoran, OTD, OTR/L

**9 Communication With Clients
and Providers, 141**
Matthew B. Garber, PT, DSc, OCS, FAAOMPT;
and Julia Hawkins-Pokabla, OTD, OTR/L

10 Leadership, 158
Sarah Corcoran, OTD, OTR/L; Tracey E. Recigno, OTD, OTR/L;
and William R. Vanwye, PT, DPT, PhD

Part III: Healthcare Management and Entrepreneurship

**11 Healthcare Management and
Administration, 177**
Scott Truskowski, PhD, OTR/L, ACUE;
and William R. Vanwye, PT, DPT, PhD

**12 Quality Assurance Performance
Improvement, 197**
Steven D. Eberth, OTD, OTR/L, CDP, CFPS;
and Amanda Scott, OTD, OTR, BCG, CADDCT-CDP, CLT

13 Fundamentals of Insurance and Billing, 207
Amanda Scott, OTD, OTR, BCG, CADDCT-CDP, CLT;
and Jamie S. Way, PhD, DPT

14 Starting a Business and Entrepreneurship, 228
Jennifer Castelli, OTD, OTR/L, CHT;
and Brett Windsor, PT, MPA, PhD

1

United States Healthcare Service Systems

EILEEN SCANLON OTD, MBA, OTR/L, CHT;
and BRANDON KOEHLER, PT, DPT, PhD, MBA

LEARNING OBJECTIVES

By the end of this chapter, the reader will be able to:

1. Differentiate health from healthcare.
2. Describe the healthcare system structure in the United States preindustrial era.
3. Recognize the influence of historical events on healthcare innovations and coverage.
4. Explain the impact of disease on United States public health policy.
5. Appreciate how political influences such as capitalism impact healthcare systems.
6. Summarize how the large insurance companies emerged in the United States.
7. Describe historical and contemporary health disparities in the United States.

CHAPTER OUTLINE

Introduction to Health and Healthcare

The World Health Organization (WHO) defines health as "a state of complete physical, mental and social wellbeing and not merely the absence of disease or infirmity" (World Health Organization, 2022). Health is heavily impacted by individual choices such as diet, exercise, smoking, alcohol consumption, seeking timely care, and avoiding risky behaviors. However, social factors have a significant impact on health as well. These factors are commonly referred to as the social determinants of health (SDOH),

which can be grouped into five domains: economic stability, education access and quality, healthcare access and quality, neighborhood and built environment, and social and community context (*Social Determinants of Health - Healthy People 2030*, n.d.). For example, factors such as access to healthy food, affordable housing, safe communities, and healthcare services can significantly impact health beyond genetics and individual choices (Table 1.1). Thus to achieve health, healthcare must move beyond the focus on medical care to a complete approach that also addresses the SDOH.

TABLE 1.1	Factors Impacting United States Healthcare	
Social Determinants of Health	• Socioeconomic factors
Affordability	• Increased costs placed on the patient
Availability and Accessibility	• Taking time off, clinic hours • Difficulty getting an appointment, finding a provider
Acceptability	• The provider would not accept health insurance
Communication	• Health literacy, culture, perception, comprehension, semantics
Disability	• Bias, inconvenient scheduling, lack of accessible equipment, lack of transportation
Race	• Race-based medicine should be replaced by race-conscious healthcare • Race is a social construct; it is not biological
Sex	• Clinical trials have not enrolled women or analyzed sex-specific differences in the data

From Cerdeña, J. P., Plaisime, M. V., & Tsai, J. (2020). From race-based to race-conscious medicine: How anti-racist uprisings call us to act. *The Lancet, 396*(10257), 1125–1128; Centers for Disease Control and Prevention (2019). *Common barriers to participation experienced by people with disabilities.* https://www.cdc.gov/ncbddd/disabilityandhealth/disability-barriers.html; Garber, M., & Boissonnault, W. G. (2021). The patient interview: the science behind the art of skillful communication. In W. G. Boissonnault & W. R. VanWye (Eds.), *Primary care for the physical therapist: examination and triage*. Elsevier; Kullgren, J. T., McLaughlin, C. G., Mitra, N., & Armstrong, K. (2012). Nonfinancial barriers and access to care for U.S. adults. *Health Services Research, 47*(1 Pt 2), 462–485; Liu, K. A., & Mager, N. A. D. (2016). Women's involvement in clinical trials: Historical perspective and future implications. *Pharmacy Practice, 14*(1), 708; US Department of Health and Human Services. *Social Determinants of Health—Healthy People 2030.* (n.d.). https://health.gov/healthypeople/priority-areas/social-determinants-health.

Healthcare Systems

A common question in the United States and worldwide is whether healthcare is a right (Fig. 1.1). Indeed, the WHO considers healthcare a fundamental human right (World Health Organization, 2017). Thus the WHO advocates for Universal Health Care (UHC) to provide access to health services for those who need them, when and where they need them, and without financial hardship (World Health Organization, 2022). UHC includes what is covered and how it is paid. What is covered in UHC includes a full range of essential health services (Box 1.1). How it is covered differs by country, but two common methods are socialized medicine and a single-payer system. Socialized medicine is government-owned and operated healthcare, while a single payer system is when one entity pays for healthcare via a tax-financed system with care provided by private nonprofit providers (Liu & Brook, 2017).

Each nation's healthcare system reflects its history, politics, economy, and national values. Learning about healthcare systems provides a background for cultural competence, advocacy, customer service, and risk management. Also, it helps to clarify differences and reduce bias. Table 1.2 provides an overview of selected global healthcare systems for comparison and the United States equivalent.

Historical Overview of the United States Healthcare System

Introduction

Healthcare in the United States is a complex system influenced by various factors such as culture, politics, science,

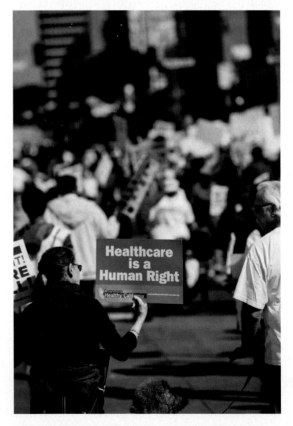

• **Fig. 1.1** Is healthcare a right? (From: https://www.flickr.com/photos/51008844@N03/35500888206)

and geography. The United States healthcare system has advanced over time and has grown into a trillion-dollar industry (American Medical Association, 2023). An overview of the evolution of healthcare is worth reviewing to gain insights into the healthcare systems in place today.

•BOX 1.1   The WHO's 16 Essential Health Services

- Reproductive, maternal, newborn, and child health:
  - family planning
  - antenatal and delivery care
  - full child immunization
  - health-seeking behavior for pneumonia
- Infectious diseases:
  - tuberculosis treatment
  - HIV antiretroviral treatment
  - use of insecticide-treated bed nets for malaria prevention
  - adequate sanitation
- Noncommunicable diseases:
  - prevention and treatment of raised blood pressure
  - prevention and treatment of raised blood glucose
  - cervical cancer screening
  - tobacco (non)smoking
- Service capacity and access:
  - basic hospital access
  - health worker density
  - access to essential medicines
  - health security: compliance with the International Health Regulations

From World Health Organization. *Universal health coverage (UHC)*. (2022). <https://www.who.int/news-room/fact-sheets/detail/universal-health-coverage-(uhc)>

United States Healthcare Origins: Part 1

Medical care was not widely available for early United States settlers, leaving many to rely on homemade preparations to treat health-related issues (McCulla, 2016). Given the difficulty in obtaining medical care, settlers may have gone long periods without physician treatment (Fig. 1.2). However, as urban centers grew due to immigration and urbanization, the accessibility of physicians improved. Health insurance was unavailable and services were purchased with currency or bartered goods. As such, it was mostly those in the professional classes who could afford the services of a physician (McCulla, 2016). In rural areas, physicians were likely to accept alternative forms of payment to currency, including agricultural staples, linens, or labor.

Resources to care for the sick and vulnerable were limited due in part to a small supply of educated physicians and few schools to teach medicine. Medical education in colonial times consisted primarily of an apprenticeship as opposed to the type of medical education found today at institutions of higher education (Rothstein, 1987). During this period, students who did receive formal training attended lectures over a few semesters and participated in apprenticeships alongside a local physician, with few clinical training requirements (Harvard Medical School, 2022). As of 1800, there were four medical schools in the United States, which included the College of Philadelphia (1765; later becoming the University of Pennsylvania School of Medicine), King's College (1767; later becoming Columbia University), Harvard Medical School (1782), and the Geisel School of Medicine at Dartmouth College (1797) (*About the Geisel School of Medicine*, n.d.; *Brief History: School of Medicine*, n.d.; *Harvard Medical School*, 2022; *The History of Columbia University*, n.d.).

The number of institutions providing medical training programs increased substantially over a 100-year period and by 1860 there were 47 medical schools in the United States (Rothstein, 1987). As the number of medical school graduates increased, the standard degree that indicated a physician's knowledge and skills became the Doctor of Medicine (MD) (Shi & Singh, 2019). Despite the growth of medical training, medical education in the early 1800s was lacking in the type of clinically based scientific training that we are familiar with today. Early United States medical schools often did not have laboratories, but rather operated out of a main building with multiple lecture halls (Rothstein, 1987). Instructors had minimal training in teaching and primarily theoretical medical education was provided, with an apprenticeship providing the clinical practice portion of the

TABLE 1.2 Global Healthcare Systems and United States Equivalent

Country, System, and Model	Who Provides	Who Pays	United States Equivalent
Canada • Single payer • National health insurance model	• Private hospitals and clinics	• Government-run insurance funded by taxes	• Medicare
Germany • Nonprofit or social insurance system • Bismarck model	• Private hospitals and clinics	• "Sickness funds" financed by employers and employees	• Employer-based insurance plans
Great Britain • Socialist • Beveridge model	• Government-owned hospitals and clinic	• Government via taxes	• Veterans Health Administration
• **Out-of-Pocket Model**	• Private providers	• The patient	• Uninsured

From *Health Care Systems - Four Basic Models* (2008). Physicians for a National Health Program. https://www.pnhp.org/single_payer_resources/health_care_systems_four_basic_models.php; Wallace, L. S. (2013). A View of Health Care Around the World. *Annals of Family Medicine*, *11*(1), 84.

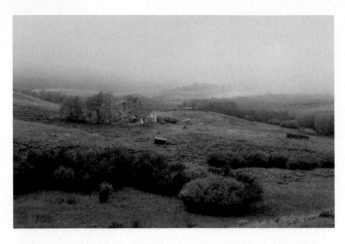

• **Fig. 1.2** Even today, rural living limits access to healthcare. (From: https://commons.wikimedia.org/w/index.php?curid=95419289)

training (Rothstein, 1987). This was not the case in Europe, as medical schools utilized laboratory-based research and professors were often expected to conduct research and teach (Shi & Singh, 2019). The curriculum of medical schools in the late 1700s and early 1800s included a number of foundational scientific subjects, including anatomy, physiology, chemistry, and possibly some other natural sciences, along with subjects related to the practice of medicine, such as medicine, surgery, midwifery, and a course that combined medical science and clinical practice called Materia Medica (Rothstein, 1987). Despite an increase in the number of medical schools, students also participated in educational activities outside of those affiliated with a medical school, including apprenticeships (which may have been required by the medical school) and private courses.

Since the early practice of medicine did not require licensing, board certification, or a degree from a medical school, there were minimal restrictions in the United States on other professions providing medical care, making entry into the medical profession relatively easy compared with today's standards of education and licensing (Shi & Singh, 2019). This created opposition between those who claimed to be medical providers. As such, the medical profession was not well organized and physicians did not necessarily have financial security and influence. It was not uncommon for physicians who could not make ends meet with their medical practices to have to take on other occupations to supplement their income.

In the early 1800s, advances in medicine, such as anesthesia, had not been developed, and tools to help with diagnosis and treatment, such as stethoscopes, thermometers, antiseptic techniques, and radiographs, were not well-known or had yet to be invented (Shi & Singh, 2017, 2019). In the early to middle part of the 1800s, the United States did not have many hospitals and those in existence were mainly found in larger urban areas. There were several types of facilities available to care for individuals who lived by themselves, had no one else to care for them in their household,

or who were homeless or poor. These facilities included the previously mentioned hospitals, as well as almshouses (poorhouses), asylums, pesthouses, and dispensaries (Rothstein, 1987). Almshouses were run by local governments and acted as places to shelter and provide basic care for a variety of individuals, including the elderly, homeless, orphaned children, ill, and individuals who were disabled. These accommodations provided patients with food, shelter, and basic medical care. Once the community in which an almshouse was located grew large enough to warrant more specialized housing and care for individuals with different medical needs, asylums, pesthouses, dispensaries, and hospitals were built (Rothstein, 1987).

State and local governments built asylums for patients who needed treatment for mental illness (Rothstein, 1987). Due to different ideas about the causes and treatment of mental illness, treatment in the 1800s took different forms, many of which proved not to be effective (Walston & Johnson, 2021). Local governments utilized pesthouses for individuals with contagious diseases to shield the population from further spread of diseases and prevent epidemics from forming in the communities (Rothstein, 1987). Dispensaries were outpatient clinics for those unable to pay for medical services. They may have been independent or associated with a hospital and tended to be rather successful in recruiting young physicians as a means of providing clinical training. Dispensaries also acted as a first resort for medical care compared with hospitals. Hospitals in early America did not have the image they do today, largely because mortality rates were exceedingly high (Pozgar, 2016). Hospitals during this time were poorly resourced, employed staff with little training, had unsanitary conditions, and lacked proper ventilation. Patients often opted to be treated in their homes or if possible in a physician's office (Rothstein, 1987).

United States Healthcare Origins: Part 2

The period from the late 1800s to the 2000s saw significant advances in the education and practice of medicine, along with an increase in the prominence of the medical profession and those who serve in it. The expansion of many urban areas in the United States, educational reform, and key scientific discoveries occurred during this time in United States history, with benefits gained in the quality of healthcare offered in the country.

The United States economy underwent a period of transition after the Civil War, with a rapid increase in technological advancement in many areas of life and changes to industry that led to the movement of people from the farmlands to the cities. Physicians also moved to urban areas, bringing them closer to the growing number of people in need of their services (Shi & Singh, 2017). As a result, the distance and effort needed to travel to be seen by a physician decreased for those living in cities and technological advancements helped make medical treatment more accessible and affordable.

As developments in science and medical-surgical care continued to advance, so did improvements in hospital sanitary practices, diagnostic techniques, and treatment practices (Shi & Singh, 2017). With this increase in scientific and technological advancements came benefits such as antiseptic surgery, anesthesia, immunology, diagnostic techniques such as radiography, and medicines such as penicillin. Further research and clinical practice with patients who had specific medical problems led to the specialization of physician practice starting in the late 1800s. The advancement of specialty practice was influenced in part by the practice in European hospitals (Rothstein, 1987). As European physicians began to be known for their specialized knowledge in certain areas of medicine, thousands of American physicians (as well as physicians from other countries) traveled to study with these renowned specialists, taking postgraduate courses. One major disadvantage of this rapid advancement was that the significant increase in specialization added to the growing cost associated with medical care.

The number of hospitals grew substantially from the late 1800s to the 2000s, from a few hospitals in the late 1800s to 6093 hospitals operating in the United States in 2020 (American Hospital Association, 2022). On August 13, 1946, a piece of legislation known as the Hill-Burton Act, or more formally called the Hospital Survey and Construction Act, was signed into law by President Harry S. Truman (Schumann, 2016). This act was intended as a way to address the need for more hospitals in the United States and in order to do so it provided a means for the distribution of federal funds to the states for the purpose of building hospitals based on the needs of the communities in each state (Longest Jr., 2016). It has been said that the Hill-Burton Act was responsible for a sizable increase in the number of hospital facilities in the United States during the 20th century.

As a result of scientific improvements and increased numbers, hospitals became centers for delivering many different healthcare services (Shi & Singh, 2017). As medical science advanced, the ability of hospitals to house expensive medical equipment helped them to become centers for the diagnosis and care of individuals in need of surgery, acute care, and specialized services. The relationship between hospitals and physicians continued to grow as they depended on each other for mutual success. Physicians needed the resources that hospitals could provide as well as a place for their patients to be treated if it was not suitable to treat them in their offices or patients' homes and the hospitals needed patient referrals from physicians (Shi & Singh, 2019).

Medical education reform began in the late 1800s and the number of medical schools and medical school graduates increased substantially between 1860 and 1900. Medical schools grew in number from 47 schools in 1860 to 160 schools in 1900 (Rothstein, 1987). Furthermore, the number of students attending and graduating from medical schools increased from less than 2000 graduates in 1870 to over 5000 graduates and 25,000 students in 1900. Admissions and licensure requirements began to change with new state licensing laws, starting around the 1880s, as a high school diploma or college degree became a prerequisite to admission and licensure examinations became more prevalent.

The structure of medical schools also changed with term lengths increasing from 4 months to 7 months and new classes and laboratory studies were added to accommodate the increased interests of students (Rothstein, 1987). Clinical faculty members who worked for hospitals, private clinics, and dispensaries were hired, although they may not have been granted the same privileges as full-time faculty at the schools. Additionally, the length of medical education increased significantly as more clinical and specialty courses that students used to seek from private instructors were added to the medical curriculum. Some medical schools began to offer 3-year graded courses starting in 1871; however, this became common practice after 1891 once the National Conference of State Medical Examining and Licensing Boards began to require students to obtain degrees from schools with 3-year graded courses for licensure (Rothstein, 1987). Shortly after, the 3-year graded course requirement was moved to a 4-year requirement. A consequence of longer terms and graded courses was an increase in the cost of medical education, thereby creating a barrier for lower-income students from being able to obtain a degree to practice medicine.

Over the first half of the 1900s, the number of medical schools decreased from 162 schools in 1906 to 77 schools in 1940, and while the number of students decreased from over 25,000 in 1906 to just under 14,000 in 1920, enrollment rebounded to over 21,000 students in 1940 (Rothstein, 1987). The curriculum was standardized starting in the early 1900s with basic science courses such as anatomy, physiology, biochemistry, pathology (basic and clinical), bacteriology, and pharmacology making up the first 2 years of schooling, and general medicine and specialty clinical courses making up the final 2 years. After 1950, the number of undergraduate medical schools and students saw a resurgence, with 127 medical schools and over 67,000 students enrolled in 1983. Affiliations between hospitals and medical schools became more common in the 1900s, largely as a means of providing educational opportunities to students and clinical practice opportunities to the faculty.

The journey of a student through the United States medical education system in the early 21st century now entails movement from premedical training that typically involves 4 years of undergraduate coursework at a college or university, followed by 3 to 4 years of medical school training in a graduate program (Mowery, 2015). The medical school curriculum is similar to that described previously, with the first 1 to 2 years devoted to basic and medical science coursework, followed by 2 years of clinical coursework and experiences in different medical specialties and fields. Medical licensure exams, residency, and specialty training are completed after medical school, with varying durations of postgraduate training based on a physician's chosen specialty.

Nursing education also underwent significant change in the 20th century, as training in theoretical subjects increased during the early part of the 1900s (Pozgar, 2016).

The American Medical Association (AMA) was founded in 1847, in some part due to the increased number of medical school graduates (Harvard Medical School, 2020;

Rothstein, 1987). The AMA's influence increased when it placed its members into county and state medical societies and began to exert control over medical education. In 1904, the AMA put together a Council on Medical Education and in 1905 this council created educational standards for medical schools that included such things as admissions, course length, and licensure examination performance standards (Rothstein, 1987; Smith, 2020). It then ranked medical schools based on an inspection of each school in relation to the standards that had been set. These reports were later published in the AMA's journal, giving descriptions and licensure examination results for each of the medical schools. Large-scale medical school inspections by the Council on Medical Education continued for a few years, but were then replaced by individual inspections that were used as a means to improve a school's functioning. Eventually, the Association of American Medical Colleges became the agency responsible for the standardization of medical education in the United States by the Federation of State Medical Boards. The AMA has been very active in the medical profession, including such activities as the pursuit of the establishment of state medical licensing laws that made it illegal to practice medicine without a state license, and supporting state laws that required students graduate from an AMA accredited school in order to obtain licensure (Johnson & Chaudhry, 2012; Shi & Singh, 2017).

Social Influences on United States Healthcare

Influence of War

The greatest changes, innovations, and practices in United States healthcare occurred out of necessity (Fig. 1.3). Wars pushed the United States government to become involved in healthcare and respond to the health-related needs of the soldiers and, eventually, the citizens. The War of 1812 resulted in the development of the first Naval Hospital in Philadelphia to care for disabled veterans (United States Department of Veterans [USDVA], 2023). This led to several other major cities developing facilities to care for veterans' health. The Civil War resulted in massive casualties that demanded a widespread response from the government. President Lincoln's second inaugural address acknowledged the need for the government to care for the injured and disabled soldiers injured in the civil war (Library of Congress, 2022). During and after the Civil War, multiple national programs arose to care for the union soldier veterans; however, the

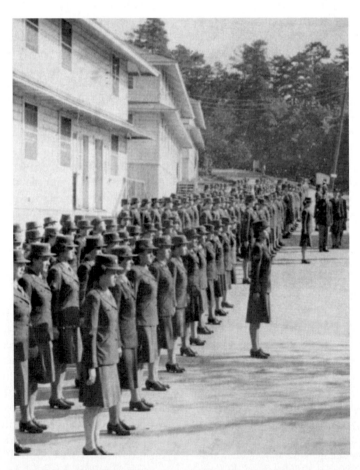

• **Fig. 1.3** Wars produced several important healthcare advances, including the creation of reconstruction aides who would become occupational and physical therapists shown. (https://www.flickr.com/photos/75426880@N06/7222897514)

focus of these programs was mainly housing (called national asylums) or pensions (Gorman, 2012; USDVA, 2021). Caring for the veterans' health arose organically in these national residential asylums, and eventually, specialized asylums emerged to care for the health of the veterans (National Park Service, 2017). Providing medical care through a government-funded policy to veterans set a precedent that would have big implications for the country's veterans and the public.

World War I (WWI) perhaps brought about the most significant and orchestrated involvement of the national government in healthcare (National Institute of Health, 2011). As discussed, there were some federally funded healthcare programs for veterans; however, veterans' programs, public health, and social welfare initiatives were managed by the city, state, church, and private organizations (Loiacono, 2017).

Shifting from local government funding to federal funding for veterans was less of an evolution and more of a rapid response. Due to advances in artillery and chemical weaponry, WWI resulted in massive illness, catastrophic casualties, and disabilities (Rett, 2017). The war resulted in 224,000 physical or mental injuries, with 40,000 amputees and thousands of burns among the United States soldiers (Rett, 2017; Mayhew, 2004). The number of burn victims alone prompted the development of veteran hospitals and medical specialties and inspired new surgical procedures

and rehabilitation methods that resulted in higher survival rates (Mayhew, 2004). There was a growing relationship between medicine and war injuries and a strengthening of the value of caring for the soldiers who risked their lives for their country. The values drove community members to increase grassroots efforts for national policy to care for the veterans and their families who were not equipped to take care of them (Maloney, 2017).

As referenced, hospitals and the growing healthcare industry with infrastructure were ignited throughout the country for veterans and the community. With the circumstances and various programs in motion, the government could not return to separating itself from funding healthcare; returning to local church and state healthcare was no longer an option. The time had finally arrived for advocacy groups (i.e., the "progressives") to see their efforts come to fruition and live in a "civilized society" with the government caring for the welfare of its citizens (Hoffman, 2003). This does not imply that the government did not attempt to stop federal funding for veterans. After WWI, the government realized that the Civil War expenses were a fraction of what they would face with WWI veterans. The American Legion and other veterans' groups fought for injured soldiers' benefits (American Legion, 2015). Healthcare shifted from local to national government care for veterans (Table 1.3).

TABLE 1.3   Healthcare From Local Care to National Care for Veterans

Survival Rate	Soldiers were now surviving due to improved medical care and life-saving capabilities. As a result, the government was placed in a position to respond to the number of men required to be integrated into society (Mayhew, 2004[a]).
Precedents	The government set multiple precedents in supporting groups of civil war veterans. At first, this was for confederate soldiers only although with time included union soldiers (Maloney, 2017[b]).
Veterans Organizations	Organizations were developed and processes were in place to support disabled veterans. This provided a foundation for growth to support WWI veterans (United States Department of Veterans Affairs, 2023[c]).
Wartime Healthcare	The government initiated sending physicians and nurses paid by the government to care for the health of the soldiers (USDVA, 2021[d]).
Reconstruction Aides	In a new government initiative, reconstruction aides were educated by the government and sent overseas to work on the physical and mental needs of the veterans. The reconstruction aides developed into physical and occupational therapy and professional organizations emerged from these specialized practice areas. Their care continued with the veterans on United States soil (Quiroga, 1995[e]).
Specialty Professions	Vocational rehabilitation, prosthetist, and psychologist specialty professions are developing alongside reconstruction aides and are tied to meeting the needs of the veterans (Schlich, 2014[f]; Bonfiglioli, 2015[g]).
Economic Growth	Opportunities for economic growth were sparked due to government-led healthcare initiatives. Prosthetic plants, rehabilitation hospitals, and medical advances were all related to caring for injured soldiers.
Values	With 4.7 million young soldiers enlisted, most families in the United States were related to or had a community member serving. The government had to develop formal policies to deal with the issue (Maloney, 2017[b]).

[a]Mayhew (2004) *Reconstruction of warriors*. Greenhill.
[b]Maloney, W. (2017, December 21). World War I: injured veterans and the disability rights movement. *Library of Congress Blog.* https://blogs.loc.gov/loc/2017/12/world-war-i-injured-veterans-and-the-disability-rights-movement/
[c]United States Department of Veterans Affairs (2023). History overview. https://department.va.gov/history/history-overview/
[d]US Department of Veterans Affairs (USDVA) (2021). *Veterans affairs history in brief.* https://www.va.gov/opa/publications/archives/docs/history_in_brief.pdf/
[e]Quiroga, V. A. (1995). *Occupational therapy: the first thirty years.* AOTA Press.
[f]Schlich, T. (2014). *The 'bionic men' of World War I.* Cable News Network. https://www.cnn.com/2014/06/26/opinion/schlich-world-war-i-prosthetics
[g]Bonfiglioli Stagni S., Tomba P., Viganò, A., Zati, A. & Benedetti M. G.(2015). The first world war drives rehabilitation toward the modern concepts of disability and participation. *European Journal of Physical Rehabilitation Medicine, 51(3)*, 331–336.

Influence of Disease

During the same period as WWI, United States soldiers were falling ill after being exposed to a novel virus, H1N1, better known as the Spanish flu. The barracks became a breeding ground for the Spanish flu, resulting in up to 40% of all soldiers becoming ill and an estimated 63,000 United States soldiers dying (Byerly, 2010). Focused solely on the war effort and the need to keep the public working to help the war, United States president Woodrow Wilson ignored pleas from the new Surgeon General Rupert Blue and censored information related to the pandemic (Barry, 2005). Surgeon General Blue ultimately relied on the American Red Cross (ARC) to help manage the pandemic (Fig. 1.4) (Barry, 2005; Jones, 2010). Though a private organization, the government temporarily controlled the American Red Cross (ARC) to assist with the war effort; however, the board members remained in their positions (Jones, 2010). The ARC, primarily made up of females, was developed in the United States to assist with wartime needs, although, at the turn of the century, its mission expanded to include care for communities during national disasters and emergencies (Jones, 2010). This quasi-government partnership inadvertently led to a merging of philosophies between the ARC and the government and the integration of female ideology into government policy (Fisher, 2015; Scott,1993).

This was one step closer to tying the national government into the healthcare of the public.

Other widespread diseases have also influenced public health policy and the government's connection to healthcare. In 1916, the first widespread polio epidemic was documented in the United States and reached its peak between 1940 and 1950 (Centers for Disease Control [CDC], 2015). The virus initially targeted young children and later attacked adults (Oshinsky, 2020). In 1921, President Franklin Delano Roosevelt contracted polio during his presidency and although he initially hid his disability from the public eye, he later became an advocate for polio and founded the National Foundation for Infant Paralysis, which became known as the March of Dimes (Fig. 1.5) (History, 2020). The March of Dimes remained separate from the government through political and celebrity figures who worked closely with the organization to raise funds and build the organization (History, 2020).

Although epidemics such as polio and the Spanish flu resulted in extensive casualties in the American public, it was not until malaria cases impacted military base operations and southern land expansion in the United States that the government stepped in. In the 1930s and 1940s, south-central and southeastern United States regions expanded and were designated year-round military training camps (CDC, n.d.). Malaria was prevalent in this region and became a persistent

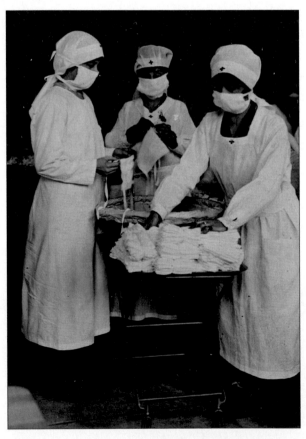

• **Fig. 1.4** Red Cross workers making masks during the Spanish flu epidemic of 1918. (Copyright © 2020 Courtesy National Archives.)

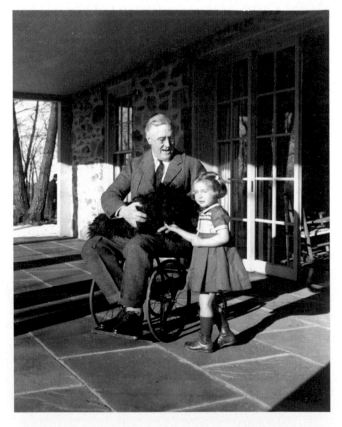

• **Fig. 1.5** President Franklin Delano Roosevelt became an advocate for the fight against polio and founded the March of Dimes. (From https://www.flickr.com/photos/54078784@N08/5813155742)

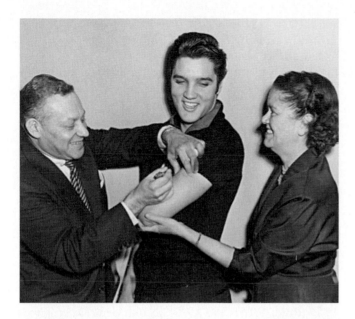

• **Fig. 1.6** Elvis Presley receiving a vaccine on television. (Courtesy Municipal Archives, City of New York.)

threat to the health of government workers and soldiers in these warmer climates. As a result, in 1947, the government established the Center for Disease Control to combat malaria (CDC, n.d.). The CDC, positioned in Atlanta, Georgia, to be close to the southern states, evolved as a government agency to manage vaccine programs for the public and soon became the "centralized authority" for United States healthcare (Fig. 1.6).

As previously discussed, values and philosophies strongly influence healthcare, including the government's involvement in healthcare. Because polio initially targeted young children, the push for a remedy and government assistance was overwhelmingly supported (History, 2020). When the acquired immune deficiency syndrome (AIDS) presented in the United States, the routine process of CDC coordination and government involvement shifted. The situation was more complex than other epidemics because it primarily targeted a marginalized population of homosexuals (Fox, 2005). The historical literature is filled with disputes on equal funding, education, control, dissemination, and prevention for those with AIDS and links the lack of successful management of the epidemic to the biases associated with homosexuality or the lack of cooperation from those affected (Fox, 2005; National Research Council, 1993; Rosenfeld, 2018). Public outcry and activism changed CDC practice from an authoritarian process to a collaborative one (National Research Council, 1993). There was the realization that healthcare coordination cannot occur without representation of the people the disease impacts and the wider impact the disease has on the population and community. This shift was an important turning point in healthcare as it included the individual and the communities in caring for their health versus a system that would manage people's health.

The COVID-19 pandemic has followed suit of the AIDS epidemic to the political divisiveness and public involvement in critiquing the CDC's recommendations. It is too early to tell the long-term impact this pandemic will have on the United States healthcare system, though the experience of the pandemic has exposed weaknesses in our healthcare system that will likely alter public healthcare delivery (Geyman, 2021).

Despite any tension related to government oversight and involvement, diseases have acted as a catalyst for government involvement in citizens' healthcare. Both federal and state governments are an integral part of healthcare for citizens although there is a growing evolution of partnering with communities to address the complex healthcare issues.

United States Healthcare Development and Reform

The movement toward federal funding of healthcare insurance in the United States is as complex and convoluted as any systemic change. Chapter 2 describes how political, economic, and social events influenced the development of government funding for healthcare. Here, an overview of people and social movements is explored concerning health insurance.

Early settlers brought the values and traditions of their countries of origin. European countries had some form of universal healthcare as early as the late 19th century or early 20th century; hence, citizens strongly pushed for national healthcare (Palmar, 1999). There were grassroots efforts to push for national healthcare; however, their efforts were largely unsuccessful (Hoffman, 2003). Legislation to pass government-funded healthcare was proposed as early as Theodore Roosevelt's time, but the Great War and the depression diverted efforts for federally funded healthcare (Starr, 2017).

During the turn of the century, labor unions formed and were proponents of joint employer and state funding for employee and family health insurance. This movement's impetus was to ensure that employees came to work and contributed to upholding business production versus an altruistic desire for improved health conditions (Hoffman, 2003). Despite motives, most physicians, nurses, social workers, and women at this time strongly supported health insurance as it served their needs and the community's (Palmar, 1999). Soon, physicians would take a different position in healthcare.

The 20th-century progressive movement had a large influence on laying a foundation for funding healthcare insurance for United States citizens. The Progressive Era in the United States (1896–1916), largely influenced by females and female ideological values of the time, supported government-funded health insurance for women, children, and the poor (Jones, 2010). While the "progressives" were not successful at this time in their advocacy efforts, their work exposed the issues surrounding healthcare and stirred visions about improving the health of society.

During his term (1945–53), President Harry Truman was intent on improving the nation's health and worked to develop a national healthcare reform for all citizens (Eldred, 2019; Library of Congress, 2020). President Truman's bill was never passed into law due to strong lobbying from the AMA, who believed they would have much to lose with this proposed system (Eldred, 2019; Roberts, 2020). Physicians who were in support of national healthcare at the turn of the century were now strongly opposed to government oversight due to the threat it imposed on private medical practice and reimbursement (Eldred, 2019; Shi & Singh, 2017). The power of the physicians and their representative association lobby reveal another shift in society toward the commodification of healthcare and the influence of capitalism on the healthcare system (Timmermans & Almeling, 2009).

Any remaining values of a decentralized government regarding healthcare were further strengthened after WWI with Germany. Publications were circulated demonizing Germany and its policies, including its universal healthcare system; the term "Prussian Menace" was used to halt further discussions about government-funded healthcare (Horning, 2009). Additionally, United States capitalistic values such as self-determination, distrust of government, and reliance on nongovernmental efforts to address social concerns were becoming more valued and ingrained. As a result, discussions and movements about anything resembling universal healthcare or socialized medicine were condemned (Starr, 2017). Despite resistance, unforeseen future social issues would again change public opinion about the government's involvement in healthcare.

Following World War II (WWII), the country was flourishing and again able to attend to societal needs and progress. Federal tax breaks for industries and businesses were given to those who offered their employees healthcare insurance (Horning, 2009). Workers' compensation benefits were one of the first health insurance plans offered to workers in the United States (Shi & Singh, 2019). At the time, workers' compensation provided reimbursements to workers for lost income as a result of disease or injury that was associated with their job. The intent was to provide temporary income to covered employees because it was thought that illness or injury as a result of working was a risk of being employed in a particular job and as such the employer should be financially responsible for the loss of income resulting from illness or injury. Medical expenses and survivor death benefits were not originally included in the plans but were added sometime later.

Disability coverage was one of the first forms of private health insurance and could be purchased individually (Shi & Singh, 2017). This provided stopgap coverage that allowed an individual to have income during times when they could not work due to illness or injury. Eventually, hospital insurance plans were formed as a result of several factors, including the increasing cost of medical care, the difficulty associated with accurately predicting future medical care needs and costs, and the economic instability faced by hospitals during the Great Depression (Shi & Singh, 2017). In 1929, Baylor University Hospital in Dallas, Texas, started a hospital healthcare plan for teachers, and shortly after, other hospitals started similar plans (Momanyi, 1994). As these plans grew, groups of hospitals formed plans that became popular by giving patients a choice of hospitals. Private health insurance corporations grew out of this movement

and the advent of third-party payers developed and eventually became a separate industry.

One of the biggest private health insurance companies, the Blue Cross Network, was developed by the American Hospital Association. Over time, the Blue Cross Commission took control of the network, later becoming the Blue Cross Association, which officially merged with Blue Shield in 1982 (Raffel, 1980; Shi & Singh, 2017). Ironically, a system that was developed to creatively provide for the healthcare of its citizens while upholding government decentralization became a platform for lobbying and financial gain.

There was no turning back from the movement of the private, commercial insurance companies. The companies began to expand by offering hospital insurance in addition to their other insurance offerings. The percentage of the United States population enrolled in private health insurance plans according to the Health Insurance Association of America (HIAA) increased from 9.3% in 1940 to 79.2% in 1964 (Reed, 1965). The Medicare and Medicaid programs were approved in 1965, which provided a public healthcare financing option for certain members of the population. As of 2021, according to the United States Census Bureau only 8.3% of people in the United States were not covered by health insurance of some kind, with 66% of the insured population covered by some type of private health insurance and 35.7% of the insured population covered by one of the publicly funded plans (Keisler-Starkey & Bunch, 2022). Therefore, a large portion of the United States population continues to be enrolled in private health insurance.

Health insurance became largely employer-based in the United States for several reasons. First, it was a response to wage freezes imposed by the United States Congress to control inflation, which was part of collective bargaining agreements between unions and employers (Teitelbaum & Wilensky, 2013). These agreements were aided by the United States Supreme Court in 1948 when it ruled that employee benefits were part of union and management negotiations (Institute of Medicine, 1993). Second, employer-paid health coverage became eligible to be paid with pretax dollars due to amendments made by Congress to the Internal Revenue Code in 1954 (Teitelbaum & Wilensky, 2013). These social and government movements would have a long-term impact on healthcare in the United States, especially for unemployed citizens.

National Health Insurance Programs

Medicare and Medicaid

As stated previously, in 1964 just over 79% of the United States population was enrolled in some form of private health insurance (Reed, 1965). However, prior to 1965, individuals and families who were unable to obtain broad-coverage health insurance were left to use their own funds to pay their healthcare bills or rely on the provision of public funds or care provided through charitable means. The healthcare needs of these individuals created a sentiment within society that was open to healthcare reforms targeted toward those who could not afford the rising cost of healthcare services.

In 1960, the Kerr-Mills Act amended the Social Security Act to help address the need for financial assistance related to healthcare costs for the elderly population (Longest Jr., 2016). The act involved grants to the states by the federal government using the state's welfare programs to provide healthcare services to low-income elderly individuals who could not afford healthcare costs (Moore & Smith, 2005). Unfortunately, this act created controversy regarding the enrollment of older individuals in welfare programs and was declared ineffective due to a lack of implementation by many states (Shi & Singh, 2017; Starr, 2017; Stevens, 1971). As a result, President Lyndon Johnson emphasized health insurance for older individuals in his Great Society program.

In 1965, Congress approved the Medicare program to provide a public health insurance option for the elderly (Fig. 1.7) (Longest Jr., 2016). This three-part program includes Parts A and B (Title XVIII of the Social Security Act of 1965) and Medicaid (Title XIX of the Social Security Act of 1965). Medicare Part A reimburses short-term acute care (i.e., hospital), long-term acute care hospitals (LTACH), home healthcare, short-term skilled nursing facilities (SNF), inpatient rehabilitation facilities (IRF), and hospice care (see Chapters 16 and 17). Medicare Part B pays for outpatient services (Chapter 15), durable medical equipment, and other healthcare services through a small patient premium and government-subsidized insurance. Medicaid was designed to provide health coverage for individuals with low incomes based on the Kerr-Mills Act (Moore & Smith, 2005). Medicaid is funded through matching funds from the federal government provided to the states based on the per capita income of each state.

The Medicare and Medicaid programs have several distinctions (Shi & Singh, 2017). While Medicare is available to anyone aged 65 years and older, Medicaid is designed to define eligibility for the program based on an individual's income level. However, based on the income level set for Medicaid eligibility, some individuals may not qualify for coverage through Medicaid despite lower incomes. Furthermore, Medicare has universal standards for eligibility and benefits regardless of which state the individual resides in since it is a federal program, while Medicaid has varied standards due to being administered separately by each state.

In 1973, Medicare was expanded to include individuals with a long-term disability (>24 months) receiving Social Security or Railroad Retirement benefits, people with end-stage renal disease who needed dialysis or a kidney transplant, and, in 2001, people with a diagnosis of Amyotrophic Lateral Sclerosis (ALS) (Longest Jr., 2016). Medicare Part C was added as part of a program included in the Balanced Budget Act of 1997; private companies approved by Medicare offered this. The Medicare Prescription Drug, Improvement, and Modernization Act (MMA) established Medicare Part D in 2003 as a prescription drug benefit plan for Medicare subscribers.

Enrollment in Medicare and Medicaid increased significantly after their creation. As an example, the number of people aged 65 years and older enrolled in Medicare was reported to be 19.1 million in 1966, 27.1 million in 1984, and 32.4 million in 1994 (Gornick et al., 1996). According to the Centers for Medicare and Medicaid Services (CMS), as of 2020, the total enrollment of individuals in Medicare was greater than 62.8 million, and the total enrollment in Medicaid was 73 million individuals, with 6.8 million children also being enrolled in the Children's Health Insurance Program (*Medicaid and CHIP Enrollment Trend Snapshot*, n.d.; *Medicare Total Enrollment*, 2022).

In 1977, the Health Care Financing Administration (HCFA) was set up to manage Medicare, Medicaid (federal portion), and the State Children's Health Insurance Program (Pozgar, 2016). This administrative office later became the Centers for Medicare and Medicaid Services (CMS). Even though the federal government finances the Medicare and Medicaid programs, services are delivered primarily through private healthcare providers (Shi & Singh, 2017). This arrangement has led to a significant increase in the regulation to oversee the delivery and reimbursement of medical care to those covered by these programs.

State Children's Health Insurance Program

The State Children's Health Insurance Program (CHIP) was passed as part of the Balanced Budget Act of 1997 and created Title XXI of the Social Security Act to assist states with funds to provide healthcare to uninsured and low income children (*History and Impact of CHIP*, n.d.; Longest, Jr., 2016; Social Security Administration, n.d.). This program allowed for health care coverage of uninsured children under the age of 19 years with a family income below 200% of the poverty level who were not covered by private insurance or eligible for Medicaid (CDC, 2022). States can expand CHIP coverage to a separate state program, increase Medicaid eligibility,

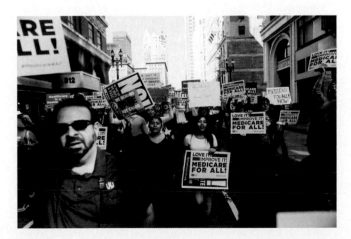

• **Fig. 1.7** Medicare is an example of a single payer system. (From https://www.flickr.com/photos/51008844@N03/35539966425)

or both. The CHIP program is available in every state and the District of Columbia; however, coverage differs depending on each state's minimum standard of benefits.

Once CHIP was enacted, the number of children without health insurance decreased significantly, while the number of uninsured adults increased. Between 1997 and 2012, the number of children without access to health insurance dropped from 10 million to under five million, and the percentage of individuals under the age of 18 years who had public health insurance increased from 21.4% to 43% (Clarke et al., 2017; *History and Impact of CHIP*, n.d.; Martinez & Cohen, 2012). A large percentage of the decline in the number of uninsured children was due to enrollment in Medicaid. The increased enrollment of children in both Medicaid and CHIP was due to efforts to improve enrollment numbers in these healthcare coverage programs (Dubay et al., 2007). Despite the program's and states' efforts, over 4 million children in the United States did not have health insurance in the calendar year 2020 (Bunch & Bandekar, 2021).

Change in systems is slow and impacted by various factors, as described. Healthcare oversight has been a dynamic process that changes based on societal needs and environmental conditions. Many presidents and special interest groups have fought for healthcare reform and the majority have not been successful. President Barack Obama is the exception and successfully passed the Patient Protection and Affordable Healthcare act (ACA) into law in 2010, which will be discussed later (United States Department of Health and Human Services, 2022). The lessons from earlier times in the history of collaborating within the communities to attend to health issues will be an important component as healthcare continues to evolve.

Health Disparity

In 1966, at a Chicago medical conference, Dr. Martin Luther King Jr. stated, "Of all the forms of inequality, injustice in health is the most shocking and the most inhuman" (Fig. 1.8) (Williams & Waters, 2017). Health injustices and health disparity have been a pervasive phenomenon in the United States (Gibbons, 2005). The early United States settlers were a mix of wealthy families, middle-class workers, and indentured servants. The poorest of this social group were the indentured servants who committed to years of hard labor in exchange for passage and work in America (Galenson, 1984). Their lack of income, extreme work conditions, poor diets, and inability to barter for services, including healthcare, resulted in a very high mortality rate for this poor class in colonial America (Galenson, 1984). The strong division between the classes and the acceptable limited access to healthcare persisted through the centuries. Other life conditions such as the type of disease, region and living conditions, age, and ethnicity have all been linked to inequity in healthcare (Baciu et al., 2017). Today it is widely accepted that access and quality of care are influenced by the type of disease, gender, sex, race, geography, education, socioeconomic status and ethnicity. (Horvath, 2022; Baciu

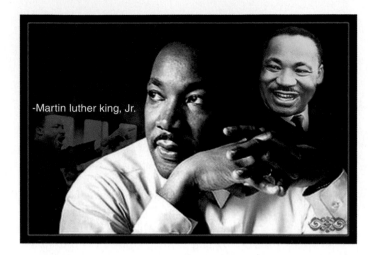

-Martin luther king, Jr.

• **Fig. 1.8** Dr. Martin Luther King Jr. battled inequality, including health disparities. (From https://www.flickr.com/photos/97328886@N00/1182295583)

et al., 2017). Although this disparity is commonly recognized, strategies to combat this inequity are in their infancy. An exploration of the inequity factors and the impact on the health of vulnerable, marginalized, and stigmatized populations is reviewed here.

Diseases related to a mental health diagnosis, AIDS, substance abuse, and visible body conditions have historically been associated with stigma, substandard care, and avoidance of medical care (Fox, 2005; National Institute on Drug Abuse [NIDA], 2021; Sartorius, 2007). Fear, ignorance, family beliefs, self-judgment, religion, and public policy have been associated with the phenomenon of stigma (Shrivastava, 2012; NIDA, 2021). The impact of societal stigma results in either substandard care or not receiving care for a health issue. This lack of care can ultimately result in high rates of societal illness, homelessness, and criminal activity (Lipari, 2017).

Health Disparity: Substance Abuse

Examining the multifactorial influences of care for substance abuse in the United States illustrates health disparities. The substance abuse death rate in the United States has now surpassed motor vehicle accidents and is ranked the fourth leading cause of death (National Safety Council, 2019). Substance use disorder and addiction are often related to poor health outcomes with strong economic and emotional costs to communities (Lipari, 2017; National Center for Health Statistics, 2017). Currently, substance use is treated as a crime in the United States as opposed to being a mental health condition, with 45% of all prison inmates serving time for a drug offense (Federal Bureau of Prisons, 2022). While healthcare is offered for some types of substances, the treatment interventions are limited and many are not covered by insurance, leaving millions of individuals and their families struggling (National Center for Health Statistics, 2017).

The trend of individuals avoiding or delaying treatment due to the stigma, denial, or the potential for criminal prosecution adds to the problem (Pauly et al., 2015). To address the rise of addiction and manage prison systems, the United States is exploring justice models and policies related to drug use (Substance Abuse and Mental Health Services Administration [SAMHSA], 2016). European countries such as Spain and Portugal have succeeded in reforming their management of drug addiction through decriminalization efforts (Bajekal, 2018). The issue is complex as it involves strong cultural mores, family values, justice, and beliefs about health. Paradigm shifts in our beliefs about health, illness, and right versus wrong will need to be challenged to support positive change and management of mental health disorders.

Health Disparity: Paradigm Shift

Constructs of health and healthcare in the United States are predominantly defined according to the biomedical model, which includes diagnosing and treatment of a disease or condition (Wilcock, 2015). Healthcare conjures up images of medicine and hospitals; however, the definition of health is much more holistic (Fig. 1.9). The WHO defines health as "a state of complete physical, mental and social wellbeing and not merely the absence of disease or infirmity" (World Health Organization, 2022). Physical wellbeing is the most integrated concept into health in the United States and includes exercise, diet, and disease prevention through avoiding excessive alcohol, smoking, and obesity (Ng et al., 2020). Mental and social wellbeing correlate with broader holistic health goals, including clean water, socialization, peace, shelter, and equity (Roth & Fee, 2010; Substance Abuse and Mental Health Services Administration [SAMHSA], 2016). Despite the adoption of the WHO and UN initiatives, holistic definitions of health have yet to be integrated into our common culture (Wilcock, 2015). It is worth considering the barriers to expanding our constructs, including the systems that we work with and how the systems and dominant models determine the focus of health. An area of health outside the traditional paradigms is explored to emphasize how emerging biological and social science is advancing and identifying factors that strongly influence health.

Neuroscience has shown that allostatic load, the cumulative psychological stress over a lifetime, is strongly correlated to health outcomes (McEwen, 2005). The psychosocial stressors associated with socioeconomic status, environmental issues, and lack of resources are perhaps stronger health indicators than the traditional biomarkers used to predict health (Guidi et al., 2021). This ideology is replicated in work on adverse childhood experiences (ACEs) (Fig. 1.10). ACEs, measured through a standardized assessment, are identified as childhood traumatic experiences that predict adult health outcomes (Bethell et al., 2017). The ACE scores are higher in minority populations and those living in poverty (Felitti, 2002; CDC, 2022). Trauma-informed care leaders are proposing to add ACEs to pediatric vital signs. Conversely, advances in social science have also led to the discovery of what supports health. Social scientists have found that socialization and social networks are essential components of health and may be equal or greater health indicators than traditional indicators (Umberson & Montez, 2010; Pinker, 2017).

Health is complex and influenced by multiple systems, both internally and externally. With new data, sharing of knowledge, and collaboration, the United States is moving toward a paradigm shift in how we perceive health, which will likely have a large impact on future healthcare and systems in healthcare. Predominant biomedical models that pushed science forward still have a place in healthcare, alongside the social sciences that explore the translation and application of health to the public.

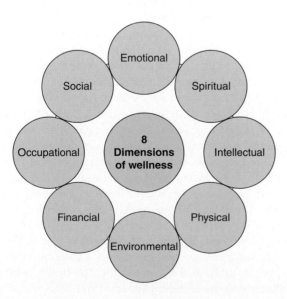

• **Fig. 1.9** A holistic approach is required to achieve optimal health.

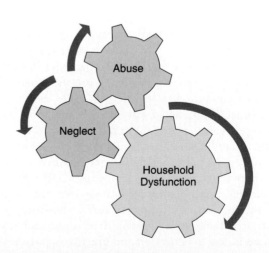

• **Fig. 1.10** Issues in childhood can affect your health in adulthood. (From https://www.cdc.gov/violenceprevention/aces/about.html)

Contemporary Public and Population Health

Corporate Era

Healthcare delivery in the United States continued to change significantly in the late 20th and early 21st centuries as technological advancements and globalization increased. Managed care, a healthcare delivery system designed to help improve healthcare quality and use, while also controlling costs, is now a significant delivery and health insurance model in the United States (*Managed Care*, n.d.). The move toward managed care started in the 1990s and allowed for the consolidation of purchasing power to slow the growing costs associated with medical care (Shi & Singh, 2017). Managed care organizations and healthcare providers formed larger organizations, which led to some benefits concerning the ability of health systems to offer a large number of services, but also brought with it the drawback of increased complexity.

The use of technology to enhance the delivery of healthcare services has been present throughout the history of medical advancement in the United States. In more recent history, medical records have been moved from paper charts to electronic records, advancements in diagnostic and treatment technologies have changed the way medicine is practiced all over the world, and an improved capacity for communication with patients remotely has allowed for greater reach of healthcare practitioners and improved access to care for patients. With regard to access, telemedicine has increased significantly since the 1990s, with the ability to transmit images and video electronically, leading to improved abilities to perform examinations and even telesurgery from and to remote locations (Shi & Singh, 2017). Providers and patients can access information from medical experts over the Internet, which has empowered patients and provided benefits to providers.

Globalization of healthcare services also increased during this period and included situations in which certain medical services began to be outsourced to other states or countries. For instance, it became possible to provide electronic images from medical practices to radiologists in other parts of the United States and other countries to be interpreted. This practice has become more common as technology improved to allow for secure and reliable transmission of patient data (McDonnell, 2006; Shi & Singh, 2017). In addition, medical tourism became more popular as services began to be sought in other countries for various reasons, including increased quality, decreased cost, and improved access to the healthcare services offered. Arrangements between United States companies and other countries allow for high-quality medical devices, healthcare services, and innovative solutions to current healthcare issues. Healthcare providers are leaving their home countries for increased access to education and practice opportunities or higher pay in other countries. Although this can be beneficial for the countries the providers are moving to, it may leave countries they are migrating from with a lack of healthcare providers.

Contemporary Health Reform Era

The term "healthcare reform" indicates major changes in how healthcare is financed, delivered, or accessed. The Patient Protection and Affordable Care Act (ACA) was signed into law on March 23, 2010 (Pozgar, 2016). The ACA had three main goals: (1) increase the availability of affordable health insurance to more people; (2) expand Medicaid eligibility for adults with income levels less than 138% of the federal poverty level; and (3) support a decrease in the costs of healthcare services through innovation (*Affordable Care Act (ACA)*, n.d.). After the ACA was passed, there were challenges to the constitutionality of several parts of the legislation (Longest Jr., 2016; Pozgar, 2016). Initial judicial decisions on lawsuits against the bill were mixed with regard to the constitutionality of certain aspects of the bill. For instance, in a decision on June 28, 2012, the Supreme Court held that the individual mandate to purchase health insurance was constitutional, but the federal government could not force states to expand Medicaid programs by withholding funds in states that did not expand Medicaid coverage. The ruling also noted that the federal government would be able to give matching funds to states that do expand Medicaid coverage, but the states that receive those funds for expansion of their Medicaid programs would have to comply with the new requirements (Longest Jr., 2016).

The ACA has provided a stimulus for change in the United States healthcare system. Since the ACA was passed, the number of uninsured nonelderly individuals in the United States decreased from 48 million in 2010 to 28 million in 2016 (Finegold et al., 2021). There was some rebound in this number between 2016 and 2020, when it was reported that 30 million nonelderly individuals were uninsured, possibly due to policy changes to coverage options under Medicaid and the ACA. Healthcare reform will continue to progress in the United States as the demand for healthcare services and the cost of healthcare continue to increase.

The United States has seen tremendous healthcare changes regarding education, access, cost, government involvement, and mode of delivery from early colonial times to the present day. These changes have led to significant improvements in medical care for society, but issues related to access, equity, and cost continue to be of concern. Each year there are numerous discussions, panels, and debates amongst healthcare professionals, private organizations, and government officials regarding proposed solutions to these issues. The next horizon in healthcare is moving toward implementing the definition of health and expanding health models to care for the ill and prevent disease. Collaboration among physicians, healthcare practitioners, public health officials, law and government officials, and economists are required to address the complexities of health and the healthcare system. Using the lessons from history is an excellent way to move forward.

Discussion and Activities

- How would you define health?
- What are some modifiable and nonmodifiable factors affecting health?
- What changes could be made to your community to improve health?
- How much does the United States spend on healthcare each year?
- How much does the United States spend on healthcare (total amount in dollars and percentage of its gross domestic product [GDP])? What about other countries?
- Why is the United States healthcare system the best? Why is it not the best?
- How does health insurance impact care?
- What are the financial risks of not having health insurance?
- What are your personal observations about receiving healthcare services and using health insurance?
- Did you notice that the United States healthcare system is a mixture of other systems used worldwide? What are some advantages and disadvantages of this approach?
- Are other countries beginning to modify their health systems?

References

About the Geisel school of medicine - Geisel school of medicine. (n.d.). Geiselmed.dartmouth.edu. https://geiselmed.dartmouth.edu/about/. Accessed December 3, 2022.

Affordable Care Act (ACA). (n.d.). HealthCare.Gov. https://www.healthcare.gov/glossary/affordable-care-act/. Accessed April 18, 2022.

American Hospital Association. (2022). *Fast facts on U.S. hospitals, 2022.* https://www.aha.org/system/files/media/file/2022/01/fast-facts-on-US-hospitals-2022.pdf.

American Legion. (2015). *Recounting the history of veterans benefits.* https://www.legion.org/washingtonconference/226244/recounting-history-veterans-benefits.

American Medical Association. (2023). *Trends in healthcare spending.* https://www.ama-assn.org/about/research/trends-health-care-spending.

Baciu, A., Negussie, T., & Geller, A., National Academies of Sciences, Engineering, and Medicine; Health and Medicine Division, Board on Population Health and Public Health Practice, & Committee on Community-Based Solutions to Promote Health Equity in the United States. (Eds.). (2017). The root causes of health inequity. In *Communities in action: Pathways to health equity.* Washington, DC: National Academies Press (US). https://www.ncbi.nlm.nih.gov/books/NBK425845/.

Bajekal, N. (2018). *Want to win the war on drugs? Portugal might have the answer.* TIME. https://time.com/longform/portugal-drug-use-decriminalization/

Barry, J. (2005). *The great influenza: The story of the deadliest pandemic in history.* Penguin.

Bethell, C. D., Carle, A., Hudziak, J., Gombojav, N., Powers, K., Wade, R., & Braverman, P. (2017). Methods to assess adverse childhood experiences of children and families: Toward approaches to promote child wellbeing in policy and practice. *Academic Pediatrics, 17*(Suppl. 7), S51–S69.

Bonfiglioli Stagni, S., Tomba, P., Viganò, A., Zati, A., & Benedetti, M. G. (2015). The first world war drives rehabilitation toward the modern concepts of disability and participation. *European Journal of Physical Rehabilitation Medicine, 51*(3), 331–336.

Brief history: School of medicine. (n.d.). University Archives and Records Center. https://archives.upenn.edu/exhibits/penn-history/school-histories/medicine/.

Bunch, L. N., & Bandekar, A. S. U. (2021). *Changes in children's health coverage varied by poverty status from 2018 to 2020.* United States Census Bureau. https://www.census.gov/library/stories/2021/09/uninsured-rates-for-children-in-poverty-increased-2018-2020.html#:~:text=In%202020%2C%204.3%20million%20children,to%20a%20report%20released%20today.

Byerly, C. R. (2010). The U.S. military and the influenza pandemic of 1918-1919. *Public Health Reports (Washington, D.C.: 1974), 125 Suppl 3*(Suppl. 3), 82–91.

Centers for Disease Control and Prevention (2005). In W. Atkinson, S. Wolfe, J. Hamborsky, & L. McIntyre, (Eds.), *Epidemiology and Prevention of Vaccine-Preventable Diseases* (13th ed.). Washington DC: Public Health Foundation.

Centers for Disease Control and Prevention. (2022). *National health interview survey.* https://www.cdc.gov/nchs/nhis/2022nhis.htm.

Centers for Disease Control and Prevention. (n.d.). *The history of malaria, an ancient disease.* https://www.cdc.gov/malaria/about/history/index.html.

Clarke, T. C., Norris, T., & Schiller, J. S. (2017). *Early Release of selected estimates based on data from the 2016 National Health Interview Survey* (pp. 1–120). US Department of Health and Human Services.

Dubay, L., Guyer, J., Mann, C., & Odeh, M. (2007). Medicaid at the ten-year anniversary of SCHIP: Looking back and moving forward. *Health Affairs, 26*(2), 370–381.

Eldred, S. M. (2019). *When Harry Truman pushed for universal health care.* https://www.history.com/news/harry-truman-universal-health-care.

Federal Bureau of Prisons (2022). *Inmate Statistics.* https://www.bop.gov/about/statistics/statistics_inmate_offenses.jsp

Felitti, V. J. (2002). The relation between adverse childhood experiences and adult health: Turning gold into lead. *The Permanent Journal, 6*(1), 44–47.

Finegold, K., Conmy, A., Chu, R. C., Bosworth, A., & Sommers, B. D. (2021). *Trends in the U.S. Uninsured Population, 2010-2020* (pp. 1–20) [Issue Brief No. HP-2021-02]. Office of the Assistant Secretary for Planning and Evaluation, US Department of Health and Human Services.

Fisher, R. (2015). *Clara Barton: CB paving.* National Park Service. https://www.nps.gov/clba/learn/historyculture/cbpaving.htm.

Fox, D. M. (2005). AIDS and the American health polity: The history and prospects of a crisis of authority. *The Milbank Quarterly, 83*(4), 7–33. doi:10.1111/j.1468-0009.2005.00432.x.

Galenson, D. W. (1984). The rise and fall of indentured servitude in the Americas: An economic analysis. *Journal of Economic History, 44*(1) 1–26.

Geyman, J. (2021). COVID-19 has revealed America's broken health care system: What can we learn? *International Journal Health Service, 51*(2), 188–194.

Gibbons, M. C. (2005). A historical overview of health disparities and the potential of eHealth solutions. *Journal of Medical Internet Research, 7*(5), e50.

Gorman, K. L. (2012). *Civil war pensions.* https://www.essentialcivilwarcurriculum.com/civil-war-pensions.html.

Gornick, M. E., Warren, J. L., Eggers, P. W., Lubitz, J. D., De Lew, N., Davis, M. H., & Cooper, B. S. (1996). Thirty years of Medicare: Impact on the covered population. *Health Care Financing Review, 18*(2), 179–237.

Guidi, J., Lucente, M., Sonino, N., & Fava, G. A. (2021). Allostatic load and its impact on health: A systematic review. *Psychotherapy and Psychosomatics, 90*(1), 11–27.

Harvard Medical School. (2020). *Perspectives of change: The creation of the National Medical Association.* https://perspectivesofchange.hms.harvard.edu/node/97.

Harvard Medical School. (2022). *The history of HMS.* https://hms.harvard.edu/about-hms/history-hms.

History. (2020). *This day in history: Franklin Roosevelt.* https://www.history.com/this-day-in-history/franklin-roosevelt-founds-march-of-dimes.

History and impact of CHIP. (n.d.). MACPAC. https://www.macpac.gov/subtopic/history-and-impact-of-chip/. Accessed April 8, 2022.

Hoffman, B. (2003). Health care reform and social movements in the United States. *American Journal of Public Health, 93*(1), 75–85.

Horning, A. (2009). *A short history of healthcare: let doctors be doctors.* Constitution Economics; Government Site Health Insurance Legal Medicine Politics Special Interest Group. https://wedeclare.wordpress.com/tag/prussian-menace/.

Horvath, L. (2022). *Health equity: Inequitable access to healthcare's racist roots.* Research Triangle Institute Health Advance. https://healthcare.rti.org

Institute of Medicine. (1993). Committee on employment-based health benefits. In M. J. Field & H. T. Shapiro (Eds.), *Employment and health benefits: A connection at risk.* Washington (DC): National Academies Press (US). https://www.ncbi.nlm.nih.gov/books/NBK235989/.

Johnson, D., & Chaudhry, H. J. (2012). The history of the Federation of State Medical Boards: Part one—19th century origins of FSMB and modern medical regulation. *Journal of Medical Regulation, 98*(1), 20–29.

Jones, M. M. (2010). The American Red Cross and local response to the 1918 influenza pandemic: A four-city case study. *Public health reports (Washington, D.C.:1974), 125, Suppl 3*(Suppl. 3), 92–104.

Keisler-Starkey, K., & Bunch, L. N. (2022). *Health insurance coverage in the United States: 2021* (P60-278). United States Census Bureau. https://www.census.gov/content/dam/Census/library/publications/2022/demo/p60-278.pdf/.

Library of Congress. (2022). *Primary documents in American history.* https://www.loc.gov/rr/program/bib/ourdocs/lincoln2nd.html.

Library of Congress. (2020). *Chronological list of presidents, first ladies, and vice presidents of the United States.* https://www.loc.gov/rr/print/list/057_chron.html.

Lipari, R. N., Ahrnsbrak, R. D., Pemberton, M. R., & Porter, J. D. (2017). *Risk and protective factors and estimates of substance use initiation: Results from the 2016 national survey on drug use and health.* Rockville, MD: CBHSQ Data Review.

Liu, J. L., & Brook, R. H. (2017). What is single-payer health care? A review of definitions and proposals in the U.S. *Journal of General Internal Medicine, 32*(7), 822–831.

Loiacono, G. (2017). Government paid for poor citizens' health care some 300 years before Obamacare. *The Atlantic.* https://www.theatlantic.com/politics/archive/2017/04/history-health-care-america-obamacare-aca/521541/.

Longest B. B., Jr. (2016). *Health policymaking in the United States* (6th ed.). Health Administration Press.

Martinez, M. E., & Cohen, R. A. (2012). *Health insurance coverage: Early release of estimates from the National Health Interview Survey, January—June 2012* (p. 36). Centers for Disease Control and Prevention. http://www.cdc.gov/nchs/data/nhis/earlyrelease/insur201212.pdf.

Mayhew. (2004). *Reconstruction of warriors.* Greenhill.

McCulla, T. (2016). *Medicine in colonial North America.* https://colonialnorthamerica.library.harvard.edu/spotlight/cna/feature/medicine-in-colonial-north-america#_edn1.

McDonnell, P. J. (2006). Is the medical world flattening? *Ophthalmology Times, 31*(19), 4.

McEwen, B. S. (2005). Stressed or stressed out: What is the difference? *Journal of Psychiatry & Neuroscience: JPN, 30*(5), 315–318.

Managed Care. (n.d.). Medicaid.Gov. https://www.medicaid.gov/medicaid/managed-care/index.html. Accessed April 22, 2022.

Medicaid and CHIP enrollment trend snapshot. (n.d.). Medicaid.Gov. https://www.medicaid.gov/medicaid/program-information/medicaid-chip-enrollment-data/medicaid-and-chip-enrollment-trend-snapshot/index.html.

Medicare total enrollment. (2022, February 3). Data.CMS.Gov. https://data.cms.gov/summary-statistics-on-beneficiary-enrollment/medicare-and-medicaid-reports/cms-program-statistics-medicare-total-enrollment.

Momanyi, B. N. (1994). *Blue cross and blue shield of Texas.* Texas State Historical Association. https://www.tshaonline.org/handbook/entries/blue-cross-and-blue-shield-of-texas.

Moore, J. D., & Smith, D. G. (2005). Legislating Medicaid: Considering Medicaid and its origins. *Health Care Financing Review, 27*(2), 45–52.

Mowery, Y. M. (2015). A primer on medical education in the United States through the lens of a current resident physician. *Annals of Translational Medicine, 3*(18), 270.

National Center for Health Statistics. (2017). Health, United States, 2016. https://www.cdc.gov/nchs/data/hus/hus16.pdf

National Institute on Drug Abuse (2021). *Addressing stigma and health disparities.* https://nida.nih.gov/nidamed-medical-health-professionals/health-professions-education/words-matter-terms-to-use-avoid-when-talking-about-addiction/addressing-stigma-health-disparities.

National Safety Council. (2019). *For the first time, we're more likely to die from accidental opioid overdose than motor vehicle crash.* https://www.nsc.org/in-the-newsroom/for-the-first-time-were-more-likely-to-die-from-accidental-opioid-overdose-than-motor-vehicle-crash.

National Research Council (US) Panel on monitoring the social impact of the AIDS Epidemic Jonsen, A. R., & Stryker, J. (Eds.). (1993). *The social impact of AIDS in the United States.* Washington (DC): National Academies Press (US).

National Park Service. (2017). *History of the national home for disabled volunteer soldiers.* https://www.nps.gov/articles/history-of-disabled-volunteer-soldiers.htm.

Ng, R., Sutradhar, R., Yao, Z., Wodchis, W. P., & Rosella, L. C. (2020). Smoking, drinking, diet and physical activity-modifiable lifestyle risk factors and their associations with age to first chronic disease. *International Journal of Epidemiology, 49(1),* 113-130.

Oshinsky, D. (2020). The epidemic that preyed on children. *The Atlantic.* https://www.theatlantic.com/ideas/archive/2020/03/when-outbreak-victims-are-children/608962/.

Palmer, K. S. (1999). A brief history: Universal health care efforts in the US. Physicians for a national health program (PHNP).

Pauly, B., McCall, J., Browne, A. J., Parker, J., & Mollison, M. A. (2015). Toward cultural safety: Nurse and patient perceptions of illicit substance use in a hospitalize setting. *Advances in Nursing Science, 38*(2), 121–135.

Pinker, S. (2017). The secret to living longer may be your social life [video]. TED conferences. https://www.ted.com/talks/susan_pinker_the_secret_to_living_longer_may_be_your_social_life/transcript?language=en

Pozgar, G. D. (2016). *Legal aspects of health care administration* (12th ed.). Jones & Bartlett Learning.

Raffel, M. W. (1980). *The U.S. health system: Origins and functions.* John Wiley & Sons.

Reft, R. (2017). *World War I: Injured veterans and the disability rights movement.* Library of Congress Blogs. https://blogs.loc.gov/loc/2017/12/world-war-i-injured-veterans-and-the-disability-rights-movement/.

Reed, L. S. (1965). Private health insurance in the United States: An overview. *Social Security Bulletin, 28*(12), 3–21, 48.

Rosenfeld, D. (2018). *The AIDS epidemic lasting impact on gay men.* https://www.thebritishacademy.ac.uk/blog/aids-epidemic-lasting-impact-gay-men/.

Roberts, N. F. (2020). 1912-2020: Presidents who changed health-care in America. *Forbes* https://www.forbes.com/sites/nicolefisher/2020/02/17/1912-2020-presidents-who-changed-health-care-in-america/?sh=adbadfb66195.

Roth G. A., & Fee, E. (2010). The United Nations and global health. *American Journal of Public Health, 100*(8), 1392.

Rothstein, W. (1972). *American physicians in the nineteenth century: From sect to science.* Johns Hopkins University Press.

Sartorius, N. (2007). Stigmatized illnesses and health care. *Croatian Medical Journal, 48*(3), 396–397.

Schumann, J. H. (2016, October 2). *A bygone era: When bipartisanship led to health care transformation.* NPR. https://www.npr.org/sections/health-shots/2016/10/02/495775518/a-bygone-era-when-bipartisanship-led-to-health-care-transformation.

Scott, A. F. (1993). *Natural allies: Women's association in American history.* University of Illinois.

Shi, L., & Singh, D. A. (2017). *Essentials of the U.S. health care system* (4th ed.). Jones & Bartlett Learning.

Shi, L., & Singh, D. A. (2019). *Delivering health care in America: A systems approach* (7th ed.). Jones & Bartlett Learning.

Shrivastava, A., Johnston, M., & Bureau, Y. (2012). Stigma of Mental Illness-1: Clinical reflections. *Mens sana monographs, 10*(1), 70–84. https://doi.org/10.4103/0973-1229.90181

Smith, T. M. (2020, March 17). *Medical education in 2020: How we got here, where we're headed.* American Medical Association. https://www.ama-assn.org/education/accelerating-change-medical-education/medical-education-2020-how-we-got-here-where-we-re.

Social Security Administration. (n.d.) *Purpose; state child health plans.* www.ssa.gov. https://www.ssa.gov/OP_Home/ssact/title21/2101.htm.

Starr, P. (2017). *The social transformation of American medicine: The rise of a sovereign profession & the making a vast industry* (Updated edition). Basic Books.

Stevens, R. (1971). *American medicine and the public interest.* Yale University Press.

Substance Abuse and Mental Health Services Administration (US), & Office of the Surgeon General (US). (2016). *Facing Addiction in America: The Surgeon General's Report on Alcohol, Drugs, and Health.* US Department of Health and Human Services.

The history of Columbia University | Columbia University in the city of New York. (n.d.). www.columbia.edu. https://www.columbia.edu/content/history-columbia-university.

Teitelbaum, J. B., & Wilensky, S. E. (2013). *Essentials of health policy and law* (2nd ed.). Jones & Bartlett Learning.

Timmermans, S., & Almeling, R. (2009). Objectification, standardization, and commodification in health care: A conceptual readjustment. *Social Science and Medicine, 69*(1), 21–27.

Umberson, D., & Montez, J. K. (2010). Social relationships and health: A flashpoint for health policy. *Journal of Health and Social Behavior, 51*, S54–S66.

United States Department of Health and Human Services (2022). *About the Affordable Care Act.* https://www.hhs.gov/healthcare/about-the-aca/index.html.

US Department of Health and Human Services. (n.d.). *Social Determinants of Health—Healthy People 2030.* https://health.gov/healthypeople/priority-areas/social-determinants-health.

United States Department of Veterans Affairs. (2023). History overview. https://department.va.gov/history/history-overview/

Walston, S. L., & Johnson, K. L. (2021). *Healthcare in the United States: Clinical, financial, and operational dimensions.* Health Administration Press.

Wilcock, A. A. & Hocking, C. (2015). *An occupational perspective of health* (3rd ed.). SLACK.

Williams, B., & Waters, M. W. (2020, Jan 17). Commentary: Martin Luther King Jr.'s fight for health care equity must continue. *Chicago Tribune.* https://www.chicagotribune.com/opinion/commentary/ct-opinion-martin-luther-king-health-inequality-20200117-way-vvwpc5rb4lpp5x3snumi2ie-story.html.

World Health Organization. (2017). *Health is a fundamental human right.* https://www.who.int/news-room/commentaries/detail/health-is-a-fundamental-human-right.

World Health Organization. (2022). *Constitution of the World Health Organization.* https://www.who.int/about/governance/constitution.

World Health Organization. (2022). *Universal health coverage (UHC).* https://www.who.int/news-room/fact-sheets/detail/universal-health-coverage-(uhc).

2

Health Legislation, Laws, Policy, and Advocacy

CRISTINA REYES SMITH, OTD, OTR/L, FAOTA; KIMBERLY ANGEL BRYANT, OTD, OTR/L; and LAUREN WENGERD, PhD, MS, OTR/L

LEARNING OBJECTIVES

By the end of this chapter, the reader will be able to:

1. Identify key legislation and factors impacting contemporary healthcare in the United States.
2. Discuss the scope and process of healthcare legislation, laws, and policies across healthcare settings.
3. Understand common healthcare laws and policies specifically related to pediatric, adult, and military settings.
4. Describe healthcare laws and policies related to liability, risk management, patient privacy, and employment.
5. Analyze legislation, laws, and policies to advocate for improvement in healthcare systems on behalf of clients, colleagues, and other stakeholders.

CHAPTER OUTLINE

Introduction

Few social systems and structures exist in the 21st century as complex, expansive, expensive, and controversial as healthcare systems. The legislation, laws, and policies that comprise these systems may vary widely from country to country. This chapter will focus primarily on healthcare systems within the United States. We will also discuss advocacy's historical and potential impact on policy and practice. Health has been defined by the World Health Organization (WHO) (2022a) as "a state of complete physical, mental and social well-being and not merely the absence of disease or infirmity." Health legislation is a branch of law that includes various aspects of health and healthcare, including the service delivery, practice, and rights of caregivers and patients (Annas, 2017). Although some legislation, laws, and policies are specific to pediatric or adult populations (these will be discussed later in this chapter), many permeate all practice settings and populations across the spectrum. We will review key legislation, laws, and policies related to various healthcare practice settings, including liability, risk management, and patient privacy. We will also discuss healthcare reform, billing, and reimbursement policies for pediatric practice settings, and those primarily serving adults and older adults. Lastly, we will discuss advocacy to promote meaningful change in local, state, national, and global care systems.

Overview of Contemporary Healthcare in the United States

The United States healthcare systems have grown more specialized, technologically advanced, and globally connected.

Despite these advancements, national health outcome indicators for the United States continue to lag distinctly behind countries worldwide (Fig. 2.1). These poor outcomes have been attributed largely to health inequities and social determinants of health (Centers for Disease Control and Prevention, 2021). Contemporary initiatives, including Healthy People 2030 (United States Department of Health and Human Services [USDHHS], n.d.), the Affordable Care Act of 2010 (USDHHS, 2022), and national and state-wide initiatives have addressed these poor health outcomes and disparities. However, continued advocacy from individuals, groups, organizations, and communities is imperative to create meaningful change to address local, state, national, and global needs.

Specialization of Healthcare Professionals and Interprofessional Teams

Healthcare has evolved from the historical all-purpose doctor-dentist to highly specialized interprofessional teams of skilled professionals across various training and educational levels, from medical assistants with associate degrees to medical scientists with doctorates. Healthcare specialization has evolved due to an aging population, increased chronic conditions, and medical advances. These factors have led to significant employment growth in healthcare and the need to diversify to respond to the needs of racial and ethnic minorities and other culturally diverse and under-represented groups (Fig. 2.2).

Diversifying the healthcare profession was punctuated by the USDHHS Office of Minority Health (2001, 2013) Standards for Culturally and Linguistically Appropriate Services (Table 2.1) and the Unequal Treatment reports of

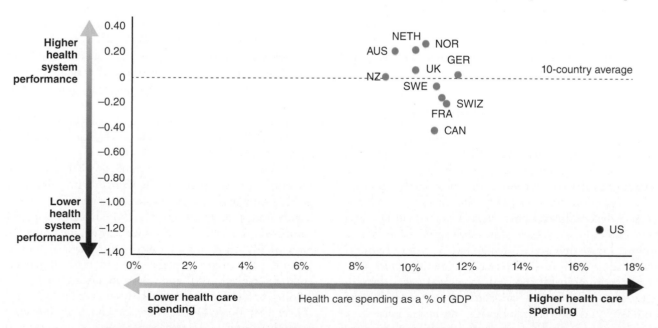

• **Fig. 2.1** United States Healthcare–High Spending. (Eric C. Schneider et al., Mirror, Mirror 2021 — Reflecting Poorly: Health Care in the U.S. Compared to Other High-Income Countries (Commonwealth Fund, Aug. 2021). https://www.commonwealthfund.org/publications/fund-reports/2021/aug/mirror-mirror-2021-reflecting-poorly)

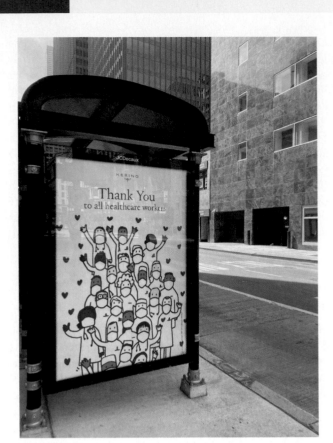

• **Fig. 2.2** Diversifying the healthcare workforce is key to improving outcomes. (From: https://www.flickr.com/photos/93084495@N04/50287703411)

the Institute of Medicine (2002). These factors are being addressed through policy changes in professional associations, healthcare organizations, and educational institutions, including the Association of American Medical Colleges (2023). Initiatives have included holistic admissions processes, recruitment and retention strategies, curriculum development, and accreditation requirements.

Transformations in Healthcare Technology

Focusing on data-driven, evidence-informed practice and service delivery started in the 1900s, which led to a new scientific discovery. Health professionals have used these discoveries to develop and utilize a robust knowledge base for healthcare practice and policy. The changes in technology and societal norms have created new challenges and opportunities for researchers, funders, and policy makers to continue innovating and evolving (Fig. 2.3). Some healthcare spending has been tied to research funding across practice areas, diagnosis groups, and age-related needs through organizations such as the National Institutes of Health, the USDHHS, and the Veterans Health Administration.

Technology has transformed the healthcare industry with the rise of the Internet and digital innovations. These technologies and advances in adaptive devices and durable medical equipment are more quickly disseminated worldwide. These advances included the development of sophisticated and increasingly available technologies such as smartphone apps, artificial intelligence, 3-D printing, virtual reality, augmented reality, and more. These tools have provided unprecedented connectivity and access to resources for low-income and other populations.

Although epidemics and pandemics have resulted in significant changes in healthcare systems throughout time, the COVID-19 global pandemic, which reached international awareness in January 2020, pushed technology to new limits. Healthcare services turned to telehealth platforms, electronic medical record systems, and online communications. These tools were catalyzed in a new age of social distancing and remote connectivity. Social media has also become a significant influencer of healthcare as health information, policy and advocacy campaigns, resources, and services have leveraged low- or no-cost tools to reach the masses like never before. Policies have been utilized to ameliorate the impact of inaccurate, uninformed, and malicious misinformation perpetuated through social media.

In the age of changing technology, patient privacy and protected information have become more vulnerable to exposure, potential misuse, and exploitation. Legislation has been enacted to protect health information as much as possible. Technology has been challenged to maintain information security in an age where information such as genetics, pregnancy status, HIV/AIDS and other sexually transmitted diseases, chronic diseases, and more can become part of a person's digital footprint or identity.

Global Connectivity and National Health Outcomes

Global connectedness has impacted healthcare system legislation, laws, and policy as subjects such as climate change, war, hunger, the water crisis, natural disasters, and other global issues have become part of everyday dialogue regarding sharing resources, personnel, and legal policy interventions. In 2021, over 300 healthcare-related organizations signed on to an open letter calling for leaders and countries to take significant action on climate change (World Health Organization, 2021).

Although socialized and accessible medicine has become the norm in most countries, the United States continues to utilize primarily privatized health insurance. Poor national health outcomes persist in the United States population compared with other countries worldwide, including lower rates of life expectancy (ranked 46), maternal mortality (ranked 129), infant mortality (ranked 174), underweight children (ranked 130), and adult obesity (ranked 12) according to the United States Central Intelligence Agency World Fact Book (2022). Poor outcomes in the United States have been attributed partly to racial and ethnic disparities and other factors. A rising focus on population health has aimed to prevent and proactively address issues through prevention policies and services for at-risk groups.

TABLE 2.1	National Culturally and Linguistically Appropriate Services Standards (CLAS)

The National CLAS Standards are intended to advance health equity, improve quality, and help eliminate healthcare disparities by establishing a blueprint for health and healthcare organizations to:

Principal Standard

1. Provide effective, equitable, understandable, and respectful quality care and services responsive to diverse cultural health beliefs and practices, preferred languages, health literacy, and other communication needs.

Governance, Leadership, and Workforce

2. Advance and sustain organizational governance and leadership that promotes CLAS and health equity through policy, practices, and allocated resources.

3. Recruit, promote, and support a culturally and linguistically diverse governance, leadership, and workforce responsive to the service area's population.

4. Educate and train governance, leadership, and workforce in culturally and linguistically appropriate policies and practices on an ongoing basis.

Communication and Language Assistance

5. Offer language assistance to individuals with limited English proficiency and/or other communication needs at no cost to facilitate timely access to all healthcare and services.

6. Inform all individuals of the availability of language assistance services clearly and in their preferred language, verbally and in writing.

7. Ensure the competence of individuals providing language assistance, recognizing that using untrained individuals or minors as interpreters should be avoided.

8. Provide easy-to-understand print and multimedia materials and signage in the languages commonly used by the populations in the service area.

Engagement, Continuous Improvement, and Accountability

9. Establish culturally and linguistically appropriate goals, policies, and management accountability, and infuse them throughout the organization's planning and operations.

10. Conduct ongoing assessments of the organization's CLAS-related activities and integrate CLAS-related measures into measurement and continuous quality improvement activities.

11. Collect and maintain accurate and reliable demographic data to monitor and evaluate the impact of CLAS on health equity and outcomes and to inform service delivery.

12. Conduct regular assessments of community health assets and needs and use the results to plan and implement services that respond to the cultural and linguistic diversity of populations in the service area.

13. Partner with the community to design, implement, and evaluate policies, practices, and services to ensure cultural and linguistic appropriateness.

14. Create conflict and grievance resolution processes that are culturally and linguistically appropriate to identify, prevent, and resolve conflicts or complaints.

15. Communicate the organization's progress in implementing and sustaining CLAS to all stakeholders, constituents, and the general public.

Adapted from United States Department of Health and Human Services Office of Minority Health, 2013. *National Standards for CLAS in health and health care: A blueprint for advancing and sustaining CLAS policy and practice.* https://www.thinkculturalhealth.hhs.gov/assets/pdfs/EnhancedCLASStandardsBlueprint.pdf

Social Determinants of Health

The Healthy People 2020 and 2030 initiatives through the USDHHS have provided guidelines, benchmarks, and resources to promote progress in these areas (USDHHS Office of Disease Prevention and Health Promotion, n.d.). The impact of social determinants of health has been explored and guidelines have been provided by leading national and international health organizations such as the Centers for Disease Control and Prevention (2021), National Academy of Medicine (2022), the USDHHS Office of Disease Prevention and Health Promotion (2018), and the World Health Organization (2022b). Social determinants of health has been defined as the impact on health from the conditions where people live, learn, work, play, and worship (Centers for Disease Control and Prevention, 2021).

Research is still emerging on how social determinants of health factors influence health, but the literature has made it evident that profound and distinct implications for health outcomes are influenced by complex social factors such as these. The COVID-19 pandemic underscored racial and ethnic health disparities and highlighted the influence of social determinants of health (Centers for Disease Control and Prevention, 2020). These disparities included an increased focus on hunger and food insecurity, which disproportionately impact children and adults in the United States

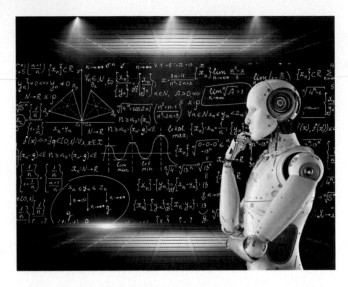

• **Fig. 2.3** How will artificial intelligence (AI) change healthcare? (From https://www.flickr.com/photos/152824664@N07/30212411048)

from racial and ethnic minority groups (Feeding America, 2021). School-based initiatives to address food insecurity have been added to the list of health policy initiatives related to oral health and hygiene, access to therapy services, visual and hearing screenings, other childhood-related illnesses and diseases screenings (e.g., learning disorders, scoliosis, mental health/trauma, abuse, and neglect) that have been integrated into public school systems across the country. These programs and services can help provide preventative care through related healthcare and social systems.

Healthcare Protections for Minority and Marginalized Groups

The United States is expected to become even more racially and ethnically diverse. By 2045, the United States Census Bureau anticipates that there will no longer be a racial/ethnic majority (Vespa et al., 2020). Hispanic Latinos make up the second-largest racial/ethnic minority group nationwide and language access, health literacy, racism, bias, and discrimination are continued challenges among multiple communities and populations. These ongoing challenges have been addressed historically through healthcare policy and legislation changes resulting in protections for minority and marginalized groups, including the Civil Rights Act of 1964 (United States National Archives and Records Administration, 2022a), Americans with Disabilities Act of 1990 (United States Department of Labor, n.d.a), Individuals with Disabilities Education Act (United States Department of Education, 2022a), and Affordable Care Act of 2010 (USDHHS, n.d.). Furthermore, a shift to de-institutionalization of individuals with disabilities was catalyzed by the United States Supreme Court decision in *Olmstead v. L.C.*, 527 United States 581 (1999), which affirmed that the unjustified segregation of individuals with disabilities is a form of discrimination prohibited by Title II of the Americans with Disabilities Act (United States Department

of Housing and Urban Development, n.d.). The United States Department of Housing and Urban Development (HUD) provides integrated housing options and long-term healthcare and support services to individuals with disabilities.

Health Legislation and the Passing of a Bill

Health legislation is typically developed and approved through a process under a governing body. It may have to go through several stages of approval from individuals and smaller committees to federal/national entities (Fig. 2.4). In the United States, this can include federal bodies related to Congress, comprised of the House of Representatives and the Senate. Federal entities such as the United States Department of Health and Human Services and Centers for Disease Control, as well as lobbying groups and others, can provide advisement and work closely with legislators in this process. State governments may have a General Assembly or other state-wide body comprised of a State House of Representatives or State Senate, which may oversee legislation for state laws. These state bodies may work closely with state-regulated entities such as a state-wide Department of Health and Human Services, Department of Health and Environmental Control, and Department of Disabilities and Special Needs.

Much healthcare legislation in the United States is developed as a "bill," which is moved forward to the governing body (Fig. 2.5). This bill may be generated by representatives (typically elected, but they may be appointed in some cases) or they may come from committees of the governing body. At times an individual, group, or organization from the public may initiate a bill; however, a governing body member will typically move the bill forward for discussion by the governing body. At that point, the bill may move forward for discussion on voting, be amended by removing or deleting words, be sent to a committee for further review, or be tabled to a future session.

Once a bill moves to a vote, members can support, disapprove, or abstain from passing the bill into law. This voting may take place through verbal affirmation ("aye" or "nay"), written ballots, or electronic systems. Votes are often confirmed publicly and recorded; however, they are sometimes provided anonymously in rare situations. These proceedings are often public with galleries where members of the general public can observe. In addition, Public Advisory Boards or Members may be established to provide stakeholder input for certain topics. At times, sessions will be held specifically for public member input. These may be called Town Halls, Public Forums, Listening Sessions, and other names. Once legislation is approved through voting, it becomes a law. It can take years to develop and implement regulations to carry out a law. For example, the Rehabilitation Act was approved in 1973; however, it took 3 to 4 years for regulations to be established and instated in response to the Act. If a piece of legislation is voted down (i.e., not approved), it may or may not be reintroduced in the future with modifications as a new bill.

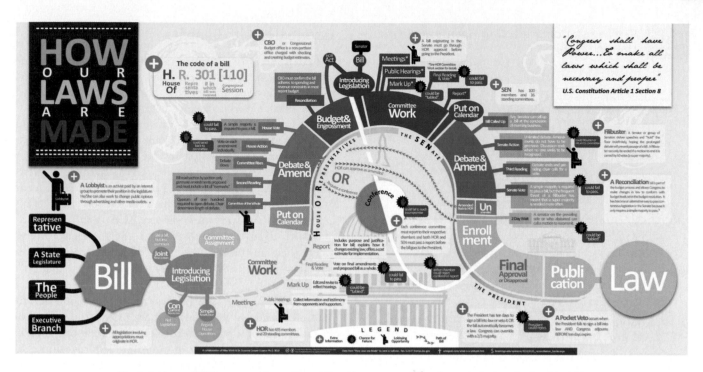

• **Fig. 2.4** How a Bill Becomes a Law. (From https://commons.wikimedia.org/w/index.php?curid=1774 5490)

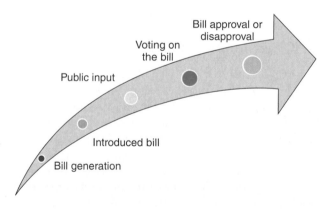

• **Fig. 2.5** Life Cycle of a Bill.

Laws can be amended or repealed through Congress or the judicial system if deemed unconstitutional. The President of the United States can also issue an Executive Order to manage the operations of the Executive branch of the government (United States Federal Register, n.d.) and interpret laws based on discretion. The President is also able to veto laws passed by Congress. This "checks and balances" system established by the Constitution supports the democratic process by preventing the three branches of government (executive, legislative, and judicial) from having too much power. The term "democracy" is derived from the Greek words meaning "the people" and "rule." The hallmark of the democratic process is social equality by voting for elected members.

In contrast to health law passed by legislation, a health policy has been defined as a statement about values related to identified goals of importance and the mechanisms

for achieving these goals (Martin, 2008). Policies are often developed to address specific problems such as disease prevention, food-born illnesses, environmental issues, and other public health or health-related issues. They may be confidential or available to the general public. Furthermore, depending on the needs being addressed, they may be short-term or longer-term in development and implementation. Laws may be utilized when developing policies (Martin, 2008).

Key Legislation Impacting Healthcare

Multiple examples of legislation have profoundly impacted healthcare services over the years (Table 2.2). These were sometimes implemented to expand access to healthcare services, protect patient or employee rights, improve quality, or reduce costs. Major laws impacting healthcare include the following in chronological order:

Healthcare Reform and the Affordable Care Act

The Affordable Care Act (ACA), also known as "Obamacare," was a landmark federal statute enacted by the United States Congress and signed into law by President Barack Obama on March 23, 2010. The ACA was enacted with three primary goals: (1) increase access to affordable healthcare, (2) expand the Medicaid program to cover adults with income below 138% of the federal poverty limit (FPL), and (3) support innovative medical care delivery methods

TABLE 2.2   Key Legislation Impacting Healthcare in the United States

- 1935: The Social Security Act
- 1964: The Civil Rights Act
- 1965: The Medicare and Medicaid Act
- 1973: The Rehabilitation Act
- 1974: The Family Education Rights and Privacy Act (FERPA)
- 1975: The Education for All Handicapped Children Act (EHA)
- 1985: The Consolidated Omnibus Budget Reconciliation Act (COBRA)
- 1990: The Americans with Disabilities Act (ADA)
- 1990: The Individuals with Disabilities Education Act (IDEA) (renamed from Education for All Handicapped Children Act)
- 1996: The Health Insurance Portability and Accountability Act (HIPAA)
- 1997: The Balanced Budget Act
- 2001: New Freedom Initiative
- 2003: The Medicare Modernization Act
- 2004: The Individuals with Disabilities Education Improvement Act (IDEA)
- 2010: The Affordable Care Act (ACA) (also known as "Obamacare")
- 2014: The Improving Medicare Post-Acute Care Transformation (IMPACT) Act
- 2018: The Bipartisan Budget Act of 2018
- 2018: The Medicare Home Health Flexibility Act

Essential Health Benefits

The ACA identifies 10 broad categories of services (including, but not limited to, rehabilitative and habilitative services and devices, preventive and wellness services, and mental health and substance use disorder services) that certain health insurance plans must cover. These services are *essential health benefits* (EHBs) (Box 2.1). It is important to note that insurance companies are not required to cover 100% of the costs associated with EHBs, except for preventative services. They are only required to include some form of coverage in their insurance plan for the services. For example, a patient with an approved ACA health insurance plan with EHB coverage may go to the emergency room, where they are billed $2000 for a visit. If a patient has a $2000 or greater deductible, they will have to pay that out-of-pocket cost.

Conversely, the same patient may receive the $2000 medical bill and have already met their deductible. However, their insurance policy may only cover 10% of the costs associated with emergency room visits. While, technically, coverage is being provided to meet the ACA requirement, it may only cover 10% of the cost and the patient would still have to pay $1800 out-of-pocket for the visit until they reach their out-of-pocket maximum for the year (which varies by plan).

Health Insurance Marketplace

The Health Insurance Marketplace was developed to streamline shopping for ACA-compliant private health insurance plans by allowing consumers to compare monthly premiums, deductibles, copayments, and out-of-pocket maximums for various insurance policies. The Health Insurance Marketplace can be accessed online at www.healthcare.gov, and individuals can enter criteria to establish eligibility for Medicaid or subsidies to offset the cost of private insurance plans based on income level. Specific details regarding Medicaid and Medicare will be discussed later in this chapter.

designed to lower healthcare costs (USDHHS, 2022) (Table 2.3). Also, under the ACA, health insurance companies cannot discriminate against individuals with a preexisting condition by refusing to cover them or charge them more for their policy (Fig. 2.6).

TABLE 2.3   Key Health Policy Terms

Policyholder	• A person who has an insurance policy and pays premiums in exchange for coverage
Deductible	• Set amount paid for medical services before health insurance policy pays any benefits
Copay	• Set rate the insured pays for prescriptions, provider visits, and other types of care (e.g., $20)
Co-insurance	• Percentage of costs the insured pays after meeting their deductible (e.g., 20%)
Out-of-pocket Maximum	• Limit the amount of money the insured pays for healthcare services in a plan year • Once met, all covered healthcare costs for the rest of the plan year are paid at 100%
Premium	• Payments to keep a healthcare plan active • Employer-based plans are deducted from the insured paychecks
Supplemental Insurance	• Additional insurance plan for healthcare costs that are not covered by an individual's primary health insurance plan

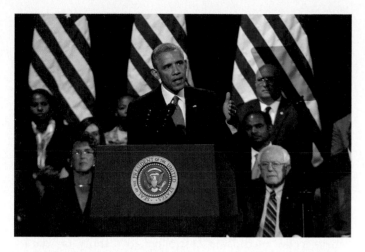

• **Fig. 2.6** A key piece of the Affordable Care Act was preventing health insurance companies from discriminating against individuals with a preexisting conditions. (From https://www.flickr.com/photos/34095168@N05/14830074316)

• BOX 2.1   10 Essential Health Benefit Categories

1. Ambulatory patient services (outpatient care you get without being admitted to a hospital)
2. Emergency services
3. Hospitalization (like surgery and overnight stays)
4. Pregnancy, maternity, and newborn care (both before and after birth)
5. Mental health and substance use disorder services, including behavioral health treatment (this includes counseling and psychotherapy)
6. Prescription drugs
7. Rehabilitative and habilitative services and devices (services and devices to help people with injuries, disabilities, or chronic conditions gain or recover mental and physical skills)
8. Laboratory services
9. Preventive and wellness services and chronic disease management
10. Pediatric services, including oral and vision care; however, adult dental and vision coverage are not considered essential health benefits)

From *Find out what Marketplace health insurance plans cover.* (n.d.) HealthCare. gov. https://www.healthcare.gov/coverage/what-marketplace-plans-cover/

The IMPACT Act of 2014 and the Push Toward Quality Improvement

In 2014, the Improving Medicare Post-Acute Care Transformation (IMPACT) Act was signed into law (United States Centers for Medicare & Medicaid Services, 2021b). This law specifically aimed to standardize data using quality measures and standardized patient assessment data elements (SPADEs) through commonly used instruments in post-acute care, including:

• Long-term care hospitals (LTCHs): long-term care hospital care data set (LCDS)
• Skilled nursing facilities (SNFs): minimum data set (MDS)

• Home health agencies (HHAs): outcome and assessment information set (OASIS)
• Inpatient rehabilitation facilities (IRFs): inpatient rehabilitation facility patient assessment instrument (IRF PAI)

These data are designed to be standardized and interoperable, allowing for data exchange and improved beneficiary outcomes among post-acute and other providers. Shared decision-making, care coordination, and enhanced discharge planning are supported through CMS "Meaningful Measures" such as effective communication, effective prevention and treatment of chronic disease, collaboration with communities to promote healthy living, affordable care, safer care, reduced costs of care, and stronger partnerships with patients and families. Reporting measures for the community and regarding resource use, hospitalization, and discharge are a part of the initiatives. Specific quality measure domains include:

• Skin integrity and changes in skin integrity;
• Functional status, cognitive function, and changes in function and cognitive function;
• Medication reconciliation;
• Incidence of major falls;
• Transfer of health information and care preferences when an individual transitions.

While these factors are directly related to post-acute patient care through the IMPACT Act, the priorities and strategies within the Act are applicable across healthcare settings and reflect a national push toward more patient-centered, safer, more cost-effective, and value-based care (United States Centers for Medicare & Medicaid Services, 2021b).

Billing and Reimbursement Policies Across Healthcare Settings

Several coding systems are utilized across pediatric and adult-serving healthcare settings. These include the International Classification of Diseases (ICD) Coding System and the Healthcare Common Procedure Coding System (HCPCS). Although ICD-10 codes and HCPCS codes are used across settings for billing and reimbursement purposes, state-regulated Medicaid systems and private insurances may have limitations in the HCPCS codes used for billing. Reimbursement by third-party payers for services heavily depends on codes utilized for initial and ongoing authorization. Healthcare agencies and practitioners should be well-versed in frequently utilized codes that are allowable for their client populations and ensure adequate measures for accurate coding and billing. In addition, accurate coding of services in documentation is critical to demonstrating the medical necessity for initial and ongoing care, including the type and duration of services delivered, participants involved, and setting. Inaccurate or insufficient coding may cause a denial of reimbursement for services already rendered. Individual providers should utilize approved and consistent abbreviations in documentation that correspond with the codes used.

Documentation should be aligned with the codes utilized and may be commonly accessed by coworkers for communication in team-based care and cases of medical supervision. Further, documentation with coding may be provided to payors, patients, families, and caregivers. Documentation with coding may also be subpoenaed in a court of law for various reasons, including licensing or ethical violations, custody cases, or malpractice lawsuits. As a result, individual providers and agencies should ensure that dates billed for service codes, duration/times, description of evaluations or interventions, and provider signatures (especially when working with assistants, technicians, aides, and students) are appropriate and accurate.

International Classification of Diseases Coding System

Healthcare practitioners are typically required to use specialized medical codes to indicate to third-party payors a patient's diagnosis and which healthcare services were provided. The International Classification of Diseases (ICD) is a system published by the WHO to indicate medical and treatment diagnoses using designated codes. As of 2022, the 10th revision of the ICD coding system was in place (i.e., ICD-10 codes). While the ICD classification system was initially developed to track mortality, it has since been updated to track morbidity (disease state/medical conditions) in what is referred to as the "ICD-10 Clinical Modification (ICD-10-CM) codes" (United States Centers for Medicare & Medicaid Services, 2021a).

The ICD-10 coding system is used to document both medical and treatment diagnoses. A medical diagnosis indicates the medical condition that caused an impairment or change in function (e.g., Parkinson disease). In contrast, a treatment diagnosis indicates the resulting impairments (e.g., signs/symptoms, deficits) that require intervention (e.g., tremors, muscle weakness) (United States Centers for Medicare & Medicaid Services, 2021a). The referring physician typically provides a medical diagnosis, while the practitioner is responsible for identifying the treatment diagnosis after conducting an evaluation. Helpful resources on coding are available from the Centers for Medicare and Medicaid and professional associations.

Healthcare Common Procedure Coding System

The Healthcare Common Procedure Coding System (HCPCS) is a collection of standardized codes based on the American Medical Association's current procedural terminology. These codes indicate to third-party payors (e.g., Medicare) the type of healthcare services, procedures, equipment, and supplies provided to a patient. In other words, the HCPCS informs the payer of the *treatment* provided, while the Medicare Physician Fee Schedule indicates the *maximum reimbursement rate* for that specific treatment. As previously mentioned, HCPCS codes bill for services payable under Medicare. However, these codes are also used for patients with different insurance coverages, including Medicaid and private insurance, as Medicare typically establishes the baseline standards for coverage and reimbursement.

The HCPCS is divided into two principal sets of codes: Level I and Level II (United States Centers for Medicare & Medicaid Services, 2022). Level I HCPCS codes, more commonly referred to as Current Procedural Terminology (CPT) codes, are numeric codes used by healthcare professionals to indicate which services were provided for billing purposes (see Chapter 13). Healthcare providers use CPT codes to document medical services and procedures (e.g., evaluation, treatment, diagnostic procedures, surgical operation). Alternatively, Level II HCPCS codes are alpha-numeric codes used across disciplines to identify products, supplies, and services not included in the CPT codes. Level II HCPCS codes include ambulance services, durable medical equipment (e.g., a bedside commode), prosthetics, orthotics, and medical supplies (e.g., catheters).

When using CPT codes (Level I HCPCS codes), it is important first to understand the difference between service-based (untimed) CPT codes and time-based CPT codes. A *service-based* CPT code cannot be billed for more than one unit, regardless of the time taken to complete it. These include services such as evaluation or unattended modalities (e.g., electrical stimulation, fluidotherapy). Whether treatment was delivered for 15 minutes or 50 minutes, both would be billed for only one untimed unit for these services. Alternatively, *time-based* CPT codes indicate the amount of time the patient spends in a direct, one-on-one, or group-based intervention. Time-based CPT codes cover all forms of constant attendance procedures. Examples include practicing bathing and dressing (CPT Code: 97535, self-care or home management training), completing lower extremity strengthening exercises (CPT Code: 97110, therapeutic exercise to develop strength, endurance, range of motion, and flexibility exercises), or addressing coordination and proprioception in preparation for functional activities (CPT Code: 97112, neuromuscular reeducation of movement, balance, coordination, posture, or proprioception for sitting or standing activities).

Time-based CPT codes are billed in 15-minute increments (i.e., 1 unit = 15 minutes) after a minimum of 8 minutes of treatment has been provided in Outpatient Medicare Part B settings; however, some other settings may also follow this guideline. This billing practice is referred to as the 8-Minute Rule, indicating that a practitioner must administer at least 8 minutes of intervention to bill for one unit of time-based services. Beyond the first 8 minutes, the provider counts in 15-minute increments to determine billable units (Table 2.4).

Liability, Risk Management, and Patient Privacy Across Healthcare Settings

Healthcare leadership, administrators, and practitioners must consider daily liability, risk management, and patient

TABLE 2.4	Medicare 8-Minute Rule Chart[a]
Time Spent (min)	Number of Billable Units
8 to 22	1
23 to 37	2
38 to 52	3
53 to 67	4
68 to 82	5
83 to 97	6

[a]This chart only applies to time-based codes.

privacy. These factors can include ethical considerations, including those related to potential fraud and abuse (including intentional or unintentional billing, erroneous documentation, and practicing without a valid license); malpractice due to negligence, error, or illegal activity; health management of individual stakeholders as well as groups, communities, and populations; and potential for death or injury for patients as well as employees. Technological advances have given rise to cyber theft and identity theft opportunities through digital pathways that did not previously exist. Cybercrimes, forgery, falsified documentation, and other "white collar crimes" are found across various industries, including healthcare.

In addition to artificial challenges, natural disasters can pose minor to catastrophic risks to patients, providers, and healthcare organizations. Natural disasters can include the threat of fire, flood, tropical events, tornadoes, earthquakes, and other naturally occurring phenomena. For example, in 2005 Hurricane Katrina spotlighted the tragedies resulting from natural disasters through shocking death counts and imagery from devastated hospitals and nursing homes. This tragedy and others have led to legislation and policies requiring clear and preventative plans for agencies and organizations that care for medically vulnerable individuals.

Other risks include theft, vandalism, and damage. While some laws are in place to protect business owners and agencies, policies can often help ameliorate the impact of these factors, such as controlled access through identification badges, security systems, video surveillance, and hiring of security personnel. When evaluating and implementing options, administrators must balance the impact of environmental modifications, sense of safety, costs, and privacy for employees and consumers.

In addition to having adequate insurance coverage for malpractice, liability, natural disasters, and other potential hazards, healthcare organizations can use additional strategies to manage liability and risk. For example, employers can provide access to training for individuals, groups, and organizations to mitigate legal, safety, and other potential risk factors. Organizations may develop plans or diagrams related to fire safety, organizational structure, chain of command, and decision trees for common processes. Individuals

are responsible for being aware of organizational and system guidelines, policies, procedures, and laws. If these resources are posted, claiming that someone "did not know" may not hold up in legal proceedings. Furthermore, individuals and organizations should be vigilant in everyday practice by developing good habits and processes for organizational skills, documentation, safety, reporting, quality assurance, and accountability. Managers and administrators have a duty to ensure that policies are adequately documented, clear, and understood; processes are implemented on regular timetables with adequate accountability; training opportunities for initial and ongoing staff are regularly available; and policies, procedures, and documents are reassessed regularly.

Employee Safety

Healthcare organizations are legally responsible for ensuring worker safety in most situations. Agencies that employ workers may be required to provide workers' compensation for employees who are injured or become disabled on the job (United States Department of Labor, n.d.c) and unemployment benefits under certain conditions. While there are federal provisions in some circumstances, these laws will vary from state to state. Companies with at least 50 full-time employees are considered applicable large employers (ALEs) and are subject to shared responsibility provisions and must report on this information when filing taxes each year (Internal Revenue Services, 2021). Under the ACA, these include full-time equivalent employees on average during the prior year. In addition to some required legal protections for employees, employers may elect to provide subsidized or fully covered disability insurance for temporary or permanent disability (these protections will frequently cover pregnancy as a temporary disability). Also, these benefits may provide additional coverage for employees' visual, dental, mental health, and other health-related needs. These policies are established at the organizational level, based on financial cost analysis, industry and geographic norms, worker risks, core values, and other factors. Benefits are typically provided for full-time W-2 employees who generally make up 20% to 30% of the salary. However, some part-time employees and 1099 independent contractors may have agreements that help cover these costs.

HIPAA, Patient Privacy, and Patient Protections

The Health Insurance Portability and Accountability Act (HIPAA) of 1996 (United States Congress, 1996) was the first federal privacy standard to protect patient medical records and other health information. This act took effect for healthcare providers, health plans, healthcare clearinghouses, and business associates on April 14, 2003, after the USD-HHS developed regulations. These standards provide patients access to their medical records and more control over how their personal health information is used and disclosed. They represent a uniform federal platform to ensure that individuals' health information is properly protected while allowing the appropriate flow of health information (Centers for Disease Control and Prevention, 2018).

These protections for patients include access to medical records, patient ability to review and obtain copies of their medical records and request corrections for any errors, and notification of privacy practices indicating how organizations may use personal medical information and patient rights. Regulations stipulate that access to patient records should be provided within 30 days; however, agencies can charge for the cost of copying and sending records. While healthcare providers are provided latitude to share information needed to treat their patients, there are limits on using personal medical information and how providers can use patient health information (PHI), which is individually identifiable.

As a part of these changes, electronic medical records have been mandated by legislation in some settings to increase accuracy, promote healthcare team communication, and reduce medical errors. Multiple software platforms are available, with varying levels of sophistication and cost. Patient health information security, accessibility, and liability are important considerations for these platforms. Newer platforms may also have telehealth secure videoconferencing capabilities to provide synchronous (i.e., live interaction between patient and provider via video camera) or asynchronous (i.e., secure video recording storing and forwarding) as other features for sharing information and communication. Additional policy considerations must be made regarding telehealth, including licensure (typically required in the state where the patient is present), state practice act considerations, Internet connectivity, and documentation of consent to treatment via telehealth.

Healthcare Legislation, Laws, and Policy in Pediatric Practice Settings

Pediatric practice refers to healthcare services provided to individuals from infancy until the age of 21 years. Pediatric healthcare services can occur in many settings, including hospitals, outpatient clinics, early-intervention agencies, home-based services, school-based services, and community-based facilities. According to a Policy Statement published by the American Academy of Pediatrics (Boudreau et al., 2022), pediatric primary care in the United States is typically provided by a medical doctor and advanced practice providers such as nurse practitioners, physician assistants, and other trained pediatric professionals. The focus is typically on preventing or ameliorating disease, illness, or disability. Pediatric primary healthcare aims to provide ongoing, comprehensive, family-centered, and coordinated care. This care can include health supervision for physical and mental health conditions, guidance and promotion of wellness, monitoring growth and development, diagnosis and treatment of acute and chronic health disorders, managing serious and life-threatening illnesses, and referring

patients with more complex conditions for specialty or medical subspecialty care. The pediatrician is typically the supervisor of primary care delivery, often through collaboration with a team and frequently through ongoing relationships with patients, which may span the entire childhood and adolescence (Boudreau et al., 2022).

Pediatric occupational, physical, and speech-language pathology practitioners provide a wide array of services for infants, children, and youth with or at risk of developmental delays, disorders, or diseases. These services include habilitation and rehabilitation of developmental milestones and skills related to behavioral, cognitive, motor, social, sensory, perceptual, self-care, and other factors. Services may be provided in a hospital, clinic, home, school, or community-based location. Health insurance typically reimburses these services when coverage is available and active. Access to specialty providers remains an ongoing challenge for some populations, particularly for individuals in rural areas and other underserved communities.

Legislation in Pediatric Practice Settings

Legislation in every healthcare practice setting drives the parameters of practice. In pediatrics, several key pieces of federal legislation drive rules, regulations, and scope of practice across pediatric settings, including inpatient, outpatient, and school-based healthcare. Federal law or legislation sets guidelines for all infants, children, and adolescents who are citizens of the United States. Thus no matter the United States state where a provider practices, the following legislation will establish basic rules and regulations for providing services to specific populations or in specific facilities.

Pediatric healthcare services provided under a medical model or in a medical institution such as a pediatric hospital, neonatal intensive care unit, outpatient clinic, or home healthcare service are under the Americans with Disabilities Act legislative regulations. For medical model settings, health and billing policies follow private or federal social insurance (i.e., Medicaid) guidelines for providing services to the pediatric population. As discussed earlier in this chapter, the Americans with Disabilities Act of 1990 (United States Department of Justice, 2016) provides comprehensive civil rights protection to individuals with disabilities. These rights include employment, state, and local government services, public accommodations, transportation, and telecommunications. Healthcare services that do not rely on federal or state funding typically fall under the general ADA guidelines for fair and equitable access, billing/cost, and treatment.

Healthcare Policy and Reimbursement in Pediatric Practice Settings

Several important policies take precedence in pediatric practice related to practice standards and billing guidelines. The state practice act outlines overarching guidelines for service provision. This legislation delineates policy requirements for clinical practice, documentation, continuing education, licensure and renewal, the scope of practice, supervision, ethics, and professional conduct.

For medically-based settings (e.g., inpatient hospitals, outpatient therapy, or home-based therapy) that are covered by private insurance, the policies for the provision of services are regulated by guidelines set forth by the Medicare Benefit Policy Manual, Medicare Chapters 5 and 16 (United States Centers for Medicare & Medicaid Services, 2015). These chapters outline the necessary components for documentation and billing for outpatient services.

At the Federal level, health policy and billing for individuals with low or no income under 18 years of age are largely determined by the United States Centers for Medicare and Medicaid Services. Medicaid and the Children's Health Insurance Program (CHIP) provide health coverage to millions of Americans, including children, pregnant women, parents, seniors, and individuals with disabilities. These programs cover all low-income adults below a certain income level in some states. CMS publishes a State Medicaid Manual as a policy guideline for how states can establish programs, eligibility, and resources for the local community.

School-Based and Early Intervention Services

Early intervention services (0 to 3 years old), school-based healthcare services (3 to 21 years old), and some state-provided outpatient healthcare services (birth to 21 years old) are regulated under the Individuals with Disabilities Education Improvement Act (IDEA) of 2004, and other legislation discussed earlier in this chapter. These services are also regulated under Section 504 of the Rehabilitation Act of 1973 (United States Department of Labor, n.d.b).

The IDEA ensures that Americans with disabilities have equal access to early intervention, special education, and related services. Originated in 1975, the Education for All Handicapped Children Act (EHA Public Law 94-142) was enacted to provide a free and appropriate public education to each disabled child in the United States by authorizing financial incentives to the states and local entities that complied with the statutes of the law (United States Department of Education, 2022a). In 1990, the Education for All Handicapped Children Act had been renamed the Individuals with Disabilities Education Act. Most importantly, the legislative definitions for developmental delay were expanded to include birth to 9 years of age, which allowed significantly more students with delayed cognitive, motor, or physical functioning to access medically appropriate intervention services. The IDEA governs how governmental agencies (national and local) provide services to eligible children with disabilities and special needs (Fig. 2.7).

In 2004 the IDEA was reauthorized with revised regulations. It is a grant-based program that provides financial assistance to local education agencies (LEAs). The Individuals with Disabilities Education Act legislation has four sections; A, B, C, and D. The four major goals of the IDEA are: (1) to provide a free and appropriate public education (FAPE) for children with disabilities, (2) to ensure that the rights of

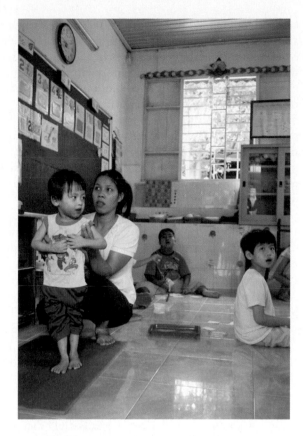

• **Fig. 2.7** IDEA governs how governmental agencies (national and local) provide services to eligible children with disabilities and special needs. (From https://commons.wikimedia.org/w/index.php?curid=22990191)

children and their families are protected, (3) to assist states and local agencies with providing education and appropriate services for ALL children with disabilities, and (4) to assess the effectiveness of the efforts to educate children with disabilities (United States Department of Education, 2021). The four parts are as follows:

• Part A outlines general provisions and guidelines. It is the foundation for the Act and defines key terms used in the language of the Act. Part A also outlines the creation of the Office of Special Education Programs (OSEP). This office provides equitable and high-quality services to improve outcomes for children with disabilities aged birth to 21 years (United States Department of Education, 2022b).

• Part B applies to individuals aged 3 to 21 years who require access to special education and related services. Related services include but are not limited to occupational therapy, physical therapy, speech-language pathology, transportation services, orientation and mobility services, interpreting services, therapeutic recreation, counseling services, and school health services (United States Department of Education, n.d.).

• Part C applies to early intervention services for infants and toddlers with disabilities ages birth to 2 years and their families. Children "age out" of early intervention on their third birthday. This funding is based on research evidence that intervening early in development is critical for the best outcomes because infants and toddlers learn and grow quickly through skills typically developing across a continuum of skills. These services are delivered in the "natural environment" whenever possible rather than in a clinical setting. A natural environment can include a home, daycare, or other location where the infant or toddler naturally spends most of their time.

- Part D recognizes the need for national activities to improve children's education with disabilities. These activities can include grants, support programs, projects, or resources that contribute meaningful and positive results to individuals with disabilities (United States Department of Education, n.d.).

Section 504 of the Rehabilitation Act of 1973 dictates that programs and activities which receive federal funding from the United States Department of Education must provide a "free and appropriate public education to each qualified student with a disability who is in the school district's jurisdiction, regardless of the nature or severity of the disability" (United States Department of Labor, n.d.b). This law includes public schools, institutions of higher education, and other state and local education agencies. The Rehabilitation Act and the IDEA intersect as they both protect the rights of students with disabilities and attempt to eliminate discrimination due to disability status across the spectrum of federal, state, and local governmental activities, programs, and services, regardless of whether a student receives federal financial assistance. The Rehabilitation Act and the ADA are nondiscrimination laws and do not administer funding.

To ensure health policy is followed, each state has contracted local education agencies (LEA) that oversee Medicaid reimbursement administration for medically necessary services (United States Department of Education, 2017). A LEA is a public board of education or authority that establishes administrative control of the public elementary and secondary schools in a local area (i.e., city, county, school district). Medicaid is designed to provide benefits as a safety net for older adults, victims of industrial accidents, unemployed individuals, dependent mothers and children, and people with disabilities (U.S. National Archives and Records Administration, 2022b). When a LEA uses Medicaid as a billing source, the policies of the Social Security Act §1903(c) apply to ensure access to children receiving services through an individualized education program (IEP) in public schools under Part B of the IDEA or individualized family services plan (IFSP) for early intervention under Part C of the IDEA (U.S. Social Security Administration, n.d.). LEA's must understand the IDEA requirements when providing Medicaid-reimbursed, school-based services to eligible children. This policy includes, but is not limited to, children under 21 years who have or are at risk of developmental delays, intellectual disabilities, sensory processing impairments, physical disabilities, behavioral challenges, or socioemotional impairments.

Privacy and the protection of client rights are of paramount importance when providing healthcare services. Privacy becomes even more important when dealing with minors who may not be able to advocate for themselves or their best interests. Two federal privacy laws that regulate pediatric practice across all settings are the Family Education Rights and Privacy Act (FERPA) of 1974 (20 USC. $1232g; 34 CFR Part 99) and the Health Insurance Portability and Accountability Act (HIPAA) of 1996. As discussed in this chapter, HIPAA is a federal law requiring a nationally standardized method of protecting confidential patient health information from being shared or obtained without the consumer's knowledge (Centers for Disease Control and Prevention, 2018). FERPA ensures the protection of the privacy of students' education records. FERPA allows parents to access their children's records (United States Department of Education, 2019). Practitioners' adherence to privacy legislation protects all entities involved and enhances consumers' trust in the healthcare system.

Healthcare Legislation, Laws, and Policy in Adult Practice Settings

Adult practice settings will primarily include organizations serving adults aged 22 years and older. These settings may occasionally have pediatric clients, especially in health professional shortage areas such as rural and low-income communities. In this section, we will focus on adult populations that may have state-regulated Medicaid if they are disabled or have low income, federally-regulated Medicare if they are 65 years or older (or have other qualifying conditions), private insurance, and military service-related insurance coverage. The related legislation, laws, and policies that govern service delivery to these populations are discussed.

Overview of Medicare and Medicaid

Medicare is a federal program that provides healthcare coverage for United States citizens aged 65 years and older and individuals who meet select eligibility requirements (Box 2.2). Although Medicare provides health coverage for qualifying individuals regardless of income, Medicaid is a joint federal and state program that provides free or low-cost health coverage to individuals and families with low or no income. The federal government establishes uniform

---

• BOX 2.2	Medicare Eligibility Requirements

- United States citizens aged 65 years or older or any of the following:
- Individuals receiving Social Security disability benefits for 24 months, regardless of age
- A diagnosis of amyotrophic lateral sclerosis (ALS), regardless of age
- A diagnosis of end-stage renal disease (ESRD) requiring regular dialysis or a kidney transplant, regardless of age

From *Who is eligible for Medicare?* HHS.gov (2014). https://www.hhs.gov/answers/medicare-and-medicaid/who-is-eligible-for-medicare/index.html

rules for Medicare at the national level, whereas individual states manage Medicaid programs. As a result, Medicare has the same eligibility requirements and coverage nationwide, whereas Medicaid eligibility and coverage can differ significantly from state to state. Therefore, what is covered by Medicaid in one state may not be paid for in another. Income eligibility requirements for Medicaid also differ state-to-state.

Furthermore, individuals with Medicare may pay for additional supplemental insurance, as described in the following section. They may also be required to pay copayments and reach a deductible before services are covered. However, Medicaid coverage will often not require copayments or deductibles. Individuals may also have healthcare coverage from Medicare and Medicaid if they meet eligibility requirements for both programs (e.g., over 65 years old living in a low- or no-income household).

The United States federal government created Medicare in 1965 to address the challenges many older Americans faced in purchasing private health insurance and accessing costly healthcare services. Medicare was originally offered with two types of coverage: Medicare Parts A and B, covering different aspects of healthcare. Since then, Medicare has evolved to include Medicare Parts C and D. A brief overview of which healthcare services are covered is given in Fig. 2.8.

Medicare Part A: Acute and Post-Acute Care

Medicare Part A provides coverage for acute and post-acute care (see Chapters 16 and 17). Acute and post-acute care includes short-term/inpatient hospital stays, long-term acute care, inpatient rehabilitation, skilled nursing care, home healthcare, and hospice. Most people do not pay for Medicare Part A if they (or their spouse) previously paid Medicare taxes for a certain amount of time while working. While there is no monthly premium for Medicare Part A, a deductible requirement is required for inpatient stays and coinsurance is required for inpatient stays longer than 60 days (United States Centers for Medicare and Medicaid Services,

n.d.a). Medical services provided under Medicare Part A are reimbursed at a predetermined, fixed amount based on diagnosis and case complexity.

Medicare Part B—Outpatient Care and Other Healthcare Services

Although Medicare Part B is a component of the original Medicare guidelines, it is considered supplemental insurance because it is voluntary to opt-in to coverage. It also typically requires the beneficiary/patient to pay a monthly premium. Many eligible recipients opt-in to Medicare Part B coverage because Part A is limited to inpatient and home health services. Medicare Part B provides coverage for medically necessary outpatient services (e.g., outpatient occupational therapy, physical therapy, speech-language pathology, doctor visits), laboratory testing, orthotics and prosthetics, durable medical equipment, mental health services, and preventive screenings. Patients with Medicare Part B coverage must also pay a deductible and often a 20% coinsurance for outpatient rehabilitation services, most doctor visits, and durable medical equipment (United States Centers for Medicare and Medicaid Services, n.d.a). Services covered under Medicare Part B are billed by healthcare providers on a fee-for-service basis using the Healthcare Common Procedure Coding System (HCPCS).

Medicare Parts C and D—Medicare Advantage and Prescription Drug Coverage

While Medicare Parts A and B provide significant healthcare coverage, several services are not covered. These include services and items such as dental care, most prescription medicines, routine eye care, and hearing exams. As such, two supplemental Medicare plans are available to individuals enrolled in Medicare to offset these additional healthcare costs: Medicare Parts C and D. Unlike Medicare Parts A and B, which are regulated entirely by the federal government, Medicare Parts C and D are managed by private insurance companies that follow the rules established by Medicare.

Medicare Part C (also known as "Medicare Advantage") is a private health insurance plan that can be selected to supplement traditional Medicare. Medicare Advantage plans typically include additional services not otherwise covered (e.g., dental care, dentures, vision care, glasses), with typical services covered under Medicare Parts A and B. In addition to monthly insurance premiums paid by beneficiaries for Medicare Advantage (Part C) plans, the federal government pays private insurers a fixed dollar amount every month for beneficiaries enrolled in their plans. Like Medicare Parts A and B, Medicare Advantage plans typically require a deductible and copayments for healthcare services and monthly premiums.

Medicare Part D is the prescription drug coverage program offered through Medicare. Part D was enacted as part of the Medicare Modernization Act of 2003 (effective January 1, 2006) and helped to pay for medications not

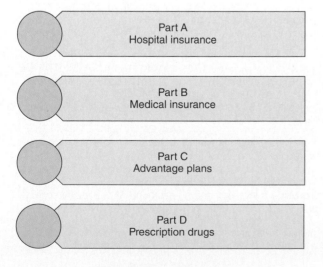

• Fig. 2.8 Parts of Medicare.

covered under Medicare Parts A or B. Monthly premiums are available for Medicare Part D plans. While the federal government pays 75% of medication costs, covered individuals must pay a deductible and copayments for prescriptions. As with Medicare Part C plans, Medicare Part D coverage is optional. These plans are managed by private insurance companies that receive funding from Medicare.

Medicare Part A Reimbursement: Prospective Payment Systems

A prospective payment system is an approach to payment for healthcare services that reimburses the healthcare provider/facility a predetermined amount based on various factors (e.g., medical diagnosis, medical complexity), regardless of the actual amount of service provided (United States Centers for Medicare and Medicaid Services, 2021c). The prepayment is based on the patient's diagnosis and standardized assessments to determine medical complexity and each covers a predefined time, such as an inpatient hospital stay or a 60-day home health episode. Prospective payment systems (PPSs) were developed by the United States Centers for Medicare and Medicaid to improve patient care quality while lowering hospital stay lengths and costs. This model enables healthcare providers to know the predetermined reimbursement amount for patient care, regardless of the volume or duration of care provided. CMS uses different PPS models across acute and post-acute care settings (Table 2.5). Reimbursement using a PPS model only applies to services covered under Medicare Part A. Healthcare services covered

under Medicare Part B are reimbursed using a fee-for-service model. Fee-for-service means payment is based on the service provided rather than a predetermined amount and that reimbursement is volume-based (e.g., reimbursed based on the amount of time spent providing treatment). The Medicare Physician Fee Schedule (MPFS) is a complete listing of the maximum allowable amount healthcare professionals can expect to be reimbursed for services covered under Medicare Part B (e.g., diagnostic services, well visits, outpatient rehabilitation visits).

Private Insurance

Private insurance options are available to qualifying individuals and families. Typically, these insurance plans will be accessed through employer plans for full-time and occasionally part-time employees as part of a benefits package. Private insurance plans are also available for those who are self-employed through some companies. These plans will typically have a deductible (an amount that must be reached before insurance will cover costs), a copayment (an amount that must be paid per visit by the patient), and an out-of-pocket maximum (the maximum amount that a beneficiary will have to pay for a given period). Insurance agencies generally offer multiple plans, including dental, vision, wellness, diagnostic, prescription, and other potential benefits. Coverage is often available for an individual, spouse, or family. Insurance authorization may have to be obtained for initial or ongoing services, and there may be caps (or maximums) for therapy services and other benefits.

TABLE 2.5	Prospective Payment Systems by Practice Setting for Medicare Part A Coverage	
Practice Setting	**Brief Description**
Short- and Long-term Acute Care Hospitals (STACH and LTACH)	• Under Inpatient Prospective Payment System (IPPS), each patient case is categorized into a diagnosis-related group (DRG). • Each DRG has a payment weight assigned based on the average resources used to treat Medicare patients in that DRG.
Home Health Agencies (HHA)	• The Patient-Driven Grouping Model (PDPM) utilizes Home Health Resource Groups (HHRGs), which are determined by an interprofessional standardized assessment called the Outcome and Assessment Information Set (OASIS). • Medicare pays a predetermined base rate adjusted for the patient's health condition and service needs, considered the case-mix adjustment.
Inpatient Rehabilitation Facilities (IRF)	• The IRF PPS utilizes information from a Patient Assessment Instrument (IRF-PAI) to classify patients into distinct groups based on clinical characteristics and expected resource needs. • Separate payments are calculated for each group, including the application of case and facility-level adjustments.
Skilled Nursing Facilities (SNF)	• The Patient-Driven Payment Model (PDPM) is used under the SNF PPS for classifying SNF patients in a covered Medicare Part A stay. • The PDPM includes a variety of functional and cognitive assessments (often referred to as 'Section GG' or 'Section GG Assessments'). • Occupational therapists, physical therapists, and nurses conduct GG assessments to establish the pre-determined amount Medicare will pay for their SNF stay.

Adapted from https://www.cms.gov/Medicare/Medicare-Fee-for-Service-Payment/AcuteInpatientPPS; https://www.cms.gov/medicare/medicare-fee-for-service-payment/homehealthpps; https://www.cms.gov/medicare/medicare-fee-for-service-payment/inpatientrehabfacpps; https://www.cms.gov/Medicare/Medicare-Fee-for-Service-Payment/SNFPPS/PDPM.

Healthcare Legislation, Laws, and Policy for Veterans and Active-Duty Service Members

United States Department of Veterans Affairs

The United States Department of Veterans Affairs (2021a), more commonly referred to as the VA, provides veterans of the United States military and their families with healthcare and other benefits and services (e.g., job placement assistance, disability compensation). The VA provides healthcare coverage to over 9 million eligible veterans and their families through the VA health plan. A person who has served in active duty for the United States military, naval, or air service—and who has been discharged or released under conditions other than dishonorable—may qualify for VA healthcare benefits. Reserve and National Guard members can qualify as well. VA healthcare plans provide coverage for most healthcare services, including outpatient medical and rehabilitation visits, inpatient medical services (e.g., surgeries, specialized care for traumatic injuries), mental health services, and emergency health (United States Department of Veterans Affairs, 2021a).

The Veterans Healthcare Administration (VHA) was established in 1946 through the VA to provide care to veterans returning from World War II (United States Department of Veterans Affairs, 2021b). It is now the largest integrated healthcare system in the country and approximately 60% of all medical residents receive some training at VA hospitals. It provides training for most medical, nursing, and allied health professionals in the United States and is one of the largest healthcare systems in the world. The medical research programs provided through the VA also benefit all members of society.

In addition to VA healthcare coverage, many veterans also have additional healthcare coverage (e.g., Medicaid, private insurance). If a veteran has a medical condition unrelated to their military service, they may still be treated at a VA medical facility. Depending on the veteran's priority group assignment, the VA may send the bill for medical services provided to the individual's additional insurance plan for reimbursement. For more information on VA health benefits, visit the VA website (va.gov) for the most up-to-date information.

TRICARE for Uniformed and Retired Service Members

TRICARE (Military Health System, n.d.) is a healthcare program operated by the United States Department of Defense Military Health System. The purpose of TRICARE is to provide comprehensive and affordable healthcare benefits to active-duty personnel and their families. TRICARE beneficiaries receive healthcare services through military treatment facilities and contracted civilian healthcare providers in the United States and abroad. According to the Military Health System, with nearly 10 million beneficiaries, TRICARE ranks among the ten largest health plans in the nation compared with civilian insurances (Military Health System, n.d.).

Employment Legislation, Laws, and Policies Across Healthcare Settings

Legislation, laws, and policies across healthcare and other industries dictate the who, what, where, when, how, and why of employment and the provision of services across settings. Although some variations may exist due to the type of organization (e.g., charitable and religious non-profits, private foundations, political organizations, sole proprietorships, partnerships, corporations), several areas of legislation, laws, and policies are commonly applicable across practice settings to ensure accountability of services and products, provider qualifications, patient rights, employee rights. These relate to licensing and credentialing, Federal Equal Employment Opportunity (EEO) laws and legal protections, employment of individuals with a disability, and sexual harassment. In addition, it is commonly understood that "ignorance of the law is no excuse" when such laws are publicly posted. Individuals and organizations must be aware of these regulations of healthcare services as governing bodies, third-party payers, workers, consumers, and the general public depend on the system's standards.

Licensing and Credentialing

Licensing is an important regulatory protection to promote professional standards, integrity, access, and stipulations for ongoing practice. In the United States, licenses are mediated at the state level and may require Governor appointments for state policy positions within the state licensure board. This process can include completing a state or national exam, submitting references, providing multiple forms of identification, and more. Some professions have sought to enhance license portability by creating compacts between states to agree on minimum qualifications and expedited applications. Individual practitioners are generally responsible for seeking initial and ongoing licensure.

Healthcare policies are often regulated by a state department of health that primarily focuses on public health, environmental control, and social services. Governing entities and organizations can require licensure and additional certifications to maintain employment. Additional requirements include cardiopulmonary resuscitation (CPR), technology education, and skills-based training certifications. In addition, individuals and organizations may be required to meet additional credentialing or mandated criteria for initial and ongoing authorization through third-party payers, including health insurance companies, grant funding entities, sponsors/donors, and other state or federal organizations. Additional documentation, training, and certifications may be required. Regulatory boards or organizations with oversight and responsibility to the public may conduct planned or random audits to ensure compliance standards are being met. Companies may also implement internal audits, designate quality assurance entities, consult with industry experts, utilize resources for worker training, and implement additional standards to evaluate and improve the quality of care on an ongoing basis. Regulatory entities may require a commonly utilized resource, the Joint Commission on Accreditation of Healthcare Organizations (JCAHO) (The Joint Commission, 2022). JCAHO is a private, not-for-profit organization founded in 1951 to evaluate healthcare organizations based on standards for patient safety. JCAHO standards are expected to be met on an ongoing basis, and the accreditation process for healthcare organizations includes evaluation by an on-site team at least every 3 years (The Joint Commission, 2022).

Federal Equal Employment Opportunity Laws and Legal Protections

Throughout the almost 400 years in the history of the United States, employment has become more accessible and more equitable, especially concerning gender, racial/ethnic, cultural, and generational norms. Much of this has been due to legislation prohibiting discrimination and bias in healthcare and other industries. See Table 2.6 for key legislation related to this topic.

Employment of Individuals With a Disability

Under the ADA, an individual with a disability is defined as someone with a physical or mental impairment that substantially limits one or more major life activities, has a record of such an impairment, or is regarded as having such an impairment (United States Department of Justice, 2016). These major life activities would be those that an average person can perform with little or no difficulty, such as walking, breathing, seeing, hearing, speaking, learning, and working. A qualified employee or applicant with a disability satisfies skill, experience, education, and other job-related requirements of the position held or desired and

who, with or without reasonable accommodation, can perform the essential functions of that position (United States Department of Justice, 2016).

Reasonable accommodations under Title I of the Americans with Disabilities Act refer to a modification or adjustment to a job, work environment, or process for hiring in order to enable an individual with a disability to have an equal opportunity to obtain and perform in employment (United States Department of Labor, 2022). These may include but are not limited to making existing facilities used by employees readily accessible to and usable by persons with disabilities; job restructuring; modification of work schedules; providing additional unpaid leave; reassignment to a vacant position; acquiring or modifying equipment or devices; adjusting or modifying exams, training materials, or policies; or providing qualified readers or interpreters. Reasonable accommodations may be necessary to apply for a job, perform job functions, or enjoy the benefits and privileges of employment that people enjoy without disabilities (United States Equal Employment Opportunity Commission, 2002). An employer is not required to lower production standards to make an accommodation. An employer generally is not obligated to provide personal use items such as eyeglasses or hearing aids. An employer must make a reasonable accommodation to a qualified individual with a disability unless doing so would impose an undue hardship on the operation of the employer's business (Fig. 2.9). An "undue hardship" is an action that requires significant difficulty or expense when considering factors such as a business' size, financial resources, and the nature and structure of its operation (United States Equal Employment Opportunity Commission, 2002).

Before making an offer of employment, an employer may not ask job applicants about the existence, nature, or severity of a disability, including a "temporary disability" such as pregnancy. However, applicants may be asked about their ability to perform job functions. A job offer may be conditional on a medical examination, but only if the examination is required for all employees in the same job category. Medical

TABLE 2.6	Legislation Impacting Employment in Healthcare Settings
1963: Equal Pay Act (EPA)	• Protects from sex-based wage discrimination when men and women perform substantially equal work in an organization.
1964: Title VII of the Civil Rights Act	• Prohibits employment discrimination based on race, color, religion, sex, or national origin.
1967: Age Discrimination in Employment Act (ADEA)	• Protects individuals who are 40 years of age or older from discrimination in the workplace.
1990: Title I and Title V of the Americans with Disabilities Act (ADA)	• Prohibits employment discrimination against qualified individuals with disabilities in the private sector as well as state and local governments.
2001: New Freedom Initiative	• Promotes the full participation of people with disabilities in all areas of society by increasing access to assistive and universally designed technologies, educational and employment opportunities, and full access to community life.

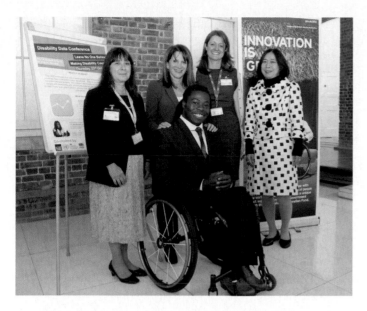

• **Fig. 2.9** Employers must make *reasonable* accommodations for qualified individuals unless doing so would impose an undue hardship on the business. (From https://commons.wikimedia.org/w/index.php?curid=38900983)

examinations of employees must be job-related and consistent with business necessities. State and federal laws also regulate the types of questions an employer can ask. Typically questions about marital status, family, or religious beliefs are not legal. However, some exceptions may exist (i.e., if individuals apply for positions in a religious organization).

The ADA does not protect employees and applicants engaging in the illegal use of drugs. Tests for illegal use of drugs are not considered medical examinations and, therefore, are not subject to the ADA's restrictions on medical examinations. Individuals who are illegally using drugs and individuals with alcoholism may be held to the same performance standards as other employees. Some state licensure applications may ask about substance abuse and history prior to licensure. Some states may also provide specialized programs for individuals in recovery.

Sexual Harassment

Title VII of the Civil Rights Act of 1964 (United States National Archives and Records Administration, 2022a) prohibits sexual harassment as discrimination. Unwelcome sexual advances, requests for sexual favors, and other verbal or physical conduct of a sexual nature constitute sexual harassment when this conduct explicitly or implicitly affects an individual's employment; interferes with an individual's work performance; or creates an intimidating, hostile, or offensive work environment. Sexual harassment can occur in a variety of circumstances, including but not limited to the following:

• The victim and harasser do not have to be of the opposite sex. Either may be a man or a woman.

• The harasser can be the victim's supervisor, an agent of the organization, a supervisor in another area, a coworker, or a non-employee.
• The victim can be anyone affected by the offensive conduct and is not limited to the individual being harassed.
• Sexual harassment may or may not occur with economic or employment impact for the victim.
• The harasser's conduct must be unwelcome.

Employers can provide sexual harassment training for employees and establish complaint or grievance processes. Employers should also take immediate and appropriate action when employees complain to prevent further issues and establish a culture of accountability and trust. It is unlawful for an employer or harasser to retaliate against an individual for opposing discrimination practices based on sex. It is also unlawful to retaliate against an individual for filing a discrimination charge, testifying, or participating in an investigation, proceeding, or litigation under Title VII.

Impact of Advocacy on Healthcare Policy and Legislation

The governing policies and legislation determine the health of individuals, groups, communities, and populations. The policies and laws that legislators and policymakers set determine the frequency, location, duration, type, recipients, providers, and more. These individuals frequently do not have a background in healthcare and rely on education and collaboration from healthcare practitioners to make the best, informed decisions regarding payment, protection, and provision of healthcare services. Healthcare practitioners, educators, and students have a professional and moral duty to advocate for improved healthcare legislation, policy, and laws on behalf of consumers, professionals, payors, and the public. The following section will discuss the role of healthcare practitioners, educators, and students and provide case examples related to advocacy.

The Role of Healthcare Practitioners, Educators, and Students in Advocacy

Advocacy is the vehicle to protect the interests of healthcare practitioners and consumers through multi-faceted outreach. A professional must advocate for the client, profession, and workforce in healthcare practice. An advocate's core role is to inform communities at large about the profession, assist clients in receiving the appropriate amount of therapy services needed for optimal progress, and help promote the improvement of healthcare systems and policies for the betterment of society.

Health policy and legislation are always evolving to respond to societal needs and the healthcare industry. For example, many state policies were quickly developed during the COVID-19 pandemic surrounding telehealth services, consumer access to services, and expanded billing practices to accommodate new methods for providing healthcare services during an unprecedented time. Clinicians must stay aware of federal and local health policy regulations while actively advocating that service delivery and reimbursement follow best practices and legal standards.

As healthcare practitioners continue to adjust to changing regulations, payment reform, and evolving service delivery models, it is vital that professionals share their unique knowledge and skills. Incorporating advocacy into everyday clinical practice helps professionals confirm their value to clients, caregivers, payers, and policymakers. Professional associations provide various resources on different legislative and policy issues relevant to healthcare practice. Health professionals may have lobbyists or Political Action Committees (PACs) to help obtain funding to support political activities (United States Federal Election Committee, n.d.). These registered PACs can effectively engage support and build professional relationships with governing individuals and entities.

Individual practitioners and groups should be involved in and promote advocacy for consumers, health professions, and healthcare improvement. Many professions offer local, state, and national advocacy events where administrators, practitioners, educators, and students are encouraged to participate in providing education and raising awareness about key issues. Many professions provide opportunities to attend in-person meetings with Congressional staff in Washington, DC, or at state legislative facilities to advocate for the profession. While important opportunities exist through in-person opportunities, other effective advocacy methods exist. These include promoting healthcare services in the community or workplace, advocating for the role of healthcare professionals in emerging practice areas and underserved communities, engaging in social media campaigns, and writing letters or emails to legislators on key issues impacting the profession. Some professions offer letter or email templates around various issues and topics of interest which are readily available to send to legislators. Engagement in these and other means of advocacy are critical for health professions' ongoing vitality, quality, and responsiveness.

Examples of Advocacy in Action

Below are three examples where advocacy initiatives from healthcare providers helped to bring about positive actions:
- In 1997 the Balanced Budget Act established annual Medicare spending limits per-beneficiary, commonly referred to as "therapy caps" for outpatient occupational therapy, physical therapy, and speech-language pathology services covered by Medicare Part B. As of 2018, the Medicare therapy cap for outpatient occupational therapy services (e.g., the maximum spending limit in a given year) was $2010 per Medicare beneficiary. Additionally, a therapy cap of $2010 is in place for combined physical therapy and speech-language pathology. These caps placed Medicare beneficiaries at risk of being denied essential rehabilitation services.
- On February 9, 2018, the President signed the Bipartisan Budget Act of 2018, which included a provision to remove existing outpatient therapy caps for occupational therapy, physical therapy, and speech-language pathology services. This Act was a significant advocacy success for these health professionals as there was no longer a maximum ceiling for outpatient rehabilitation as long as services continued to be deemed medically necessary.
- The Medicare Home Health Flexibility Act and the Bipartisan Budget Act of 2018 are just a few recent examples of how professional associations, healthcare practitioners, educators, and students have advocated for meaningful change to maximize patient outcomes and quality of life.

Conclusion

The US healthcare system is complex and ever-changing due to societal needs and the socio-political climate. Although policy impacts practice, practice can impact policy when practitioners, students, organizations, and other stakeholders advocate and collaborate for meaningful change. Individuals and organizations can use the resources discussed in this chapter to enhance their knowledge, raise awareness, and provide critical information to educate gatekeepers, stakeholders, and colleagues to build a better healthcare system for the future.

References

Annas, G. J. (2017). *Health law*. Encyclopedia Britannica. https://www.britannica.com/science/health-law.

Association of American Medical Colleges. (2003). *Equity, Diversity, & Inclusion*. https://www.aamc.org/about-us/equity-diversity-inclusion.

Boudreau, A., Hamling, A., Pont, E., Pendergrass, T. W., & Richerson, J. (2022). Committee On Pediatric Workforce, Committee on Practice and Ambulatory Medicine, Pediatric Primary Health Care: The central role of pediatricians in maintaining children's health in evolving health care models. *Pediatrics, 149*(2), e2021055553.

Centers for Disease Control and Prevention. (2018). *Health Insurance Portability and Accountability Act of 1996 (HIPAA)*. https://www.cdc.gov/phlp/publications/topic/hipaa.html.

Centers for Disease Control and Prevention. (2020). *COVID-19 racial and ethnic health disparities*. https://www.cdc.gov/coronavirus/2019-ncov/community/health-equity/racial-ethnic-disparities/index.html.

Centers for Disease Control and Prevention. (2021). *Social Determinants of health: Know what affects health*. https://www.cdc.gov/socialdeterminants/index.htm.

Feeding America. (2021). *The impact of the coronavirus on food insecurity in 2020 & 2021*. https://www.feedingamerica.org/sites/default/files/2021-03/National%20Projections%20Brief_3.9.2021_0.pdf.

Institute of Medicine. (2002). *Unequal treatment: What health care system administrators need to know about racial and ethnic disparities in healthcare.* https://nap.nationalacademies.org/resource/10260/disparities_admin.pdf.

Internal Revenue Services. (2021). *Determining if an employer is an applicable large employer.* https://www.irs.gov/affordable-care-act/employers/determining-if-an-employer-is-an-applicable-large-employer.

Joint Commission. (2022). *Facts about the joint commission.* https://www.jointcommission.org/about-us/facts-about-the-joint-commission/.

Martin, R. (2008). Law, and public health policy. *International Encyclopedia of Public Health,* 30–38. https://doi.org/10.1016/B978-012373960-5.00236-7.

Military Health System. (n.d.). *Elements of the Military Health System.* The official website of the military health system. https://health.mil/About-MHS/MHS-Elements.

National Academy of Medicine. (2022). *Social determinants of health archives.* https://nam.edu/tag/social-determinants-of-health/.

US Centers for Medicare and Medicaid Services. (n.d.a). *Medicare costs at a glance.* https://www.medicare.gov/basics/costs/medicare-costs.

US Centers for Medicare & Medicaid Services. (2015). *Medicare benefit policy manual.* https://www.cms.gov/Regulations-and-Guidance/Guidance/Manuals/downloads/bp102c15.pdf.

US Centers for Medicare & Medicaid Services. (2021a). *ICD-10 codes.* https://www.cms.gov/Medicare/Coding/ICD10.

US Centers for Medicare & Medicaid Services. (2021b). *IMPACT act of 2014 data standardization & cross setting measures.* https://www.cms.gov/Medicare/Quality-Initiatives-Patient-Assessment-Instruments/Post-Acute-Care-Quality-Initiatives/IMPACT-Act-of-2014/IMPACT-Act-of-2014-Data-Standardization-and-Cross-Setting-Measures.

US Centers for Medicare & Medicaid Services. (2021c). *Prospective payment systems—general information.* https://www.cms.gov/Medicare/Medicare-Fee-for-Service-Payment/ProspMedicareFeeSvcPmtGen.

US Centers for Medicare & Medicaid Services. (2022). *HCPCS - General information.* https://www.cms.gov/medicare/coding/medhcpcsgeninfo.

US Central Intelligence Agency World Fact Book. (2022). *Explore all countries: United States.* https://www.cia.gov/the-world-factbook/countries/united-states.

US Congress. (1996). *Health Insurance Portability and Accountability Act of 1996.* https://www.congress.gov/104/plaws/publ191/PLAW-104publ191.pdf.

US Department of Education. (n.d.). *Individuals with Disabilities Education Act: Statute and regulations.* https://sites.ed.gov/idea/statuteregulations/.

US Department of Education. (2017). *Sec. 303.23 Local educational agency.* https://sites.ed.gov/idea/regs/c/a/303.23.

US Department of Education. (2019). *What is FERPA? Protecting student privacy.* https://studentprivacy.ed.gov/faq/what-ferpa.

US Department of Education. (2021). *Department Submits 42nd Annual Report to Congress on the IDEA.* Individuals with Disabilities Education Act. https://sites.ed.gov/idea/department-submits-the-42nd-annual-report-to-congress-idea.

US Department of Education. (2022a). *A History of the Individuals with Disabilities Education Act.* https://sites.ed.gov/idea/IDEA-History.

US Department of Education. (2022b). *About OSEP.* https://www2.ed.gov/about/offices/list/osers/osep/about.html.

US Department of Health and Human Services (USDHHS). (2022). *About the Affordable Care Act.* https://www.hhs.gov/healthcare/about-the-aca/index.html.

US Department of Health and Human Services (USDHHS) Office of Disease Prevention and Health Promotion. (n.d.). *Healthy people 2030.* https://health.gov/healthypeople/about.

US Department of Health and Human Services Office of Disease Prevention and Health Promotion. (2018). *Social Determinants of Health.* https://www.healthypeople.gov/2020/topics-objectives/topic/social-determinants-of-health.

US Department of Health and Human Services Office of Minority Health. (2001). *National standards for culturally and linguistically appropriate services (CLAS) in healthcare: Executive summary.* http://minorityhealth.hhs.gov/assets/pdf/checked/executive.pdf.

US Department of Health and Human Services Office of Minority Health. (2013). *National Standards for CLAS in health and health care: A blueprint for advancing and sustaining CLAS policy and practice.* https://www.thinkculturalhealth.hhs.gov/assets/pdfs/EnhancedCLASStandardsBlueprint.pdf.

US Department of Housing and Urban Development. (n.d.). *Providing integrated, community-based settings for individuals with disabilities.* https://www.hud.gov/program_offices/fair_housing_equal_opp/integrated_community_based_settings.

US Department of Justice. (2016). *Americans with Disabilities Act Title II Regulations.* https://www.ada.gov/regs2010/titleII_2010/titleII_2010_regulations.htm#a35103.

US Department of Labor. (n.d.a). *Americans with Disabilities Act.* www.ada.gov/2010_regs.htm.

US Department of Labor. (n.d.b). *Section 504, Rehabilitation Act of 1973.* www.dol.gov/agencies/oasam/centers-offices/civil-rights-center/statutes/section-504-rehabilitation-act-of-1973.

US Department of Labor. (n.d.c). *Workers' compensation.* https://www.dol.gov/general/topic/workcomp.

US Department of Labor. (2022). *Accommodations.* https://www.dol.gov/agencies/odep/program-areas/employers/accommodations.

US Department of Veterans Affairs. (2021a). *About VA health benefits.* https://www.va.gov/health-care/about-va-health-benefits/.

US Department of Veterans Affairs. (2021b). *VHA history.* https://www.va.gov/vha-history/.

US Equal Employment Opportunity Commission. (2002). *Enforcement guidance on reasonable accommodation and undue hardship under the ADA.* https://www.eeoc.gov/laws/guidance/enforcement-guidance-reasonable-accommodation-and-undue-hardship-under-ada.

US Federal Election Committee. (n.d.). *Political action committees (PACs).* https://www.fec.gov/press/resources-journalists/political-action-committees-pacs/.

US Federal Register. (n.d.). *Executive Orders.* https://www.federalregister.gov/presidential-documents/executive-orders.

US National Archives and Records Administration. (2022a). *Civil Rights Act of 1964.* https://www.archives.gov/milestone-documents/civil-rights-act.

US National Archives and Records Administration. (2022b). *Social Security Act (1935).* https://www.archives.gov/milestone-documents/social-security-act.

US Social Security Administration. (n.d.). *Compilation of the Social Security Laws: Payment to states.* https://www.ssa.gov/OP_Home/ssact/title19/1903.htm.

Vespa, Medina, Armstrong. (2020). *Demographic turning points for the United States: Population projections for 2020 to 2060.* https://www.census.gov/content/dam/Census/library/publications/2020/demo/p25-1144.pdf.

World Health Organization. (2021). *WHO's 10 calls for climate action to assure sustained recovery from COVID-19.* https://www.who.int/news/item/11-10-2021-who-s-10-calls-for-climate-action-to-assure-sustained-recovery-from-covid-19.

World Health Organization. (2022a). *Constitution.* https://www.who.int/about/governance/constitution.

World Health Organization. (2022b). *Social determinants of health.* https://www.who.int/teams/social-determinants-of-health.

3

Proposal and Grant Writing

SARAH DOERRER, PhD, OTR/L, CHT, CLT;
and ROSE L. McANDREW, OTD, OTR/L, CHT

LEARNING OBJECTIVES

By the end of this chapter, the reader will be able to:

1. Describe how to target a problem for a proposal
2. Explain how program theory is used in proposal development
3. Describe the role of logic models in program theory
4. Describe the grant proposal process, including searching for relevant grants
5. List the pertinent components of a grant proposal

CHAPTER OUTLINE

Introduction
Creating A Proposal
    Identifying and Targeting the Problem
    Needs Assessment
        Data Mining
    Program Theory
    Logic Models
    Context Analysis
    Theories of Change and Action
        Theory of Change
        Theory of Action
Grant Writing
    Formulating a Competitive Idea
    Finding a Mentor
    Searching for a Grant
    The Grant Proposal
    Introduction/Problem Statement
    Writing the Aims

Institutional Review Board
Preliminary Data
Letter of Intent/Abstract/Cover Letter
Criteria for Evaluation of Grants
Background/Significance
Approach
    Design Overview
    Methods
    Data Analysis
    Timeline
Environment
Innovation
Applicant
Budget
Dissemination
After the Grant Award
Conclusion

Imagine you are a healthcare provider at a community hospital. As providers and observers, you have spent time on many floors and in the outpatient gym. Recently, you noticed an increase in otherwise healthy older adults needing treatment for fall-related injuries requiring surgical intervention and nonsurgical rehabilitation. You begin to wonder if something could be done *to prevent* these falls from happening in the first place. Your training as a healthcare provider gives you some basic ideas. Still, you are unsure how to develop and implement this program, to know whether your program is working, whether your supervisors will approve your program, and even how to pay for this program to help decrease falls in older adults in your community (Fig. 3.1). The whole process appears to be both exciting and overwhelming. This chapter provides evidence-informed and systematic proposal and grant writing methods to help move your idea into a working program that improves healthcare outcomes.

Introduction

Like a marriage proposal, a proposal for a program should be thoughtfully crafted to create a "yes" response from the receiver. However, the similarities with a marriage proposal end there, with a proposal seeking to solve an established or observed problem. At the least, a proposal must (1) establish a need, (2) demonstrate that an idea will meet the need using the methods proposed, and (3) indicate which data will be collected and the outcomes to be achieved. A proposal may also function as a way of communication to those who will provide consultation, give consent, or disburse funds.

Creating A Proposal

Throughout this section, creating a proposal is further refined and explored in depth under each subheading. This

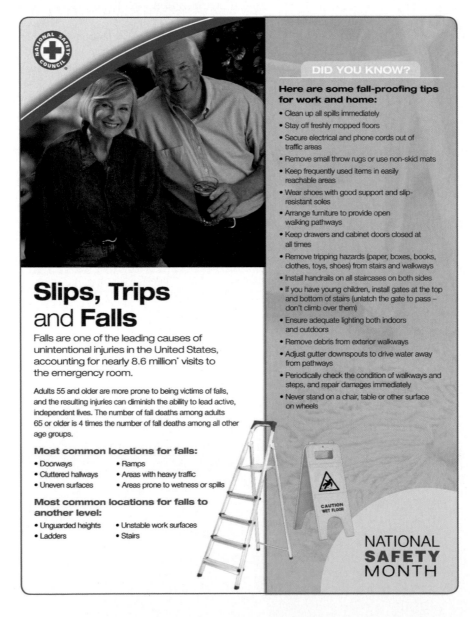

• **Fig. 3.1** Fall Prevention. (From: https://www.flickr.com/photos/51640646@N04/5786856474).

process will systematically progress an observed problem and possible idea into a functional, outcome-focused proposal. The proposal steps include identifying and targeting the problem, needs assessments, program theory, logic models, context analysis, and theories of change and action.

Identifying and Targeting the Problem

The first part of writing a proposal is deciding on a topic and the problem to be solved. In establishing the problem, you need to be clear and concise. A problem should have the ability to be solved within the available resources. At this early stage, the problem should be just that—no proposed solutions. Most likely, simple observation has identified a problem, such as the increased number of fall-related injuries at the hospital. However, most casual observations have many causes and managing them at the same time is impossible. Thus narrowing down the problem into smaller, more manageable components presents a problem that is clear, concise, and solvable within available resources. A fishbone diagram, also called a cause-effect or Ishikawa diagram, provides a method for narrowing down a problem into something the proposal can address.

In a fishbone diagram, start with the significant, observed problem—the effect (Centers for Medicare & Medicaid Services, n.d.). Then, move backward by identifying major categories of the causes of issues and creating a diagram that connects each arrow to the problem (creating the body of the fish) (Centers for Medicare & Medicaid Services, 2014). In Fig. 3.2, several broad categories were chosen, including (1) demographics of the people experiencing the falls, (2) the built environment of the home and community, and (3) resources available to the people having the falls. Once major categories are established, further exploration identifies root causes. Asking, "*why does this problem happen?*" under each category can help at this stage (Centers for Medicare & Medicaid Services, 2014). For example, "*What is occurring in the environment leading to an increase in falls?*" Perhaps it is the community's infrastructure or maybe the individuals have poor lighting in their homes. These answers are a new branch of the major category, further creating the fish's body.

Needs Assessment

Although a needs assessment is not required to identify the narrowed problem or create a proposal for a program, it is recommended because it assists in giving preliminary data. It may identify causes and different points of view regarding the observed problem. A needs assessment is an informal or formal evaluative process to assess an individual, group, and community for gaps in service or other unmet physical, emotional, or psychological needs (Bolduc & Robnett, 2019). For example, suppose the idea is a fall prevention program. In that case, a survey of the local geriatric community to assess how many falls they have had, if they have been hospitalized due to a fall, and what fall prevention programs they have participated in or are currently participating in, are all questions to help define the need for the fall prevention program. Data collection tools for needs assessment may include but are not limited to interviews, surveys, and focus groups. Seeking out multiple stakeholders in the needs assessment gives insight into the problem through others' lived experiences and can help create and add details to the categories of the fishbone diagram.

Data Mining

A needs assessment can include data mining, a means to retrospectively collect data to add depth and help answer the question, "*why does this problem happen?*" Data mining can occur in the clinic or could be pulled from larger databases. For example, to establish a need for the community-based falls prevention program, some data to explore might be if a medical condition contributed to the fall, where the fall occurred, how the fall occurred, and if hospitalization or surgery was required. If this information is unavailable, prospectively collecting data in the clinic is another viable option. Note that Institutional Review (IRB) approval is typically needed for data mining. Please refer to the Grant Writing section in this chapter for more information on IRB.

The needs assessment's utility does not end once the cause of the problem to target is decided. It informs the entire proposal and grant writing process outlined in this chapter.

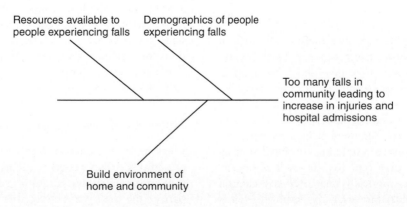

• **Fig. 3.2** Example of fishbone diagram to target problem for fall prevention program.

Program Theory

Program theory is a systematic way to develop your proposal to show stakeholders how the proposed idea will work (Issel, 2022). Like theory in the sciences, program theory is a hypothesis on what will happen given certain parameters and outlines the relationships among the problem statement, interventions to address the problem, and intended outcomes. It is difficult to ascertain whether the interventions led to the observed outcome without program theory. The lack of program theory blurs the cause-effect relationship and decreases the ability to generalize results across populations and contexts. If undesirable outcomes are observed, program theory helps determine if the interventions did not work as intended, if the implementation went awry, or if the lack of success could be attributed to external factors.

Program theory provides guidance and provides a logical foundation for understanding the program. Like a road-map, it outlines the steps to move successfully from the start (idea or problem) to the end (outcomes and overall impact). Typically, several stakeholders have a vested interest in the program. Stakeholders include the individuals benefiting from the program, people creating the program, people implementing the program, and those financially supporting the program, among others. Sometimes, the program creators implicitly understand the relationships, given their background and training. However, a financer of the program or an administrator may have limited to no training in this field. Program theory makes explicit what people mistakenly assume is implicit or intuitive due to their professional experience.

Using program theory is not just for the original implementation of the program. Well-developed program theory allows program evaluation after implementation and makes iterative changes as necessary. If a program's outcomes differ from expected, the program theory allows stakeholders to focus on the components and modify them as necessary instead of starting the program from scratch. For example: if the number of falls in the community after 2 months of your programming has not decreased, look at the program theory to determine what might have gone wrong.

Logic Models

Logic models provide a visual representation of program theory to tell the story of how a program is supposed to work. Where narrative explanations may give detail, the graphic nature of a logic model proves helpful in communicating the program to the many stakeholders listed earlier, mainly if there is limited time for a deep explanation. Users develop logic models representing an outcomes chain, a pipeline, or a realist matrix. The authors recommend additional reading regarding the nuances of each type (e.g. Funnell & Rogers, 2011). A critique of logic models is that they lack enough detail to make them usable. However, the level of detail is simply up to the user on how they want to create their logic

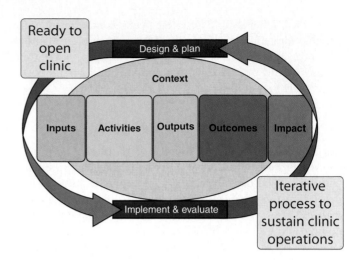

• **Fig. 3.3** Example of a pipeline logic model by McAndrew and Kaskutas (2020) used for a community-based pro bono occupational and physical therapy clinic. (Figure used with permission).

model. More than one logic model designed for a particular audience might be necessary. For example, individuals funding a project or administrators of a large organization are looking for elevator speeches with a logic model that is clear and to the point.

Conversely, stakeholders responsible for day-to-day operations may need a more thorough explanation, including narrative descriptions of each component to support the logic model for those stakeholders accountable for operations. Planners use logic models for a variety of situations, with the most robust usage appearing in community programming; authors describe successful program implementation using logic models for pro bono health care clinics (McAndrew & Kaskutas, 2020), service learning for college students (Lowery et al., 2006) and driving programs for indigenous people (Cullen et al., 2016) to name a few. An example of a pipeline logic model is presented in Fig. 3.3.

Context Analysis

The context of a logic model affects all aspects of programming. These parts of the environment are immutable or at least not easily modifiable and are not an aim of the program itself. Examples include general programming location, local, state, and national policies and regulations, cultural expectations, or socioeconomic status of the targeted audience. The needs assessment completed to target the problem also provides robust context analysis.

Theories of Change and Action

Breaking logic models into theories of change and theories of action clarifies program theory components. Although some program theory guides suggest that context analysis is part of the theory of action, this is debatable. Performing the theory of change before the theory of action can help avoid pitfalls or faulty assumptions. The needs assessment used to narrow down the problem provides a great deal of data for the contextual analysis.

Theory of Change

The theory of change, also known as effect theory, designates the outcomes as measures of success leading to the impacts, as noted on the right side of the logic model in. Although the terms outcomes and impact seem similar, they have distinct differences. An impact of a program is broad, long-term, and wide-reaching. Impacts are long-term, often 5 to 10 years or longer. Often, many different programs share the same impact, while the remaining components of the pipeline logic model are unique to each program, including the outcomes. Outcomes are shorter in length than the impact and are the specific and measurable changes, progress, and successes that developers assume lead to an impact. You may also consider breaking down the outcomes into short-term and long-term outcomes. This decision is based on necessity, such as differences in outcome measures, participation with stakeholders, and observable changes within the community. It is recommended to state outcomes in the form of SMART goals: Specific, Measurable, Achievable, Relevant, and Time-bound (Centers of Disease Control and Prevention, 2022). Some examples of SMART goals to focus on include change in outcome measures, participation of the stakeholders, or overall positive change within the community.

While the pipeline logic model is read left to right, the theory of change portion of the logic model (the right side) is developed first. Because a logic model is based on cause-effect assumptions, the theory of change states that achieving outcomes will lead to the program's overall impact. Defining these causal assumptions is a necessary and perhaps frustrating component of the theory of change. It is helpful to draw assumptions from the literature, strengthening the case; however, emerging programs may have little to no scholarship available for support. When stakeholders verbalize the assumptions, they can further refine the cause-effect relationship. For example, in a fall prevention program, creators assume an improvement in a person's balance leads to decreased falls. A decrease in falls leads to a decrease in hospital admissions in this population.

Theory of Action

Theory of action, also known as process theory, is what the program does to enact the theory of change. In the logic model, the theory of action involves the left-side components of inputs, activities, and outputs. Outputs include raw data on program reach and the tangible products or services that arise from the program's activities. Whereas outcomes are measurable changes expected to occur due to work done, outputs ensure the target audience is accessing the program. Consistent with rigorous research, too few participants may lead to faulty conclusions on the outcomes.

Activities and inputs are the programs themselves. What is needed and what is being done to achieve the chosen

---

• BOX 3.1 Key Strategies in Proposal Development

1. Target the problem by narrowing down an idea using a strategy such as a fishbone diagram.
2. Perform a needs assessment of various stakeholders involved with potential proposal, using a variety of methods like interviews, surveys, and focus groups.
3. Undergo retrospective data mining of clinic or larger databases to add additional information to needs assessment.
4. Develop a logic model to represent program theory, and divide into theory of change and theory of action.
5. Begin with theory of change by identifying long-term impacts and shorter-term outcomes, using SMART method to establish goals.
6. Move to theory of action, which includes the outputs, activities, and inputs of the program itself, using if-then statements to link to outcomes and impacts established in theory of change.
7. Continue to use developed program theory for program evaluation, making iterative changes as necessary for longevity.

---

outcomes? Common missteps occur when the activities are planned before the theory of change, including intended outcomes, long-term impact, and assumptions about the cause-effect relationship. It is helpful to think of the relationship between activities and outcomes as if-then statements: If this *activity* is implemented, then this *outcome* occurs. If program developers create an activity without a targeted outcome (i.e., create the logic model left to right), the activity may be useful. However, it may lead to an unintended effect, wasted time, or harm to the participants. Conversely, there may be an outcome with no activity leading to that change.

Using program theory is not just for designing the program. Well-developed program theory also allows program evaluation, enabling iterative changes as necessary. If the program's outcomes differ from expected, the program theory allows stakeholders to home in on components and modify or change as necessary instead of starting the entire program from scratch. It may be discovered that the inputs needed to carry out the activities to achieve the outcomes are no longer feasible. For example, a loss of staffing (input) directly affects the outcome because most activities cannot be completed as written. At this point, the program theory can be assessed to determine where changes need to be made. The modification may need to be with the input (e.g., number of people carrying out the intervention), the activity (the intervention itself), or the outputs (number of people reached with the intervention). It is also possible that the outcome(s) need to be modified. For a review of key strategies in proposal development discussed in this chapter, please refer to Box 3.1.

Grant Writing

Clinicians seek grant funding to initiate a program or project such as those created from the planning process outlined earlier in this chapter. However, they also use grant funding to conduct a research study, expand clinical education opportunities, enhance their institution's prestige, or advance their professional career (Gitlin et al., 2021). Obtaining a grant can be challenging and should be taken with knowledge of the grant writing process. One of the first steps is to develop an idea that matches the grant writer's interests and has funding potential. The idea must be novel and should address a problem that has been identified as important. The idea should bridge a gap somehow, meaning that the program or project should offer a solution to a problem identified as important to solve. Success in obtaining grant funding depends on having an innovative idea, matching the proposed project to the funding agency's mission, having a clear approach, and producing a well-written proposal. Some elements of the grant proposal were described earlier in the chapter and included targeting the problem and collecting preliminary data. This chapter section will further explore the areas of the grant proposal that will contribute to a successful grant application.

Formulating a Competitive Idea

There are various ways to create a competitive idea for a grant application. What is observed with patients in the clinic can be one way to start an innovative idea for what is to be studied or a program that needs grant funding. Examining the evidence for a gap in the literature could assist in formulating a competitive idea. Conversations with colleagues can help identify problems that can develop into fundable projects, or speaking with individuals who have already received funding can also further inform ideas. The competitive idea could come from creating an interdisciplinary team to brainstorm. Innovation frequently comes from multiple perspectives.

Government initiatives or hot topics can also provide competitive grant proposal ideas. Implementation science and health services research are areas that have grown tremendously, and many grants specifically support these areas of research. Federal government initiatives such as Healthy People 2030 can help cultivate the ideas and win more federal grant money. Community-based programs are another area of grant funding, and stakeholders can facilitate a competitive idea. Grant agencies like to see that research or programs benefit the communities they serve.

Finding a Mentor

Once a novel idea has been identified, opportunities should be investigated, which requires funding. New grant writers may find this part extremely difficult and overwhelming due to the many grant opportunities available. One way to address this is to find a mentor. When identifying an individual for mentorship, consider their experience with prior grant funding, their sources of grant funding, their availability to meet, and if their research interests are similar. Some doctoral programs offer these opportunities as part of their curriculum. Consider enrolling in these programs if research and grant funding are career goals. Additional options include reaching out to professional organizations to

see whether mentoring opportunities are available. Granting agencies may also have mentors available for inexperienced grant writers. Grant writing workshops are another resource that can support a new grant writer.

Searching for a Grant

Before searching for a grant, a few items are important to address. First, consider experience level. Choosing a grant that fits the writer's level of expertise is essential. Second, you should consider the approximate funding needed for the project or research study. If the grant chosen does not offer enough funding, there may be problems fully implementing the project or research study. Third, you should consider which items the grant will or will not cover. If there is a need for the grant to cover personnel, the grant must include that item, as many are explicit that they do not. Fourth, it is helpful to consider all the grant agency's requirements once awarded. You need to ensure there are time and resources to fulfill those requirements. Examples of requirements are further explored in the After the Grant Award section. Finally, you must choose a grant agency that will be interested in the chosen project or research study (Fig. 3.4). One way to decide whether the grant is a good fit is by carefully reading the request for proposal, which is a call that grant agencies make public to encourage applications for funding (Doll, 2010). These notices vary in detail but should provide the eligibility, grant application requirements, due dates, amount of funding, and program requirements (Doll, 2010).

Before identifying a funder, clinicians should be familiar with different types of grants. Research grants provide money to a researcher and their team to conduct a research study. Training or education grants are used for educating students, clinicians, educators, or other practitioners (Gitlin et al., 2021). Finally, demonstration grants support programs or projects and highlight healthcare delivery or community healthcare needs.

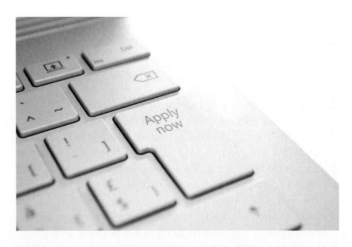

• **Fig. 3.4** Important Point! Avoid investing a significant amount of time applying for a grant that is not attainable. (From: https://www.flickr.com/photos/189262541@N04/50096480067).

A clinician should identify a funder early in the process so that they may structure the grant proposal based on the funder's guidelines. Identifying the funder can be challenging, and experienced program planners and researchers note a learning curve in finding and selecting the appropriate sources to finance their proposals (Gitlin et al., 2021). Health professionals have five key grant funding sources: intramural, federal agencies, private foundations, professional organizations, and private industry (Gitlin et al., 2021). These funding agencies all have specific areas that they want to fund. Intramural funding opportunities are through the institution where one works, such as through a large hospital system. These grant opportunities can generally be accessed on the institution's website and should not be ignored. These grants offer a chance to work with and potentially receive mentorship from individuals at the sponsoring institution. Intramural grants can help develop a track record at the institution (Gitlin et al., 2021).

The federal government is full of grant opportunities and includes different departments, agencies, institutes, bureaus, and centers. Searching for a federal government grant can be extremely difficult for an inexperienced grant writer to navigate. Grants can be searched via www.grants.gov (n.d.a) (Fig. 3.5). Registration on this site is required, but thousands of grants can be viewed once registration is complete. Multiple agencies offer grants to clinicians, such as the National Institute of Health, The Department of Health and Human Services, or The Department of Veterans Affairs. One way to look for rehabilitation research grants is by using a CFDA number. Once the CFDA number is entered, all grants associated with that organization can be viewed. For example, the CFDA number is 93.433 for the National Institute on Disability, Independent Living, and Rehabilitation Research, part of the Administration for Community Living. This specific funding agency has given grants to fall prevention programs similar to the one discussed in this chapter.

Private foundations and public charities are excellent resources and include organizations such as the American Association of Retired Persons (AARP) Foundation or the Michael J Fox Foundation. Foundation grants are an excellent way to start for inexperienced grant writers because they are relatively brief and straightforward compared with federal grants (Holtzclaw et al., 2018). Professional organizations are an additional resource for inexperienced grant writers, including organizations such as AOTA's American Occupational Therapy Foundation or APTA's Foundation for Physical Therapy. Professional organizations frequently post all grant opportunities on their website. Private industry grants include equipment companies or other healthcare companies related to healthcare. These companies can fund small projects which may relate to the company's interests. For example, this could include a study funded by a company that provides bathroom modification. They may ask the receiver to study the effect of installing grab bars in the bathroom on falls.

The Grant Proposal

Once a novel idea has been determined, addresses a gap, has the potential to make an impact, and matches a priority or interest of a funding agency, it is time to write the grant proposal. A grant proposal should discuss what is to be done, how it will be done, why it is significant and innovative, what the cost is and what the cost includes, and justify why the requestor and team are the best fit to complete the project (Gitlin et al., 2021). When writing a grant proposal, it is vital that it is written within the granting agency's guidelines and includes all areas in which it will be evaluated. Sections of the grant proposal may vary but generally include: title, introduction/problem statement, goals/aims, background/significance, project/study approach, environment, budget, dissemination, and references. The authors of this chapter will thread the falls prevention program throughout this section. A fictional county called North

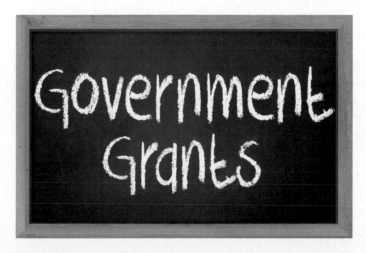

• **Fig. 3.5** Government grants can be searched at https://www.grants.gov/web/grants/search-grants.html. (From https://www.flickr.com/photos/86530412@N02/8224546207).

Plains, AR, will be used as the location for the fall prevention program to fund.

Introduction/Problem Statement

The introduction section makes a case for the suggested program or study and gives its purpose (Funk & Tornquist, 2015). The introduction should be short and summarize the areas of the grant proposal. In this section, the problem the project or study is designed to solve should be summarized, the need of the project or study for the target population should be stated, the purpose of the project or study should be described, and the methods by which the project or study will be performed should be outlined (Funk & Tornquist, 2015). The introduction paragraph should draw interest from the grant agency and demonstrate how innovative the suggested program of study is. The problem statement should identify the problem being addressed and why it is important or discuss the importance of the problem for a specific population and the need for a solution to it (Funk & Tornquist, 2015). An example of a problem statement that could be used in a grant proposal for the fall prevention program would be: A needs assessment performed with the senior community members of North Plains, AR, has found that a high percentage of community members have experienced more than one fall, and many of these falls have resulted in high admissions to the local hospital. Most falls in North Plains, AR, have occurred in our community and there are currently no community-based fall prevention programs available to our community members. Falls contribute to higher mortality (Center of Disease Control, 2021) and increased health care costs (Florence et al., 2018). Community-based fall prevention programs effectively decrease falls in communities (Kulinski et al., 2017). There is a need to develop a fall prevention program that will serve the community members in the county of North Plains, AR.

Writing the Aims

The aims section of a proposal is the most important part and can be the most difficult to write. Aims should identify what will be accomplished in the project, program, or study. Each aim should describe what is to be done, why, and how (Gitlin et al., 2021). This proposal section should also state the project's purpose and long-term goal. The purpose statement should be related to the problem statement. For example, the fall prevention program's purpose statement would be to develop a community-based falls prevention program. A long-term goal would be to decrease falls in the community and decrease hospital admissions due to falls. The aims could address the development of the program and the evaluation plan. For example, one aim could be to develop specific fall prevention programs based on interviews with seniors. Under this aim, it will be important to describe various causes of falls and create programs based on each client's needs to support long-term goals. Those programs may include a home visit, a community

outing, or a balance and musculoskeletal assessment. Explaining that seniors will be screened and then carry out these specific programs will be important details to include under this aim. A second aim could be improving Berg Balance Scale scores for individuals in the program. For this aim, details will need to be provided on how these metrics will be evaluated over time.

Aims for a grant proposal should be written to align with the grant's goals and objectives or the grant agency's mission. Gitlin et al. (2021) summarized some conventions for aims statements that include that each aim should be measurable, each aim should support the overarching goal of the project, each aim should lead to a particular methodology and set of activities, and the grant proposal should include at least two or three aims. Common pitfalls include aims that are unfocused, conflicting, inconsistent, too ambitious, or too interdependent (Gitlin et al., 2021). Each aim is elaborated for a research grant with a hypothesis or question (Holtzclaw et al., 2018).

Institutional Review Board

If the program or study involves human subjects research, it needs to be examined by an IRB. Universities and large medical facilities typically already have a human subject protection office and an IRB. Do not speculate whether the program or research requires an IRB review; human subjects protection offices are helpful in this area. Smaller facilities that do not have an IRB in place can pair with local ones or consider paying for institutional review through a company such as Western IRB. If a grant does not directly support human subject research, IRB review and approval are not needed unless the funding agency requires it; requirements should therefore be read closely. In addition to obtaining IRB approval, clear descriptions of procedures for protecting subjects' rights and obtaining informed consent in the grant proposal must be included.

Preliminary Data

Earlier in the chapter, the authors discussed how to collect preliminary data to support the need for a program. The National Institute of Health requires grant applicants to include this information in a separate proposal section. Other resources suggest including this information in the background/significance section. Preliminary data should be included in the grant proposal based on the guidelines of the grant agency and provide evidence of the magnitude or significance of the problem. A pilot study is one avenue to provide preliminary data. A pilot study is a smaller scale study done before performing a larger one that pilots the procedures, methods and evaluates feasibility.

Letter of Intent/Abstract/Cover Letter

Depending on the grant agency, several things may be required, including a letter of intent, abstract, and cover letter.

The letter of intent asks whether the grant agency is interested in funding the project and is a shortened grant proposal that may include the description of the grant agency and a brief description of the proposed program or research study (Doll, 2010). The grant agency may use this letter to decide whether they are interested in inviting the applicant to apply for funding. The abstract summarizes the project or research study, and when implementing a program, it is used to describe the program briefly (Doll, 2010). For a research study, the abstract should include the general purpose of the research, the specific goals/aims, research design, methods, and significance. Some abstracts will need to include estimated costs of the program or study and it is therefore important to read the grant agency's instructions. A cover letter is required for some government and foundation grants. A cover letter should be brief and include one or two statements on what is requested in the proposal and one or two reasons why that grant from that specific foundation or government agency is needed (Karsh & Fox, 2019). If an abstract is not included in the proposal, a cover letter may be used to describe the need for the program or study, the objectives, a summary of the program or study, collaborators, program evaluation, cost, and the amount requested in the budget (Karch & Fox, 2019).

Criteria for Evaluation of Grants

The focus of a grant writer is to prove to an agency and its reviewers that the proposed idea is sound, that it is feasible, that the applicant is the best person/team to carry out the proposed project and is located in an environment that can support the proposed efforts (Gitlin et al., 2021). It is important to read the guidelines the grant agency sets before putting the grant proposal together. A peer review panel will review the grant proposal. A peer review panel is a group of experts selected to evaluate the grant proposals submitted to that specific grant funding agency and decide whether to fund them or not. The peer review panel evaluates and scores each proposal according to the agency's evaluative criteria (Gitlin et al., 2021). The evaluative criteria differ between funding agencies; however, typical areas of evaluation include significance, approach, environment, innovation, applicant, and budget.

Essential elements of a grant that reviewers look for include:
- Meaningful question (significance, impact, and scientific premise)
- Good science (approach and innovation)
- Careful attention to the application (approach, environment)
- Qualified applicant (investigators)
(Holtzclaw et al., 2018).

Background/Significance

Background information identifies the current state of the problem and the evidence to support the proposed solution. A literature review is an avenue to explore the problem further and give more context; it is the part of the proposal showing the significance of the problem and a critical knowledge gap. The significance of a grant proposal is not the importance of the topic or clinical problem; instead, it is established by citing literature that summarizes the magnitude of the problem and its health and societal consequences (Gitlin et al., 2021). The grant proposal must have clear evidence that a gap in quality exists. The funding agency wants to know whether a quality gap exists and why the project is necessary and whether it will have an impact. The impact is the likelihood that a project will have a sustained, powerful influence in a specific field (Holtzclaw et al., 2018). For example, suppose a literature review on falls in the geriatric population is needed. In that case, the background should examine the frequency of falls in the geriatric community, which variables contribute to falls, which environments falls occur in, and which interventions are currently being used to reduce falls and their effectiveness. A gap may be that community-based fall prevention programs are effective but have not been implemented in rural communities and there is no evidence of rural fall prevention program outcomes. Additionally, identifying why this specific fall prevention program fills a quality gap and how this program will directly impact the community served further supports the need for proposal and grant funding.

Approach

The approach section of the grant proposal serves as a framework or implementation plan for the planned work and will include all the strategies to achieve the study's or program's aims (Holtzclaw et al., 2018). This section should discuss the design overview, sample description, selection, procedures, intervention (if performed), data collection, data analysis, and timeline.

Design Overview

A design overview should serve as a strategic plan to accomplish the aims or test the research questions (Holtzclaw et al., 2018). If a research study is chosen, this section is where quantitative or qualitative design is described. If a program is being designed, such as the falls prevention program, the program's overall design should be described and include items such as a logic model. This description will give the grant reviewer a visual picture of how the program's components come together to produce an outcome. Fig. 3.6 presents a logic model for our fall prevention program. Please note that the examples provided under each column are not exhaustive.

Methods

The sample or population included in the project or research study is important for the grant proposal. A research study should include inclusion/exclusion criteria and sampling and recruitment strategies. A program should include who the target population is, including the demographics of that population. This section should detail a methodology that includes a

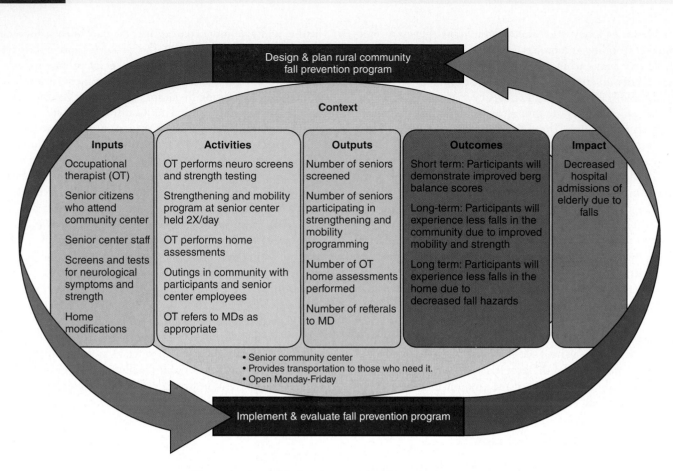

• **Fig. 3.6** Logic model of rural community falls prevention program.

diverse population from differing socioeconomic areas and not exclude individuals based on their sex/gender, race, or ethnicity. These details strengthen the grant proposal and give grant reviewers evidence that equity and inclusivity are priorities.

Research studies must ensure rigor and reproducibility. This rigorous description includes details on the intervention and outcome measures. The approach section should include the validity and reliability of the outcome measures and the periods when data will be collected. A program needs to describe both an implementation plan and an evaluation plan. The implementation plan is all the activities that will occur as part of the program and who is carrying out each activity. In the evaluation plan, information should be provided on how the achievement of the program objectives or aims will be evaluated, what data will be collected, when the data will be collected, how the data will be collected, and who will collect the data (Doll, 2010). Within the context of grants, the evaluation plan can act as a resource for tracking outcomes that must be reported to funding agencies (Doll, 2010, p. 278). Evaluation plans can act as a method for quality improvement and exploring the feasibility of sustainability (Doll, 2010). Any program development project needs to describe the evaluation plan over the first year regarding meeting outcomes, evaluating partnerships, community buy-in, and developing a reimbursement system to produce revenue.

Data Analysis

The data analysis section of a grant proposal should include data preparation and data analysis procedures. As described earlier in the chapter, each aim of a research grant should have a research question attached to it (Fig. 3.7). The approach section should refer to the aim and research question to describe explicitly the analysis intended to be performed based on the type of data collected. For a program development grant, aims may not all be related to data analysis; however, the evaluation plan should include an analysis of either qualitative or quantitative data. For example, the second aim is to improve Berg Balance Scale scores for individuals in the community program for the falls-prevention program. Data analysis could include a paired samples t-test to examine differences in mean scores between different time points for program participants' Berg Balance Scale scores. A long-term goal may include an analysis to determine whether there was a significant reduction in falls over the year in which the program was implemented. All analysis would be within the fall prevention program group because there is no control group. Any statistical or qualitative data analysis software should also be included in the data analysis section.

Timeline

A timeline gives the grant agency step-by-step guidelines of when each part of the project will be completed. Timelines

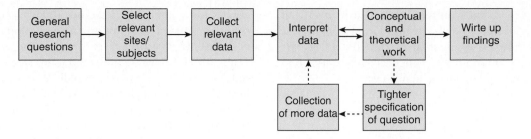

• **Fig. 3.7** Research Steps. (From https://www.flickr.com/photos/96691515@N00/3006848456).

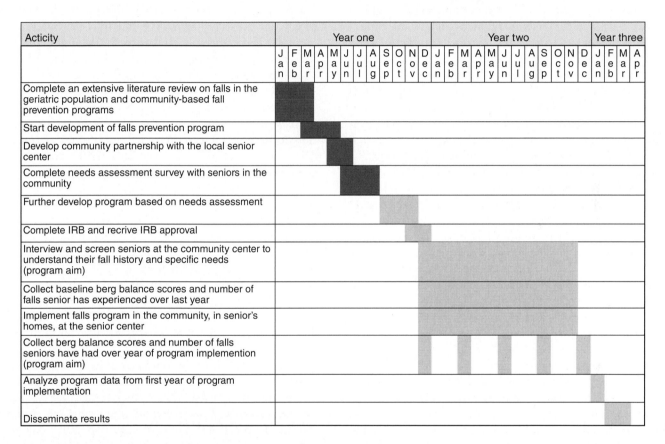

• **Fig. 3.8** Example of a timeline for the fall prevention grant application. The dark gray shading includes activities that are in process or already completed. The light gray shading indicates future activities.

do not have to give specific dates but should give a timeframe for when completion of that specific project piece will be completed. This timeline gives grant agencies a framework for activity completion if grants are awarded. Fig. 3.8 outlines a potential timeline for this program.

Environment

The environment section of the grant proposal will describe the setting where the project, program, or study will occur. The environments to be used and the resources available within those environments, including financial resources, should be described in detail. The benefits of the environment where the research or program takes place should be discussed. Any aspects that make the environment unique such as the socioeconomic population it serves, should also be discussed. Building a program where resources are provided to vulnerable populations is important in the grant application. In addition, information should be provided on the setting's readiness or capacity for change. Grant funders do not want to fund projects if they feel they are not sustainable. Existing partnerships or those to be built should be included. For example, in the falls prevention program, discuss the senior center, who funds it, and who manages it. Discuss the resources used within the community center, including staff, equipment, and transportation services. Many community-based fall prevention programs serve urban communities. This sample program is unique because it serves a rural community with a high rate of hospital admissions due to falls. In addition, it is important to talk about how environmental barriers differ between urban and rural communities. This difference can signify innovation, which will be talked about next.

Innovation

Some grant applications may not require this section to be included in the grant proposal; however, it serves in the best interest of a proposal to include a paragraph that describes how the idea is innovative. This section should include a logical, clear, and compelling argument on how this project or study represents a new and creative approach (Gitlin et al., 2021). Innovation proposes solving a problem in a new way by either generating new ideas or applying existing ideas to a new situation that improves healthcare outcomes (Holtzclaw et al., 2018, p. 17). The following questions should be considered when writing this grant proposal section: *What is new about this work? Does this project or study seek to challenge or shift current research or clinical practice? Is this an implementation of an improvement to what is already being done?* For example, many fall prevention programs occur in the artificial environment of the outpatient rehabilitation clinic, which is not where falls occur. The innovation of the suggested fall prevention program involves multiple innovative pieces, but the program is designed to meet the individual needs of each client that attends the program. This program also works with clients in environments where they have falls.

Applicant

To be considered for a grant, applicants must show they are qualified. Multiple areas can be included in the applicant section of the proposal. A grant agency may require the applicant section to include the applicant's research program, publications, previous funding, and collaborators' biographical sketches or curriculum vitae. Grant review panels also want to see a career trajectory on a common theme, meaning that each grant application is a stepping stone for the next grant submission. Pilot and preliminary work that has led to the present project can also be included here. The applicant may not have prior experience running a community-based fall prevention program; however, this does not mean they are not a candidate for a grant award. Collaborators can make a big difference in the potential of a grant proposal. The grant application can be improved by including collaborators such as the senior center program manager, a local therapy program faculty member, and a local hospital administrator.

Budget

The budget in a grant proposal acts as a map for funding and aids in the implementation process of when the money will be spent (Doll, 2010, p. 219). Funding is why someone applies for a grant, but it can be difficult to estimate what funds are needed. It is important to develop a project idea with realistic objectives from a funding perspective (Gitlin et al., 2021). If ideas require monies outside what the grant funding agency can provide, it will be necessary to identify how these additional monies will be secured. Granting agencies will not want to award a grant if it is unclear that the program or study can be implemented because of insufficient funds. The grant application will also detail which budget items the grant agency will cover and not cover. For example, some grant agencies will pay for a salary only during the grant activities; therefore, only the applicable percentage of the salary should be put into the budget. For example, if the therapist's salary is $75,000 and the falls prevention program will require 25% of their time, $25,000 should be budgeted in the grant application.

The budget plan should start by identifying every resource needed for the project or research study, then categorizing each resource as a direct or indirect cost. *Direct costs* are necessary to carry out the project or research study. These costs could include specific activities that require personnel, travel, equipment, and supplies necessary for the project aims (Gitlin et al., 2021). *Indirect costs* are hidden costs that an institution absorbs, such as administration support or electricity. Indirect costs must be factored into the grant and negotiated with the funding agency. The grant may or may not cover indirect costs, which is important to consider when applying. The indirect costs that the community partner or institution can cover before applying for the grant should be discussed to understand the resources needed for funding. See Table 3.1 for an example of direct and indirect costs for the fall prevention program.

After a list of direct and indirect costs of the project or research study is created, the budget needs to be justified and the funds reported for each budget item. Budget justification involves a brief explanation and rationale for each item in the budget (Gitlin et al., 2021, p. 208). The budget justification also provides the opportunity to explain where estimated costs come from and why they are essential (Doll, 2010, p. 225). The budget justification is an important part of the grant proposal, and a lack of budget justification may be why the grant proposal is rejected. When asking for funds for each item, it is important to avoid padding the budget or underestimating the cost of items. For example, the Medicare and Medicaid billing personnel budget item is justified because Medicare and Medicaid will need to be billed for therapy services for the program to be sustainable. Billing personnel may be contractors who bill by the hour or part of a larger affiliate health care system. It may be difficult to estimate the time they will need to provide this service and, once the program is profitable, it may be possible to pay for these services from the revenue. One way to estimate the funding needed would be to discuss with billing experts or interview billing personnel with experience billing for community-based programs.

TABLE 3.1	Examples of Direct and Indirect Costs of the Fall Prevention Program	
Direct Costs		**Indirect Costs**
• Therapist salary (25% effort in the proposed program) • Exercise equipment • Transportation to and from the client's home for home modification visits • Website development with scheduling capability • Training for therapists and senior center staff • Documentation system/laptop • Medicare and Medicaid billing personnel		• Senior center space • Utilities in senior center • Senior center staff • Senior center transportation for community outings and for seniors to access community center • Senior center telephone

---

• BOX 3.2   Key Strategies in Grant Writing

1. Develop an idea that is novel and has the potential to make an impact.
2. Perform a literature review to explore the problem in more depth.
3. Use preliminary data to support the need for the program.
4. Write a problem statement that reflects the importance of the problem and why it is important to solve the problem.
5. Choosing a funding agency should be based on experience, budget, grant project topic, and how the topic fits the grant funder's interests.
6. Aims should be measurable and support the long-term goal.
7. IRB approval should be documented in the grant proposal if this is human subjects research.
8. Logic models are effective ways to provide a visual representation of the program implementation.
9. Structure the grant proposal based on the funder's guidelines.
10. Areas of grant evaluation typically include significance, approach, environment, innovation, applicant, and budget, and each of these areas should be written about in detail in the proposal.

Developing a budget can be very difficult, depending on the size of the grant. It is recommended that mentors, funding specialists, fiscal specialists, or other collaborators be utilized to develop this section of the grant proposal. For a review of key strategies in grant writing discussed in this chapter, please refer to Box 3.2.

Dissemination

Some granting agencies require dissemination as part of the grant proposal and designate funding in the budget to support it (Doll, 2010, p. 218). Dissemination is the targeted distribution of information to public health organizations or clinical practices with the intent to spread knowledge and associated evidence-based interventions (Glasgow et al., 2012). It provides information, such as outcome data, to community members and other practitioners (Doll, 2010). Also, dissemination is a way to create excitement about the research or program and to facilitate future funding.

Dissemination via publication in a peer-reviewed journal is an important part of the grant process for individuals with a research agenda. Also, findings can be disseminated by presenting at state and national conferences, allowing engagement with other professionals, including feedback on the research or project. Another dissemination option is publishing an article in a practice magazine or peer-reviewed journal. For community-based programs, dissemination should be provided on a local level. For example, the outcomes of the falls prevention program should be disseminated to sustain community support with both seniors and the senior center. The program results can be written up for a local paper or a flyer can be created to distribute at the community health fair. Disseminating the data to local hospitals where hospital admissions have been high due to falls may assist in finding partnerships and additional funding.

After the Grant Award

Once awarded a grant, communication with the grant agency is required periodically. The post-award phase encompasses significant work throughout the award dates, including implementing the grant, reporting progress, and completing closeout requirements (grants.gov, n.d.b). The awarding agency typically has a grants officer assigned to the project and its facilitator over the life of the grant. This individual will review reports and may conduct a site visit (grants.gov, n.d.b). Reports generally include a financial report and performance in meeting metrics established in the grant application. Closeout requirements are completed once the grant process ends and may include final financial and programmatic reports (grant.gov, n.d.b). Based on the submitted financial reports, funding not spent may need to be returned to the granting agency. There are also cases where grantors allow a no-cost extension that occurs when money is left over after the program has been implemented (Doll, 2010). The grantor can award the grantee time to spend the remaining funds (Doll, 2010).

Conclusion

Healthcare providers are well-suited to implement programs in their clinics and community. This chapter provides a systematic way to create a strong proposal from an idea and demonstrates how to support a program through funding, listing the important steps needed to secure a grant. Program theory is an important part of proposal development because it demonstrates to stakeholders how the program will work by clearly stating the short-term and long-term outcomes and the impact the program hopes to achieve. Program theory also outlines the processes needed to achieve the outcomes and impact. Grants are available to support healthcare programs financially but require diligence from applicants to ensure that criteria from funding agencies are met and that the program to be funded is supported by literature, meets a need, and is innovative.

References

Bolduc, J. J., & Robnett, R. (2019). Grant Proposal writing. In K. Jacobs & G. McCormack (Eds.), *The occupational therapy manager* (6th ed., pp. 427–434). Bethesda, MD: AOTA Press.

Center for Medicare and Medicaid Services. (n.d.). *How to use the fishbone tool for root cause analysis.* https://www.cms.gov/medicare/provider-enrollment-and-certification/qapi/downloads/fishbonerevised.pdf.

Center of Disease Control and Prevention. (2021). *Older adult fall prevention.* https://www.cdc.gov/falls/facts.html.

Center of Disease Control and Prevention. (2022). *Writing smart objectives.* https://www.cdc.gov/dhdsp/evaluation_resources/guides/writing-smart-objectives.htm.

Cullen, P., Clapham, K., Byrne, J., Hunter, K., Senserrick, T., Keay, L., & Ivers, R. (2016). The importance of context in logic model construction for a multi-site community-based Aboriginal driver licensing program. *Evaluation and Program Planning, 57,* 8–15.

Doll, J. D. (2010). *Program development and grant writing in occupational therapy: Making the connection.* Jones & Bartlett Publishers.

Florence, C. S., Bergen, G., Atherly, A., Burns, E., Stevens, J. & Drake, C. (2018). Medical costs of fatal falls and fall injuries among older adults. *Journal of the American Geriatrics Society,* 66(4), 693–698. https://doi.org/10.1111/jgs.15304

Funk, S. G., & Tornquist, E. M. (2015). *Writing winning proposals for nurses and health care professionals.* Springer Publishing Company.

Funnell, S. C., & Rogers, P. J. (2011). *Purposeful program theory: Effective use of theories of change and logic models* (Vol. 31). John Wiley & Sons.

Gitlin, L. N., Kolanowski, A., & Lyons, K. J. (2021). *Successful grant writing: Strategies for health and human service professionals.* Springer Publishing Company.

Glasgow, R. E., Vinson, C., Chambers, D., Khoury, M. J., Kaplan, R. M., & Hunter, C. (2012). National Institutes of Health approaches to dissemination and implementation science: current and future directions. *American Journal of Public Health,* 102(7), 1274–1281.

Grants.gov. (n.d.a). *Grants 101: Post award phase.* https://www.grants.gov/web/grants/learn-grants/grants-101/post-award-phase.html.

Grants.gov. (n.d.b). *Search grants.* https://www.grants.gov/web/grants/search-grants.html.

Holtzclaw, B., Kenner, C., & Walden, M. (2018). *Grant writing handbook for nurses and health professionals.* Springer Publishing Company.

Issel, L. M., Wells, R., & Williams, M. (2022). *Health program planning and evaluation: A practice, systematic approach for community health* (5th ed.). Jones & Bartlett Learning.

Karsh, E., & Fox, A. S. (2019). *The only grant-writing book you'll ever need.* Basic Books.

Kulinski, K., DiCocco, C., Skowronski, S., & Sprowls, P. (2017). Advancing community-based falls prevention programs for older adults—the work of the administration for community living/administration on aging. *Frontiers in Public Health, 5,* 4.

Lowery, D., May, D. L., Duchane, K. A., Coulter-Kern, R., Bryant, D., Morris, P. V., Pomery, J. G., & Bellner, M. (2006). A logic model of service learning: Tensions and issues for further consideration. *Michigan Journal of Community Service Learning,* 12(2), 47–60.

McAndrew, R., & Kaskutas, V. (2020). A logic model for planning, implementing, and evaluating a student-run free clinic. *Journal of Student-Run Clinics,* 6(1). https://journalsrc.org/index.php/jsrc/article/view/132.

4

Current Issues in Healthcare: Barriers and Strategies

STEVEN D. EBERTH, OTD, OTR/L, CDP, CFPS; PATRICIA LAVERDURE, OTD, OTR/L, BCP, FAOTA; DEBORAH ELGIN BUDASH, PhD, OTR/L; TAMMY BRUEGGER, OTD, MSED, OTR/L, ATP; AMBER RICHARDSON, OTR/L, CHES, OMS; and WILLIAM R. VANWYE, PT, DPT, PhD

LEARNING OBJECTIVES

By the end of this chapter, the reader will be able to:

1. Define healthcare trends and emerging practice settings.
2. Interpret the importance of understanding current trends to be ahead of the curve.
3. Identify barriers to change and explain how the stages of change and team development can promote awareness of the change process.
4. Apply strategies to facilitate successful service delivery.
5. Identify the pros and cons of social media for healthcare providers.
6. Discuss the importance of interprofessional collaboration.

CHAPTER OUTLINE

Introduction

This chapter identifies current trends in healthcare and explores the barriers and strategies to consider when addressing practice change. The contributing authors wish to identify opportunities to advocate, promote change, collaborate with colleagues, and promote interprofessional practice whenever possible. To be prepared to act upon opportunities, it is advantageous to appraise fully both the barriers and the strengths related to current trends. The United States healthcare system is large and complex, with governmental regulators and competing providers that can create challenges and opportunities for innovative change. Change requires knowledge, insight, communication and problem-solving skills, and a willingness to collaborate and seize opportunities when working with individuals and groups. Understanding how change can be facilitated and how group development works are essential. When the process of change is understood, it can be used to customize a message when advocating. Understanding the dynamic change that occurs regarding group development, you can appreciate, anticipate, and respond to the dynamics that may support or impede collaboration. All healthcare professions collaborate to provide their unique services, but there are times when it can be helpful to recognize the readiness for change and group dynamics that influence change. Common ground is necessary to support one another in providing equitable access to high-quality healthcare.

The Institute for Healthcare Improvement Triple Aim (IHI, 2022) is a framework designed to optimize health system performance by focusing on the efforts of healthcare providers to address patient quality and satisfaction, improve the health of populations, and reduce the cost of healthcare. The United States healthcare system considers the Triple Aim an integral component of the national healthcare strategy for quality improvement. Consequently, healthcare providers need tools to collaborate to promote quality improvement and two such tools are the stages of change and group development.

The Transtheoretical Model of Health Behavior Change (TTM) provides a framework for understanding the continuum of stages of behavior change (Fig. 4.1) (DiClemente & Prochaska, 1982; Prochaska & DiClemente, 1983; Prochaska & Velicer, 1997). Knowing each stage of an individual's readiness to change may make a difference in their willingness to agree with the issue you are advocating for. For example, if an individual is in a precontemplative stage, they do not believe in the need to change and may downplay the issue, but someone in the contemplation stage is willing to weigh the benefits and costs of change and is amenable to it. Contemplation provides an opportunity for advocacy. Likewise, the stages of group development can provide insights into the development of a group when they are addressing a topic. For example, if a group is forming, they are coming together to understand a topic and it is an opportune time for advocacy versus storming, where group members are claiming roles and responsibilities. Both TTM and the group development model can assist in understanding key individuals or groups in the effort of advocacy to promote change.

The Transtheoretical Model

The stages of change begin with precontemplation when there is no awareness of the need for change and no intended actions are planned within the next 6 months. For

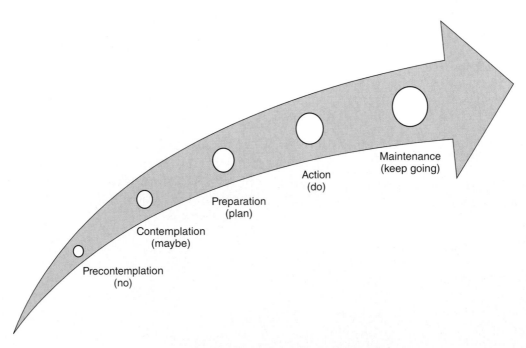

• **Fig. 4.1** Stages of the Transtheoretical Model.

example, a leader may have no awareness of the need to change their perspective on an issue until they are made aware. The contemplation stage occurs when you conceptualize action within the next 6 months. This occurs when the leader is made aware of another perspective. Preparation occurs when you intend to take action within the next 30 days and have already taken behavioral steps toward change, occurring when the leader determines a need to change and begins the process. Action is when overt behavioral change is demonstrated for less than 6 months. At this point, the change process is new and is subject to alteration. The maintenance stage demonstrates the engagement in change for more than 6 months. The leader and organization are engaged in long-term change that is a part of the new culture. Termination occurs when confidence is at its highest level and the culture change has shifted by evidence in practice.

Group Development

The stages of group development include forming, storming, norming, performing, and adjourning (Fig. 4.2) (Tuckman, 1965). The *forming* stage is characterized by individuals coming together and testing interpersonal relationships. At this stage, task behaviors include orientation to the work. An example may be a group of clinicians who wish to advocate for change. The *storming* stage is characterized by establishing roles within the group and each person bringing their perceived expectations to the interaction. The task activity elicits an emotional response to the demands of the work. The storming stage is a critical point in team development that can either "make or break" a group; either a group will congeal and share roles and responsibilities or fracture. Group members must adjust their roles to accommodate the other team members so they can help each other with the task demands. The team may have difficulty if members cannot share in the effort and negotiate for control.

The *norming* stage comes after team members feel a sense of cohesiveness and new standards evolve as new roles are adopted (Tuckman, 1965). Task activities result from open communication and the exchange of information becomes less inhibited. The *performing* stage is characterized by

increased role flexibility after resolving structural barriers. Task activities receive the greatest attention and productive solutions can occur. The final stage of team development is *adjourning*, characterized by the ending of the work with the primary task of reflecting on the experience.

Considering the stages of change and team development, this chapter will begin to highlight current issues facing occupational and physical therapists, delve into their background, and recommend addressing the barriers with strategies for change.

Technology

History and Background

According to the Pew Research Center, 100% of young adults 18–29 years report using the Internet or other technology daily, while only 27% of adults over 65 years report using the Internet (Hitlin, 2018), largely due to many older adults requiring assistance setting up and learning to use technology. It is so common for children and younger adults that it is difficult for them to participate in daily occupations without technology. Lastly, access to digital technology is an issue for six out of ten rural Americans and in a 2015 survey, 43% of adults did not have broadband access for socioeconomic reasons.

The use of technology has increased every year up to 2016, but since 2018 it has not increased significantly due to "saturation" (Hitlin, 2018). This saturation has resulted in many available forms of technology, such as fitness watches, smartphones, applications (apps), robotics, the Internet of Things (IoT), artificial intelligence (AI), 3-D printing, virtual reality, autonomous vehicles, smart home technology, and many more. The IoT is a system of wireless, interrelated, and connected digital devices that can collect, send, and store data over a network without requiring human-to-human or human-to-computer interaction. With this rapid increase in technology in everyday life, there will be an increase in the opportunities to utilize technology in healthcare.

Technology is used in many areas of practice for occupational and physical therapy and is required content in entry-level

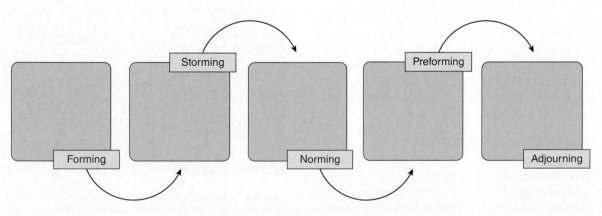

• **Fig. 4.2** Stages of Group Development.

occupational and physical therapy programs (ACOTE, 2018, CAPTE 2022). Technology in practice includes electronic documentation systems, virtual reality, robotics, and telehealth technology. According to the Individuals with Disabilities Education Act (IDEA), "Assistive technology device means any item, piece of equipment, or product system, whether acquired commercially off the shelf, modified, or customized, that is used to increase, maintain, or improve functional capabilities of a child with a disability" (IDEA, 2014, 300.5 Assistive Technology Device).

Assistive Technology

Assistive technology (AT) is the term commonly used to describe the use of technology or assistive devices to improve the function, independence, and quality of life of people with disabilities (Individuals with Disabilities Education Act, 1990; Technology-Related Assistance for Individuals with Disabilities Act, 1988; World Health Organization, 2018). This term is intentionally broad and includes equipment and devices that are custom-made or mass-produced. AT service delivery also spans multiple disciplines. Occupational, speech, and physical therapists, rehabilitation engineers, durable medical equipment suppliers, and educators use assistive technology to impact change (Rehabilitation Engineering and Assistive Technology Society of North America [RESNA], 2015). The wide scope of assistive technology services provided by various healthcare and educational professionals to meet various goals results in difficulty in reaching a consensus on a detailed definition for AT.

The use of AT allows enhancement or enablement of client engagement in occupation (AOTA, 2016) and activities of meaning for the client. This is always client-centered and evidence-based. Through the evaluation process, assistive technology may be one solution to the client's needs, as documented in the evaluation. The therapist then designs, fabricates, applies, modifies, and provides training with various assistive technologies and tools as part of the intervention process to enable access and participation in the daily occupations of the patient or client (AOTA, 2016). The Vision Statement for the Physical Therapy Profession (APTA, 2019) asserts that adopting innovation with interprofessional collaboration is critical to care provision and to advance the profession, including technology. The use of assistive technology is used in practice for occupational and physical therapy, as well as speech-language pathology, in the form of low technology adaptive devices such as dressing sticks, reachers, adaptive feeding aides, orthotics, and high technology devices such as power wheelchairs and speech generating devices, and digital tablets.

Electronic Documentation Systems

Electronic documentation systems include electronic medical records (EMR) and electronic health records (EHR). An EMR is a digital copy of a patient's paper chart containing the care provided within an organization. An EHR serves as an EMR and allows healthcare providers and organizations to share medical information. Electronic documentation systems vary by organization and setting but have similar formats and structures. Many include dropdown menus that have diagnoses, billing and diagnostic codes, goals, and templates for evaluations and intervention categories.

Electronic documentation systems were developed to save time and provide more accurate, effective, evidence-based healthcare documentation (McVeigh et al., 2018). Wroten and associates (2020) compared handwritten and electronic notes for quality and other properties and found that therapists wrote accurate notes, provided more rationale for therapy, and completed more areas of the note when using the electronic documentation system. In addition, therapists could send progress notes directly to the physician and referral source from the electronic documentation system, saving additional time.

Virtual Reality

Virtual reality (VR) refers to interactive simulations created with computer hardware and software to present users with opportunities to engage in environments that appear and feel similar to real-world objects, locations, contexts, and events (Fig. 4.3). VR has been used in stroke rehabilitation (Corbetta et al., 2015), assessment of clients with traumatic brain injury (Lamargue-Hamel et al., 2015; Zhang et al., 2003), training for power wheelchair use (Nunnerley et al., 2017), rehabilitation for clients with Parkinson's disease (Albiol-Pérez et al., 2017) and hand injuries (Huang et al., 2018).

Although contemporary low-cost video capture gaming systems were not developed specifically for rehabilitation, they offer an easy-to-setup, fun, and less-expensive alternative to costly VR systems. Numerous digital tablet applications can access virtual or augmentative reality and even tactile responses to provide multiple sensory experiences. These options for therapy may provide more motivating experiences for individuals with mobility issues or dementia, improving outcomes in rehabilitation.

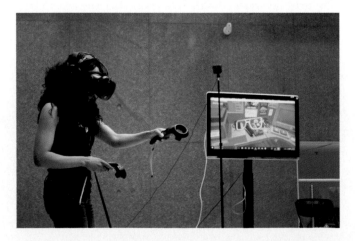

• **Fig. 4.3** Virtual reality offers interactive simulations that can be used for rehabilitation. (From https://www.flickr.com/photos/46300592@N02/28951455421.)

Telehealth

Technology provides opportunities for engagement in daily occupations where physical challenges make those same in-person tasks seem insurmountable. It also permits us to connect remotely to others anywhere in the world, thereby preventing isolation and promoting social engagement in ways not available even a decade ago. Telehealth is another technology innovation defined as healthcare provision with a remote healthcare provider using Internet access through a computer or mobile device (United States Department of Health and Human Services [USDHHS], 2022b). Telehealth often refers to video conferencing, but other information and communication technologies are also used, including telephone, email, text messaging, and remote monitoring systems. Telehealth has long been recognized as a way to provide care to individuals who may not be able to get to a provider's office (Tenforde et al., 2017) and for those who cannot access in-person care promptly (Chen et al., 2021; Tenforde et al., 2020).

At no other time has telehealth's value been more apparent than during the COVID-19 pandemic, when individuals were restricted by isolation and social distancing policies (Tenforde et al., 2020). Telehealth services were offered before the pandemic, but persistent issues with reimbursement, professional licensing, and other regulations, as well as workflow and related technology issues, were obstacles to full adoption (Chen et al., 2021). Many of these regulatory and financing concerns were temporarily eased during the pandemic, prompting unparalleled growth during a time when the usual methods of accessing healthcare services were restricted or eliminated (Koonan et al., 2020; Malliaras et al., 2021; Miller et al., 2021; Tenforde et al. 2020; USDHHS, 2021).

Telehealth provides flexibility for both the provider and the client. Telehealth services can be completed synchronously, asynchronously, or by a mix of the two (Malliaras et al., 2021). Synchronous telehealth is simultaneous consultation between the provider and the client. Asynchronous telehealth is characterized by the care provider and client collaborating using technology at different times. A mix of these two methods could include a client uploading a document, image, or video for the provider to review and once the provider has reviewed the documents, a synchronous appointment is set for consultation.

A benefit of telehealth services includes access to care for individuals living in areas where services are not readily available. Access can also be timelier for follow-up appointments, as online meetings do not involve travel or other considerations. In addition, online platforms facilitate consultation with experts, making access to expertise easier. Lastly, the inherent flexibility of telehealth services can also provide care after traditional office hours, further improving access to care (Malliaras et al., 2021).

Similarly, telehealth services can make interdisciplinary collaboration easier, providing more comprehensive care (Tenforde et al., 2017, 2020). Continuity of care can be enhanced with telehealth, occurring between in-person visits, lessening the burdens associated with being seen in-person (e.g., travel, time off from work, and the need for childcare) (Chen et al., 2021; Tenforde et al., 2020). Telehealth may also be a viable tool for managing chronic healthcare needs by allowing more frequent monitoring of clients' conditions at a distance (Koonan et al., 2020; Malliaras et al., 2021; Tenforde et al., 2017).

Telehealth services can be provided to the care recipient in their natural environment. This provides advantages that in-person or office, or clinic visits do not. The home environment can be viewed, providing insights into accessibility and safety issues. Equipment recommendations can permit problem-solving in the home environment (Chen et al., 2021). In addition, caregivers may be present in the home environment permitting educational opportunities, collaborative brainstorming, and a glimpse into the nature of the relationships in the home environment (e.g., how supportive they are) (Onal et al., 2021; Tenforde et al., 2020). Gaining insights into the home environment can also provide clues to more effective and authentic treatment planning tailored to the client's unique contextual needs. Telehealth is a useful and flexible tool that addresses many of the challenges associated with in-person care and seems to have a role in meeting those needs well into the future (Fig. 4.4).

The remote nature of telehealth services also presents limitations in care provision, and any honest assessment of this method's usefulness must incorporate these considerations. There are times when telehealth services are ethically not the best care option. A common criticism of telehealth is the lack of human touch (Chen et al., 2021; Koonan et al., 2020). The inability to palpate and feel the client's response to stimuli can be perceived as an obstacle that can hinder diagnosis, limit the treatments offered, and impede the therapeutic relationship (Malliaras et al., 2021; Tenforde et al., 2020). Particularly as it relates to interventions with children, keeping young clients engaged in online endeavors can be difficult for extended periods (Tenforde et al., 2020).

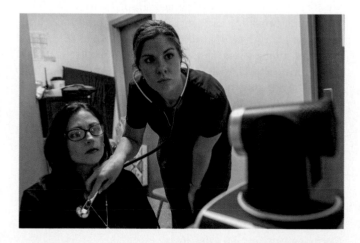

• **Fig. 4.4** A licensed practical nurse examines a patient while instantly transmitting the physical assessment back to an off-site nurse practitioner. (From https://www.flickr.com/photos/41284017@N08/43923099875.)

Other challenges associated with telehealth services include the expertise required to troubleshoot technology issues, the need for new and evolving equipment, and the associated workflow for this new approach (HRSA, n.d.). Workflow issues include considering which platform to use, accommodating accessibility issues of clients, such as hearing impairments and completing the associated follow-up tasks identified as a consequence of the telehealth session. Cybersecurity, specifically phishing, malware, and safeguarding client information, are also concerns for telehealth providers, as such disruptions can seriously affect patient care (AMA, 2017). Cybersecurity is ethically required for online health services, that is, safeguarding client health information, but many clinicians are not fully equipped and prepared to ensure full security (AMA, 2017; AOTA, 2020; APTA, 2019c). There are also limiting concerns related to bandwidth and the technology available from the client's perspective that can impact telehealth services, which are out of the clinician's control (Chen et al., 2021; Malliaras et al., 2021). Given the changing and uncertain landscape related to reimbursement, licensing issues, malpractice insurance, and other associated regulations, full buy-in to this mode of care is perceived as a venture that carries risk. It seems reasonable that the full implementation of telehealth services will be hindered until these important considerations are negotiated and resolved.

Telehealth has been demonstrated to be of value to remote clients and there is evidence of success in many different arenas (Cahill, 2021; Lew et al., 2020; Mercier et al., 2015; Miller et al., 2021; Rimmer et al., 2013). The absence of in-person services during the COVID-19 pandemic has been detrimental (Sutter et al., 2021), making telehealth a viable solution. Ultimately, the future of telehealth services will be determined by continuing to grow the body of evidence supporting these services, the establishment of clarity and regulations in terms of reimbursement and funding of these services, licensing issues, and malpractice insurance concerns (Chen et al., 2021). At the time of writing, both the American Physical Therapy Association (APTA) and the American Occupational Therapy Association (AOTA) are lobbying for the Expanded Telehealth Access Act (AOTA, 2021; APTA, 2021b). Healthcare students and clinicians also need to learn about this way of providing care. It will ultimately need to include curricular content in healthcare professional programs and educating current clinicians in telehealth best practices (Miller et al., 2021), including in practice frameworks such as PACE (i.e. Population and Health Outcomes; Access for All Clients; Costs and Cost Effectiveness; and Experiences of Clients and Occupational Therapy Practitioners) (Little et al., 2021) and continued training related to evolving technologies and techniques, such as the APTA Telehealth Certificate Course (APTA, 2021a). Telehealth is an effective option for meeting clients' needs in many circumstances and presents a great opportunity for healthcare professionals to be open and willing to work with clients in new and different ways.

Remote Patient Monitoring

Telemonitoring, or remote patient monitoring (RPM), is commonly used in the medical model for chronic disease management and involves the transmission of a client's vital signs (e.g., blood pressure, heart rate, oxygen levels) and other health data (e.g., blood sugar levels, weight, activity of daily living [ADL] performance, fall events) for review by a clinician to assure more timely monitoring (Walthers et al., 2020). This type of monitoring can prevent health crises, emergency department use, and hospitalization and promote health and wellness. Monitoring like this may be done with a Smartwatch, applications on a Smartphone or digital tablet, and other wearable technology.

Robotics

Robotics have been increasingly used in physical rehabilitation for increasing upper and lower extremity movement or trunk control, strength, manipulation, and balance (Fig. 4.5). A robot is an "actuated mechanism programmable in two or more axes with a degree of autonomy, moving within its environment, to perform intended tasks" (Cook et al., 2020). Robots are typically used to provide manipulation in environments where it is not safe for a person or to enable a person to participate in daily activities. Generic manipulation by a device requires it to be able to move in three-dimensional space and to adapt its action according to the specific task.

Robotics use "freedom of motion," the degree of motion in a particular plane or movement. Exoskeletal instruments cover the limb, following and replicating its movement characteristics and guiding each segment involved in the

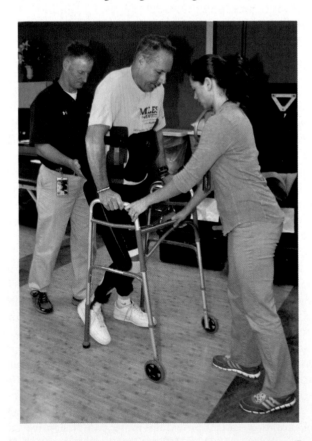

• **Fig. 4.5** An individual walks with the aid of an exoskeleton. (From https://www.flickr.com/photos/95597328@N08/27822290366.)

movement (Giansanti, 2020). Another type is end-effector robotics, in which the input for carrying out the rehabilitation exercise comes directly from the distal part of the limb, allowing the natural activation of the movement without unnatural constraints (Giansanti, 2020). Several companies are offering these types of devices. One such robotic system offered by Saebo uses robotics to simulate or take a client through various movements with a variation in assistance in the movements or resistance, based on individual setup and the client's needs. In addition to rehabilitation robotics, or rehabilitation technical tools (RTT), robotic arms serve as a substitute for movements that the person does not have due to a neurological condition. These include the Jaco robotic arm by Kinovo and the Manus manipulator. The Jaco arm and Manus manipulator have an articulated arm that can be mounted on a wheelchair, bed, or table with a "hand" piece that is operated by adaptive switching or a joystick to enable a person to participate in work, play, or leisure tasks requiring manipulation.

Other rehabilitation technology uses a screen, such as the BITS system by Biotech/Bioness, which incorporates visual and cognitive neurorehabilitation with UE, LE, and trunk balance activities (Stephenson et al., 2019). The BITS uses progressively more complex visual/cognitive activities while challenging reaction time and balance. It is often used in Driver's rehabilitation programs in occupational therapy.

Wheelchair Seating and Mobility

Wheelchair seating and mobility is an area of assistive technology that occupational and physical therapy practitioners may be involved with, along with an assistive technology practitioner (ATP) or seating and mobility specialist (SMS) employed through a durable medical equipment company. Medicaid, Medicare, and most insurance companies require that a professional certified as an ATP by the Rehabilitation and Engineering Society of North America (RESNA) be involved when evaluating a client for a wheelchair. Proper wheelchair seating and mobility involves positioning the client and identifying the seating system and the wheelchair base (Owens & Davis, 2022). Positioning is the practice of determining the optimal body position for a client, while the wheelchair seating system is used to maintain that identified position. Seating systems are used on manual or power wheelchair bases. All wheelchair mobility bases require a seating system that uniquely meets the user's needs. Both occupational and physical therapists may achieve additional certification as an ATP or SMS through RESNA.

Alternative and Augmentative Communication

Alternative and augmentative communication (AAC) are methods, strategies, and speech-generating systems to improve the communication of individuals with disabilities (Fig. 4.6). Practitioners should consider optimum positioning, physical access, visual, cognitive, and functional participation when using AAC devices. Using alternative access such as eye gaze technology, adaptive switches, speech-to-text, and other assistive devices for communication requires

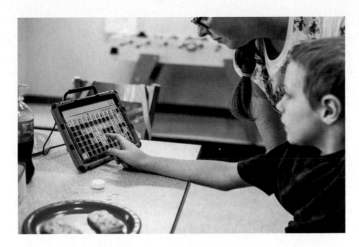

• **Fig. 4.6** Alternative and augmentative communication methods help individuals with disabilities communicate. (© 2022 PRC-Saltillo. Image used with permission. All rights reserved.)

additional training to develop the skills needed to work with high-tech devices.

Health Informatics

Health or medical informatics, also known as Health Information Systems (HIT), began during World War II when the complexity of healthcare expanded, the need for information management increased, and the first computational system (i.e., computer) was developed (Cesnik & Kidd, 2010). The early efforts to integrate and store diverse medical records were developed to enhance communication and coordination of care among healthcare systems and providers. However, HIT has evolved into a system of resources and tools that are useful to providers and consumers of healthcare services as well as healthcare systems, researchers, payers, and government agencies and policymakers (American Medical Informatics Association [AMIA], 2022; Eysenbach, 2000; Jen 2021). At the intersection of information/data science and healthcare, this rapidly expanding interprofessional field focuses on integrating computational, cognitive, and social sciences to improve healthcare effectiveness and efficiency and improve healthcare outcomes for service users (Fig. 4.7).

A now widely interconnected field, HIT addresses the resources, devices, and methods required to optimize the acquisition, storage, retrieval, and use of information in health and wellness (AMIA, 2022). It includes data management (e.g., privacy, security, provider and consumer health information access), technology and communication ethics (e.g., healthcare education [health literacy], telemedicine, homecare, global health), translational and decisional support resources and systems (e.g., predictive measures, genomic data, artificial intelligence), and research and policy resources. HIT relies upon the development of subspecialty expertise in:

- Data mining and information analysis (e.g., collection, analysis, and visualization of complex data).
- Internet informatics and information architecture (e.g., design and access of websites, software, intranets, and online communities and the data within them, use of the

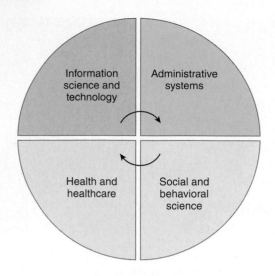

• **Fig. 4.7** Health informatics combines technology and management strategies to improve healthcare effectiveness, efficiency, and outcomes.

Internet to map and solve complex problems, and the interaction of humans and computers).
• Life, social, and public health informatics (e.g., identify and analyze components of ecosystems and organisms and their interactions and health surveillance, prevention, preparedness, and health).

Perhaps the most relevant to occupational and physical therapy providers are clinical informatics, the application of informatics, and information technology to deliver healthcare services (AMIA, 2022; Jen et al., 2021). Clinical informatics blends information technologies and HIT with clinical practice that advances healthcare research, improves healthcare delivery and outcomes, and increases healthcare delivery's value (Jen et al., 2021).

In 2004, President George W. Bush signed Executive Order 13335, the Incentives for the Use of Health Information Technology, and established the position of National Health Information Technology Coordinator. This order paved the foundation for developing a nationwide health information exchange across healthcare systems, hospitals, and providers (Jen et al., 2021). It was not until 2009, however, with the passage of the Affordable Care Act that required healthcare systems to transition from paper to EMR systems, that clinical informatics became more widely used. That same year, the Health Information Technology for Economic and Clinical Health (HITECH) Act was passed by Congress as part of the American Recovery and Reinvestment Act of 2009 to incentivize providers to adopt EMR use and to integrate electronic records across institutions to improve healthcare quality, safety, and efficiency (Jen et al., 2021). With the development of large data sets, called Big Data, researchers could collate large quantities of data across a wide array of healthcare systems and providers to identify trends, to predict illness and care trajectories, and to improve healthcare treatment protocol and outcomes.

The measure of quality healthcare service delivery and outcomes is of central importance to occupational and physical therapy practitioners and managers. Clinical informatics may be a valuable tool to promote the value of our practice and professions. In a study of the use of data extraction from EHRs for the quality measurement of the physical therapy process, Scholte and colleagues (2016) found that analysis of EMR data can provide valuable information regarding the quality of service delivery outcomes and these data can lead to the development of recommendations for quality improvements. Today service delivery and healthcare outcomes not only benefit from the extraction and aggregation of Big Data from EMRs, but they also benefit from consumer informatics research that continually codifies consumers' needs, values, and preferences. This information is leading to improvements in health literacy and healthcare education, consumer advocacy, and improvements in patient experience design (Meloncon, 2017).

Strengths and Opportunities

Technology use in healthcare can improve effectiveness, save time, and provide data collection and storage options. In addition, it could allow therapists to spend more time working with patients instead of collecting data or completing documentation. Technology also has the potential to provide novel and motivating interventions with built-in positive reinforcement that could improve the outcomes of occupational and physical therapy services. There are many opportunities for therapists to partner with engineers and information technology professionals in developing these new devices to improve usability and application in therapy practice.

Barriers and Considerations

Barriers and considerations to using technology in therapy practices and healthcare include considering ease of use, equity due to cost or other reasons, and time needed to maintain current knowledge on technological advances. Implementation of technology and IoT in healthcare will rely on a clear and robust code of practice for the management of data, privacy, confidentiality, and cybersecurity concerning the supply and use of technology, including the IoT and devices in healthcare (Kelly et al., 2020).

Future Directions

With nearly 41.1 million people in the United States with a disability, there is a great incentive for businesses, education settings, and the government to invest in accessible technology to ensure that working environments are inclusive and available to all user groups (United States Census, 2021). The use of universal design in the built world, learning environments, and healthcare is increasing to allow access for all individuals (CDC, 2020).

Universal Design is based on seven principles:
1. Equitable use: The design is useful and marketable to people with diverse abilities.

2. Flexibility in use: The design accommodates a wide range of individual preferences and abilities.
3. Simple and intuitive use: The design is easy to understand, regardless of the user's experience, knowledge, language skills, or current concentration level.
4. Perceptible information: The design communicates necessary information effectively to the user, regardless of ambient conditions or the user's sensory abilities.
5. Tolerance for error: The design minimizes hazards and the adverse consequences of accidental or unintended actions.
6. Low physical effort: The design can be used efficiently, comfortably, and with minimum fatigue.
7. Size and space for approach and use: Appropriate size and space are provided for approach, reach, manipulation, and use regardless of the user's body size, posture, or mobility (CDC 2020).

Occupational and physical therapy practitioners use everyday technology such as reachers, built-up eating utensils, nonslip grip mats, and pencil grips. They also use digital tablets, smartphones, computer software, game consoles, and more complex rehabilitation technologies that require additional training. These more complex rehabilitation technologies include robotics, complex computer access configurations (e.g., access through eye gaze), complex augmentative communication systems (e.g., integrated multifunction devices with dynamic display), powered mobility, complex seating and positioning systems, and complex home modification systems (e.g., smart home technology).

The use of technology in rehabilitation in multiple areas with occupational and physical therapy will most likely continue to increase as new technologies develop using universal design for mainstream technology access. The additional types of technology will be developed to meet a need for access, to reduce barriers, and to enable participation in all occupations. Therefore, occupational and physical therapy practitioners and other health professionals must learn about and use technology and assistive technology.

Discussion and Activities

The use of technology in healthcare is continuing to increase to provide more effective healthcare services and to utilize time more efficiently. This increase comes with ethical considerations regarding patient information, artificial intelligence, data storage, and usage. With the rapid expansion of technology, laws, policies, and procedures must be implemented to provide appropriate safeguards for the misuse of technology and data in healthcare. Occupational and physical therapy practitioners must ensure they possess the necessary knowledge and skills in technology and environmental interventions to support their clients effectively in the evaluation, intervention, and outcomes measurement processes. Reflect on your comfort with technology and consider the following:
1. Describe how technology has changed the provision and outcomes of rehabilitation services. How has the public

health emergency (COVID-19) changed the use of technology in your state?
2. How might you incorporate technology in the evaluation and treatment of clients? Consider how technology use may differ among populations (i.e., gender, age, diagnoses, outcome expectations).
3. Examine the differences between technological treatment modalities (e.g., Bioness), assistive technology (adaptive devices), and AAC.

Health Literacy

Background and Current State

Communication between healthcare providers and their clients is essential to providing effective client-centered care and achieving optimal health outcomes (Fig. 4.8). Health literacy is defined by the United States Health Resources and Services Administration (HRSA) as the extent to which individuals receiving healthcare have the "capacity to obtain, process, and understand basic health information needed to make appropriate health decisions" (HRSA, 2019). An individual's ability to interpret, to make decisions, and to act on the health information they receive plays a significant role in health maintenance and disease prevention, illness and injury care, and health advocacy for self and others. Achieving and maintaining health is increasingly complex in today's healthcare market and having the ability to access the healthcare systems, to describe health attributes and symptomatology, to read labels on food and medicines, and to engage in healthy behaviors are essential skills of healthcare consumers.

Personal health literacy refers to how an individual can access and understand healthcare information required to make healthcare decisions. Literacy skills include the ability to read, write, speak, listen, calculate, problem solves, and use current technology (Harvard T.H. Chan School of Public Health, 2022). It is estimated that at least 88% of adults living in the United States have inadequate health literacy levels to navigate the healthcare system (Lopez et al., 2022). Lopez and colleagues (2022) report that adults with low health literacy are more likely to have difficulty completing intake forms and assessments and accurately reporting

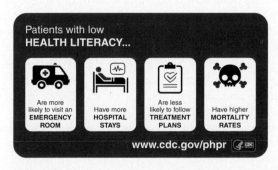

• **Fig. 4.8** Communication between healthcare providers and their clients is essential to achieving optimal health outcomes. (From https://www.cdc.gov/cpr/infographics/healthliteracy.htm.)

medical histories and symptomology. Also, these individuals are more likely to miss appointments and neglect follow-up visits. Paasche-Orlow and his colleagues (2005) argue that health literacy prevalence data generally focus on reading, readability (the ease at which written information can be read), and numeracy (read and interpret numbers) and often fail to address other important domains of health literacy such as listening, speaking, writing, or comprehension (the ability to understand what is read). Adding to this complexity, Samerski (2019) describes health literacy as being influenced by the social elements of a situation where an individual may seem literate in one circumstance and less so in another. Second, much of the literature focuses on the health literacy of English-speaking consumers. Language barriers pose a significant health literacy obstacle to many non-English speaking clients and are often excluded from health literacy prevalence data. The prevalence of low health literacy is consistently associated with levels of education, socioeconomic status, ethnicity, and age (Paasche-Orlow et al., 2005; Taylor et al., 2017, White et al., 2008).

Clients with low to marginal health literacy are less likely to engage in preventative healthcare and more likely to engage the healthcare system only under emergent conditions (Balakrishnan et al., 2017). Clients with low to marginal health literacy are two to three times more likely to visit the emergency room to manage their healthcare needs. That low to marginal health literacy is associated with higher mortality (Peterson et al., 2011) is not hard to imagine. These individuals have less knowledge of managing chronic diseases, struggle to follow multiple-step instructions, take medications according to dosage and frequency, and have poorer mental and physical health (Bostock & Steptoe, 2012).

An important aspect inherent to health literacy is digital health literacy (Smith & Magnani, 2019). With the advent of the Internet as the main information source coupled with technology-facilitated tools such as electronic medical records, digital health literacy requires additional skills related to technology use, specifically the ability to identify quality information and navigate patient portals to evaluate information. There are personal implications, such as access to technology and the ability to use it, and broader considerations, such as how intuitive online tools are to use (Smith & Magnani, 2019).

On the other hand, organizational health literacy refers to how healthcare organizations and providers support individuals to access, understand, and use health information to make informed decisions about their healthcare needs (Bregga et al., 2019; Farmanova et al., 2018). Several key components of organizational health literacy have been identified and include (Bregga et al., 2019; Farmanova et al., 2018; Sentell, 2021):

- Understanding and advocacy for health literacy among the healthcare workforce through leadership, prioritization, and training.
- Client access to and navigation of the healthcare system (e.g., attention to reading, numeracy, listening, and speaking literacy).

- Client engagement in the continuum of services offered throughout the healthcare process.
- Effective communication with clients and their families/caregivers.

Strengths and Opportunities

The Healthy People initiative began in 1979 after the United States Surgeon General identified and prioritized health promotion and disease prevention strategies for the population (USDHHS, 2022a). The Healthy People 2030 Framework builds on the knowledge of four decades of research on population health and health outcomes in the United States and it represents the fifth revision of the Healthy People initiative (USDHHS, 2022a). For the first time in its 40-year history, USDHHS has prioritized personal and organizational health literacy in its health goals and objectives for the population and includes as one of its central aims to "eliminate health disparities, achieve health equity, and attain health literacy to improve the health and well-being of all" (USDHHS, n.d.). The following objectives are included in the initiatives:

- Increase the proportion of adults whose healthcare provider checked their understanding.
- Decrease the proportion of adults who report poor communication with their healthcare provider.
- Increase the proportion of adults whose healthcare providers involved them in decisions as much as they wanted.
- Increase the proportion of people who say their online medical record is easy to understand.
- Increase the proportion of adults with limited English proficiency who say their providers explain things clearly.

By prioritizing health literacy in the Healthy People 2030 Framework, USDHHS is increasing public awareness of the influence of determinants of health, disease, and disability and outlining opportunities for progress for all healthcare providers. The Centers for Disease Control and Prevention (CDC) established the National Action Plan to Improve Health Literacy in 2010 (CDC, 2019). Based on goals of increasing personal and organizational health literacy, the plan ensures that healthcare information is accessible and understandable and empowers consumers to make informed decisions about their health and healthcare. The Healthy People 2030 Framework and the National Action Plan to Improve Health Literacy align with occupational and physical therapy ethical and practice guidance to deliver person-centered care, provide thorough, understandable, and actionable health information, and deliver an educational intervention that promotes health, well-being, and quality of life. AOTA Societal Statement on Health Literacy and the APTA Position on Health Literacy emphasize that health literacy is essential for optimal health outcomes and promote opportunities for practitioners to develop knowledge and skills to create a more health-literate society (AOTA, 2017; APTA, 2019e). With a focus on advancing health literacy, occupational and physical therapy practitioners can encourage clients to become active members of the healthcare team and empower informed decision-making (Attard et al., 2021).

Valuable health literacy assessments are increasingly available to support client access to health information and informed decision-making. Two common assessments include the Rapid Estimate of Adult Literacy in Medicine, Revised (REALM-R) (Arozullah et al., 2007; Davis et al., 1991), and the Test of Functional Health Literacy in Adults (TOFHLA) (Parker et al., 1995). The REALM-R was developed to assess reading levels and comprehension in English speakers and the TOFHLA measures both reading comprehension and numeracy in English and Spanish speakers. The Agency for Healthcare Research and Quality (AHRQ) has developed four tools to assess reading comprehension of health-related terminology in English and Spanish speakers (AHRQ, 2019). The Short Assessment of Health Literacy–Spanish and English (SAHL-S&E) (Lee et al., 2010), one of the tools developed by the AHRQ, can be administered in approximately three minutes and yields information about a client's ability to comprehend health terms. The Newest Vital Sign is another tool that can be easily administered in two or three minutes and uses labels and images to assess health literacy (Powers et al., 2010). Finally, the National Institutes of Health's National Library of Medicine funds the Health Literacy Tool Shed, an online collaboratively developed database of health literacy measures that assess a range of health literacy domains such as communication, comprehension, numeracy, and media literacy (Health Literacy Tool Shed, 2022). A criticism of health literacy assessments is that there is no single comprehensive assessment that can be used globally; rather, many tools assess an aspect of health literacy (Liu et al., 2018). The results provide valuable information but not a complete assessment across varied circumstances.

Barriers and Considerations

Complex changes in healthcare systems (e.g., shorter hospital stays, increased medications, and more self-management requirements for healthcare) and client demographics (e.g., aging population, a growing number of clients with limited English proficiency) require that organizations and healthcare providers regularly examine and improve their health literacy resources and supports. The National Action Plan to Improve Health Literacy provides an evidence-based pathway to improve health literacy in organizations and healthcare consumers (CDC, 2019). Table 4.1 illustrates how occupational and physical therapy providers can address health literacy in their practice.

Future Directions

The prioritization of health literacy in healthcare promises to achieve the Healthy People 2030 goal to increase personal and organizational health literacy in the United States. Occupational and physical therapy practitioners will play an important role in their interprofessional teams in promoting health literacy, cultural competence, and behavior change principles. Though health literacy is not a new concept, incorporating health literacy principles into team

TABLE 4.1 Strategies to Improve Health Literacy

National Action Plan to Improve Health Literacy Goal (CDC, 2019[a])	Strategies to Improve Health Literacy
Develop and disseminate health and safety information that is accurate, accessible, and actionable.	• Simplify language in patient education materials. The CDC Simply Put resource is a valuable tool to help create easy-to-understand materials (CDC, 2010[b]). • Use graphics, pictures, and videos (note that the use of icons can be difficult or have different cultural meanings). Be sure videos have closed captioning for those with hearing or information processing difficulties. • Check reading levels of written material. The Patient Education Materials Assessment Tool (PEMAT) and User's Guide assess patient education materials' understandability (AHRQ, 2020[c]). • Establish guidelines for appraising and modifying patient education materials (Attard et al., 2021[d]). • When making written education materials in print or digital formats, consider changes due to aging, such as decreased vision or slower cognitive processing. The Centers for Medicare and Medicaid have a Toolkit for Making Written Material Clear and Effective (CMS, 2021[e]), which helps design written materials.
Promote changes in the healthcare delivery system that improve information, communication, informed decision-making, and access to health services.	• Assess the physical facility for effective navigation for clients with low health literacy (Rudd, 2010[f]). • Provide training to ensure that the workforce is knowledgeable about the influences of social determinants of health on health literacy. The National Library of Medicine (NLM) Clinical Conversations Program offers a seven-module series on health literacy promotion (NLM, 2022[g]). • Engage patient advocates and language/ hearing interpreters to support client communication and health literacy. • Offer assistance completing written and digital forms.

Continued

TABLE 4.1	Strategies to Improve Health Literacy—cont'd

National Action Plan to Improve Health Literacy Goal (CDC, 2019[a])	Strategies to Improve Health Literacy
Incorporate accurate and standards-based health and developmentally appropriate health and science information and curricula into child care and education through the university level.	• Ensure occupational and physical therapy education programs offer training on health literacy and client educational intervention at the individual, group, and population levels (Hildenbrand, 2020[h]). • Provide training to increase digital health literacy to clients. The NLM offers various digital health literacy resources to support training initiatives (NLM, 2021[i]). • Engage students in interprofessional learning activities to empower clients' access to relevant health information and informed decision-making. • Provide health literacy training to pre-professional students (pre-occupational and physical therapy clubs, high school students). The University of Maryland's (UM) Project SHARE Curriculum addresses health literacy and equity in its six-module curriculum (UM, 2020[j]).
Support and expand local efforts to provide adult education, English-language instruction, and culturally and linguistically appropriate health information services in the community.	• Identify individuals with low literacy using evidence-based assessment tools. • Offer training and resources to support healthy lifestyles for individuals with chronic illnesses.
Build partnerships, develop guidance, and change policies.	• Develop professional guidelines and standards of care for clients with low health literacy (Attard et al., 2021[d]).
Increase basic research and develop, implement, and evaluate practices and interventions to improve health literacy.	• Collaborate with the team to build knowledge of effective health literacy assessment and educational interventions with clients.
Increase the dissemination and use of evidence-based health literacy practices and interventions.	• Avoid making assumptions. • Simplify language and define all technical terms. • Speak more slowly (note that individuals with low literacy may need additional time to process complex descriptions and instructions). • Supplement instructions with appropriate patient education materials. • Ask open-ended questions to assess client comprehension of verbal and written information. • Start a client healthcare journal or review information in the patient healthcare portal. • Uses Teach Back (Centrella-Nigro & Alexander, 2017[k]) and Show Back methods to ensure understanding.

[a]Centers for Disease Control and Prevention (CDC). (2019). *National action plan to improve health literacy.* https://www.cdc.gov/healthliteracy/planact/national.html
[b]Centers for Disease Control and Prevention (CDC). (2010). *Simply put; a guide for creating easy-to-understand materials.* https://stacks.cdc.gov/view/cdc/11938/ Agency for Healthcare
[c]Agency for Healthcare Research and Quality (AHRQ). (2020). *The patient education materials assessment tool (pemat) and user's guide.* https://www.ahrq.gov/health-literacy/patient-education/pemat.html#:~:text=The%20Patient%20Education%20Materials%20Assessment%20Tool%20(PEMAT)%20is%20a%20systematic,understand%20and%20act%20on%20information
[d]Attard, E., Musallam, A., Vaas, K., Chaney, T., Fortuna, J. K., & Williams, B. (2021). Health literacy in occupational therapy research: A scoping review. *The Open Journal of Occupational Therapy, 9*(4), 1–18.
[e]Centers for Medicare and Medicaid Services (CMS). (2021). *Toolkit for making written material clear and effective.* https://www.cms.gov/Outreach-and-Education/Outreach/WrittenMaterialsToolkit
[f]Rudd, R. (2010). *The health literacy environment activity packet: First impressions and walking interview.* https://cdn1.sph.harvard.edu/wp-content/uploads/sites/135/2012/09/activitypacket.pdf
[g]National Library of Medicine (NLM). (2022). Clinical conversations training program: Health literacy. https://nnlm.gov/guides/clinical-conversations-training-program
[h]Hildenbrand, G. M., Perrault, E. K., & Keller, P. E. (2020). Evaluating a health literacy communication training for medical students: Using plain language. *Journal of Health Communication, 25*(8), 624–631
[i]National Library of Medicine (NLM). (2021). Digital Health Literacy. https://allofus.nnlm.gov/digital-health-literacy
[j]University of Maryland (UM). (2020). Project SHARE Curriculum. https://guides.hshsl.umaryland.edu/c.php?g=76220&p=1538472
[k]Centrella-Nigro, A. M., & Alexander, C. (2017). Using the teach-back method in patient education to improve patient satisfaction. *Journal of Continuing Education in Nursing, 48*(1), 47–52.

practices requires intentionality and attention to the team development process (Tuckman, 1965).

In the forming phase, the team members orient themselves to the influences of health literacy on client outcomes and examine discipline-specific considerations. Occupational and physical therapists can be instrumental in the storming phase by using their leadership and advocacy skills to develop training and collaboration methods to empower clients as team members and informed decision makers. As team members begin to work closely with one another, valuable evidence will emerge of effective health literacy and educative interventions aimed at helping clients learn not just about their illness or injury but how to navigate the healthcare system effectively to achieve better health outcomes and quality of life. At the final team development stage of performing, team members will have collaboratively addressed organizational health literacy, developed competencies in culturally responsive client communication, and established an array of accessible resources to support client healthcare education needs.

Discussion and Activities

In order to provide effective client-centered care, occupational and physical therapy practitioners must know their clients' factors and cultural backgrounds, including their health literacy. Reflect on the role of occupational and physical therapy and consider the following questions:

1. What is the health literacy of the populations you serve? Examine your patient population's health literacy prevalence data for your geographical region. What do the data suggest relative to the needs of your client population?
2. Which tools or resources are available to assess your population's health literacy? Examine the tools available in the Health Literacy Tool Shed (Health Literacy Tool Shed, 2022) and practice administering them to a peer. Discuss the advantages and limitations of using a structured measure to assess health literacy. Conduct an organizational health literacy assessment of your workplace.
3. Are the patient educational materials available at your facility accessible and actionable? Evaluate the readability of patient education materials and modify them with accessible language. Develop an accessible fact sheet on a health-related topic.
4. Do you modify your interactions with clients to accommodate their level of health literacy? Practice communicating with a peer using simple language and open-ended questions, avoiding jargon and culturally stigmatizing language, and using teach-back and show-back methods.

Social Media

Background and Current State

Social media is a popular destination for Internet users, with most United States adults reporting they use YouTube or Facebook (Auxier & Anderson, 2021). Many individuals utilize the Internet, including social media, for health information (Finney Rutten et al., 2019; Prestin et al., 2015). Social media is a popular format for seeking and sharing health information regarding diagnosis, treatment, and support (Gupta et al., 2020). Thus due to social media's powerful influence on modern healthcare, providers must be familiar with the potential benefits and risks of using social media to inform or interact with consumers.

Strengths and Opportunities

Social media can be used as a tool by providers to answer questions or consult, provide health information on various conditions, promote healthy behaviors, educate, and facilitate dialogue. In addition, social media can increase interaction for peer, social, and emotional support and increase the ability to make information available, accessible, shared, and individualized. Lastly, social media can be a powerful tool for networking, professional education, and marketing yourself or a business (Moorhead et al., 2013; Ventola, 2014).

Barriers and Considerations

A major concern is that the information posted on social media lacks quality and reliability or that the author of the content is not credible. Poor quality information could discourage care and result in negative health beliefs or behaviors (Fig. 4.9). Inaccurate information could lead to adverse outcomes (Moorhead et al., 2013; Ventola, 2014).

Interacting with consumers online or via social media could jeopardize confidentiality and privacy. The Health Insurance Portability and Accountability Act (HIPAA) states that healthcare providers must protect sensitive patient health information. Even accidental breaches can involve legal ramifications (Health Insurance Portability and Accountability Act of 1996 [HIPAA] CDC, 2019). Beyond damage to one's professional image, violating a provider's code of ethics and state or federal laws could lead to discipline (Moorhead et al., 2013; Ventola, 2014).

Future Directions

The American Medical Association (AMA) was the first to publish an opinion regarding physicians' use of social media. The AMA recognizes the benefit of social media for

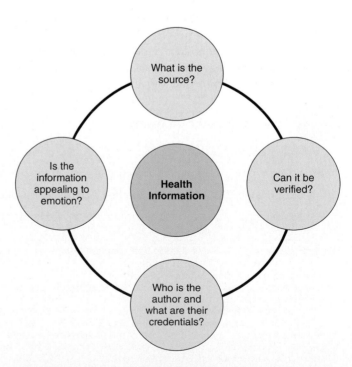

• **Fig. 4.9** A major concern with health information posted on social media is quality and accuracy.

quick, widespread dissemination of information. However, the AMA stresses the importance of patient privacy and confidentiality. Also, physicians must maintain professionalism when interacting with patients and other professionals. Inability to conduct oneself professionally online, either in actions or content, one's reputation could be negatively affected (AMA, 2016).

The APTA agrees that social media can be an effective tool for networking, education, and marketing; however, inappropriate behavior could damage the profession and a person's reputation (APTA, 2019, September 2). In agreement with AMA, the APTA recommends that physical therapists conduct themselves ethically and professionally, maintain patient privacy and confidentiality, and provide accurate information. Advice for occupational therapists includes avoiding unprofessional behavior, ensuring client confidentiality, respecting boundaries, following social media platforms' rules, and monitoring accounts for breaches (Wong, 2015). Overall, therapists must recognize that their actions can affect their reputation, employer, and profession (APTA, 2019, September 2).

The following are tips for successful social media use:
- Protecting patient privacy and confidentiality
- Being professional in all communications
- Knowing your code of ethics and the professional licensure requirements for your state
- Reviewing your employer's policies
- Sharing information from credible sources
- Refuting inaccurate information
- Establishing a brand with a clear message by defining your goals and objectives
- Avoiding impulsive social media behavior
- Respecting copyright laws
- Not engaging anonymously
- Thinking carefully before establishing separate personal and professional identities on social media platforms (i.e., separate accounts do not guarantee separation of personal and professional images)
- Monitoring your online identity

Discussion and Activities

- List other potential benefits of social media for providers.
- List other potential risks of social media for providers.
- Are there more pros or cons for providers who use social media?
- How could you post success stories on your website or social media without violating HIPAA?
- Should your personal social media activity have any impact on your professional life?
- Can your employer discipline or fire you for your personal social media activity?

Interprofessional Collaboration

Background and Current State

In healthcare, interprofessional collaboration (see Chapters 7 and 21) occurs with numerous professionals, including occupational and physical therapists (Table 4.2). According to the World Health Organization, interprofessional collaboration is defined as "when multiple health workers from different professional backgrounds work together with patients, families, [caregivers], and communities to deliver the highest quality of care" (WHO, 2010). In addition, collaborative care improves health outcomes and client satisfaction, optimizes health services, and strengthens health systems (WHO, 2010).

Interprofessional care requires that healthcare providers set aside time to meet and establish trusting relationships based on mutual respect, understand each other's roles, and have shared decision-making with equal voices (Johnson, Hermosura, Price & Gougeon, 2021). Although there is a great deal of evidence to support interprofessional collaboration, there are barriers to interprofessional care. These include a uniprofessional mindset, organizational challenges, and a lack of training in teamwork (Johnson, et al, 2022). A "turf war" may occur when these barriers are too

TABLE 4.2 Types of Healthcare Teams

Interprofessional[a]	Collaboration among a team of professionals from different professions.
Intraprofessional[a]	Collaboration among a team of professionals from the same profession.
Interdisciplinary[b]	Analyzes, synthesizes, and harmonizes links between disciplines into a coordinated and coherent whole.
Transdisciplinary[b]	Integrates the natural, social, and health sciences in a humanities context and transcends their traditional boundaries.
Multidisciplinary[b]	Knowledge from different disciplines but remaining within their boundaries.

[a]Professional is the preferred terminology in healthcare.
[b]Disciplines are described as individual sciences that study different subjects independently of each other to develop theories as a means of scientifically understanding the world.
Information from Chamberlain-Salaun, J., Mills, J., & Usher, K. (2013). Terminology used to describe healthcare teams: An integrative review of the literature. *Journal of Multidisciplinary Healthcare, 6*, 65–74; Choi, B. C. K., Pak, A. W. P. (2006). Multidisciplinarity, interdisciplinarity and transdisciplinarity in health research, services, education and policy: 1. Definitions, objectives, and evidence of effectiveness. *Clinical and investigative medicine. Medecine clinique et experimentale, 29*(6), 351–364; Mahler, C., Gutmann, T., Karstens, S., & Joos, S. (2014). Terminology for interprofessional collaboration: definition and current practice. GMS *Zeitschrift fur medizinische Ausbildung, 31*(4):Doc40.

great. A turf war is a dispute between competing groups. In healthcare, the dispute is typically centered around what is within a person's scope of practice and if it infringes upon another's practice. For example, physical therapists performing dry needling may be viewed as infringing on acupuncturists' practice. These debates are, at times, necessary to protect a person's profession and to protect the public from unsafe practices. However, turf wars can develop merely for one group of professionals to maintain power over another, sometimes even to the detriment of the patient.

Although turf wars may occur, it is important to consider why. Evidence shows that the main reasons for a turf war may be because students are often taught in an unprofessional manner with little knowledge of other disciplines or their roles or training (Johnson, et al, 2022). This approach may affect their attitudes toward other healthcare professionals. The Interprofessional Educational Program (Johnson, 2017) has developed four tenants for interprofessional collaboration, including values/ethics, roles/responsibilities, interprofessional communication, teams, and teamwork. Occupational and physical therapy students should seek to understand the values and ethics of each professional, find out what each professional's training entails, utilize effective communication skills, consider the client first, pursue training on teamwork, and be a professional team member (Fig. 4.10). Involving the client in the team and ensuring that all team members have an equal voice can facilitate a culture of transparency and the ability to discuss issues openly with those involved. This transparency fosters a trusting therapeutic relationship rather than focusing on individuals' power or control in the relationship.

Strengths and Opportunities

Using the Interprofessional Educational Program will benefit patients and maintain a client-centered approach for occupational and physiotherapists and other healthcare

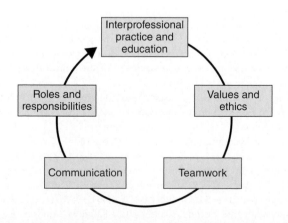

• **Fig. 4.10** Interprofessional practice and education is important for client-centered care and optimal outcomes.

providers on teams (WHO, 2010 and 2012). Educational benefits of interprofessional education include students gaining insight from and learning to work with other practitioners. Clinical benefits of interprofessional collaboration include:

- Better access to healthcare
- Enhanced communication
- Improved coordination of care
- Improved outcomes and quality of care
- Improved patient safety and satisfaction
- Reduced medical errors
- Reduced hospitalizations and readmissions
- Improved productivity and staff morale

Barriers and Considerations

Common barriers to interprofessional collaboration are lack of time, medical hierarchies, and a lack of knowledge regarding other professionals' scope of practice (WHO, 2012). In addition, professionals may be reluctant (precontemplation or contemplation stage of change) to share information due to role release (the storming phase of group development), but communicating clearly with other professionals respectfully can counteract these issues related to role release. Unlike the historic system of working in silos, physical therapists, occupational therapists, and speech-language pathologists collaborate with various other disciplines, including nursing, case management, social work, and recreation therapists. This benefits practitioners and patients; however, integrating disciplines and creating allies with other professionals comes with some challenges. One notable challenge is profession-specific language, models, and theories.

Research supports using a common model for clarity in communication, team building, and collaboration. The Kawa model is a culturally neutral occupational therapy model that has also been applied to professional team building. Kawa is a metaphysical representation of a river with rocks, driftwood, and riverbanks representing assets, liabilities, physical and social environments, and circumstances affecting river flow. In a pilot study that involved rehabilitation, nursing, administration, social work, and activities personnel, 10/10 people reported that the Kawa model provided a common language for interprofessional communication (Lape, 2019). In an acute care rehabilitation team study, 100% of participants reported that the Kawa model could improve team collaboration (Ober, 2019). Using existing interprofessional collaboration models and a common language is a viable opportunity for interdisciplinary teams.

Future Directions

Interprofessional collaboration will become increasingly important, especially with expanding physical (PT) occupational therapists' (OT) roles in healthcare. For example, therapists

TABLE 4.3	Potential Interprofessional Issues	
Professionals	**Entry-level Training**	**Potential Issues**
ABA	Master's or Doctorate	Behavior analysis
Acupuncturist	Master's	Dry needling
Athletic Trainers	Bachelor or Master's	Rehabilitation services Concussion
Chiropractors	Doctorate	Sensory processing Manipulation Use of the term "physical therapy"
Exercise Professionals	Largely unlicensed, certifications available	Health and wellness Use of "PT" designation by personal trainers
Nursing (RN)	Associates or Bachelor's	Wound and ostomy care
Nursing (APRN)	Master's or Doctorate	Primary care
Physicians	Doctorate with required residency	Imaging Primary care POPTS
Prosthetists and Orthotists	Master's	Furnishing and fabricating orthotics and prosthetics
Speech-Language Pathologists	Master's	Dysphagia/feeding Cognition

ABA, Applied behavior analyst; *APRN,* advanced practice registered nurse; *POPTS,* physician-owned physical therapy services: *RN,* registered nurse.
Information from APRNs in the U.S. (2022). NCSBN. https://www.ncsbn.org/aprn.htm; Board Certified Behavior Analysts (BCBA). (2022). Behavior Analyst Certification Board. https://www.bacb.com/bcba/; Board of Nursing Professional Licensure Requirements. (2022). NCSBN. https://www.ncsbn.org/nursing-regulation/education/board-of-nursing-professional-licensure-requirements.page; Chiropractic: In Depth. (2022). NCCIH. https://www.nccih.nih.gov/health/chiropractic-in-depth; Obtain Certification. (2021). NATA. https://www.nata.org/about/athletic-training/obtain-certification; Orthotist & Prosthetist—Eligibility. (2022). Abcop.Org. https://www.abcop.org/individual-certification/get-certified/exam-dates-deadlines/orthotist-prosthetist; Planning Your Education in Communication Sciences and Disorders. (2022). American Speech-Language-Hearing Association; American Speech-Language-Hearing Association. https://www.asha.org/students/planning-your-education-in-csd/; Training Requirements for Family Physicians. (2022). https://www.aafp.org/students-residents/medical-students/explore-career-in-family-medicine/training-requirements.html; Why Choose a Board-Certified Acupuncturist? NCCAOM. (2022). https://www.nccaom.org/about-us/why-choose-national-board-certified-practitioner/

are beginning to take on primary care roles and gaining privileges to order imaging (Boissonnault & VanWye, 2021; Keil et al., 2021). Thus, therapists must consider how these emerging roles may impact other professionals.

Overall, collaborative practice is important for client satisfaction and optimizing health services. Providers should learn more about their colleagues to improve their understanding of what that individual brings to each setting professionally and utilize their strengths to improve patient care. In addition, collaborative care improves health outcomes and client satisfaction, optimizes health services, and strengthens health systems (WHO, 2010).

Discussion and Activities

- Refer to Table 4.3 for the following questions:
  - Why do you think these issues exist?
  - What issues might arise from the expansion of a profession's practice act?
  - How might traditional primary care providers perceive physical and occupational therapists advertising themselves as primary care providers?
- What are some potential positives and negatives to physical and occupational therapists ordering imaging?
- How could OTs and PTs collaborate with other professionals to address these potential issues?
- What potential issues might there be between OTs and PTs?

References

Accreditation Council for Occupational Therapy Education. (2018). 2018 *Accreditation council for occupational therapy education (acote) standards and interpretive guide.* https://acoteonline.org/accreditation-explained/standards/.

Agency for Healthcare Research and Quality (AHRQ). (2019). *Health literacy measurement tools (revised).* https://www.ahrq.gov/health-literacy/research/tools/index.html.

Agency for Healthcare Research and Quality (AHRQ). (2020). *The patient education materials assessment tool (pemat) and user's guide.* https://www.ahrq.gov/health-literacy/patient-education/pemat.html#:~:text=The%20Patient%20Education%20Materials%20Assessment%20Tool%20(PEMAT)%20is%20a%20systematic,understand%20and%20act%20on%20information.

Albiol-Pérez, S., Gil-Gómez, J. A., Muñoz-Tomás, M. T., Gil-Gómez, H., Vial-Escolano, R., & Lozano-Quilis, J. A. (2017). The effect of balance training on postural control in patients with Parkinson's disease using a virtual rehabilitation system. *Methods of Information in Medicine, 56*(2), 138–144.

American Medical Association (AMA). (2017). *8 in 10 doctors have experienced a cyberattack in practice.* https://www.ama-assn.org/practice-management/sustainability/8-10-doctors-have-experienced-cyberattack-practice.

American Medical Association. (2016). *Professionalism in the use of social media.* https://www.ama-assn.org/delivering-care/ethics/professionalism-use-social-media.

American Medical Informatics Association (AMIA). (2022). *Informatics: Research and practice.* American Medical Informatics Association. https://amia.org/about-amia/why-informatics/informatics-research-and-practice.

American Occupational Therapy Association (AOTA). (2016). Assistive technology and occupational performance. *American Journal of Occupational Therapy, 70,* 7012410030.

American Occupational Therapy Association (AOTA). (2017). AOTA's societal statement on health literacy. *American Journal of Occupational Therapy, 71*(Suppl. 2), 7112410065.

American Occupational Therapy Association (AOTA). (2020) Occupational therapy in the promotion of health and well-being. *American Journal of Occupational Therapy, 74,* 7403420010.

American Occupational Therapy Association (AOTA). (2021). *Occupational therapy via telehealth for Medicare beneficiaries support the expanded telehealth access act (H.R. 2168/S. 3193).* https://cqrcengage.com/aota/file/Z6wpbsnLGaG/Expanded-Telehealth-Access-Act-One-Pager.pdf.

American Physical Therapy Association (APTA). (2019, September 2) *Succeeding on Social Media.* https://www.apta.org/social-media/succeeding-on-social-media.

American Physical Therapy Association (APTA). (2019c). *Health literacy.* https://www.apta.org/siteassets/pdfs/policies/health-literacy.pdf.

American Physical Therapy Association (APTA). (2019d). *Physical therapists' role in prevention, wellness, fitness, health promotion, and management of disease and disability.* https://www.apta.org/siteassets/pdfs/policies/pt-role-advocacy.pdf.

American Physical Therapy Association (APTA). (2019e). *Vision statement for the physical therapy profession: Policies and bylaws.* https://www.apta.org/apta-and-you/leadership-and-governance/policies/vision-statement-for-the-physical-therapy-profession.

American Physical Therapy Association (APTA). (2021a). *APTA telehealth certificate course ready to roll.* https://www.apta.org/news.

American Physical Therapy Association (APTA). (2021b). *Expanded telehealth access act of 2021 (H. R. 2168/S. 3193).* https://www.apta.org/advocacy/issues/telehealth/expanded-telehealth-access-act-of-2021.

Arozullah, A. M., Yarnold, P. R., Bennett, C. L., Soltysik, R. C., Wolf, M. S., Ferreira, R. M., Lee, S. Y., Costello, S., Shakir, A., Denwood, C., Bryant, F. B., & Davis, T. (2007). Development and validation of a short-form, rapid estimate of adult literacy in medicine. *Medical Care, 45*(11), 1026–1033.

Attard, E., Musallam, A., Vaas, K., Chaney, T., Fortuna, J. K., & Williams, B. (2021). Health literacy in occupational therapy research: A scoping review. *The Open Journal of Occupational Therapy, 9*(4), 1–18.

Auxier, B., & Anderson, M. (2021, April 7). *Social media use in 2021.* Pew Research Center. https://www.pewresearch.org/internet/2021/04/07/social-media-use-in-2021/.

Balakrishnan, M. P., Herndon, J. B., Zhang, J., Payton, T., Shuster, J., & Carden, D. L. (2017). The Association of Health Literacy with preventable emergency department visits: A cross-sectional study. *Academic emergency medicine. Journal of the Society for Academic Emergency Medicine, 24*(9), 1042–1050.

Boissonnault, W. G., & VanWye, W. R. (Eds.). (2021). *Primary care for the physical therapist: Examination and triage.* Elsevier.

Bostock, S., & Steptoe, A. (2012). Association between low functional health literacy and mortality in older adults: Longitudinal cohort study. *The BMJ, 344,* e1602.

Brega, A. G., Hamer, M. K., Albright, K., Brach, C., Saliba, D., Abbey, D., & Gritz, R. M. (2019). Organizational Health Literacy: Quality Improvement Measures with Expert Consensus. *Health Literacy Research and Practice, 3*(2), e127–e146. https://doi.org/10.3928/24748307-20190503-01.

Cahill, S. (2021). *Research update on telehealth: Client outcomes and satisfaction, occupation-based coaching, and stroke rehabilitation.* https://www.aota.org/publications/ot-practice/ot-practice-issues/2021.

Centers for Disease Control and Prevention (CDC). (2010). *Simply put; A guide for creating easy-to-understand materials.* https://stacks.cdc.gov/view/cdc/11938/.

Centers for Disease Control and Prevention (CDC). (2019). *National action plan to improve health literacy.* https://www.cdc.gov/health-literacy/planact/national.html.

Centers for Disease Control and Prevention (CDC). (2020). *Disability and health inclusion strategies.* https://www.cdc.gov/ncbddd/disabilityandhealth/disability-strategies.html.

Cesnik, B., & Kidd, M. R. (2010). History of health informatics: A global perspective. *Studies in Health Technology and Informatics, 151,* 3–8.

Chen, Y., Kathirithamby, D. R., Candelario-Velazquez, C., Bloomfield, A., & Ambrose, A. F. (2021). Telemedicine in the coronavirus disease 2019 pandemic. *American Journal of Physical Medicine and Rehabilitation, 100*(4), 321–326.

Commission on Accreditation in Physical Therapy Education (CAPTE), (2022). *Standards and Required Elements for Accreditation of Physical Therapist Education Programs.* https://www.capteonline.org/

Cook, A. M., Polgar, J. M., & Encarnac, P. (2020). *Assistive technologies: Principles & practice* (5th ed.). St. Louis, MO: Elsevier/Mosby Inc.

Corbetta, D., Imeri, F., & Gatti, R. (2015). Rehabilitation that incorporates virtual reality is more effective than standard rehabilitation for improving walking speed, balance and mobility after stroke: A systematic review. *Journal of Physiotherapy, 61*(3), 117–124.

Davis, T. C., Crouch, M. A., Long, S. W., Jackson, R. H., Bates, P., George, R. B., & Bairnsfather, L. E. (1991). Rapid assessment of literacy levels of adult primary care patients. *Family Medicine, 23*(6), 433–435.

DiClemente, C. C., & Prochaska, J. O. (1982). Self change and therapy change of smoking behavior: A comparison of processes of change in cessation and maintenance. *Addictive Behavior, 7,* 133–142.

Eysenbach, G. (2000). Consumer health informatics. *The BMJ* (Clinical research ed.), *320*(7251), 1713–1716. https://doi.org/10.1136/bmj.320.7251.1713.

Farmanova, E., Bonneville, L., & Bouchard, L. (2018). Organizational health literacy: Review of theories, frameworks, guides, and implementation issues. *Inquiry, 55,* 46958018757848.

Finney Rutten, L. J., Blake, K. D., Greenberg-Worisek, A. J., Allen, S. V., Moser, R. P., & Hesse, B. W. (2019). Online health information seeking among US adults: Measuring progress toward a healthy people 2020 objective. *Public Health Reports, 134*(6), 617–625.

Giansanti, D. (2020). The rehabilitation and the robotics: Are they going together well? *Healthcare, 9*(1), 26.

Gupta, P., Khan, A., & Kumar, A. (2022). Social media use by patients in health care: A scoping review. *International Journal of Healthcare Management, 15*(2), 121–131. doi: 10.1080/20479700.2020.1860563.

Harvard, T. H. Chan, School of Public Health. (HCSPS). (2022). *Health literacy studies.* https://www.hsph.harvard.edu/healthliteracy/overview-2-2/.

Health Insurance Portability and Accountability Act of 1996 (HIPAA) | CDC. (2019, February 21). Centers for Disease Control and Prevention. https://www.cdc.gov/phlp/publications/topic/hipaa.html.

Health Literacy Tool Shed. (2022). *About the health literacy tool shed.* http://healthliteracy.bu.edu/.

Health Resources & Services Administration. (n.d.). *Plan your telehealth workflow: A tip sheet for making telehealth part of your practice.* https://th-site-downloads.s3.us-east-2.amazonaws.com/Telehealth_Workflow_07-15-2021.pdf.

Health Resources & Services Administration (HRSA). (2019). *Health literacy.* https://www.hrsa.gov/about/organization/bureaus/ohe/health-literacy/index.html.

Hitlin, P. (2018). *Internet, social media use and device ownership in U.S. have plateaued after years of growth.* Pew Research Center. https://www.pewresearch.org/fact-tank/2018/09/28/internet-social-media-use-and-device-ownership-in-u-s-have-plateaued-after-years-of-growth/.

Huang, X., Naghdy, F., Naghdy, G., Du, H., & Todd, C. (2018). The combined effects of adaptive control and virtual reality on robot-assisted fine hand motion rehabilitation in chronic stroke patients: A case study. *Journal of Stroke and Cerebrovascular Diseases: The Official Journal of National Stroke Association, 27*(1), 221–228.

Individuals with Disabilities Education Act (IDEA) of 1990, Pub. L. 101-476, 104 Stat, 1142.

Institute for Healthcare Improvement [IHI]. (2022). *The IHI triple aim.* http://www.ihi.org/Engage/Initiatives/TripleAim/Pages/default.aspx.

Jen, M. Y., Mechanic, O. J., & Teoli, D. (2021). *Informatics.* https://www.ncbi.nlm.nih.gov/books/NBK470564/.

Johnson, J. M., Hermosura, B. J., Price, S. L. & Gougeon, L. (2021). Factors influencing interprofessional team collaboration when delivering care to community-dwelling seniors: A metasynthesis of Canadian interventions. *Journal of Interprofessional Care, 35*(3), 376–382. doi:10.1080/13561820.2020.1758641.

Keil, A. P., Hazle, C., Maurer, A., Kittleson, C., Watson, D., Young, B., Rezac, S., Epsley, S., & Baranyi, B. (2021). Referral for imaging in physical therapist practice: Key recommendations for successful implementation. *Physical Therapy, 101*(3), pzab013.

Kelly, J., Campbell, K., Gong, E., & Scuffham, P. (2020). The internet of things: Impact and implications for health care delivery. *Journal of Medical Internet Research, 22*(11), e20135 https://www.jmir.org/2020/11/e20135.

Koonan, L. M., Hoots, B., Tsang, C. A., Leroy, Z., Farris, K., Jolly, B., Antall, P., McCabe, B., Zelis, C. B. R., Tong, I., & Harris, A. M. (2020). Trends in the use of telehealth during the emergence of the COVID-19 pandemic- United States, January-March 2020. *Morbidity and Mortality Weekly Report, 69*(43), 1595–1599.

Lamargue-Hamel, D., Deloire, M., Saubusse, A., Ruet, A., Taillard, J., Philip, P., & Brochet, B. (2015). Cognitive evaluation by tasks in a virtual reality environment in multiple sclerosis. *Journal of Neurological Science, 359*(1-2), 94–99. doi:10.1016/j.jns.2015.10.039.

Lape, J., Lukose, A., Ritter, D., &; Scaife, B. (2019). Use of the Kawa model to facilitate interprofessional collaboration: A pilot study. *Internet Journal of Allied Health Sciences and Practice. 17*(1), 3.

Lee, S. Y., Stucky, B. D., Lee, J. Y., Rozier, R. G., & Bender, D. E. (2010). Short Assessment of Health Literacy-Spanish and English: A comparable test of health literacy for Spanish and English speakers. *Health Services Research, 45*(4), 1105–1120.

Lew, H. L., Oh-Park, M., & Cifu, D. X. (2020). The war on COVID-19 pandemic: Role of rehabilitation professionals and hospitals. *American Journal of Physical Medicine and Rehabilitation, 99*(7), 571–572.

Little, L. M., Cason, J., Pickett, K. A., & Proffitt, R. (2021). *Keeping PACE with the new normal: A framework for telehealth practice, research, and policy.* http://www.aota.org/publications/ot-pactice-issues/2021.

Liu, H., Zeng, H., Shen, Y., Zhang, F., Sharma, M., Lai, W., Zhao, Y., Tao, G., Yuan, J., & Zhao, Y. (2018). Assessment tools for health literacy among the general population. A systematic review. *International Journal of Environmental Research and Public Health, 15*, 1711–1727.

Lopez, C., Bumyang, K., & Sacks, K. (2022). *Health literacy in the United States: Enhancing Assessments and reducing disparities.* Milken Institute. http://dx.doi.org/10.2139/ssrn.4182046

Malliaras, P., Merolli, M., Williams, C. M., Caneiro, J. P., Haines, T., & Barton, C. (2021). It's not hands-on therapy, so it's very limited: Telehealth use and views among allied health clinicians during the coronavirus pandemic. *Musculoskeletal Science and Practice, 52*, 102340.

McVeigh, K. H., Arnold, S. M., & Banta, C. (2018). *Utilization of lean methodology to improve quality and efficiency of rehabilitation electronic health record documentation.* https://www.semanticscholar.org/paper/Utilization-of-Lean-Methodology-to-Improve-Quality-McVeigh-Arnold/9a9c8e4c3ea52460d74619d75b8ae3c85165a5bc?p2df.

Meloncon, L. K. (2017). Patient experience design: Expanding usability methodologies for healthcare. *Communication Design Quarterly, 5*(2), 19–28. https://doi.org/10.1145/3131201.3131203.

Mercier, H. W., Ni, P., Houlihan, B. V., & Jette, A. M. (2015). Differential impact and use of a telehealth intervention by persons with MS or SCI. *American Journal of Physical Medicine and Rehabilitation, 94*(11), 987–999.

Miller, M. J., Pak, S. S., Keller, D. R., & Barnes, D. E. (2021). Evaluation of pragmatic telehealth physical therapy implementation during the COVID-19 pandemic. *Physical Therapy & Rehabilitation Journal, 101*, 1–10.

Moorhead, S. A., Hazlett, D. E., Harrison, L., Carroll, J. K., Irwin, A., & Hoving, C. (2013). A new dimension of health care: Systematic review of the uses, benefits, and limitations of social media for health communication. *Journal of Medical Internet Research, 15*(4), e85.

Nunnerley, J. L., Gupta, S., Snell, D. L., & King, M. (2017). Training wheelchair navigation in immersive virtual environments for patients with spinal cord injury – end-user input to design an effective system. *Disability and Rehabilitation Assistive Technology, 12*, 417–423.

Ober, J., & Lape, J. (2019). Cultivating acute care rehabilitation team collaboration using the Kawa model. *Internet Journal of Allied Health Sciences and Practice, 17*(3), 9. https://nsuworks.nova.edu/ijahsp/vol17/iss3/9/.

Onal, G., Guney, G., Gun, F., & Huri, M. (2021). Telehealth in paediatric occupational therapy: A scoping review. *International Journal of Therapy and Rehabilitation, 28*(7), 1–16. https://doi.org/10.12968/ijtr.2020.0070.

Owens, J., & Davis, D. (2022). Seating and Wheelchair Evaluation. In: *StatPearls* [Internet]. Treasure Island (FL): StatPearls Publishing. https://www.ncbi.nlm.nih.gov/books/NBK559231/#_NBK559231_pubdet_.

Paasche-Orlow, M. K., Parker, R. M., Gazmararian, J. A., Nielsen-Bohlman, L. T., & Rudd, R. R. (2005). The prevalence of limited health literacy. *Journal of General Internal Medicine, 20*(2), 175–184.

Parker, R. M., Baker, D. W., Williams, M. D., & Nurss, J. R. (1995). The Test of Functional Health Literacy in Adults: A new instrument for measuring patients' literacy skills. *Journal of General Internal Medicine, 10*, 537–541.

Peterson, P. N., Shetterly, S. M., Clarke, C. L., Bekelman, D. B., Chan, P. S., Allen, L. A., Matlock, D. D., Magid, D. J., & Masoudi, F. A. (2011). Health literacy and outcomes among patients with heart failure. *JAMA, 305*(16), 1695–1701.

Powers, B. J., Trinh, J. V., & Bosworth, H. B. (2010). Can this patient read and understand written health information? *JAMA, 304*(1), 76–84.

Prestin, A., Vieux, S. N., & Chou, W. Y. S. (2015). Is online health activity alive and well or flatlining? Findings from 10 years of the health information national trends survey. *Journal of Health Communication, 20*(7), 790–798.

Prochaska, J. O., & DiClemente, C. C. (1982). Transtheoretical therapy: Toward a more integrative model of change. *Psychotherapy Theory Research & Practice, 19*(3), 276–288.

Prochaska, J. O., & DiClemente, C. C. (1983). Stages and processes of self-change of smoking: Toward an integrative model of change. *Journal of Consulting and Clinical Psychology, 51*(3), 390–395.

Prochaska, J. O., & Velicer, W. F. (1997). The transtheoretical model of health behavior change. *American Journal of Health Promotion, 12*(1), 38–48.

Rehabilitation Engineering and Assistive Technology Society of North America. [RESNA]. (2015). https://www.resna.org/.

Rimmer, J. H., Wand, E., Pellegrino, C. A., Lullo, C., & Gerber, B. S. (2013). Telehealth weight management intervention for adults with physical disabilities: A randomized controlled trial. *American Journal of Physical Medicine and Rehabilitation, 92*(12), 1084–1094.

Rudd, R. (2010). *The health literacy environment activity packet: First impressions and walking interview.* https://cdn1.sph.harvard.edu/wp-content/uploads/sites/135/2012/09/activitypacket.pdf.

Samerski, S. (2019). Health literacy as a social practice: Social and empirical dimensions of knowledge on health and healthcare. *Social Science & Medicine, 226*, 1–8.

Scholte, M., van Dulmen, S. A., Neeleman-Van der Steen, C. W., van der Wees, P. J., Nijhuis-van der Sanden, M. W., & Braspenning, J. (2016). Data extraction from electronic health records (EHRs) for quality measurement of the physical therapy process: Comparison between EHR data and survey data. *BMC Medical Informatics and Decision Making, 16*(1), 141.

Sentell, T., Foss-Durant, A., Patil, U., Taira, D., Paasche-Orlow, M. K., & Trinacty, C. M. (2021). Organizational health literacy: Opportunities for patient-centered care in the wake of COVID-19. *Quality Management in Health Care, 30*(1), 49–60.

Smith, B., & Magnani, J. W. (2019). New technologies, new disparities: The intersection of electronic health and digital health literacy. *International Journal of Cardiology, 292*, 280–282.

Stephenson, S., Anderson-Tome, A., Fischer, S., Guzman, A., Meredith, W., & Somers, C. (2019). Pilot study: Using the bioness integrated therapy system (BITS) to examine the correlation between skills and success with on-the-road driving evaluations. *American Journal of Occupational Therapy, 73*(4_Supplement_1), 7311515280p1.

Sutter, E. N., Francis, L. S., Francis, S. M., Lench, D. H., Nemanich, S. T., Krach, L. E., Sukal-Moulton, T., & Gillick, B. T. (2021). Disrupted access to therapies and impact on well-being during the COVID-19 pandemic for children with motor impairment and their caregivers. *American Journal of Physical Medicine and Rehabilitation, 100*(9), 821–830.

Taylor, D. M., Fraser, S., Bradley, J. A., Bradley, C., Draper, H., Metcalfe, W., Oniscu, G. C., Tomson, C., Ravanan, R., Roderick, P. J., & ATTOM investigators. (2017). A systematic review of the prevalence and associations of limited health literacy in CKD. *Clinical Journal of the American Society of Nephrology, 12*(7), 1070–1084.

Technology-Related Assistance for Individuals with Disabilities Act of 1988, Pub. L. 100-407, 100 Stat. 2561.

Tenforde, A. S., Borgstrom, H., Polich, G., Steere, H., Davis, I. S., Cotton, K., O'Donnell, M., & Silver, J. K. (2020). Outpatient physical, occupational, and speech therapy synchronous telemedicine: A survey of patient satisfaction with virtual visits during the COVID 19 pandemic. *American Journal of Physical Medicine and Rehabilitation, 99*(11), 977–981.

Tenforde, A. S., Hefner, J. E., Kodish-Wachs, J., Iaccarino, M. A., & Paganoni, S. (2017). Telehealth in physical medicine and rehabilitation: A narrative review. *Clinical Informatics in Physiatry, 9*(5), S51–S58.

Tuckman, B. W. (1965). Developmental sequence in small groups. *Psychological Bulletin, 63*(6), 384–399. https://psycnet.apa.org/doi/10.1037/h0022100.

US Census Bureau, (2021). *Anniversary of Americans with Disabilities Act: July 26, 2021.* https://www.census.gov/newsroom/facts-for-features/2021/disabilities-act.html

US Department of Health and Human Services (USDHHS). (2021). *Consolidated appropriations and American rescue plan acts of 2021 telehealth updates.* https://telehealth.hhs.gov/providers/policy-changes-during-the-covid-1.

US Department of Health and Human Services (USDHHS). (2022a). *Healthy people 2030.* https://health.gov/our-work/national-health-initiatives/healthy-people/healthy-people-2030.

US Department of Health and Human Services (USDHHS). (2022b). *What is telehealth?* https://telehalth.hhs.gov/patients/understanding-telehalth/#what-does.

US Department of Health and Human Services (USDHHS). (n.d.). *Healthy people 2030.* Office of Disease Prevention and Health Promotion. https://health.gov/healthypeople.

Ventola, C. L. (2014). Social Media and Health Care Professionals: Benefits, risks, and best practices. *Pharmacy and Therapeutics, 39*(7), 491–520.

Walthers, K. M., Zimmer, J. N., & Graves, C. (2020). The utility of smart home technology within OT practice. *American Journal of Occupational Therapy, 75*(Suppl. 2), p.7512505108-7512505108p1.

White, S., Chen, J., & Atchison, R. (2008). Relationship of preventive health practices and health literacy: A national study. *American Journal of Health Behavior, 32*(3), 227–242.

World Health Organization. (2010). *Framework for action on interprofessional education and collaborative practice.* http://www.who.int/hrh/resources/framework_action/en/.

World Health Organization. (2012). *Being an effective team player.* https://www.who.int/publications/m/item/course-04-being-an-effective-team-player.

World Health Organization. (2018). *Assistive Technology.* https://www.who.int/news-room/fact-sheets/detail/assistive-technology.

Wong, B. (2015, July 10). *How to use social media as a professional development tool.* AOTA. https://www.aota.org/publications/student-articles/career-advice/social-media.

Wroten, C., Zapf, S., & Hudgins, E. (2020). Effectiveness of electronic documentation: A case report. *The Open Journal of Occupational Therapy, 8*(3), 1–10.

Zhang, L., Abreu, B. C., Seale, G. S., Masel, B., Christiansen, C. H., & Ottenbacher, K. J. (2003). A virtual reality environment for evaluation of a daily living skill in brain injury rehabilitation: Reliability and validity. *Archives of Physical Medicine and Rehabilitation, 84*(8), 1118–1124.

5

Core Values and Ethical Implications

DAVID L. BELL, PT, DPT, PhD, OCS, MTC, Cert DN; and AMY L. BRZUZ, OTD, OTR/L

LEARNING OBJECTIVES

Upon completion of this chapter, the reader will be able to:

1. Describe core values and explain how they link to an organization's mission and vision.
2. Define ethics-related definitions and historical concepts such as the Hippocratic Oath.
3. Compare and contrast the four main ethical theories that support professional codes of ethics.
4. Apply the American Physical Therapy Association and the American Occupational Therapy Association codes of ethics to real-world ethical dilemmas.
5. Identify resources for continuing competency in the area of core values and ethics.

CHAPTER OUTLINE

Introduction

Healthcare students spend much time learning discipline-specific procedures and skills in their respective programs. These practices are based on evidence and current practice trends. As these students become new practitioners and enter the workforce, they use this procedural-like information to make decisions. This thought process is called procedural reasoning (O'Brien & Hussey, 2018). Sometimes, however, practitioners face problems whose answers cannot be found in the current evidence and usual procedures. Without specific standards, reflection on personal and professional core values and ethics can be helpful. This thought process is called ethical reasoning (O'Brien & Hussey, 2018). This chapter will help improve confidence and competence with ethical reasoning and describe core values and ethics and their implications for interdisciplinary practice.

Core Values, Mission, and Vision

Core values are the fundamental beliefs of a person or organization. In our personal lives, core values are the ideas that

TABLE 5.1	Core Values	
Family	Freedom	Loyalty
Creativity	Respect	Integrity
Love	Kindness	Teamwork
Spiritualism	Wealth	Affection
Patience	Wellness	Grace
Fun	Happiness	Peace

a person can "get behind," feel deeply, and will support in everyday situations. They help guide personal behaviors and decisions. For example, when faced with a difficult decision to help a family member move into a new home on your only day off from work, you may reflect upon your core values of family and loyalty and decide to help. Examples of core values can be found in Table 5.1 (White, 2022).

People reveal their core values by their attitudes, decisions, and actions, and most do this subconsciously. At the organization level, however, core values must be identified so that all members of the organization can share a common purpose. Core values are the fundamental beliefs on which an organization bases its mission and vision statements. These values, coupled with a profession's beliefs, truths, and principles, help guide an organization's education, scholarship, practice, and members (O'Brien & Hussey, 2018).

Most healthcare professions are represented by professional organizations with their own set of core values that guide the actions and behaviors of their members. These core values represent the foundational ideas that all organization members can agree are of utmost importance for the organization to represent. An organization's core values help guide everyone's interactions with others, such as clients, coworkers, family members, students, and the public.

The vision statement of an organization describes what the organization ultimately hopes to achieve. The mission statement defines how it will get there. Neither the vision nor mission statements can exist without core values. An organization's core values form the soil from which vision and mission spring.

For example, the American Medical Association (AMA) represents physicians in the United States. The AMA holds leadership, excellence, integrity, and ethical behavior as its core values (American Medical Association, 2021). These core values are essential components of their vision and mission statements that guide the decision-making of their membership. The AMA's mission and vision statements can be found in Fig. 5.1. There is a clear link between the AMA's core value of "excellence" and their mission element of "betterment of public health." If all AMA members provide excellent healthcare to their clients, this care will facilitate the betterment of public health, which is their mission.

Another example of how core values are applied within a professional healthcare organization can be found in the World Health Organization (WHO). The WHO is an international interdisciplinary public health organization that assists in responding to worldwide health emergencies, promoting wellbeing and disease prevention, and increasing healthcare access (World Health Organization, 2022). The WHO holds integrity, professionalism, and respect for diversity as its core values. These core values inform their vision of a world "in which all peoples attain the highest possible level of health" and their mission to "promote health, keep the world safe and serve the vulnerable, with a measurable impact for people at country level" (World Health Organization, 2022). For example, the link between their core value of respect for diversity, their mission of serving the vulnerable, and their vision of a world where all people attain the highest level of health is clear. If all WHO members demonstrate high respect for diversity, they will be able to serve all clients regardless of their background or socioeconomic status and, thus, help facilitate the WHO vision of serving all people (see Fig. 5.2).

The Interprofessional Education Collaborative (IPEC) is another healthcare organization where the application of core values can be found. The IPEC's purpose is to promote and encourage interprofessional learning to help prepare future healthcare professionals for collaborative practice (Interprofessional Education Collaborative, 2022). Although

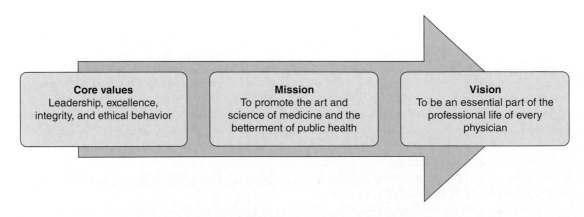

• **Fig. 5.1** American Medical Association core values, mission, and vision.

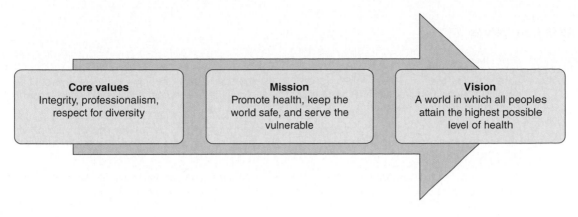

• **Fig. 5.2** World Health Organization core values, mission, and vision.

TABLE 5.2	IPEC Core Competencies for Interprofessional Practice
1. Values/Ethics: Work with individuals of other professions to maintain a climate of mutual respect and shared values.	
2. Roles/Responsibilities: Use the knowledge of one's own role and those of other professions to appropriately assess and address the health care needs of patients and to promote and advance the health of populations.	
3. Interprofessional Communication: Communicate with patients, families, communities, and professionals in health and other fields in a responsive and responsible manner that supports a team approach to the promotion and maintenance of health and the prevention and treatment of disease.	
4. Teams and Teamwork: Apply relationship-building values and the principles of team dynamics to perform effectively in different team roles to plan, deliver, and evaluate patient/population-centered care and population health programs and policies that are safe, timely, efficient, effective, and equitable.	

the IPEC does not explicitly state its organization's core values, these values can be inferred from its mission and vision statements. The IPEC's mission is to "promote, encourage and support efforts to prepare future health professionals so that they enter the workforce ready for interprofessional collaborative practice that helps to ensure the health of individuals and populations" (Interprofessional Education Collaborative, 2022). Their vision is that "interprofessional collaborative practice drives safe, high-quality, accessible, person-centered care and improved population health outcomes" (Interprofessional Education Collaborative, 2022). Upon reviewing the IPEC's mission and vision statements, and their core competencies for interprofessional collaborative practice (Table 5.2), we can deduce that they value respect, advocacy, communication, and teamwork. We can conclude that if all IPEC members share the core value of teamwork, they will be able to help promote the organization's vision of "high-quality collaborative practice" while living out the IPEC's mission element of "preparing future health professionals for interprofessional collaborative practice."

Core Values, Mission, and Vision of the American Physical Therapy Association

The American Physical Therapy Association (APTA) is the primary professional organization for the physical therapy

profession in the United States. Established in 1921, it represents 100,000 member physical therapists, physical therapist assistants, and physical therapy students. The APTA has identified nine core values to guide physical therapist and physical therapist assistant practice (see Table 5.3) (American Physical Therapy Association, 2021).

As seen with other organizations, the APTA's vision statement sets the direction for the profession, while the mission statement sets the direction for the association (American Physical Therapy Association, 2022b):

• Vision Statement for the Physical Therapy Profession: "Transforming society by optimizing movement to improve the human experience."
• Mission Statement for the Association: "Building a community that advances the profession of physical therapy to improve the health of society."

Thus the APTA hopes to advance the profession of physical therapy such that society is transformed through the optimization of human movement (see Fig. 5.3).

Core Values, Mission, and Vision of the American Occupational Therapy Association

The American Occupational Therapy Association (AOTA), founded in 1917, is the primary professional organization for the occupational therapy profession in the United States. Its membership consists of occupational therapists,

TABLE 5.3	APTA Core Values	
Core Value	**Definition**	
Accountability	Active acceptance of the responsibility for the diverse roles, obligations, and actions of the physical therapist and physical therapist assistant including self-regulation and other behaviors that positively influence patient and client outcomes, the profession, and the health needs of society.	
Altruism	The primary regard for or devotion to the interest of patients and clients, thus assuming the responsibility of placing the needs of patients and clients ahead of the physical therapist's or physical therapist assistant's self-interest.	
Collaboration	Working together with patients and clients, families, communities, and professionals in health and other fields to achieve shared goals. Collaboration within the physical therapist-physical therapist assistant team is working together, within each partner's respective role, to achieve optimal physical therapist services and outcomes for patients and clients.	
Compassion and Caring	Compassion is the desire to identify with or sense something of another's experience; a precursor of caring. Caring is the concern, empathy, and consideration for the needs and values of others.	
Duty	The commitment to meeting one's obligations to provide effective physical therapist services to patients and clients, to serve the profession, and to influence the health of society positively.	
Excellence	Excellence in the provision of physical therapist services occurs when the physical therapist and physical therapist assistant consistently use current knowledge and skills while understanding personal limits, integrate the patient or client perspective, embrace advancement, and challenge mediocrity.	
Inclusion	Inclusion occurs when the physical therapist and physical therapist assistant create a welcoming and equitable environment for all. Physical therapists and physical therapist assistants are inclusive when they commit to providing a safe space, elevating diverse and minority voices, acknowledging personal biases that may impact patient care, and taking a position of antidiscrimination.	
Integrity	Steadfast adherence to high ethical principles and professional standards, being truthful, ensuring fairness, following through on commitments, and verbalizing to others the rationale for actions.	
Social Responsibility	The promotion of a mutual trust between the profession and the larger public that necessitates responding to societal needs for health and wellness.	

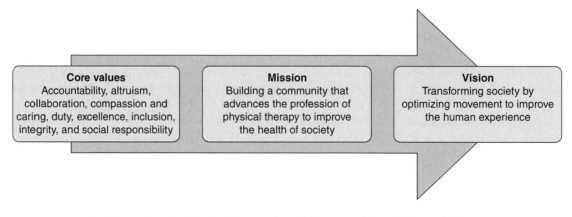

• **Fig. 5.3** American Physical Therapy Association core values, mission, and vision.

occupational therapy assistants, occupational therapy students, and organization members. AOTA represents the concerns of occupational therapy practitioners and students and aims to improve the quality of occupational therapy services for clients (American Occupational Therapy Association, 2022a).

AOTA's mission is "to advance occupational therapy practice, education, and research through standard setting and advocacy on behalf of its members, the profession, and the public" (American Occupational Therapy Association, 2022a). Their vision states, "As an inclusive profession, occupational therapy maximizes health, wellbeing, and quality of life for all people, populations, and communities through effective solutions that facilitate participation in everyday living" (American Occupational Therapy Association, 2022a). The mission and vision statements of AOTA were created partly upon the profession's core concepts and core values. Core concepts of the occupational therapy

TABLE 5.4	AOTA Core Values
Core Value	**Definition**
Altruism	Demonstration of the unselfish concern for the welfare of others.
Equality	All persons have fundamental human rights and the right to the same opportunities.
Freedom	Valuing each person's right to exercise autonomy and demonstrate independence, initiative, and self-direction.
Justice	Occupational therapy personnel should provide occupational therapy services for all persons in need of these services and maintain a goal-directed and objective relationship with recipients of service.
Dignity	The importance of valuing, promoting, and preserving the inherent worth and uniqueness of each person.
Truth	Occupational therapy personnel in all situations should be faithful to facts and reality.
Prudence	The ability to govern and discipline oneself through the use of reason.

profession are specific to occupational therapy and include holism, occupation as means and end, and client-centeredness (O'Brien & Hussey, 2018). AOTA's core values are broader concepts that the occupational therapy profession might share with other professions. AOTA's core values help guide practitioners' interactions with others. These core values are found in AOTA's Code of Ethics document and are listed in Table 5.4 (American Occupational Therapy Association, 2020).

While there are many links between AOTA's core values and its mission and vision, we can see a clear link between AOTA's core values of equality and justice and its vision statement elements of "maximizing health for all people, populations, and communities." There is also a link between the core value of altruism and the mission element of public advocacy. See Figs. 5.4 and 5.5 for visual depictions of how AOTA's core values inform its mission and vision.

Ethics

Core values drive mission and vision and provide a foundation for ethical decision-making. Therefore, identifying core values is only the first step in ethical decision-making. Ethics/ethical theories tell us how to apply the values we hold dear. Core values tell us "what" we value; ethics tell us "how" we value them. Thus understanding ethics-related definitions and historical concepts are beneficial.

Morality

Morality is the concept of right and wrong. All people and all societies have ideas about what constitutes right behavior and wrong behavior, although those social mores may vary widely according to culture and time. Objective morality refers to an external standard of behavior applicable to everyone. Laws that govern a society provide an objective reference for behavior (crime and punishment) that all citizens are obligated to follow. Various religions and theocracies

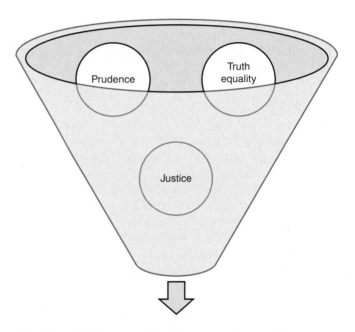

• **Fig. 5.4** Link between American Occupational Therapy Association's mission and core values.

may look to a deity to provide them with an objective standard of morality, as is given in the Ten Commandments (Gabard & Martin, 2011). Subjective morality, also known as moral relativism, looks to an internal standard of right and wrong. In other words, the individuals themselves determine what is right and wrong according to their moral compass (Rae, 1995).

Not surprisingly, many people operate with objective and subjective moral standards, often granting themselves the freedom to determine right and wrong for themselves but expecting others to conform to an objective standard; for example, Rebecca claims to be a moral relativist until someone steals her phone. When someone objects to our behavior, we often say, "It's a free country." However, when we object to others' behavior, we often say, "There ought to be a law..."

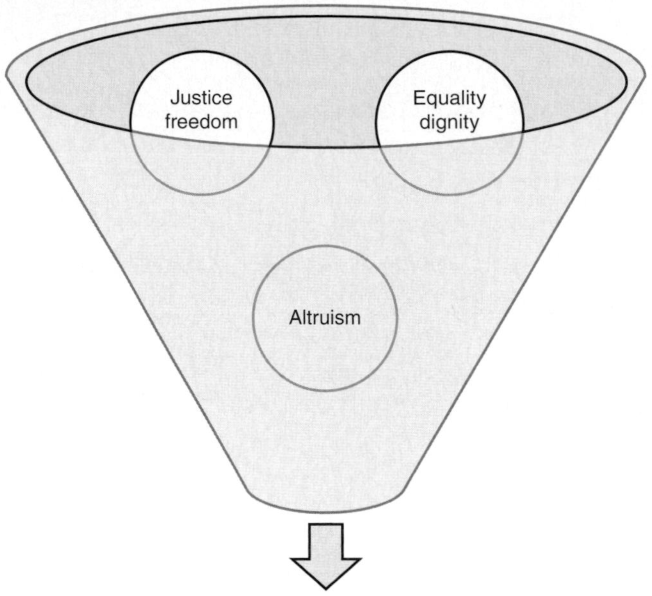

• **Fig. 5.5** Link between American Occupational Therapy Association's vision and core values.

Ethics

Ethics is applied morality. It applies moral principles to govern behavior or conduct an activity. Within healthcare professions, a code of professional ethics is a formal code that reflects ethical principles applied to issues arising in each healthcare setting. Most professions have a written code of ethics developed by professional organizations (Gabard & Martin, 2011). The code of ethics of the APTA and AOTA are discussed later in this chapter. Perhaps the oldest known example of a medical code of ethics is found in the Hippocratic Oath.

Hippocratic Oath (400 BCE)

Medical ethics traces its roots at least as far back as Hippocrates, known as the "Father of Medicine." While the original Hippocratic Oath has been modified several times to align better with current times, the spirit of the oath remains relevant in modern healthcare (Fig. 5.6). Its timeless message of ethical morals and principles still informs ethical theories and healthcare professions' codes of ethics. Several principles may be derived from his original oath, which is still applicable to contemporary healthcare:

- Do not cause any harm to the patient.
- Do only those things that are designed to benefit the patient.
- Use your best judgment and abilities.
- Live an exemplary professional and personal life.
- Teach others to do the same.

Do Not Cause Any Harm to the Patient

This idea reflects the principle of nonmaleficence (Beauchamp & Childress, 2019). The Latin root *mal* means "bad" or "evil." We see this root in words such as "malice," "malfunction," and

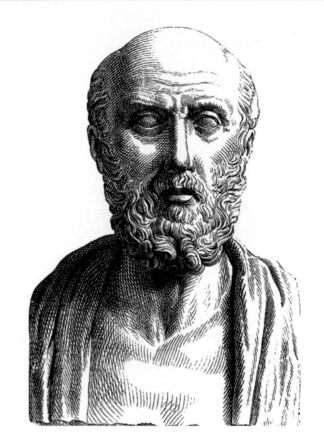

• **Fig. 5.6** Nonmaleficence and beneficence are two principles of the Hippocratic Oath that remain relevant today. https://en.wikipedia.org/wiki/Hippocratic_Oath

"malpractice." What constitutes "harm" in the clinical setting? Most obviously, healthcare providers must not render procedures designed to harm the patient or make the patient worse. However, other types of harm must be considered: subjecting them to unnecessary pain or discomfort, wasting their time or causing them unnecessary inconvenience, charging them for unnecessary expenses, or committing fraud.

Harm can also come to our patients through negligence or omission. Failure to recognize "red flags" and make the proper referral to other practitioners could lead to unnecessary or critical medical care delays. A "red flag" indicates the patient's medical history, signs, or symptoms may warrant a medical referral. Similarly, a failure to render proper care, through either ignorance or incompetence, within our scope of practice could potentially harm patients by delaying their recovery.

Do Only Those Things That Are Designed to Benefit the Patient

This idea reflects the principle of beneficence – to act in the best interests of and improve our patients' welfare (Beauchamp & Childress, 2019). It comes from the Latin *beneficentia,* which means "to do good" or "to do well." This can be seen as a root in words such as "benefit" and "bene-factor." The principle of beneficence means that healthcare providers will act in the patient's best interests and are morally obligated to help the patient to the best of their ability.

Use Your Best Judgment and Abilities

This idea is well-reflected in clinical reasoning, i.e., applying the science and art of healthcare. Clinical reasoning is the decision-making process by which clinicians determine the best course of action for the individual patient. It applies the science of the provider's particular field within the context of the provider's experiences and clinical skills. Students first learn to practice clinical reasoning under the watchful eyes of experienced clinical instructors. Then, as licensed clinicians, they are ethically obligated to remain lifelong learners by staying up-to-date on advancements regarding best practices and seeking opportunities to expand their clinical skills through continuing education (Swisher & Page, 2005). It is unethical for clinicians to remain stagnant while their profession advances.

Live an Exemplary Professional and Personal Life

Healthcare professionals have a fiduciary duty to their patients. "Fiduciary" is derived from the Latin *fide*, which means "faith" or "trust." *Fide* is seen as a root in words such as "fidelity" (faithfulness) or "bona fide" (in good trust or the genuine article). A licensed professional is someone who is held in the public trust. Healthcare providers should seek to be people of good reputation, above reproach both personally and professionally. To paraphrase Proverbs 22:1, "a good reputation is more valuable than gold." Providers should be of such high moral character that no one would suspect wrongdoing and no one will believe it if we are accused. Our professional "core values" (discussed elsewhere in this chapter) act as a guide to exemplary conduct that brings honor to our profession and serves our patients' best interests.

Teach Others to Do the Same

If we have lived up to these ethical principles, we owe it to our profession and society to pass on our knowledge, skill, and ethical standards to our contemporaries and the next generation of professionals. We can all set an example to our fellow students and coworkers. As students, our professors and clinical instructors make the necessary sacrifices to pass on these professional ethics to us. As licensed clinicians, we will pay it forward by passing the baton to the next generation.

Ethical Theories

Before we discuss the professional codes of ethics of the APTA and AOTA, we need a foundational understanding of various ethical theories that lead to such codes. Additionally, our coworkers and patients operate according to these various theories or some combination of them, even though the individuals may be unaware of them. Even though most people may not be aware of (or able to articulate or defend) their ethical beliefs, if we can recognize the theories upon which they make decisions, we can better understand their positions and arrive at solutions to ethical dilemmas. To that end, we will consider four major ethical theories: consequentialism, deontology, virtue ethics, and principlism (Fig. 5.7).

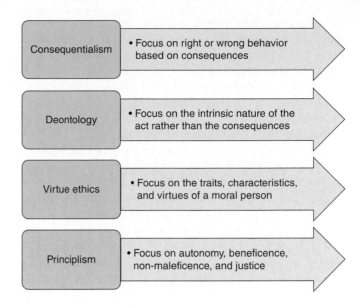

• **Fig. 5.7** Ethical theories.

Consequentialism

Consequentialism determines right and wrong behavior based on outcomes, or predicted outcomes, of the behavior (Beauchamp & Childress, 2019; Rae, 1995). It is also called consequence-oriented theory or teleology (Greek *telos*: end, purpose, or goal). In this case, the ends justify the means. When faced with an ethical dilemma, the behavior itself, lying, for example, may be considered immoral when viewed in isolation. When viewed within the context of the dilemma, however, an ordinarily immoral behavior may be considered moral or justifiable if the outcome of the behavior produces a good or moral result. The classic example is lying to the Gestapo to protect Jews hiding in the attic. A problem with consequentialism is our inability to predict the outcomes of our behaviors with certainty. Unintended consequences could compound the error of already questionable behavior.

A particularly problematic form of consequentialism is utilitarianism. In utilitarianism, decisions are made according to the "greater good," or what is intended to produce the most good for the most people (Beauchamp & Childress, 2019; Gabard & Martin, 2011). In this case, the human rights of minorities or individual liberties may be violated "for the greater good." In Nazi Germany, authorities used a utilitarian argument to justify executing Jews, other ethnic minorities, the mentally disabled, and homosexuals in concentration camps. However, utilitarian arguments are used not only to justify such horrific atrocities but also to justify the violation of human freedoms on a much smaller scale. Every time a government or authority violates someone's freedom, it is always according to a "greater good" or "common good" argument, whether the action is mass genocide or compulsive vaccination.

Deontology

In deontology, the rightness or wrongness of an act is based on the intrinsic nature of the act rather than on its consequences (Rae, 1995). It is also called duty-oriented theory (Greek *deon*: obligation, or duty). Following established rules, living up to obligations, and performing duty are all signs of ethical behavior (Gabard & Martin, 2011). The appeal of deontology is the equitable treatment of individuals. The American criminal justice system is based on this concept with "equal protection of the laws" enshrined in the Constitution's 14th Amendment and the motto, "justice is blind." It is symbolized by the statue of Lady Justice, who is blindfolded, holding the sword of justice in one hand and the balance scales of justice in the other. Legislators and policymakers must then work to define moral actions that address ethical issues.

Students in occupational and physical therapy programs will recognize deontology at work in their student handbooks, where policies and procedures are outlined. Those policies and procedures define proper (moral) student conduct and the consequences of failure to meet those standards. The obvious benefit to students is that they are treated equitably when the policies are followed. Faculty do not favor one student in an ethical situation but disfavor another student in that same situation. By predicting and addressing ethical issues *before ethical dilemmas arise*, deontology avoids the clouded judgment and impact of emotions that may arise during the heat of an ethical dilemma.

One disadvantage of deontology is our inability to predict all the issues and nuances that may arise. We may face an ethical dilemma for which no policy exists or for which the policy is unclear. Consequently, we must look to other theories to arrive at a moral decision. It is a common joke among faculty that every policy has a student's name on it. Such policies are often written *after* an ethical decision has been reached to guide similar situations in the future. Another disadvantage is that this theory may not allow the "authority" to consider all the various factors that may have been at play in violating the law or policy. In this case, the person may be technically guilty of violating the policy but have a very good reason for doing so, which was not envisioned when the policy was generated. According to a strict application of deontology, the authority may not have the freedom to consider the reasoning behind the perpetrator's violation of policy. Thus the human element may be excluded if we operate according to strict deontology.

Virtue Ethics

Virtue ethics focuses on the person making the decision rather than on the decision itself (Rae, 1995). This theory emphasizes the traits, characteristics, and virtue that a moral person should have (Gabard & Martin, 2011). It trusts that someone with these virtues, wisdom, and experience will make the right decision. Healthcare providers should be aware that many patients hold to this theory when trusting a provider with their care. We recognize that patients possess the power of informed consent regarding decisions that affect their health. However, many patients lack the medical foundation to make fully informed decisions; therefore, they trust their providers to make those decisions on their behalf. They may express such trust as, "What do you think I should do, Doc?" or "Do whatever you think is best." This level of trust is a direct expression of the fiduciary role that licensed providers hold in society. As healthcare professionals, we must not violate that trust and must work to ensure that our patients have adequate information to partner with us in making those decisions.

Virtue ethics may be a valid and effective means of determining the right course of action in an ethical dilemma if the person entrusted with making ethical decisions is truly virtuous. However, not even the most virtuous person is all-knowing. No one person or group has comprehensive knowledge of all the circumstances and possible outcomes involved in every situation. Patients may err in placing blind trust in a physician or other healthcare provider under the false assumption that the provider has the knowledge and skills to render the best care possible. Additionally, trust can be wrongly placed. Although thankfully rare, there are healthcare providers who do not operate according to their patient's best interests. More commonly, however, patients may trust providers who have good motives but are nonetheless incompetent. Physical and occupational therapists who work in an area long enough will often develop a good knowledge of the best—and worst—providers in the area. For example, we may feel sorry for patients who ignorantly place their trust in the hands of the worst surgeon in the area and consequently receive substandard care and poor outcomes compared with more skilled surgeons. Similarly, certain physical and occupational therapists may offer substandard care and produce poorer outcomes than skilled therapists. See Box 5.1 for practice in identifying and applying these theories.

Principlism

Principlism is a contemporary model to guide healthcare ethics (Beauchamp & Childress, 2019). It rests on four principles: autonomy, beneficence, nonmaleficence, and justice.

• BOX 5.1 Ethics in Practice

Ethics in Practice

The hospital Board of Directors is discussing a difficult situation in which a physical therapist (PT) has broken hospital policy but had good intentions in doing so. Jessica argues that the PT has violated the policy and should be held accountable; otherwise, there is no reason for having a policy. Travis argues that holding the PT accountable in this circumstance would lead to a bad result; after all, the PT had good intentions behind their actions. Elizabeth knows the PT personally and believes that they are a good person and can be trusted to do the right thing in this situation.

Imagine you are on the Board of Directors. What ethical theory guides your decision-making process in such circumstances? Identify the ethical theories that guide Jessica, Travis, and Elizabeth. What are the advantages and disadvantages of each of those ethical theories in this scenario? How could understanding your own ethical decision-making process as well as those of others help you navigate such situations?

Autonomy

Autonomy (Greek *auto–*: self; *nomos*: ruled or governed) is the capacity to think, decide, and act freely and independently (Beauchamp & Childress, 2019). In the healthcare setting, it refers to a patient's right to make their own decisions regarding their care (Swisher & Page, 2005). It is closely tied to the requirement for informed consent (Gabard & Martin, 2011). Does the patient understand the condition being treated, the intervention's risks and benefits, and the consequences of the decision? Healthcare providers are obligated to fill in such gaps in the patient's knowledge to the best of their ability.

Is the patient free from coercion? Family and employers are often coercive influences on the patients seen by occupational and physical therapists. Well-intentioned but overzealous family members may push patients into receiving unwanted services or achieving goals not set by the patients themselves. Employers may often be a coercive force in terms of financial or occupational impacts if the patient does not meet goals or expectations set by the employer.

Therapists must also avoid the temptation to coerce patients or make them believe they will damage the therapeutic relationship if they do not agree to our proposed plan of care (Gabard & Martin, 2011). Respect for patient autonomy demands that we partner with our patients to develop an agreeable plan of care that is consistent with our knowledge and experience and reflects the patient's own goals, values, and preferences.

Beneficence and Nonmaleficence

As healthcare providers, we are morally obligated to act in our patients' best interests, do them as much good as possible, and refrain from harming them. These principles were discussed earlier under the Hippocratic Oath.

Justice

There are three forms of justice considered in principlism. They are not mutually exclusive and are regularly overlapping. All three forms of justice may be identified in any discussion of ethics and are well-represented in professional codes of ethics such as those developed by the APTA and AOTA.

- *Procedural justice*: obeying the relevant laws. Physical and occupational therapists are legally obligated to follow their state practice act. The practice act is often composed of laws passed by the state legislature and regulations written by the state board.
- *Rights-based justice*: respect for human rights. At a minimum, healthcare providers must respect and not violate basic human rights. Advocates of rights-based justice often advocate for healthcare policies and programs designed to provide all individuals with the highest quality care and outcomes that can be achieved.
- *Distributive justice*: concerned with issues of fairness, equity, and equality (Beauchamp & Childress, 2019). Healthcare providers are obligated to provide fair and equitable treatment to all patients regardless of age, gender, race, or religion (among others) (Papanikitas, 2015; Wilkinson et al., 2020). Advocates of distributive justice look for solutions to address disparities in healthcare provision and outcomes experienced by minorities and underrepresented populations.

Additional Principles Applied in Healthcare

The ethical theories and principles covered thus far are by no means exhaustive. Any text on ethics in general or healthcare ethics, in particular, will include more principles and a more nuanced discussion of those principles than is provided here. However, at least three more principles should be considered: confidentiality, veracity, and role fidelity. Confidentiality and veracity are cornerstones of healthcare ethics (Beauchamp & Childress, 2019). Role fidelity is included as a special consideration for nonphysician providers.

Confidentiality

Healthcare providers must follow strict measures to protect the privacy of their patients (Beauchamp & Childress, 2019). The Health Insurance Portability and Accountability Act (HIPAA) outlines such measures at the federal level. HIPAA is discussed in detail in Chapters 2 and 9. Healthcare organizations often have additional policies designed to guarantee patient confidentiality. When treating friends and relatives, occupational and physical therapists must be mindful of confidentiality.

Veracity

Veracity means to tell the truth. (Latin *veritas*: truth. This root is in words such as "verified" and "verdict.") It seems obvious that veracity is inseparable from the fiduciary responsibility of healthcare professionals (Beauchamp & Childress, 2019). How can we be trustworthy if we are not truthful? However, this principle may occasionally pose dilemmas in healthcare: What if telling the truth is not in the patient's best interests? We may use the *placebo* as an example of this dilemma. Healthcare providers may try to navigate this conundrum by distinguishing between stating falsehoods versus withholding certain information that may harm the patient or inhibit recovery – a "benevolent deception" (Beauchamp & Childress, 2019). A physician may offer a placebo to a patient stating, "This pill may help you" (a truthful statement) while withholding the fact that the pill is composed of sugar and has no medicinal value.

Role Fidelity

This principle requires healthcare providers to be faithful to our scope of practice, i.e., we must not make decisions or perform interventions outside our scope of practice. For example, physical and occupational therapists must not attempt to make medical diagnoses on our patients. We are obligated to screen our patients for referral to medical providers, but we must avoid the temptation to make medical diagnoses ourselves or suggest such diagnoses to medical providers. For example, we must avoid the temptation to offer pharmacological advice to our patients if such advice falls outside our scope of practice. State legislatures and state boards of physical and occupational therapy define the scope of practice within the practice acts regulating those professions.

Role fidelity also requires that we not misrepresent ourselves to our patients. This principle is particularly important for physical and occupational therapists with a clinical or academic doctorate. While we may rightly introduce ourselves as doctors, we must be careful not to mislead our patients into believing that we are physicians. A proper introduction might be, "I am Dr. Jane Smith. I am a physical therapist." However, consider a case involving a clinician with a Ph.D. in their field. This clinician regularly misrepresented themselves to their patients, introducing themselves as a doctor without clarifying their role. They parked in the physician lot and used the physician lounge. They wrote in the physician section of paper charts rather than the therapy section and ordered tests and procedures outside their authority. The hospital quietly tolerated and accommodated this behavior for many years until a patient's family discovered the deception and filed a complaint. The hospital paid the consequences and the clinician lost all of their hospital privileges (Fig. 5.8).

Professional Codes of Ethics

Ethical theories and principles can be considered moral guidelines that govern behavior. These principles help inform us about what is *good* and *right* and help us answer the question, "How should we live?" (Papanikitas, 2015) or in health professions, "How should we act in this difficult situation?" The core values and ethical principles are used as a basis for professional codes of ethics. The American Physical Therapy Association and the American Occupational Therapy Association have created codes of ethics to guide their professions.

APTA Code of Ethics

The Preamble for the Code of Ethics for the Physical Therapist (see Table 5.5) states,

"The Code of Ethics for the Physical Therapist (Code of Ethics) delineates the ethical obligations of all physical therapists as determined by the House of Delegates of the American Physical

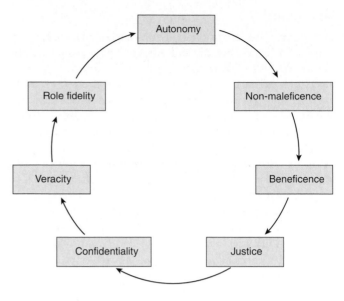

• **Fig. 5.8** Ethical principles in healthcare—could you define each and provide an example?

Therapy Association (APTA). The purposes of this Code of Ethics are to:

1. *Define the ethical principles that form the foundation of physical therapist practice in patient/client management, consultation, education, research, and administration.*
2. *Provide standards of behavior and performance that form the basis of professional accountability to the public.*
3. *Provide guidance for physical therapists facing ethical challenges, regardless of their professional roles and responsibilities.*
4. *Educate physical therapists, students, other health care professionals, regulators, and the public regarding the core values, ethical principles, and standards that guide the professional conduct of the physical therapist.*

TABLE 5.5	Code of Ethics for the Physical Therapist	
	Principles	**Core Values**
	1: Physical therapists shall respect the inherent dignity and rights of all individuals.	Compassion, integrity
	2: Physical therapists shall be trustworthy and compassionate in addressing the rights and needs of patients/clients.	Altruism, compassion, professional duty
	3: Physical therapists shall be accountable for making sound professional judgments.	Excellence, integrity
	4: Physical therapists shall demonstrate integrity in their relationships with patients/clients, families, colleagues, students, research participants, other health care providers, employers, payers, and the public.	Integrity
	5: Physical therapists shall fulfill their legal and professional obligations.	Professional duty, accountability
	6: Physical therapists shall enhance their expertise through the lifelong acquisition and refinement of knowledge, skills, abilities, and professional behaviors.	Excellence
	7: Physical therapists shall promote organizational behaviors and business practices that benefit patients/clients and society.	Integrity, accountability
	8: Physical therapists shall participate in efforts to meet the health needs of people locally, nationally, or globally.	Social responsibility

5. *Establish the standards by which the American Physical Therapy Association can determine if a physical therapist has engaged in unethical conduct.*

No code of ethics is exhaustive, nor can it address every situation. Physical therapists are encouraged to seek additional advice or consultation in instances where the guidance of the Code of Ethics may not be definitive. This Code of Ethics is built upon the five roles of the physical therapist (management of patients/clients, consultation, education, research, and administration), the core values of the profession, and the multiple realms of ethical action (individual, organizational, and societal).

Seven core values guide physical therapist practice: accountability, altruism, compassion/caring, excellence, integrity, professional duty, and social responsibility. The primary core values supporting specific principles are indicated throughout the document in parentheses. Unless a specific role is indicated in principle, the duties and obligations being delineated pertain to the five roles of the physical therapist. Fundamental to the Code of Ethics is the special obligation of physical therapists to empower, educate, and enable those with impairments, activity limitations, participation restrictions, and disabilities to facilitate greater independence, health, wellness, and enhanced quality of life" (AMERICAN PHYSICAL THERAPY ASSOCIATION, 2020).

All eight principles are illustrated with actionable steps that physical therapists may take to apply the principles and core values in real-world situations. For example, Principle 8 has four actionable steps, one of which is 8A: "Physical therapists shall provide pro bono physical therapist services or support organizations that meet the health needs of people who are economically disadvantaged, uninsured, and underinsured."

The Ethics and Judicial Committee of the APTA has also developed a Guide for Professional Conduct. The Guide is closely related to the Core Values and Code of Ethics. The Guide lists topics and specific guidance on ethical dilemmas common in physical therapist practice. Those topics and their related principles are listed in Table 5.6.

TABLE 5.6 APTA Guide for Professional Conduct

Topic	Principles
Respect	Physical therapists shall act in a respectful manner toward each person regardless of age, gender, race, nationality, religion, ethnicity, social or economic status, sexual orientation, health condition, or disability.
Altruism	Physical therapists shall adhere to the core values of the profession and shall act in the best interests of patients/clients over the interests of the physical therapist.
Patient Autonomy	Physical therapists shall provide the information necessary to allow patients or their surrogates to make informed decisions about physical therapy care or participation in clinical research.
Professional Judgment	Physical therapists shall be accountable for making sound professional judgments. Physical therapists shall demonstrate independent and objective professional judgment in the patient's/client's best interest in all practice settings. Physical therapists shall demonstrate professional judgment informed by professional standards, evidence (including current literature and established best practice), practitioner experience, and patient/client values.
Supervision	Physical therapists shall provide appropriate direction of and communication with physical therapist assistants and support personnel.
Integrity in Relationships	Physical therapists shall demonstrate integrity in their relationships with patients/clients, families, colleagues, students, research participants, other health care providers, employers, payers, and the public.
Reporting	Physical therapists shall discourage misconduct by healthcare professionals and report illegal or unethical acts to the relevant authority, when appropriate.
Exploitation	Physical therapists shall not exploit persons over whom they have supervisory, evaluative or other authority (e.g., patients/clients, students, supervisees, research participants, or employees). Physical therapists shall not engage in any sexual relationship with any of their patients/clients, supervisees, or students.
Colleague Impairment	Physical therapists shall encourage colleagues with physical, psychological, or substance-related impairments that may adversely impact their professional responsibilities to seek assistance or counsel. Physical therapists who have knowledge that a colleague is unable to perform their professional responsibilities with reasonable skill and safety shall report the information to the appropriate authority.
Professional Competence	Physical therapists shall achieve and maintain professional competence.
Professional Growth	Physical therapists shall cultivate practice environments that support professional development, life-long learning, and excellence.
Charges and Coding	Physical therapists shall be aware of charges and shall ensure that documentation and coding for physical therapy services accurately reflect the nature and extent of the services provided.
Pro Bono Services	Physical therapists shall provide pro bono physical therapy services or support organizations that meet the health needs of people who are economically disadvantaged, uninsured, and underinsured.

Due to length constraints, the reader is encouraged to consult the full text of the Guide for those specific examples of guidance (American Physical Therapy Association, 2019b). A Guide for Ethical Conduct for the Physical Therapist Assistant is also available (American Physical Therapy Association, 2019a).

AOTA Code of Ethics

The American Occupational Therapy Association has created a Code of Ethics document that "sets forth Core Values and outlines Standards of Conduct the public can expect from those in the profession" (American Occupational Therapy Association, 2020). The document, first published in 1975, is updated regularly and has a dual purpose: first, to describe the Core Values of the profession that guide decision-making; and second, to delineate ethical principles and enforceable standards of conduct (American Occupational Therapy Association, 2020). The Code of Ethics provides guidance in unclear situations in the clinic, in the classroom, or when engaging in research. It is to be utilized by practitioners and students.

The AOTA Code of Ethics document begins with defining the profession's core values, described previously in this chapter. The core values are altruism, equality, freedom, justice, truth, and prudence. Then, the document continues with an explanation of the profession's ethical principles. These ethical principles that guide practitioners' decision-making were chosen with the profession's core values in mind and included beneficence, nonmaleficence, autonomy, justice, veracity, and fidelity. These principles are described in Table 5.7.

The answer can sometimes be unclear when using these core values and ethical principles to guide decision-making. Therefore, AOTA has created a third section of the code. This section is the Standards of Conduct section that provides concrete professional behavior examples of how the core values and ethical principles can be applied to actual occupational therapy situations in various contexts. The Standards of Conduct are enforceable by the AOTA Ethics Commission. There are seven sections of Standards of Conduct:

1. Professional Integrity, Responsibility, and Accountability
2. Therapeutic Relationships
3. Documentation, Reimbursement, and Financial Matters
4. Service Delivery
5. Professional Competence, Education, Supervision, and Training
6. Communication
7. Professional Civility

It is recommended that occupational therapy students and practitioners become familiar with the entire Code of Ethics document. The Code of Ethics is reviewed and updated every five years (American Occupational Therapy Association, 2020). It can be found on the AOTA website, and all versions are published in the *American Journal of Occupational Therapy*.

Ethical Dilemmas

A dilemma is a situation in which you have to make a difficult choice. Perhaps your choice involves your plan of care for a client. For example, the client wants to continue treatment even though progress has plateaued despite all your efforts. Do you choose to keep the client on your caseload

TABLE 5.7	AOTA Ethical Principles	
Principle	**Definition**	**Example**
Beneficence	Occupational therapy personnel shall demonstrate a concern for the wellbeing and safety of persons	Providing a client with access to a call bell when leaving their hospital room.
Nonmaleficence	Occupational therapy personnel shall refrain from actions that cause harm	Not using a physical agent modality on a client where it is contraindicated (e.g., using paraffin on a client with an open wound).
Autonomy	Occupational therapy personnel shall respect the right of the person to self-determination, privacy, confidentiality, and consent	Not forcing a client to participate in a therapy session when they have refused due to not feeling well.
Justice	Occupational therapy personnel shall promote equity, inclusion, and objectivity in the provision of occupational therapy services	Referring your client to a pro bono clinic for continued services when their insurance runs out and they cannot pay out-of-pocket for your services.
Veracity	Occupational therapy personnel shall provide comprehensive, accurate, and objective information when representing the profession	Ensuring your consulting business advertising is accurate and truthful regarding the services you offer and the specializations you hold.
Fidelity	Occupational therapy personnel shall treat clients (persons, groups, or populations), colleagues, and other professionals with respect, fairness, discretion, and integrity	Do not speak poorly of your coworkers when talking with your client.

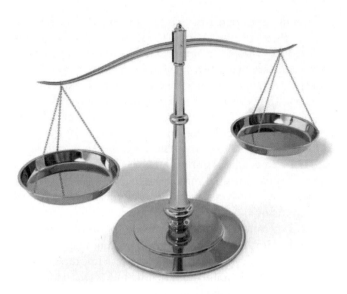

• **Fig. 5.9** Ethical dilemmas often involve weighing competing values. https://www.flickr.com/photos/86530412@N02/7953227784

or discharge them? That is your dilemma. Maybe you must choose whether to report an ethical violation you witnessed in your work or school environment. For example, perhaps you observed a colleague arrive at work intoxicated or you witnessed a colleague billing for a service not provided. Do you choose to ignore these behaviors hoping they were each a one-time lapse in judgment by your colleague? Do you address this directly with the colleague, or do you report your colleague to someone with authority to investigate further? The difficult choice you must make is an ethical dilemma. When we face these dilemmas, we can reflect on our values and the values and ethics of our profession to guide our decision-making (Fig. 5.9).

The process we go through when addressing ethical dilemmas regarding our decision-making differs from addressing ethical concerns we witness in others. This section of the chapter will focus on what to do if you witness an ethical concern in your setting (e.g., school, practice setting). First, when we become aware of a potential ethical violation by others, we must decide whether to do anything. This determination will likely be made, at least in part, by our ethical compass. The consequentialist may weigh the risks, benefits, and potential outcomes of a response. The virtue ethicist may carefully consider the character of the person who committed the potential violation before deciding if/how to proceed, whereas the deontologist may feel compelled to respond in any case. Second, we must decide whether to respond alone or involve a third party.

A crucial component of that decision is whether or not we can gather all the relevant facts. Do some relevant facts lie with a patient with whom we do not have a relationship? If that patient is not under our care, do we have the authority to approach that patient to gather facts? Unless we are in

management, the likely answer is "no." Do some relevant facts lie with an insurance company or other outside institution? Do we have access to all the relevant laws, policies, and procedures to determine whether what we think might be an ethical violation is even an ethical violation? Those considerations are just some examples.

Depending upon the severity of the apparent violation, the best first response may be to approach the person involved. That person may be able to provide context, reasoning, or additional information that clarifies and resolves the whole issue. This is the best possible outcome of an ethical dilemma.

In the case of the PT or OT student facing an ethical dilemma on a clinical rotation, the best response is almost always to approach the clinical instructor (CI) or fieldwork educator (FWE) first. Students often lack the requisite insight, knowledge, or experience to process an ethical dilemma in the clinic adequately. The student should be respectful and humble, seeking guidance and understanding rather than accusatory. In most cases, the CI/FWE can provide the relevant information and reasoning to clarify and resolve the dilemma. If the CI/FWE's response is unsatisfactory, the student should consult the Director of Clinical Education (DCE) or Academic Fieldwork Coordinator (AFWC) at their educational institution as the next step (in most cases). There are some cases, however, where the student should not consult the CI/FWE first. If the CI/FWE makes unwelcome or inappropriate advances, for instance, the student should seek assistance from a third party.

If we decide to involve a third party in resolving an ethical dilemma, we have several options depending upon the circumstances. The following options are adapted from the APTA document "Resolving Disputes or Complaints" (American Physical Therapy Association, 2018). A more complete list of options and the rationale for choosing them can be found in that document.

- **Employer or organizational grievance department**
  Most healthcare organizations and larger corporations have a formal process by which employees, patients, clients, or customers may file a complaint. The employee handbook often outlines how such complaints against employees are handled. A phone number or website is often provided for complaints to be registered for patients or others.
- **State board of physical or occupational therapy**
  The state boards are the agencies responsible for governing their respective professions. Although the process varies by state, those boards have a means of receiving complaints, determining whether the complaint is within their jurisdiction, assigning an investigator(s), gathering relevant facts, and presenting findings to the board. The board then has the legal and regulatory authority to dismiss the complaint or remedy the situation. The remedy may be nothing more than a private admonition of the offender or as severe as permanently revoking a license to practice.

- **Legal counsel**

  Depending on the nature of the offense, it may be advisable to seek the opinion of someone who is well-versed in the relevant statutes and regulations and can provide guidance on the specific situation. Legal counsel may also guide whether criminal or civil proceedings are warranted.

- **Law enforcement**

  A criminal investigation may be in order if the ethical dilemma includes the possibility that a crime has been committed. As healthcare professionals, we must remember that we do not have the authority, resources, or experience to investigate criminal matters. We must also remember that healthcare providers are "mandatory reporters," meaning that we are legally obligated to report suspected abuse (among other things) to law enforcement or another agency (such as state social services) who have the jurisdiction to investigate those matters.

- **Federal agency**

  If the matter involves a potential violation of federal law, consider reporting the complaint to the appropriate agency. Although this list is by no means exhaustive, a few examples are listed below:

  - United States Department of Labor: complaints regarding worker protection laws.
  - United States Department of Health and Human Services: complaints regarding privacy laws, such as HIPAA (Health Insurance Portability and Accountability Act); complaints regarding Medicare fraud.
  - Equal Employment Opportunity Commission (EEOC): complaints regarding discrimination.

Ethical dilemmas can be difficult to navigate, but we need not do them alone. Most professions have a process to help identify, address and report ethical concerns that may arise in various contexts. The APTA and AOTA offer several resources dedicated to ethical decision-making and a place to report potential ethical violations by *members*. Those resources may be accessed by APTA members at https://www.apta.org/your-practice/ethics-and-professionalism and by AOTA members at https://www.aota.org/practice/practice-essentials/ethics.

Process for Handling Ethical Complaints

Although the APTA (American Physical Therapy Association, 2022a) and AOTA (American Occupational Therapy Association, 2022b) have a process by which ethical concerns may be received and investigated, they do not have the jurisdiction of the state boards. The APTA and AOTA are voluntary organizations. As such, they may remove offenders from membership, but they may not mandate remediation, place restrictions on practice, or revoke or suspend a license.

Although both organizations have processes for handling ethical complaints, the AOTA process is provided here. The American Occupational Therapy Association has two documents that can assist students and practitioners in identifying, addressing, and reporting ethical concerns. First, refer to section three of the AOTA Code of Ethics Standards of Conduct. These standards contain seven sections of observable actions described previously in this chapter. These standards help practitioners live the Code of Ethics in all contexts. They can help in identifying an ethical concern. For example, the Code outlines 15 standards of conduct for practitioners to follow in the Professional Integrity, Responsibility, and Accountability section. Also, each standard is linked to ethical principles, such as Standard 1I, which states, "Report impaired practice to the appropriate authorities [Principle: Non-maleficence]" (American Occupational Therapy Association, 2020, p. 5). Being familiar with this standard of conduct could help in the previously described ethical dilemma regarding an intoxicated colleague.

Another example that would help in the improper billing ethical dilemma is standard 3A: "Bill and collect fees justly and legally in a manner that is fair, reasonable, and commensurate with services delivered. [Principle: Justice]" (American Occupational Therapy Association, 2020, p. 6). Overall, identifying an ethical violation is not enough. Practitioners must make the difficult choice to act on the concern and address or report it. Attempting to resolve the ethical concern directly with the student or colleague would be preferred, but sometimes a resolution cannot be found. In this case, you may need to report your concern.

Second, if you cannot resolve the ethical concern directly with the individual, you should file your concern via the *Enforcement Procedures for the AOTA Occupational Therapy Code of Ethics* document. This document outlines the steps followed by the Ethics Commission as it enforces the code and follows up on reports. It is important to note that the code of ethics and enforcement procedures are "not intended to address private business, legal, or other disputes for which there are other, more appropriate forums for resolution" (American Occupational Therapy Association, 2019, p. 1). Additionally, enforcement of the Code of Ethics applies only to students and clinicians who are AOTA members or were members of AOTA at the time of the incident in question (American Occupational Therapy Association, 2019).

If the decision is made to file a complaint with the ethics commission, all participants in the process are bound by confidentiality. Confidentiality protects the person filing the complaint and the person who is the subject of the complaint. Four steps are taken when a complaint is filed. These steps are described in a general way in Table 5.8. For more detailed information about this process, refer to the *Enforcement Procedures for the AOTA Occupational Therapy Code of Ethics* document (American Occupational Therapy Association, 2019).

Continuing Competency in Core Values and Ethics

Because healthcare is constantly evolving, continuing competency is required for healthcare professionals to

TABLE 5.8	Ethics Enforcement Process
Step 1: FILING	A complaint is filed with the Ethics Office using the Formal Statement of Complaint Form. The complaint is reviewed by AOTA Ethics Office staff.
Step 2: REVIEW BY ETHICS COMMISSION	The complaint is reviewed by the Ethics Commission and either dismissed or investigated further. If investigated further, a decision is made and disciplinary (e.g., suspension of AOTA membership) or non-disciplinary (e.g., educative letter) actions are taken. The respondent can respond to the action and accept the decision, request a reduction in sanction, request a hearing, or decide not to respond. Case closes if there is no request for appeal.
Step 3: APPEAL	The respondent can appeal a decision or sanction. An appeal board is assembled. Hearing is held. Decision is made by an Ethics Panel to uphold, modify, or reverse the decision.
Step 4: REPORTS, RECORDS, PUBLICATIONS	The respondent is notified of all procedures in writing. Case files are maintained in the Ethics Office. Public sanctions are published in AOTA's official publications.

Adapted from American Occupational Therapy Association. (2019). Enforcement procedures for the AOTA occupational therapy code of ethics. *The American Journal of Occupational Therapy, 73*(Supplement_2), 7312410003p1-7312410003p12.

maintain certain national certifications and state licensure. Pursuing continuing education opportunities and resources in core values and ethics allows practitioners to increase their knowledge in this area and improve confidence in the ethical decision-making and reporting process. The following is a list of resources that can be utilized for this purpose:

- Professional organizations: The APTA and AOTA, along with their state affiliates, offer continuing education courses, or conference sessions, at their annual assemblies. Look for opportunities to attend courses on ethics and professionalism. The ethics pages of the APTA and AOTA (see website addresses above) have specific examples of ethical scenarios. The APTA website has a page called "Ethics and Professionalism." The AOTA website has a list of ethics resources for educators and a list of ethics advisory opinions.
- Journals: Professional journals often provide examples of ethical dilemmas and how those dilemmas were resolved.
- Online courses: Several online organizations offer physical and occupational therapists continuing education. Some organizations may allow participants to take a specific course for a fee, while others offer an annual membership that allows participants to take all course offerings. (Specific online organizations are not named here to avoid the appearance of endorsement.)
- Books: Several books address professionalism and ethics in both healthcare in general as well as discipline-specific texts.

References

American Medical Association. (2021). *Core values.* https://policysearch.ama-assn.org/policyfinder/detail/core%20values?uri=%2FAMADoc%2FHODGOV.xml-0-109.xml.

American Occupational Therapy Association. (2019). Enforcement procedures for the AOTA occupational therapy code of ethics. *The American Journal of Occupational Therapy, 73*(Supplement_2), 7312410003p1-7312410003p12.

American Occupational Therapy Association. (2020). AOTA 2020 occupational therapy code of ethics. *The American Journal of Occupational Therapy, 74*(Supplement_3), 7413410005p1-7413410005p13.

American Occupational Therapy Association. (2022a). *About AOTA.* https://www.aota.org/about.

American Occupational Therapy Association. (2022b). *How to file an ethics complaint | AOTA.* https://www.aota.org/practice/practice-essentials/ethics/how-to-file-an-ethics-complaint.

American Physical Therapy Association. (2018). *Resolving disputes or complaints.* APTA. https://www.apta.org/your-practice/ethics-and-professionalism/resolving-disputes-complaints.

American Physical Therapy Association. (2019a). *APTA Guide for conduct of the physical therapist assistant.* APTA.

American Physical Therapy Association. (2019b). *APTA Guide for professional conduct.* APTA.

American Physical Therapy Association. (2020). *Code of ethics for the physical therapist.* APTA.

American Physical Therapy Association. (2021). *Core values for the physical therapist and physical therapist assistant.* APTA.

American Physical Therapy Association. (2022a). *File a complaint with APTA's ethics and judicial committee.* APTA. https://www.apta.org/your-practice/ethics-and-professionalism/file-a-complaint.

American Physical Therapy Association. (2022b). *Vision, mission, and strategic plan*. APTA. https://www.apta.org/apta-and-you/leadership-and-governance/vision-mission-and-strategic-plan.

Beauchamp, T. L., & Childress, J. F. (2019). *Principles of biomedical ethics* (8th ed.). Oxford University Press.

Gabard, D. L., & Martin, M. W. (2011). *Physical therapy ethics* (2nd ed.). F A Davis.

Interprofessional Education Collaborative. (2022). *About us*. https://www.ipecollaborative.org/about-us.

O'Brien, J. C., & Hussey, S. M. (2018). *Introduction to occupational therapy* (5th ed.). Elsevier, Inc.

Papanikitas, A. (2015). *Medical ethics and sociology* (2nd ed.). Elsevier, Inc.

Rae, S. B. (1995). *Moral choices: An introduction to ethics*. Zondervan Publishing House.

Swisher, L. L., & Page, C. G. (2005). *Professionalism in physical therapy: History, practice, & development*. Elsevier, Inc.

White, M. G. (2022, May 26). *Examples of core values: 100 powerful principles*. Your Dictionary. https://examples.yourdictionary.com/examples-of-core-values.html.

Wilkinson, D., Herring, J., & Savulescu, J. (2020). *Medical ethics and law: A curriculum for the 21st century* (3rd ed.). Elsevier, Inc.

World Health Organization. (2022). *Who we are*. https://www.who.int/about/who-we-are.

6

Professionalism, Professional Development, and Mentorship

MELISSA GOODMAN, PT, DPT, NCS, CARLA; FLOYD-SLABAUGH, DOT, OTR/L, CBIS;
KAREN MUELLER, PT, DPT, PhD, NBC-HWC; DIANNA LUNSFORD, OTD, MEd, OTR/L, CHT;
and WILLIAM R. VANWYE, PT, DPT, PhD

LEARNING OBJECTIVES

By the end of this chapter, the reader will be able to:

- Explore the evolution of the occupational therapy and physical therapy professions
- Compare and contrast an occupation versus a profession
- Explain how a theoretical body of knowledge is necessary for a profession
- Differentiate autonomy and accountability and their role within the professions
- Define professionalism
- Identify the characteristics of professionals
- Explore evidence-based practice and its relationship to professionalism
- Explain the importance of lifelong learning and professional development

- Compare and contrast structured versus unstructured learning opportunities
- Discuss the specialist and advanced certification pathways available to therapists
- Examine the importance and benefits of mentorship, belonging, professional socialization, and professional identity formation
- Evaluate methods to find and connect with a mentor
- Compare and contrast the different models of mentorship
- Analyze why mentoring relationships fail

CHAPTER OUTLINE

Introduction

An occupation is any work or regular activity performed to earn a living. The work typically does not require any specific educational qualifications or skills. In contrast, a profession requires a high degree of knowledge and expertise in a specific field. It is a calling or vocation consisting of individuals (i.e., professionals) who are highly trained, motivated, committed, and ethical (Swisher & Page, 2005). At one time, physical and occupational therapists would have been more accurately labeled as technicians or paraprofessionals; however, over the past 100 years, occupational and physical therapists have evolved into professionals.

Evolution of the Occupational Therapy Profession

Occupational therapy has evolved into a widely known profession that evaluates and treats people to live full and meaningful lives. Throughout the past 100 years, the use and concept of occupation have been the philosophical underpinning of the various areas of the profession of occupational therapy (Bing, 1981; Nelson, 1997; Schwartz, 2009; Trombly, 1995). As noted by Nelson (1997), "occupational therapy was founded for one reason: To use occupation as a therapeutic method" (p. 12). The history of occupational therapy is rich in evolution and influences. This section provides a broad overview for the reader to understand the events and paradigm shifts that make occupational therapy the profession it is today.

The occupational therapy perspective began with a history of mental illness in the 18th century. Those who had a mental illness were often ostracized and locked away. The Moral Treatment Movement was born from the need to provide a humane approach to treating this population using "occupations" or purposeful activities (Bing, 1981). This social justice issue and the traditional view of work, which valued work from an economic perspective, were performed by patients in psychiatric facilities for these facilities' successful day-to-day operations (Harvey-Krefting, 1985; Trombly, 1995). Before occupational therapists were recognized professionals, the use of work and occupations was increasingly appreciated and acknowledged as a therapeutic tool.

The term occupational therapy was first formally introduced in 1915 by Dr. William Rush Dunton Jr., a psychiatrist, in his book *Occupational Therapy, A Manual for Nurses*. Dunton and others went on to write additional publications related to occupational therapy, setting forth principles of the profession (AOTA, 1925, Dunton, 1918;). Although occupational therapy was formalized in 1915 and the National Society for the Promotion of Occupational Therapy was created in 1917, the first formal occupation training occurred before 1915 given by Susan Tracy, an occupational health nurse and educator. Another founding member, Eleanor Clarke Slagle, originally a social worker and later seen as the mother of occupational therapy, opened the first

school for occupational therapy in 1912 (Slagle, 1927). Maxwell and Maxwell (1984) noted that other individuals from various professions influenced the development of occupational therapy. Additional founding members of the society included Adolph Meyer, a psychiatrist; George Edward Barton, an architect; Isabel G. Newton, who worked as the assistant to George Barton and later became his wife; Susan Johnson, a designer and arts and crafts teacher; and Thomas Kidner, the vocational secretary of the Canadian Military Hospital. This organization became, in 1923, the American Occupational Therapy Association (AOTA). However, due to the breadth of influence, the identity of the occupational therapy profession was unclear.

Following World War I, in the 1920s, there was an increased focus on returning injured or disabled soldiers to productive work (Anderson & Reed, 2017). With this focus came the need for more rehabilitation workers and facilities. Women were recruited, and many courses and programs were established throughout the United States to educate those recruited and support the efforts (Anderson & Reed, 2017). While some trained "reconstruction aides," as these first occupational therapists were known, used crafts for the treatment of "shell shock" to occupy the minds of soldiers, others focused on orthopedics and exercise (Anderson & Reed, 2017; Harvey-Krefting, 1985; Matheson et al., 1985).

Dr. Dunton and Dr. Adolph Meyers posited that daily occupations and routines could positively influence mental health. Dr. Dunton was instrumental in moving the profession forward, as he was the founding editor of the profession's first journal. He also assisted in standardizing the education of early occupational therapists, which continued to advance in the mid-1930s and 1940s, supported and mostly led by physicians in the American Medical Association (AMA) (Quiroga, 1995).

In the 1930s, vocational and industrial rehabilitation aided injured soldiers to reach a normal level of function for return to work which continued with the return of soldiers from World War II (Fig. 6.1) (Harvey-Krefting, 1985; Matheson et al., 1985). Throughout the 1930s, this focus on vocation expanded to include individuals who sustained orthopedic injuries unrelated to the war (Matheson, et al., 1985). Also, the AMA created educational standards for occupational therapy certification for consistency in the training of occupational therapists. In the 1940s, the United States Army classified occupational therapy as a profession; thus, a shift to a more scientific view of occupational therapy emerged (McLoughlin Gray,1998).

From the 1940s through the 1960s, occupational therapists became more involved with returning soldiers' mental and physical rehabilitation. Due to this high demand for occupational therapists, who were now required to complete 4 years of training, the certified occupational therapy assistant (COTA) position was created. COTA education required less training, thus increasing access to occupational therapy services (AOTA, 1958). With this medical influence, occupational therapists began implementing biomechanical constructs such as motion and strength into their treatment. The collaboration between AOTA and the AMA

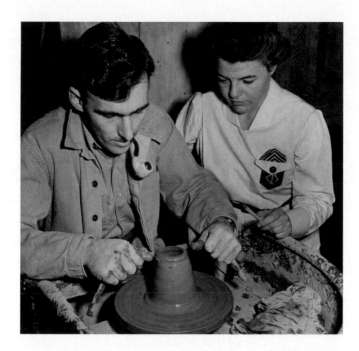

• **Fig. 6.1** Vocational and industrial rehabilitation aided injured soldiers to reach a normal level of function for return to work. (From https://www.flickr.com/photos/28853433@N02/36689269526).

remained. It would not be until the 1990s that the educational standards for occupational therapists were recognized separate from the AMA by the United States Department of Education (AOTA, 1993b).

During the 1960s and 1970s, occupational therapy continued to be influenced by the medical model. However, other occupational therapists called for the profession to return to the use of occupation. When discussing occupational history and addressing life skills, the environment, personal factors, culture, attitudes, and values, were also emphasized (Klavins, 1972; Maurer, 1971; Moorehead, 1969). In 1970, occupational therapy transitioned to a bachelor's degree. Other major influences in the 1970s were regulation and the push for state licensure (AOTA, 1974; Johnson, 1975), occupational therapy becoming a reimbursable service (AOTA, 1974), and protection for those with disabilities, including children in schools (American Occupational Therapy Association, n.d.). As occupational therapy developed into a profession, its philosophy, beliefs, and values were identified through a uniform language, which later became the Occupational Therapy Practice Framework and a document known as the occupational therapy Code of Ethics (AOTA, 1977; 1980; 1984).

In 1979, AOTA released a document requested by the federal government called the *Occupational Therapy Product Output Reporting System and Uniform Terminology for Reporting Occupational Therapy Services*. This document was intended as a means to unify the language used in reporting on therapy (AOTA, 1979). There were two additional versions of this document, with the name shortened to *Uniform Terminology for Occupational Therapy* (version II & III; AOTA, 1989; 1994) which further identified the "areas of

concern for occupational therapy" (*Framework IV;* AOTA, 2018). The current document in use at the time of this publication is the fourth revision, which outlines the practice of occupational therapy, called the *Occupational Therapy Practice Framework IV* (OTPF IV). This document is revised every 5 years for relevance and to include current trends. The *OTPF-IV* serves as a guide for students and therapists to "clearly articulate the occupational therapy domain and process, it builds on a set of values that the profession has held since its founding in 1917" (*Framework IV;* AOTA, 2018). Another document guiding professional practice is the *Occupational Therapy Code of Ethics* (AOTA, 2020).

The 1980s expanded occupational therapy practice under specified reimbursement systems, including Medicare for home health, skilled nursing, and the early education system (Health Insurance Association of America, 1984; Salend & Garrick Duhaney, 2011). The debate over occupational therapy focusing on the medical model, becoming specialists or generalists, persisted (Gillette & Kielhofner, 1979; Yerxa, 1979). It was determined that AOTA, as a professional organization, should not also control the accreditation of occupational therapy educational programs. By the mid-1980s, AOTA and what is known today as the National Board for Certification in Occupational Therapy (NBCOT) became separate organizations (AOTA, 1986). The initial NBCOT certification and membership in AOTA were separated and many states also required licensure. At the same time, other professionals continued to be confused about the role of occupational therapists and it was clear that there was a need for an understanding of occupational therapists' unique professional level of practice (Reed & Peters, 2010; Yerxa, 1998).

Into the 1990s, occupational therapy was identified as a profession and the need for research and scholarship was recognized (AOTA, 1984). The occupational therapy education requirements moved from a baccalaureate level toward an entry-level master's degree, which all accredited schools required by 2007. Since then, there has been much debate regarding increasing the entry-level of occupational therapy to a doctoral degree (Table 6.1).

Although the AOTA Board of Directors (2014) provided reasons for the support for moving to this degree advancement, many argued that there would be consequences and limited benefits. Benefits identified included autonomy, evidence-based practice, leadership, practice specialization, competition with other professionals, and overall advancement of the profession of occupational therapy. Some concerns regarding the entry-level doctorate mandate revolved around decreased program enrollment, potential negative impact on diversity, increased student debt, and an increased burden on fieldwork sites due to the doctoral capstone internship experience. There were also questions about who made the decision and whether enough research had been reviewed. After much opposition and discussion, the mandate was reconsidered and a dual entry into the profession of occupational therapy remained (AOTA, 2019).

Increased reimbursement coverage, specialty area certifications, an advanced entry-level doctoral degree, and evolving

TABLE 6.1	Potential Pros and Cons of Entry-Level Doctoral Degree for Occupational and Physical Therapists	
Potential Pros		**Potential Cons**
• Therapists are recognized by colleagues and by the public as a truly autonomous profession • Prepare graduates for autonomous practice at the entry-level • The changing clinical environment requires a higher level of knowledge and skills upon entry into the profession • A doctoral program offers a greater number of (clinical) internship hours • A doctoral-level education may be associated with an increase in salary • Doctoral-level graduates would be more likely to continue to develop science and evidence for practice		• A change in "title" may confuse the public and other health professional colleagues • Many believe using the title doctor in hospital or community health settings is inappropriate • It may be viewed as trying to gain legitimacy by awarding graduates a higher credential for fulfilling the same entry-level requirements • If the doctoral degree does result in higher salaries, employers may choose to hire paraprofessionals • A doctoral level of education may be associated with greater student debt

From American Occupational Therapy Association. (Feb. 2019). *Special task force report: Executive summary.* https://www.aota.org/~/media/Corporate/Files/AboutAOTA/BOD/Special-Task-Force-February-2019-Summary-Report.pdf; AOTA Board of Directors. (2014). *Position statement on entry-level degree for the occupational therapist.* https://www.aota.org/AboutAOTA/Get-Involved/ BOD/OTD-Statement.aspx; Mathur, S. (2011). Doctorate in physical therapy: Is it time for a conversation? *Physiotherapy Canada, 63*(2), 140–142.

healthcare perspectives continue to influence the profession of occupational therapy. AOTA has developed and modified the practice framework on which the profession of occupational therapy practice is based. Over 100 years of accomplishments have made occupational therapy a unique and widely varied profession (Fig. 6.2).

Evolution of the Physical Therapy Profession

Physical therapists are movement experts who examine, diagnose, and design treatment plans to manage pain, improve function, and prevent disability (Becoming a Physical

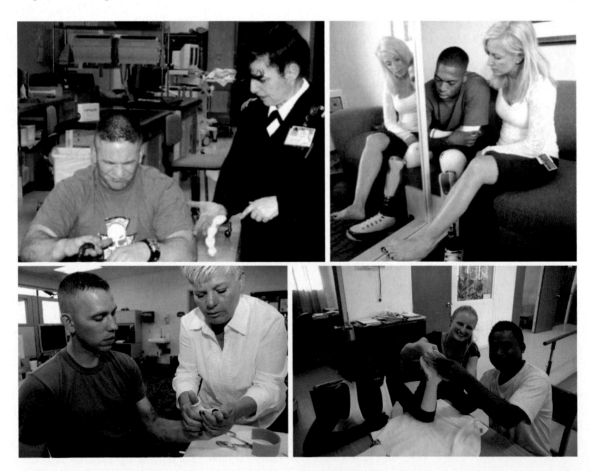

• **Fig. 6.2** Occupational therapists help people of all ages participate in their desired occupations such as making meals, dressing, driving, going to school or work, playing, or caring for family members. (From https://commons.wikimedia.org/w/index.php?curid=59183867; https://www.flickr.com/photos/106853342@N04/10681196793).

Therapist, 2021). Over the past 100 years, many significant events have shaped the profession. Thus gaining a historical perspective is critical to understanding fully the professionalization of physical therapists, who have progressed from their early days as technicians to professionals.

The creation of the physical therapy profession centered around two major events in the early 1900s: World War I and the polio epidemic. Early physical therapists were known as reconstruction aides. They were primarily women with a physical education background with additional training in therapeutic exercise, manual therapy, hydrotherapy, and electrotherapy. In 1921, a pioneer reconstruction aide named Mary McMillan founded what is known today as the American Physical Therapy Association (APTA). Her training consisted of a degree in physical education and postgraduate training in physical therapy science. She later became a United States Army Medical Corps member as a reconstruction aide at Walter Reed General Hospital. She was the first President of the APTA and was instrumental in establishing the early standards for training other reconstruction aides (APTA, 2020; Barrett, 2021; Swisher & Page, 2005).

By the late 1920s, the APTA established a minimum standard curriculum for physical therapy schools, which recommended at least 9 months of PT-related training. Up to the 1950s, physical therapists' training remained consistent at around 12 months; however, by the late 1950s, over half of the accredited programs offered 4-year degrees. Thus physical therapists focused on professional and educational development to expand their knowledge base and skill set, which led them to today's doctoring profession (APTA, 2020; Barrett, 2021; Swisher & Page, 2005).

The profession saw substantial growth from the 1940s to the 1970s. In the 1940s, during World War II, physical therapists expanded their skills to treat many of the conditions they do today. Their skills were sought for various complex conditions such as burns, amputations, wounds, fractures, and neuromusculoskeletal conditions. During the 1950s and 1960s, physical therapy demand increased due to the Korean War and the introduction of Medicare and Medicaid programs. In the late 1960s, the APTA created the role of physical therapist assistant, which extended physical therapists' roles to supervisors. In the 1970s, during the Vietnam War, United States military physical therapists became primary care providers for neuromusculoskeletal conditions as a wartime effort to support orthopedic surgeons (Fig. 6.3). These events were critical in shaping physical therapists' autonomy and expertise in clinical reasoning (APTA, 2020; Barrett, 2021; Greathouse et al., 2021; Musolino & Jensen, 2020).

Although physical therapists were improving their curricula and expanding the scope of practice, initially, they remained tightly connected with and controlled by physicians. The link to physicians extended into the 1960s when physicians peaked their political power. During this period, physicians controlled all healthcare providers' training and scopes of practice and any provider who did not accept this physician dominance risked being labeled

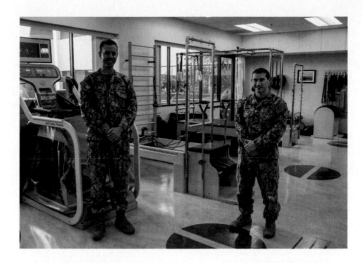

• **Fig. 6.3** During the Vietnam War, United States military physical therapists became primary care providers for neuromusculoskeletal conditions, which continues today. (From https://www.flickr.com/photos/61270229@N05/50489789872).

fraudulent. Thus many healthcare professionals, including physical therapists, relinquished autonomy to maintain legitimacy within the medical profession (Barrett, 2021; Sandstrom, 2007).

However, during the 1970s, 1980s, and 1990s, physical therapists began taking measures to break away from this physician dominance and establish themselves as professionals through the expansion of United States state licensure laws, the promotion of direct access, the opening of private practices, the creation of specialty boards, and doctorate-level education. In 1996, Creighton University became the first professional Doctor of Physical Therapy (DPT) program in the nation to graduate its first class of students. Although there has been much debate regarding increasing the entry-level degree of physical therapists to a doctoral degree (Table 6.1), in 2016, the DPT became the only degree conferred by CAPTE-accredited educational institutions (APTA, 2021). Ultimately, each milestone helped physical therapy become the profession it is today.

What is a Profession?

A profession is characterized by autonomy, accountability (including a code of ethics), and a theoretical body of knowledge (Swisher & Page, 2005; Tipton, 2017). Professionals practice consistently with these characteristics to carry out their various professional roles and responsibilities (Table 6.2). The following sections will detail the characteristics of a profession along with the responsibility for professional growth through lifelong learning.

Autonomy and Accountability

Autonomy, or unfettered practice, is the ability to have a high degree of decision-making and control over one's work (APTA, 2012; Fritz & Flynn, 2005; Johnson & Abrams,

TABLE 6.2	Therapists' Professional Roles and Responsibilities
Professional	• Therapists practice in an ethical and legal manner • Therapists are responsible for individual professional development • Therapists supervise physical and occupational therapy assistants, aides, and students • Therapists recognize that supervision guidelines and laws differ among the APTA, AOTA, state licensure, and payor (e.g., Medicare)
Patient manager	• The therapist is responsible for all aspects of the examination, evaluation, and reevaluation process • Therapists incorporate evidence-based practice by integrating the best available research evidence, clinical expertise, and an individual's values
Administrator	• Therapists are guided and informed by positions, standards, guidelines, policies, and procedures
Educator and consultant	• Therapists provide education and consultation to consumers, peers, health services providers, and students
Advocate	• Therapists participate in advocacy for patients' and clients' rights
Researcher or critical inquirer	• Therapists apply research findings to practice and encourage, participate in, and promote activities that establish the outcomes of patient and client management
Community member	• Therapists demonstrate community responsibility by participating in community and community agency activities, educating the public, formulating public policy, and providing pro bono services

AOTA, American Occupational Therapy Association; *APTA*, American Physical Therapy Association
From American Occupational Therapy Association. (2021). Standards of practice for occupational therapy. *The American Journal of Occupational Therapy*, 75(Supplement_3), 7513410030; American Physical Therapy Association. (2019). *Code of ethics for the physical therapist*. http://www.apta.org/uploadedFiles/APTAorg/About_Us/Policies/Ethics/CodeofEthics.pdf; American Physical Therapy Association. (2020, August 12). *Standards of practice for physical therapy*. https://www.apta.org/siteassets/pdfs/policies/standards-of-practice-pt.pdf.

2005; Rothstein, 2002, 2003; Sandstrom, 2007; Swisher & Page, 2005). Professionals exercise independence and self-determination within their scope of practice (Moffat, 2003; Swisher & Page, 2005). This freedom is typically based on accountability, ethical conduct, and knowledge (Fritz & Flynn, 2005; Swisher & Page, 2005). Unfettered practice requires therapists to follow their profession's codes and standards and act in the patient's best interest. They must collaborate by referring and consulting with other healthcare providers to enhance patient/client management. As professionals, therapists are responsible for all patient/client management aspects.

Therapists are accountable to numerous stakeholders, including patients, employers, hospitals, payors, investors, the APTA and AOTA, the states, and the courts. Subsequently, ethical and legal standards are in place to ensure accountability. A code of ethics (Chapter 5) is a collective document or professional consensus that articulates standards for practice. Self-regulation is an important aspect of a profession, which requires avenues for reporting ethical and legal breaches (AOTA, 2021; APTA, 2019; Swisher & Page, 2005). Accordingly, the APTA, the AOTA, and state licensing boards have processes to handle ethical breaches and disciplinary actions (AOTA, 2021; APTA, 2018; FSBPT, 2009).

Theoretical Body of Knowledge

A theoretical body of knowledge speaks to what is widely known as an evidence-based practice (EBP) (Fig. 6.4). A

• **Fig. 6.4** Evidence-based practice serves as an avenue for creating and maintaining a theoretical body of knowledge. (From https://www.flickr.com/photos/92675621@N00/2956927902).

profession's theoretical body of knowledge should be broad and generalizable to guide professionals in utilizing effective techniques (Swisher & Page, 2005). To achieve this, the APTA created the Guide to Physical Therapist Practice. This comprehensive guide provides educators, students, and clinicians with a description of physical therapist practice (APTA, 2021). To support knowledge translation and EBP, occupational therapy's AOTA created an evidenced-based toolkit that includes resources for evidence-informed interventions, connecting with others, and practice guidelines in various settings (Skaletski, 2021).

Given the complex and ongoing changes in healthcare, therapists need to remain informed within their field to meet the needs of their patients, the profession, funders, and the greater society (Juckett et al., 2021). Indeed, Johnson et al. (2021) stated, "Our society's welfare depends on healthcare practitioners' abilities to adapt to changes in clinical practice" (p. 2). This section will investigate the steps of EBP, the therapist's perspective, evidence to guide practice, and professional responsibility.

Evidence-Based Practice

Evidence-based medicine began in the 1970s with the development of a "problem-based" medical program by Dr. David Sackett, an epidemiologist, and his colleagues at McMaster University in Ontario, Canada (Law & MacDermid, 2014). The often-quoted definition of evidence-based medicine by Sackett et al. is "The conscientious, explicit and judicious use of current best evidence in making decisions about the care of individual patients" (Holm, 2000). The colleagues continued to collaborate and disseminate key principles of evidence-based medicine (Law & MacDermid, 2014). Over time the evidence-based process expanded and evolved into EBP, which is now used worldwide by various fields and disciplines and thereby incorporated into professional education programs (Law & MacDermid, 2014). While evidence-based medicine remains a preferred term by physicians, the field of rehabilitation typically uses the term EBP (Law & MacDermid, 2014). The overall goal of EBP is the integration of three perspectives: the best research evidence, the therapist's experience, and the client's preferences, values, and circumstance (Brown, 2017; Fetters & Tilson, 2012). This goal is reflected in both occupational and physical therapy professions, with each professional organization stating its commitment to EBP. Both professions explicitly state they promote EBP to integrate the evidence, the professional's expertise, and the client's values (AOTA, 2020; APTA, 2022).

EBP is known to improve professional performance, reduce healthcare costs, and improve patient outcomes (Crable et al., 2020). Individuals can use the evidence in daily practice, organizations, and policy-making (Crable et al., 2020; Granger, 2020). The evidence can also be used for scientific inquiry, establishing best practice standards, developing quality improvement processes, and engaging in EBP (Juckett et al., 2021). Scientific inquiry, also known as research, is the generation of new knowledge using a systematic process to gather and synthesize data (Crable et al., 2020). Based on this new knowledge, the literature is used to establish best practice standards and create quality improvement processes (Crable et al., 2020; Juckett et al., 2021). Also, the existing literature is used to engage in EBP.

EBP is a dynamic, complex, and iterative process of integrating the best available evidence with the therapist's clinical experience, knowledge of the client's unique characteristics, and knowledge of the healthcare organization's culture with the patient's perspective. Most importantly, the patient's perspective is integrated. The patient and their family's values and preferences are honored, along with the patient's specific needs. Moreover, EBP improves professional performance and reduces healthcare costs (Atler & Stephens, 2020; Crable et al., 2020; Vingerhoets et al., 2020).

Evidence-Based Practice Steps

To engage in EBP, the therapist will use a step-by-step process to create a clinical question, search for the evidence, appraise the evidence, apply the best available evidence, and reflect (Brown, 2017; Fetters & Tilson, 2012; Law & MacDermid, 2014).

Step 1: Question

The first step of the EBP process is to write a clinical question that is answerable, focused, and searchable. One method to create a clinical question is to develop a PICO question; PICO stands for patient/population, intervention, comparison, and outcomes. Variations of the PICO question are the PIO question which does not contain a comparison, and the PICOT, which adds time (Brown, 2017; Fetters and Tilson, 2012; Granger, 2020).

Step 2: Search

The next step of the EBP process is to search for the evidence, which entails gathering reliable published evidence (Brown, 2017; Fetters and Tilson, 2012; Law & MacDermid, 2014). Databases commonly used include the Cumulative Index of Nursing and Allied Health (i.e., CINHAL), MEDLINE, PubMed, PsycINFO, Ovid, ERIC, PEDro, OTseeker, and Cochrane. CINHAL indexes nursing and allied health literature (CINHAL, 2022). MEDLINE, part of PubMed, is the National Library of Medicine's database for life sciences (MEDLINE, 2022; PubMed, n.d.). PsycINFO is a database for literature in the field of psychology (PsycINFO, 2022). Ovid contains medical, nursing, and allied health articles and resources (Ovid, 2022). ERIC is an education research database (ERIC, n.d.). The Physiotherapy Evidence Database, commonly known as PEDro, is a database of systematic reviews, randomized trials, and clinical practice guidelines particularly relevant to physical therapy (PEDro, 2022).

Similarly, OTseeker is a database of systematic reviews, randomized trials, and resources particularly relevant to occupational therapy (OTSeeker, n.d.). Lastly, the Cochrane database contains systematic reviews and metaanalyses with a summary and interpretation of the results (Cochrane, 2022). Information management skills are needed to select keywords and apply search strategies; however, librarian assistance may be needed to navigate the intricacies of each database (Brown, 2017; Fetters and Tilson, 2012; Law & MacDermid, 2014).

Step 3: Appraise

The search may result in obtaining quantitative, qualitative, and mixed-method studies. Quantitative studies best answer clinical questions that seek to identify the effectiveness of an intervention, whereas qualitative studies best answer clinical questions that seek to understand a culture, experience, process, or phenomenon (Fig. 6.5). Whether the search results produce quantitative or qualitative studies, an appraisal requires critically analyzing each article section (Brown, 2017). Appraisal of the evidence is a four-step process to critique a study's relevance, quality or trustworthiness, results, and clinical significance (Fig. 6.6 and Table 6.3).

Step 4: Apply

Therapists must use their judgment to complete the fourth step of the process to discern the evidence's clinical application. Even though the evidence rarely answers a clinical question directly, the therapist's use of EBP enables the evidence to be implemented. Step 4 of this process requires the therapist to use the evidence, their expertise, and the client's values. The therapist will continue to employ critical thinking to balance the critically appraised research evidence and their clinical expertise while also incorporating the client's values. Furthermore, therapists must communicate the evidence with their clients, caregivers, managers, and funders (Fetters & Tilson, 2012; Vingerhoets et al., 2020).

Step 5: Reflect

Although reflective thinking is used throughout the EBP process, the last step of the EBP process is reflection (Fetters & Tilson, 2012). Therapists with higher self-reflective behaviors were found to have higher rates of implementing EBP (Krueger et al., 2020b). Honorees showcase the importance of reflection within the fields of physical and occupational therapy: Gail Jensen, PT, the 2011 McMillan Lecture honoree, and Margo Holm, OT, the 2000 Slagle Lecture honoree. These distinguished representatives of their fields each emphasized the importance of reflection, a concept created by John Dewey, a renowned educational theorist (Holm, 2000; Jensen, 2011; Krueger et al., 2020b). The therapist engages in reflection-on-action and deeper critical self-reflection (Jensen, 2011). The therapist reflects on the process of asking a clinical question, locating the evidence, navigating the databases, then critically thinking about and appraising the evidence (Holm, 2000; Jensen, 2011). At the same time, deeper critical self-reflection is required to identify the skills needed to be a continually competent therapist (Jensen, 2011). This deep critical self-reflection is also required to consider if the evidence was implemented correctly and effectively (Holm, 2000). Finally, this deeper level of self-reflection is needed for the therapist to consider the impact of their EBP (Holm, 2000). Did the EBP expand beyond an individual case to the development of clinical guidelines? If so, is this project being monitored from varying perspectives for cost-effectiveness, patient outcomes, patient satisfaction, and therapist satisfaction? (Holm, 2000).

The Therapist's Perspective

Evidenced-based medicine, EBP, evidence-informed practice, and evidence-based care relate to questioning, searching, applying, evaluating, or reflecting (Brown, 2017; Fetters & Tilson, 2012). Likewise, professional occupational and physical therapy organizations have also declared their commitment to EBP (AOTA, 2020; APTA, 2022). Challenges remain with EBP, despite the billions of dollars spent on research and development in the United States medical and health sector (Bauer et al., 2015; Li et al., 2018; Tucker et al., 2021). While advances have been made in the generation of knowledge for EBP, implementation of EBP has been less successful, with a surprising 17-year evidence-to-practice time lag (Li et al., 2018).

To be actionable, knowledge has to be translated and then implemented. First, knowledge translation is defined by the Canadian Institutes of Health Research as "a dynamic and iterative process that includes synthesis, dissemination, exchange and ethically sound application of knowledge" (Bennett et al., 2018, p. 156). In knowledge translation, the evidence is implemented using a multi-stage process to change clinical practice (Barrimore et al., 2020; Bennett et al., 2018; Eames et al., 2018). Knowledge translation can include integrating new interventions into practice and no

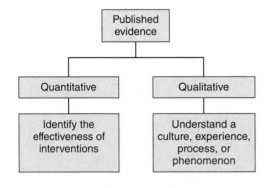

• **Fig. 6.5** Types of Evidence.

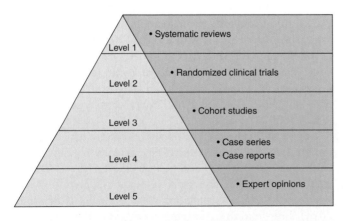

• **Fig. 6.6** Levels of Evidence. (Howick, J., Chalmers, I., Glasziou, P., Greenhalgh, T., Heneghan, C., Liberati, A., Moschetti, I., Phillips, B., & Thornton, H. *The 2011 Oxford CEBM Evidence Levels of Evidence [Introductory Document]*. Oxford Centre for Evidence-Based Medicine. https://www.cebm.ox.ac.uk/resources/levels-of-evidence/levels-of-evidence-introductory-document).

TABLE 6.3	Evidence Appraisal	
	Quantitative	**Qualitative**
Research design	Quantitative studies best answer clinical questions that seek to identify the effectiveness of an intervention.	Qualitative studies best answer clinical questions that seek to understand a culture, experience, process, or phenomenon.
Step 1 Critique the study's relevance	Consider whether the study is relevant to the clinical question.	

Step 2 Critique the study's quality or trustworthiness	Critique the study's quality Determine the level of evidence
	• Use a hierarchy of evidence to rank research designs based on the study's validity or rigor:
	  • Level 1 studies are the most rigorous study designs, randomized controlled trials (RCTs), and systematic reviews
	  • Levels 2, 3, and 4 are cross-sectional, cohort, and case-series, respectively
	  • Level 5, expert opinion, is the lowest
	-Critique the study's methodology and procedures
		Critique the study's trustworthiness Determine the type of design
		• Phenomenological designs describe a lived experience
		• Ethnographic designs describe patterns of behavior and customs
		• Grounded designs are used to develop a theory based on the participants' views
		• Participatory action research involves researchers and participants working together in a cycle of research, data collection, reflection, and action
		Analyze the study's design, methods, ethical practice, theoretical connections, data analysis, and limitations.
		Trustworthiness:
		• Is the study's design appropriate for the research question?
		• Is the study credible?
		• Credibility: the sense of confidence that the data is believable. The equivalent of internal validity in quantitative research. Can be increased with:
		  • Transferability: describes the reader's ability to transfer the results to another context, dependent upon the researcher providing a "thick description"
		  • Dependability: reliability of the research findings, which can be enhanced with thorough documentation of research procedures
		  • Confirmability: the sense of confidence that the data is believable
		    • Member checking: confirm the researcher's interpretation of the participants' words for accuracy
		    • Data triangulation: gathering different perspectives

Step 3 Critique the study's results	• Descriptive statistics: describe the participants in the study
	• Inferential statistics: allows for predictions from a sample to generalize about the population
	• Low P-value:
	  • **statistically significant**
	  • less than or equal to 0.05 ($P \leq .05$)
	  • a low probability that the results occurred by chance
	  • higher confidence that the sample results can be **generalized** to the population
	• Confidence interval: the probability that the characteristics of the sample represent the population
	• Effect size: how much or the degree an intervention affected the study's participants
	• Studies with a larger effect size hold more practical significance and may be more meaningful in clinical practice
		• The data analysis expectations are a vivid description of the site, participants, and events and analytical rigor and audibility.
		• Judge the study's limitations, if the conclusions are reasonable, and if the implications are appropriate.
		• What are the study's overall reasonableness and usefulness?

Continued

TABLE 6.3	Evidence Appraisal—cont'd	
	Quantitative	**Qualitative**
Step 4 Weigh the clinical significance	Requires the therapist to use the evidence, their expertise, and the client's values.	

From Baum, F., MacDougall, C., & Smith, D. (2006). Participatory action research. *Journal of epidemiology and community health, 60*(10), 854-857;Brown, C. (2017). *The evidence-based practitioner: Applying research to meet client needs.* FA Davis; Creswell, J. W. & Creswell, J. D. (2018). *Research design: Qualitative, quantitative, and mixed methods approaches.* 5th edition. SAGE; Evans, D. (2003). Hierarchy of evidence: A framework for ranking evidence evaluating health-care interventions. *Journal of Clinical Nursing, 12*, 77-84; Fetters, L. & Tilson, J. (2012). *Evidence based physical therapy.* F.A. Davis Company; Korstjens, I., & Moser, A. (2018) Series: Practical guidance to qualitative research. Part 4: Trustworthiness and publishing. *European Journal of General Practice, 24*(1), 120-124; *OCEBM Levels of Evidence Working Group.* (2011). *The Oxford levels of evidence 2.* Oxford Centre for Evidence-Based Medicine. https://www.cebm.ox.ac.uk/resources/levels-of-evidence/ocebm-levels-of-evidence.

longer utilizing interventions ascertained to be ineffective (Bennett et al., 2018). Moreover, translating knowledge into practice is imperative to improve outcomes for therapy clients (Bennett et al., 2018).

There are several barriers to therapists engaging with the evidence. Some of these barriers are individual, while others are organizational (Crable et al., 2020; Li et al., 2018). The individual barriers include a lack of time, a lack of skill, a lack of professional development, and limitations with the use-ability of the information (Barrimore et al., 2020; Krueger, et al., 2020a). The lack of time is often cited as a barrier for individuals engaging in evidence-informed practice (Fetter & Tilson, 2012). Gathering and appraising evidence requires time and reflection (Bennet et al., 2018). Also, individual therapists may lack skills in locating the evidence and understanding the statistics (Fetter & Tilson, 2012).

Moreover, the useability of information may be a barrier for individual therapists. Two issues arise with the useability of information. First, scholarly peer-reviewed journal articles are not translated into clinically relevant findings for the therapist (Law & MacDermid, 2014). Second, publications with lower levels of evidence may fit the therapist's clinical question yet lack generalizability (Juckett et al., 2021). While at the same time, individual therapists may also lack the time and financial funding to conduct a high-quality study in the workplace (Juckett et al., 2021). Translating research to fill the research-to-practice gap is a time-consuming and complex task (Tucker et al., 2021). Hence, a new field of study, Implementation Science, has emerged to "facilitate the spread of EBPs, in-cluding both psychosocial and medical interventions for mental and physical health concerns" with a broad focus from patient and provider levels to organization and policy levels (Bauer, 2015, p. 1).

The organizational barriers include the lack of organiza-tional structure, a lack of organizational support, and limi-tations in the organizational culture. A limitation in the organizational structure may require a therapist to engage in evidence-informed practice *in addition* to their clinical work instead of facilitating the therapist to engage with the evidence *as part of* their clinical work (Law & MacDermid, 2014). Likewise, the organization may not support infor-mational resources, such as access to a medical library and professional journals. Other informational resources are re-search activities, membership in professional organizations, and reimbursement for evidenced-based continuing educa-tion (Fetter & Tilson, 2012; Hissong et al., 2015).

Given the importance of EBP, there is a need to over-come barriers. To overcome barriers, individual therapists and managers can exert leadership, as leadership is key for implementation effectiveness (Li et al., 2018). Managers, in particular, can be influential in enabling knowledge transla-tion (Bennett et al., 2018). Transformative leaders serve as role models by setting and abiding by expectations on a mi-cro level and strategically influencing the organization on a macro level. (Bennett et al., 2018). Leaders may also need to engage in capacity building. Capacity building can occur "at four levels: structures, systems and roles; staff and infra-structure; skills; and tools" (Eames et al., 2018, p. 480). In clinical practice, therapists could address research-practice gaps once the knowledge translation capacity building is in place (Eames et al., 2018). Furthermore, there may be a need to create or organize education sessions, departmental professional development, or identify resources (Barrimore et al., 2020). Notably, an evidence-based culture and men-torship have been deemed vital to individuals developing competency and implementing evidence-based care as a large part of professional practice (Li et al., 2018; Melnyk et al., 2021).

Using Evidence to Guide Practice

As professionals, therapists use evidence to guide all aspects of their practice, beginning with the evaluation. The therapist utilizes evidence-based information to choose assessment tools and critique the assessment tool's validity and reliability (Chisholm & Schell, 2019). Furthermore, the therapist utilizes the best evidence to determine interventions (Brown, 2017; Fetter & Tilson, 2012).

Therapists also use the evidence to create and establish best practice standards (Juckett et al., 2021). Additionally, there may be opportunities for the therapist to optimize quality measures. These quality measures are tracked by the Center for Medicare and Medicaid Services (CMS) as part of the quality and payment programs (Juckett et al., 2021). Likewise, therapists can conduct an EBP project whereby there is a literature review, generation of critically-appraised papers (CAPs) and critically appraised topics (CAT), and synthesis of the results, which are turned into clinical practice guidelines (Hissong et al., 2015). A critically-appraised paper is a summarized, in-depth analysis and critique of a published research study, including interpretation of the results for clinical application (Brown, 2017). Similarly, a critically appraised topic focuses on a single topic and includes a collection of critically appraised papers with summarized pertinent information (Hissong et al., 2015). APTA and AOTA provide CAPs and CATs as evidence-based resources for therapists' use.

Professional Responsibility for EBP

"Evidence-based practice implementation has been associated with the provision of high-quality healthcare including improved patient outcomes; reduced costs; and higher levels of health practitioner engagement, teamwork, and job satisfaction" (Krueger et al., 2020a, p. 254). To translate the evidence into practice—knowledge translation—the therapist must possess strong EBP skills (Atler & Stephens, 2020; Juckett et al., 2021). There is a practical and ethical need for the therapist to use EBP skills to remain current, requiring the therapist to sift through a large volume of evidence and then determine the quality (Holm, 2000; Vingerhoets et al., 2020). To meet this practical and ethical need, ongoing continued competence is needed (Hachtel & Plummer, 2015). Furthermore, a professional may need mentorship, education, and training to develop EBP skills (Staffileno et al., 2022).

A healthcare professional carries the responsibility to meet the expectations of several stakeholders. Professionals are obliged to society, funders, the profession, and our patients (AOTA 2020; Jensen, 2011). In order to satisfy the many stakeholders, therapists need to generate knowledge and translate that knowledge into practice (Atler & Stephens, 2020; Holm, 2000). Engaging in EBP requires time to analyze, implement, and reflect, which are all higher-order cognitive skills (Bloom's Taxonomy, n.d.; Staffileno et al., 2022). Given the ongoing critical thinking required to engage in EBP, it is understandable that EBP is perceived as a high-level cognitive task (Halle et al., 2021).

EBP requires the therapist to possess many skills, such as information management and specialized EBP skills. The therapist combines these skills with the ongoing application of high-level cognitive skills to discern, judge, appraise, critique, and reflect. Notwithstanding the therapist's depth of skill and judgment, leadership is also needed. Leaders also serve as role models by promoting EBP and creating an environment supporting EBP. Moreover, leaders

support others in engaging in reflective practice. To engage in reflective practice, therapists reflect on the actions and participate in deeper critical self-reflection. The deeper critical self-reflection is part of being a continually competent therapist. Continually competent therapists identify the skills *they* need. Deeper critical self-reflection is also needed to contemplate how the evidence can be used with a broader scope, beyond the individual patient, to more enduring knowledge products like clinical guidelines. Alas, the development of clinical guidelines also requires deep reflection. Extensive planning is needed to investigate the evidence and create the necessary processes and tools. The creation of processes and tools is needed to monitor key factors important to stakeholders and the therapist.

To create an environment that supports EBP, a leader may need to engage in capacity building of structures, systems, staff, and skills. Therapists may need time and skill development. Further, therapists benefit greatly from mentorship and a supportive environment (Li et al., 2018; Melnyk et al., 2021); therefore, leaders facilitate therapists to identify their EBP professional development needs. Likewise, leaders can support the creation of more enduring uses of the evidence in the form of a critically appraised paper, a critically appraised topic, or clinical guidelines.

Healthcare has ever-changing models, payment structures, and client needs. However, occupational and physical therapists are well-suited to adapt to change as they earn advanced degrees with EBP in professional education programs. A state of ongoing change in the healthcare system and with the patient's needs can be anticipated. Therapists can use EBP to improve professional performance, decrease healthcare costs, and facilitate better patient outcomes, affecting individual patients, policy, and society. With EBP, therapists can mobilize their education, training, professionalism, and leadership to translate the written words in scholarly publications into improved patient lives.

Professionalism

Professionalism is often hard to define, thus the adage, "I know it when I see it." Professionalism can be defined as adhering to values, attitudes, and beliefs with a commitment to excellence, altruism, and service (Tipton, 2017). Professional actions or behaviors are not necessarily inherent; therefore, established core values and a code of ethics must be present and emphasized during entry-level education, clinical experiences and practice, and professional development (Ditwiler et al., 2021; Lecours et al., 2021). The AOTA and APTA established core values and codes of ethics to define the specific professional behaviors required for occupational and physical therapists, respectively (Chapter 5). Consequently, failing to abide by these professional behaviors will result in being labeled unprofessional (Tipton, 2017).

Developing Professionalism

Professionalism is not perfectionism because no one is completely or consistently professional (Tipton, 2017). Thus professionalism is ongoing and developmental. Developing professionalism begins with entry-level training and continues throughout a person's career via lifelong learning, professional development, and mentorship. Entry-level professional programs typically focus on foundational skills and clinical practice. However, students need time and energy to devote to personal growth. Personal growth must precede professional growth because personal actions cannot be separated from professional ones.

A major aspect of growth is reflection. Reflection includes introspection and self-awareness related to one's strengths, challenges, and biases (Foronda et al., 2016; Lecours et al., 2021; Reiter et al., 2018). By aligning reflective practice with ethical and value-based principles, training, and experience, students and new therapists can alter attitudes and behaviors to create change. When added to evidence-based practice, these professional precursors create a professional who can be a trusted advocate for the client and community.

To facilitate reflective practice, individuals need structured feedback. Recognizing this, Ditwiler et al. (2021) developed the RISE tool to assess and facilitate student professional development. This tool has four categories of professionalism that are scored and ranked by the student and the clinical instructor. Each area is scored as "exemplary," "satisfactory," or "needs improvement." The student and clinical instructor provide examples of the student's positive and negative behaviors to support the scores and rankings. See Table 6.4 for an overview of the RISE Tool Categories and Sample Behaviors.

Lifelong Learning and Professional Development

Graduates of an accredited program must pass the national license examination and meet individual state requirements to become licensed. Although these newly licensed therapists have completed numerous hours of guided, rigorous education, they have ethical and legal obligations for ongoing professional development (Box 6.1). A professional development plan should focus on lifelong learning to maintain contemporary expertise (i.e., continuing competence) (Table 6.5). Developing a professional development plan is part of the transition to becoming a self-directed learner, a key characteristic of adult learners.

Professional development plans are fluid and will change as the therapist's career develops. Overall, the plan should be based on previous education, current interests, practice areas, gaps in knowledge, and organizational needs. Continued competence is a lifelong process, as healthcare practices are consistently evolving, and as evidence emerges, therapists must be committed to learning and utilizing new information. Thus lifelong learning via a professional development plan is part of being a professional. Although there are numerous continuing education opportunities for therapists, it is important to realize that these opportunities offer varying levels of structure. These opportunities are categorized as structured and unstructured.

TABLE 6.4	RISE Tool Categories and Sample Behaviors	
Professional Behavior	**Sample Positive Behaviors**	**Sample Negative Behaviors**
Respect for Others Demonstrates regard for and consideration of others	• Respectful verbal and non-verbal communication • Empathic interactions • Sensitivity to cultural and religious differences	• Overly informal behavior • Crossing professional boundaries • Discrimination
Integrity and Compliance Demonstrates trustworthiness and ability to follow laws, rules, and regulations	• Honesty • Following all laws, rules, and regulations • Admitting mistakes or omissions	• Misrepresenting self or qualifications • Cheating • Not following institutional policies and procedures
Self-awareness and Commitment to Development Demonstrates awareness of professional identity and commitment to improving performance	• Accepting and seeking feedback • Taking responsibility for actions • Seeks to fill gaps in knowledge	• Defensive behavior • Blaming external factors for actions • Poor insight into strengths and weaknesses
Engagement and Work Ethic Actively participates in and attends to tasks	• Timeliness for assigned activities • Performing to a high standard • Responsibility	• Tardiness • Not fulfilling academic or clinical course expectations • Escaping teamwork

From Ditwiler, R., Wagner, B., Swisher, L., & Anderson, S. (2021). DPT student professional behaviors in academic and clinical settings: Introducing a novel tool (RISE). *APTA CSM*, Virtual.

- License renewal is required biennially
- Continuing education requirements to maintain licensure
  - 20–40 biennially
- Approval or authorization required for courses
- Specified allotments of hours that can be completed online
- Required hours for legal and ethical principles of practice

From Licensing Authorities Contact Information. (2022). Federation of State Boards of Physical Therapy. https://www.fsbpt.org/Free-Resources/Licensing-Authorities-Contact-Information; Occupational therapy profession-continuing competence requirements. (2022). https://www.aota.org/-/media/corporate/files/advocacy/licensure/stateregs/contcomp/continuing-competence-chart-summary.pdf.

Structured Opportunities: Residencies and Fellowships

Unlike physicians, therapists must elect to complete a residency. Residencies facilitate the development of novice practitioners to enhance their skills and, ultimately, achieve recognition as a specialist via advanced certification (see Specialist or Advanced Certification section). Residency training has been emphasized in the physical therapy literature as residencies provide *structured mentorship* that continuing education courses cannot (Godges, 2004). Residencies help new clinicians acquire additional clinical skills and knowledge, as well as exposure to education techniques, research, and leadership (American Board of Physical Therapy Education Residency and Fellowship [ABPTRFE], 2020). Table 6.6 provides examples of residencies.

An additional postprofessional opportunity for therapists is fellowship training. Fellowships utilize structured mentorship to facilitate the development of advanced practitioners around competencies such as knowledge, critical reasoning, interpersonal abilities, performance skills, and leadership (ABPTRFE. 2020; AOTA, 2005). Fellowships go beyond residencies to help more experienced clinicians focus on subspecialty areas of clinical practice, education, or research. Overall, fellows-in-training are afforded focused time to acquire expertise and hone their leadership skills in their subspecialty. Table 6.6 provides examples of fellowships.

Structured Opportunities: Postprofessional Degrees

A postprofessional degree is a structured educational experience attained after professional training (APTA, 2021). Professional degrees help students prepare for careers such as medicine (e.g., MD, DO), law (JD), or education. Occupational and physical therapists graduate with professional degrees (e.g., MOT, OTD, DPT). In contrast, advanced academic degrees typically focus on a specific field of study, are research-oriented, and require a thesis or dissertation to graduate (e.g., MS, PhD). Common advanced academic degrees that therapists seek are highlighted in Table 6.7.

The highest degree earned in a profession or field is a *terminal degree* (e.g., a master's or doctoral degree). For example, common terminal academic degrees are the doctor of philosophy (PhD) and a doctorate in education (EdD). In contrast, common terminal professional degrees are doctorates such as the DPT, OTD, MD, DDS, PharmD, or a master's degree for professionals such as physician assistants.

Unstructured Opportunities

Unstructured activities are driven by the professional. These include completing academic courses not part of a degree program, journal clubs, on-the-job training, mentoring, working on professional committees, or acting as a clinical instructor. One of the most common unstructured professional development activities among practicing therapists is continuing education courses. In addition, it is not uncommon for therapists to seek certification as part of their professional development.

Continuing Education Courses

The most cited barrier to nonparticipation in continuing education activities is a lack of money or time (Merriam et al., 2007). To address these concerns, some facilities host continuing education courses onsite, while others may contract with online healthcare continuing education companies

TABLE 6.5	Professional Development, Lifelong Learning, and Continuing Competence	
Competence	• The possession and application of contemporary knowledge, skills, and abilities commensurate with an individual's role within the context of public health, welfare, and safety
Continuing Competence	• The ongoing possession and application of contemporary knowledge, skills, and abilities commensurate with an individual's role within the context of public health, welfare, and safety and defined by a scope of practice and practice setting
Lifelong Learning	• The ongoing maintenance and improvement of knowledge, skills, and abilities through one's professional career or working life
Professional Development	• The ongoing self-assessment, acquisition, and application of knowledge, skills, and abilities that meet or exceed contemporary performance standards

TABLE 6.6 Examples of Occupational and Physical Therapist Residencies and Fellowships

PT Residencies	PT Fellowships	OT Fellowships
• Acute Care	• Critical Care	• Acute and Critical Care
• Cardiovascular & Pulmonary	• Hand Therapy	• Assistive Technology
• Clinical Electrophysiology	• Movement System	• Burns
• Geriatrics	• Neonatology	• Dysphagia
• Neurology	• Orthopedic Manual Physical Therapy	• Gerontology
• Oncology	• Performing Arts	• Hand Therapy and Upper Extremity
• Orthopedics	• Spine	• Lymphedema
• Pediatrics	• Sports Division 1	• Mental Health
• Sports	• Upper Extremity Athlete	• Neurology
• Women's Health	• Higher Education Leadership	• Pediatrics
• Wound Management		• Physical Rehabilitation

OT, Occupational therapist; *PT*, physical therapist.
From American Occupational Therapy Association (AOTA). (2022). *Fellowship directory*. https://www.aota.org/career/career-center/fellowship-program/fellowship-directory; American Board of Physical Therapy Education Residency and Fellowship. (2022). *For physical therapist residency and fellowship participants or prospective participants*. https://abptrfe.apta.org/for-participants

TABLE 6.7 Examples of Advanced Academic Degrees

Master of Business Administration (MBA)	• Study of finance, accounting, marketing, economics, and management
Master of Health Administration (MHA)	• Study of legal, technical, and ethical of the healthcare industry
Master of Public Administration (MPA)	• Study of organizational theory, policy, budgeting, human resources, management, strategic planning, and statistics
Doctor of Philosophy (PhD)	• Study of skills to perform research within and outside academic institutions
Doctor of Education (EdD)	• Study of education, curriculum, and educational leadership
Doctor of Health Science (DHS) Doctor of Science (ScD or DSc)	• Academic doctorates similar to PhD and EdD

(O'Neil et al., 2009). Although these strategies save time and money, they may limit educational opportunities.

Overall, therapists and organizations need to be cautious when selecting continuing education courses. The quality of continuing education courses (i.e., evidence-based) should be thoroughly vetted before any potential investments, especially considering how these educational activities will impact therapists, the facility, and their patients (Leahy et al., 2017; Peterson et al., 2022).

Unfortunately, numerous poor-quality continuing education courses exist, including predatory courses, conferences, and journals that target unsuspecting consumers (*Questionable Conferences*, 2021). The APTA and AOTA sponsor and endorse conferences throughout the year. Therapists unsure of a course or conference's validity are encouraged to utilize the resources within their national organizations.

Specialist or Advanced Certification

The AOTA has identified board certification and specialty certification options for occupational therapists. The purpose of board certification is recognition of an advanced skill set and experience in a particular practice area beyond entry-level (Table 6.8). In order to establish this board certification, you must be certified or licensed for at least 3 years as an occupational therapist in good standing and have obtained at least 3000 hours within 5 years in a particular practice area, with 500 of those hours acquired with direct service delivery to clients. The occupational therapist must apply for the certification and, in most instances, take a board exam. This process has changed; those interested should verify current requirements via AOTA.org.

Specialty certifications for the occupational therapist established a commitment to developing an advanced skill set and experience in a particular practice area (Table 68). The requirements for these specialty certifications are under review, and professional certificates and microcredentials are being considered. Therapists interested in more information should refer to AOTA.org.

The American Physical Therapy Association recognizes board-certified clinical specialists in 10 practice areas governed by the American Board of Physical Therapy

TABLE 6.8	AOTA and APTA Certifications	
AOTA	**APTA Specialist Certification - Governed by ABPTS**
Advanced Certifications • Board certification in gerontology • Board certification in mental health • Board certification in pediatrics • Board certification in physical rehabilitation	**Board-Certified Clinical Specialists** • Cardiovascular and pulmonary physical therapy • Clinical electrophysiologic physical therapy • Geriatric physical therapy • Neurologic physical therapy • Oncologic physical therapy • Orthopedic physical therapy • Pediatric physical therapy • Sports physical therapy • Women's health physical therapy • Wound management physical therapy
Specialty Certifications • Driving and community mobility • Environmental modification • Feeding, eating and swallowing • Low vision • School systems	

AOTA, American Occupational Therapy Association; *APTA*, American Physical Therapy Association; *ABPTS*, American Board of Physical Therapy Specialty Certification.
From American Occupational Therapy Association (AOTA). (2022). *AOTA's advanced certification program.* AOTA. https://www.aota.org/career/advanced-certification-program; *Become a board-certified specialist.* (2022). APTA Specialist Certification - Governed by ABPTS. https://specialization.apta.org/become-a-specialist; American Occupational Therapy Association (AOTA). (2022). *Specialty certified occupational therapy practitioners.* https://www.aota.org/career/advanced-certification-program/specialty-certified-practitioners.

Specialties (ABPTS) (*Become a Board-Certified Specialist*, 2022). Board certification is a voluntary process that allows therapists to demonstrate advanced knowledge and skill within their chosen specialty beyond that of an entry-level clinician. A physical therapist must hold a current license to practice within the United States to obtain certification. The certification process requires a candidate to demonstrate evidence of a minimum of 2000 hours of clinical practice within their specialty area or complete an APTA-accredited postprofessional clinical residency within the specialty area. Once these requirements are complete, the candidate may apply to take the board examination.

These board examinations are designed to test advanced knowledge, clinical skills, and reasoning, including patient care, teaching, administration, consultation, communication, and interpretation of research. Once obtained, board certification is valid for 10 years. During those 10 years, board-certified specialists are expected to participate in activities for the maintenance of specialist certification (MOSC). MOSC requires specialists to meet requirements every three years with evidence of continued patient care, continuing education, publications, presentations, clinical supervision, research, clinical instruction, or teaching. In year 10, specialists must pass an exam to maintain their certification. Board-certified physical therapists can use the credentials listed in Table 6.8. The APTA no longer recognizes the use of abbreviations for board-certified clinical specialists (e.g., CCS, OCS). See Table 6.9 for the APTA's House of Delegates policy for appropriate use of designations.

Other Certifications

Many nationally and internationally recognized specialty certifications exist, open to occupational and physical therapists and, in some instances, other disciplines (Table 6.10). It is imperative that therapists thoroughly investigate the specialty and certification for recognition and legitimacy. Due to the rigor of physical and occupational therapists' entry-level education, most certifications do not expand their ability to practice beyond what is already included in their license. That is, the certification may offer recognition and expansion of one skill set; however, individuals could perform the same skills without certification, putting the legitimacy of many certifications for physical and occupational therapists in question.

Some states require additional training, certification, or endorsement for things such as spinal manipulation, dry needling, telehealth, imaging, physical agent modalities and direct access. Therapists should refer to their state practice act to identify practice areas requiring additional education or training. Lastly, some programs require therapists to complete their training and become certified through their organization to advertise the use of a proprietary treatment method or materials.

Mentoring

Mentoring in healthcare is characterized by an interpersonal relationship between a more experienced professional and a willing protégé. This relationship may include knowledge sharing, guidance, and emotional support. Mentoring in physical and occupational therapy is vital to personal and

TABLE 6.9	APTA's House of Delegates Policy for Appropriate Use of Designations

- 1st designation: symbolizes you are a licensed PT
  - PT
- 2nd designation: highest earned physical therapy-related degree
  - DPT, MPT, MSPT, BSPT
- 3rd designation: other regulatory designation(s) issued by government entities
  - APN, ATC, CRNP, LMSW, NP, OTR/L, RN, SLP
- 4th designation: other earned academic degree(s)
  - PhD, EdD, MBA, MS, MA
- 5th designation (optional): FAPTA
  - APTA no longer recognizes ABPTS abbreviations (e.g., OCS, CCS)

Compliant With House Policy	Noncompliant With House Policy
• William VanWye, PT, DPT, PhD Board-Certified Clinical Specialist in Cardiovascular and Pulmonary Physical Therapy	• William VanWye, PT, DPT, PhD, CCS
• Holly Fowler, PT, DPT, FAPTA Certified Hand Therapist	• Holly Fowler, PT, DPT, CHT, FAPTA
• Melissa Goodman, PT, DPT	• Melissa Goodman, DPT

TABLE 6.10	Other Selected Certifications

Certification	Organization and Notes
Certified wound specialist	• American Board of Wound Management
Certified hand therapist	• Hand Certification Commission
Certified lymphedema therapist	• Lymphology Association of North America • Academy of Lymphatic Studies
Assistive technology professional	• Rehabilitation Engineering and Assistive Technology Society of North America
Certified driver rehabilitation specialist	• Association of Driver Rehabilitation Specialists

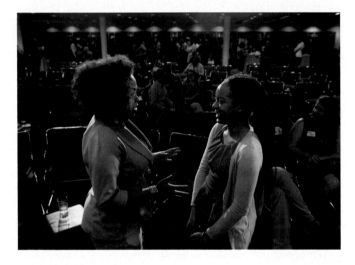

• **Fig. 6.7** Mentorship is vital to personal and professional growth. (From https://www.flickr.com/photos/100836534@N04/34717248966).

professional growth and advances the professions (Fig. 6.7). Several other benefits to mentoring and the mentoring process have been identified in the literature across disciplines. There is an increase in overall job satisfaction, organization loyalty, discipline retention, and socialization into the respective professions. Mentoring aids in professional competency, socializes a new or recent graduate into their chosen profession, and can foster a sense of belonging.

Professional Socialization, Belonging, and Mentorship

"Begin with the end in mind."

This quote from Stephen Covey, author of the acclaimed book *"7 Habits of Highly Effective People,"* speaks to the intentional process of identifying the specific outcome of a personal or professional pursuit (Covey, 2013). Applying this quote for yourself, imagine that you are nearing the end of your professional career, having spent a considerable portion of your life navigating the educational process, developing expertise, scaling the promotional ladder, and accruing an arsenal of memorable experiences and meaningful relationships. You are encouraged to write down your answers to the questions in Box 6.2, giving your mind free range to think boldly and courageously.

Answering such questions may seem frivolous; however, the findings from neuroscience suggest that persons who write down their goals are 1.2–1.4 times more likely to achieve them (Murphy, 2018). Writing creates a visual record of your goals, enabling you to picture what is important to you. Putting your goals on paper further cements them in your memory, generating motivation and commitment while enhancing the consistent attentional focus needed for goal attainment.

• BOX 6.2   Personal or Professional Pursuit Questions

- What specific accomplishments would you like to achieve in your career?
- What challenges might you face along the way?
- How will you measure your success?
- What do you hope your patients and colleagues would say about your interactions?

• BOX 6.3   Professional Identity Essay (PIE)

Instructions: Please answer these questions as fully as possible in 1 hour. Write at least a paragraph for each question.
1. What does being a member of the physical or occupational therapy profession mean to you? How did you come to this understanding?
2. What do you expect of yourself as you work towards becoming a full-fledged physical or occupational therapist?
3. What will the profession expect of you?
4. What conflicts do you experience or expect to experience between your responsibility to yourself and others—patients, family, and profession? How do you resolve them?
5. What would be the worst thing for you if you failed to live up to the expectations you have set for yourself?
6. What would be the worst thing for you if you failed to live up to your patients' expectations?
7. What would be the worst thing for you if you failed to live up to what society expects of physical or occupational therapists? How did you come to this understanding?
8. Think of a physical or occupational therapist you consider an exemplar of professionalism. Describe why you chose this person, illustrating an incident or pattern of decisions or actions that support your choice.
9. Reflect on your experiences in physical or occupational therapy school or in the community that have been critical in fostering change in your understanding of what it means to be a professional physical or occupational therapist.
   You are invited to reflect on these questions, returning to them at the end of your educational journey.

How will you reach these goals? More importantly, how will you do so with the positivity, engagement, and relational support needed for a meaningful career that promotes pride and a sense of accomplishment? These elements, positivity, engagement, relationships, meaning, and accomplishment, have a wealth of evidence supporting their value as elements of human flourishing (Seligman, 2011). Your health profession's career will be devoted to fostering the optimal wellbeing of your patients and clients, and this process begins the moment you meet. How will you show up?

Professional Identity Formation

As an emerging health professional, questions about your career aspirations reflect the journey of assuming a profession's roles, privileges, and responsibilities. Inherent in this journey is the transformational process of claiming the profession's core values, behaviors, and beliefs as your own. This process, known as *professional identity formation*, has gained considerable attention in health professions education (Holden et al., 2012). Defined as the "the complex and transformational process of internalizing a profession's core values and beliefs," professional identity formation speaks to the intentional and gradual processes of aligning the individual and the professional as an inseparable whole, thus supporting the highest levels of expertise and ethical integrity in all interactions.

This professional identity journey enables a sense of professional agency through which your healthcare role is societally recognized, sought after, and valued. Successful navigation through this journey engenders the individual sense of pride and professional belonging that brings meaning and purpose to a professional career. In becoming a professional in today's healthcare system, therapists often face challenging ethical decisions around providing optimal personalized patient care amid organizational productivity requirements, third-party payor restrictions, and staff shortages. The stress of addressing such conflicts can lead to practitioner burnout, poor patient outcomes, and "ethical fading," the gradual lowering of one's moral standards (Edwards & Dirette, 2010; Tenbrunsel & Messick, 2004). A strong sense of professional identity (which includes the expectation for the highest levels of moral reasoning and ethical practice) measures our professional vision to "transform society by optimizing movement to improve the human experience" (APTA, 2019).

Professional identity formation can be assessed through 9 questions, collectively known as the professional identity essay (PIE) (Kalet et al., 2018). The PIE is a valid instrument, originally developed by Kegan (1982) to assess professional military cadets and recently adapted by Bebeau and Monson (2012) for use by medical students. The following PIE questions have been adapted for physical therapy students and practitioners and are illustrated in Box 6.3.

Belonging

A key element of your professional identity formation process is establishing a sense of belonging, characterized by feelings of acceptance and the affirmation of one's value by others in a group (Hirsch & Clark, 2019). As a future physical or occupational therapist, establishing belonging is a critical first step in validating your role as a healthcare professional, evolving through interpersonal connections. Far beyond the inherent satisfaction of developing relationships with like-minded individuals, the ability to secure meaningful connections is one of the most important predictors of lifelong health and wellbeing.

The Harvard Study of Adult Development (Harvard Second Generation Study, 2015) is one of the longest research projects on human wellbeing and continues as of this writing. This research sought to identify behaviors predicting healthy aging and wellbeing over time, beginning in 1938 with a cohort of 268 Harvard sophomores (and now their spouses and offspring). While many of the study's participants were highly successful in their chosen careers, this success came with high costs for some, including divorce, alcoholism, and mental illness.

What was the difference for those who could maintain productive careers without sacrificing their wellbeing and overall happiness? Strong social connections. What is the result of strong social connections? A sense of *belonging*.

The pathways to belonging as a healthcare professional or member of any group are multi-faceted, providing numerous opportunities to begin your professional identity formation journey. Hirsch and Clark (2019) describe four pathways to belonging, each providing the opportunity to develop a sense of worth and validation. These paths collectively reinforce and can be easily pursued in your educational journey. These pathways include *group memberships, communal relationships, minor sociability,* and *general approbation*. The following story can illustrate the manifestation of each pathway.

The Case of Len

Len has just begun physical therapy school. Having moved from another state to begin his education, he wants to fit in and feel accepted by his classmates. Friendly and outgoing, he tries to speak to his classmates in the first weeks of class. As these conversations ensue, Len feels at home among his class group. His classes further enhance this sentiment on professionalism, whereby Len begins to feel a sense of belonging to the physical therapy profession.

Feelings of belonging in a group with common interests and goals are examples of the *group membership pathway*, involving intentional membership, such as classmates in a physical therapy or occupational therapy program, or unintentional, such as finding common interests among neighbors. In the healthcare profession, joining your professional organization is a powerful example of the group membership pathway, whereby such membership provides further opportunities to strengthen the other routes to belonging. Many of us find our closest friends (and even our spouses) in the context of our group memberships, and these connections often begin during our health professions education, as our continuing story regarding Len illustrates.

As Len interacts with his classmates, he connects with Rachel and John, two classmates who share Len's passion for hiking and outdoor sports. Len invites Rachel and John for a weekend hike and they quickly become friends. Later in the semester, when Len's dad is unexpectedly hospitalized after a minor stroke, Rachel and John encourage him to return home for a visit, assuring him that they will take notes from their classes and offering help with studying for an upcoming exam. As the school year progresses, the three become each other's support system, enhancing Len's sense of belonging through the *communal relationship* pathway.

Considerable evidence supports the value of the communal relationship pathway as a facilitator of improved life satisfaction, high subjective wellbeing, and better overall health (Le et al., 2018). Communal relationships are typically developed over time and are characterized by "mutual responsiveness," an abiding and reciprocal concern for the welfare of those involved. Consider the friends you would do anything for in your life, whose accomplishments you celebrate, and whose disappointments evoke your deepest compassion. A wealth of evidence supports the value of close relationships as a health-enhancing behavior. A landmark systematic review of the health benefits of a strong social network among older adults was conducted in 2010 (Holt-Lunstad et al., 2010). The findings indicated that a network of close friends had a 50% greater likelihood of survival than those with poor or insufficient close connections.

Moreover, strong social connections provided equal benefits to quitting smoking and greater health protection than being obese or sedentary. The Gallup organization conducts regular national surveys of the factors associated with work engagement, characterized by employee involvement, enthusiasm, and commitment (Mann, 2018). One of the most important drivers of such engagement is having a "best friend" at work. Given that your current job is to engage in your professional studies, these findings are likely applicable in the educational setting. Now, back to Len.

Len continues to interact with other classmates through participation in laboratory sessions and various group projects. His classmates come to see him as a valued class member, electing him to serve as their class representative. The high esteem of Len's classmates is an example of the *general approbation pathway*, where belonging is enhanced by the admiration of his classmates and the recognition of Len's capacity for leadership.

Persons who strive for belonging through the general approbation pathway are often accomplishment-driven and skilled at connecting with other successful individuals. Many persons seek general approbation by posting their accomplishments on social media, seeking membership in prestigious groups, and acquiring material goods advertising their success. Successful politicians are well versed in their ability to secure general approbation, even without the ability to form close communal relationships. While some of these approaches may seem vain or superficial, self-awareness of one's intent (i.e., impressing others by showing off vs. getting the support of others to expand positive influence), an identified set of personal values, high moral standards, and a dose of humility can help us utilize this pathway in a healthy manner that empowers positive outcomes.

Finally, as Len becomes settled into his educational experience, his sense of belonging increases his self-esteem, another recognized indicator of belonging (MacDonald, 2012). Len now brings this increased self-esteem to the simplest interactions, making small talk with an increasing scope of mere acquaintances, smiling and chatting with the barista at the campus coffee shop, students in other educational fields, and people standing in line at the grocery store.

These day-to-day interactions are examples of the *minor sociability pathway*. The mutual exchange of these simple pleasantries has gained increasing evidence for its value in

---

BOX 6.4 Putting the Belonging Pathways in Action

Using Len as an example, will you consider making a concerted effort to:

- Become an active contributing member of your class community by reaching out to classmates beyond those you already know.
  - Explore common interests and seek opportunities to strengthen your class community.
- Join your professional organization (The APTA or AOTA).
  - In each organization, there are many opportunities for student involvement. Each organization sponsors numerous conferences and community activities as well. Explore these opportunities and set a goal for at least one specific professional activity each year.
- Make at least one close friend among your classmates.
  - These friendships often last a lifetime, sometimes providing professional growth opportunities. The physical and occupational therapy professions are relatively small, often relying on collegial connections for work references, promotions, and nominations for professional awards. Ask yourself what you hope your classmates will say about you after graduation.
- Approach everyday interactions with kindness and positivity.
  - Even the simplest questions, such as asking about someone's day, coupled with eye contact and a smile, can lift your spirits and those of others. More importantly, positively interacting with various people will be an essential skill for developing a therapeutic alliance with your future patients.
- Be humble in the face of accomplishments.
  - Few successes occur in a vacuum. Consider the persons who supported your efforts and share your gratitude. Connect your accomplishments to a greater good for the persons you are called to serve.

---

increasing general happiness and wellbeing. On a practical level, the ability to form a therapeutic bond with your patients generally begins through the minor sociability pathway, eventually expanding to the communal relationship essential for shared decision-making within the plan of care. You are encouraged to explore these four pathways to belonging, perhaps challenging yourself to engage in pathways that will positively support your self-efficacy as an engaged professional.

Putting the Belonging Pathways in Action

Awareness creates choice. By acknowledging the four pathways of belonging, you are now better positioned to integrate these into your professional identity formation process. How will you proceed (Box 6.4)?

The Importance of Mentorship

As you settle into your evolving physical or occupational therapist identity, you will likely interact with future colleagues in your classes, clinical settings, and professional meetings. As all humans do, you will likely engage in a subconscious assessment of these individuals, identifying their admirable traits and relating these to your ideal of the therapist you want to become.

Question 8 of the PIE addresses these traits by inviting you to think of a physical or occupational therapist you consider a model of professionalism. Furthermore, you are asked to describe why you chose this person, illustrating an incident or pattern of decisions or actions that support your choice. How did you answer this question? What traits or observed skills most resonated with your inner ideal? How can you integrate these in an authentic and meaningful way in the service of your future career?

Mentorship provides a powerful and often lifelong opportunity for such integration. By interacting with a more experienced individual whose traits and skills you admire, you may grow in ways you never thought possible. As you progress in your career, you may also mentor new professionals as a clinical instructor, where your impact can be a key motivator for selecting a clinical specialty or practice. Moreover, serving as a clinical instructor is a powerful way to develop your teaching skills, provide supervision, and enhance your clinical reasoning. Aristotle purportedly once said, "*Those who know, do. Those that understand, teach*" (Shulman, 1986). This statement underscores the rich learning that occurs in sharing your knowledge.

"Mentor" arises from Greek mythology described in Homer's *Odyssey*. In this epic story, Mentor, an older warrior, was too old to fight in the Trojan war. Odysseus, another hero in Homer's tale, sends his young son, Telemachus, to Mentor's palace to learn the ways of valiant warriors. Hence comes the concept of a more experienced "mentor" supporting a less experienced one.

Mentorship is described as "a process through which an experienced person (mentor) guides another individual (mentee or protégé) in the development of skills and knowledge that enhance their professional development (Burgess et al., 2018). Although mentorship has existed for years, it has recently become an essential element of health professions education. There are many compelling reasons for this interest in mentorship.

First, the subtle complexities of the current healthcare system can be confusing and overwhelming to new professionals. These complexities are part of what is known as the "hidden curriculum," which relates to the set of spoken and unspoken influences affecting an organization and its culture (Lawrence et al., 2018). These influences can be positive, such as a culture that supports collaboration and learning to enhance patient care, or negative, such as a culture that values productivity and high revenue at the expense of patient care. In either case, these influences may not be obvious, and an experienced mentor can be instrumental in clarifying expectations and providing support when organizational assumptions are not in line with personal ones.

Second, an effective mentor can assist in developing and pursuing clear and attainable career goals, fostering their achievement by acting as a teacher, coach, counselor, and role model. By observing a skilled mentor in action, a new professional can begin to incorporate the expert skills that elevate the value of our interventions, the relational skills that enhance patient efficacy and wellbeing, and the execution of transformative leadership that inspires positive change.

Third, a good mentor can expedite the journey of professional identity formation by instilling values and by orienting mentees to the cultural, social, and relational elements of their profession. An effective mentor illuminates the privileges and opportunities in professional practice, bringing them to the forefront and generating excitement for realizing these possibilities.

Benefits of Mentorship

There is a significant body of evidence supporting the benefits of mentorship for both parties (Burgess et al., 2018). The mentor and mentee grow and develop throughout the mentoring process, suggesting a bidirectional impact that can be enjoyed at any point in one's career. Benefits to the mentee include increased self-efficacy (i.e., pursuing a goal confidently), increased work satisfaction, enhanced networking opportunities, improved productivity, and protection against burnout. Studies of medical students in mentoring programs demonstrated greater personal growth, career satisfaction, and a higher passing rate on medical board exams. Mentors have been shown to play a critical role in choosing a specialty, a factor often cited by physical and occupational therapy students. Mentors also benefit through greater personal and professional satisfaction, often learning new skills (i.e., the use of emerging interventions and technologies). These benefits are so valuable that mentorship has been identified as a wellness intervention among physicians (Shanafelt et al., 2017).

Connecting With a Mentor

Like any satisfying relationship, strong evidence suggests that mentorship works best when there is a genuine connection between mentor and mentee. This connection is based on similar values, interests, and personality traits. Kilgallon and Thompson (2012) identify three key considerations; attraction, affect, and action in selecting a mentor.

First, the mentee must feel *attracted to their mentor, acknowledging a set of traits and behaviors* they want to emulate. For example, when Karen was in physical therapy school, she had no idea about the direction of her career in an area of specialization. This perception changed during her first rehabilitation internship, where Karen was captivated by the vivacious personality of her clinical instructor Julie. This sentiment was enhanced as she observed Julie's passion for each patient encounter, using her warmth and humor to encourage their progress. Not surprisingly, Julie's patients achieved outcomes Karen never thought possible, expanding her appreciation for physical therapy intervention's life-changing possibilities. As a mentor, Julie approached her interactions with the same purposeful energy, leading Karen to choose neurologic rehabilitation as a clinical specialty.

The second consideration in selecting a mentor is *affect.* Mentors should be approachable and encouraging. As you identify potential mentors, it can be helpful to engage them in an area of mutual interest. For example, after Sheila presented a guest lecture on hand splinting in one of Mary's occupational therapy school courses, Mary sent Sheila an email sharing her appreciation for the presentation and asking a thoughtful question about the topic. Sheila responded enthusiastically, beginning a mentoring relationship that resulted in an offer of employment that enabled Mary and Sheila to interact more directly. Years later, they count each other among their closest friends.

The third element is *action.* In a successful mentoring relationship, both parties take an active role. Mentors need to be willing to invest the time and energy needed to support the mentee's development. They must be able to provide a safe and comfortable learning environment, involving the mentee in their activities as appropriate and identifying helpful resources needed for the mentee to achieve their goals. Mentors should advocate for their mentees when needed, offering networking opportunities and introductions to colleagues for mentee follow-up if desired. Good mentors engage their mentees in self-reflection, providing useful feedback and suggestions for continued development. They also encourage their mentees to set high but realistic standards for themselves while providing the resources, guidance, and advice needed for their achievement (Fulton, 2013).

The mentee should also be an active participant in the mentoring process. They should demonstrate a willingness to learn, a desire to grow, and a positive, growth-minded perspective. Good mentees respect the mentor's time, clearly identifying their goals, expectations, and ideas for how they will meet these. They should take the initiative to prepare for discussions with their mentor, offering their ideas and resources and following up on any commitments.

Finding a Mentor

Your didactic and clinical education experiences will offer numerous opportunities to interact with bright, passionate, and deeply engaged clinicians. Pay attention to whatever excites you; this could be new content presented in a class or conference, a faculty member or speaker who teaches in a style you admire, or a clinical instructor who seamlessly connects with their patients even in the most challenging situations. Let these individuals know how they captured your interest and what you admired; ask a thoughtful question and provide your insights; offer a resource that may be helpful. Let them know your goals and interests. Initial overtures like these may lead to thoughtful interactions and a mentoring relationship.

Knowing the importance of mentorship, you are encouraged to ask about related opportunities after graduation when seeking your first professional position. Specifically, how are new professionals supported when they join the practice? What mentorship opportunities exist in the organization? You should also consider active membership in your professional organization (i.e., APTA or AOTA). Both of these organizations provided numerous opportunities for networking and connecting with colleagues from a wide range of backgrounds. Many state chapters of these organizations have special interest groups (SIGS) or special interest sections (SIS) for new professionals (defined as 0–5 years of experience). These SIGS/SIS often sponsor webinars and podcasts on various important topics that provide a form of collective mentorship and the opportunity to share helpful experiences and resources.

Models of Mentorship

Although an ideal mentoring relationship is based on a shared attraction and subsequent connection, other valuable forms can yield similar benefits. In the classic mentoring model, there is an intentional pairing between experienced and lesser experienced individuals to achieve a specific outcome for the mentee. For example, residencies and fellowships are valuable pathways toward developing expertise. In such experiences, there are shared responsibilities for both mentors and mentees. Consistent communication, mentee accountability, initiative, and self-reflection are all essential for the success of this model.

Many organizations also utilize *group mentorship* models, involving one or more mentors working with several individuals. These models are often used as an efficient way to onboard new employees while providing support for the challenges involved. *Peer-to-peer mentorship* is often used in clinical education, where two or more students work under the same clinical instructor. In this model, the students support and coach each other, sharing their knowledge and skills. Health professions students often form peer study groups that enable a broader range of perspectives that enhance collective learning. You may have found yourself involved in such groups, and success depends on sustained, focused attention to the required learning. Many study groups fail when side conversations or social agendas interfere. *Reverse mentorship* started in the 1990s when Jack Welch, the CEO of General Electric, decided to have younger employees mentor older ones on the effective use of technology. One of the most valuable benefits of serving as a clinical instructor is learning about the emerging content being delivered in professional education programs. Lastly, in *speed mentoring*, the mentor and mentee meet briefly to focus on a specific skill. Meetings are centered on the task to be accomplished, the information needed, and the best strategies for achievement. No matter the model, mentorship can provide a tremendous advantage to your professional identity development, and you are encouraged to seek such opportunities throughout your career.

Why Mentoring Relationships Fail

Besides poor communication, personality differences, and lack of commitment, competition between mentor and mentee can become problematic, typically when the mentee's skills begin to eclipse the mentor's, resulting in feelings of threat. Having clear goals and expectations for the mentoring relationship can help set boundaries. When challenges arise, noting this objectively and early can forestall further difficulties. Given the value of mentorship, it is no surprise that the APTA House of Delegates passed a 2018 motion outlining best practices for mentorship (Box 6.5) (APTA, 2018).

• BOX 6.5   APTA Best Practices for Mentorship

- Acclimating the mentee into the culture and values of physical therapy;
- Actively promoting to physical therapist colleagues the importance of the Code of Ethics for the Physical Therapist and Core Values for the Physical Therapist as critical components of a doctoring profession;
- Actively promoting to physical therapist assistant colleagues the importance of Values-Based Behaviors for the Physical Therapist Assistant as a model of expected behaviors;
- Being open to working as a mentor to the mentee;
- Clarifying expectations and instilling accountability for support of APTA's positions, standards, guidelines, policies, and procedures;
- Creating a collegial atmosphere that provides responsiveness and respect for the mentee;
- Consistently demonstrating best practices in physical therapy;
- Seeking training and education to further skills in mentoring;
- Modeling and promoting the importance of membership and active participation in APTA and its components;
- Encouraging leadership development in the mentee's chosen arena.
- The responsibilities of mentees include, but are not limited to:
  - Identifying knowledge and skill gaps;
  - Establishing career goals for lifelong learning, both short term, and long term;
  - Identifying specific experiential opportunities (e.g., presentation, clinical research); and,
  - Identifying potential junior and senior mentors who may be physical therapists, physical therapist assistants, or others who have compatible interest.

Discussion and Activities

1. What were the major factors affecting the evolution of occupational and physical therapy professions?
2. What characteristics make up a profession? A professional?
3. Make a side-by-side list comparing an occupation with a profession.
4. Why does it take nearly 20 years for evidence to change practice?
5. Discuss the pros and cons of structured and unstructured learning opportunities.
6. Do you think mentorship is important?
7. What might prevent you from seeking mentorship?
8. Develop a professional development plan.

References

American Board of Physical Therapy Education Residency and Fellowship. (2020, January 1). *Part III: Quality standards for clinical physical therapist residency and fellowship programs.* https://abptrfe.apta.org/for-programs/clinical-programs/quality-standards-clinical.

American Board of Physical Therapy Education Residency and Fellowship (ABPTRFE). (2022). *For physical therapist residency and fellowship participants or prospective participants.* https://abptrfe.apta.org/for-participants.

American Occupational Therapy Association. (n.d.). *OT's role in shaping contexts and environments.* Retrieved from August 28,

2023. https://www.aota.org/advocacy/everyday-advocacy/ots-role-in-shaping-contexts-and-environments.

American Occupational Therapy Association. (1925). An outline of lectures on occupational therapy to medical students and physicians. *Occupational Therapy and Rehabilitation, 4*(3), 280–281.

American Occupational Therapy Association (AOTA). (1958). Report of the project committee on recognition of OT assistants. *The American Journal of Occupational Therapy, 12*, 38–39.

American Occupational Therapy Association. (1974). Medicare coverage for occupational therapy services. American Journal of Occupational Therapy, 28, 109–110.

American Occupational Therapy Association. (1977). 1977 Representative Assembly—Resolution A, Principles of occupational therapy ethics. *American Journal of Occupational Therapy, 31*, 594.

American Occupational Therapy Association. (1986). RA Minutes: Autonomous certification board resolution adopted. *American Journal of Occupational Therapy, 40*, 852.

American Occupational Therapy Association (1993). RA Minutes: Independent accreditation agency. *American Journal of Occupational Therapy, 47*, 1123.

American Occupational Therapy Association (AOTA). (2005). Standards for continuing competence. *The American Journal of Occupational Therapy, 59*(6), 661–662.

American Occupational Therapy Association. (2019). *Special task force report: Executive summary.* https://www.aota.org/-/media/Corporate/Files/AboutAOTA/BOD/Special-Task-Force-February-2019-Summary-Report.pdf

American Occupational Therapy Association. (2020). Occupational therapy practice framework: Domain and process (4th ed.). *The American Journal of Occupational Therapy, 74*(Suppl. 2), 7412410010.

American Occupational Therapy Association (AOTA). (2021). Standards of practice for occupational therapy. *The American Journal of Occupational Therapy, 75*(Supplement_3), 7513410030.

American Occupational Therapy Association (AOTA). (2022). *AOTA's advanced certification program.* AOTA. https://www.aota.org/career/advanced-certification-program.

American Physical Therapy Association (APTA). (2012). *Professional development, lifelong learning, and continuing competence in physical therapy.* https://www.apta.org/uploadedFiles/APTAorg/About_Us/Policies/HOD/Professional_Development/ProfessionalDev.pdf.

American Physical Therapy Association. (2018). *Disciplinary action procedural document.* https://www.apta.org/apta-and-you/leadership-and-governance/policies/disciplinary-action-procedural-document.

American Physical Therapy Association. (2019, September 25). *Vision statement for the physical therapy profession.* https://www.apta.org/apta-and-you/leadership-and-governance/policies/vision-statement-for-the-physical-therapy-profession.

American Physical Therapy Association (APTA). (2020a). *Appropriate use of designations.* https://www.apta.org/apta-and-you/leadership-and-governance/policies/appropriate-use-of-designations.

American Physical Therapy Association (APTA). (2020b) *100 Milestones of physical therapy – APTA centennial.* https://centennial.apta.org/centennial-timeline/.

American Physical Therapy Association (APTA). (2021a). *APTA centennial: The clinical doctorate (or "DPT") becomes the only degree conferred by CAPTE-accredited educational institutions.* https://centennial.apta.org/timeline/the-clinical-doctorate-or-dpt-becomes-the-only-degree-conferred-by-capte-accredited-educational-institutions/.

American Physical Therapy Association (APTA). (2021b). *APTA guide to physical therapist practice.* https://guide.apta.org/.

American Physical Therapy Association (APTA). (2021c). *Post-professional degree.* https://www.apta.org/your-career/career-advancement/postprofessional-degree.

American Physical Therapy Association (APTA). (2022*). Evidence-based practice resources.* https://www.apta.org/patient-care/evidence-based-practice-resources.

Anderson, L., Reed, K. (2017). The history of occupational therapy: The first century. Thorofare, NJ: Slack Incorporated.

AOTA Board of Directors. (2014). *Position statement on entry-level degree for the occupational therapist.* https://www.aota.org/AboutAOTA/Get-Involved/ BOD/OTD-Statement.aspx

Atler, K., & Stephens, J. (2020). Pilot use of the adapted Fresno test for evaluating evidence-based practice knowledge in occupational therapy students. *American Journal of Occupational Therapy, 74*, 7404205100.

Autonomous Physical Therapist Practice. (2012, August 8). *Autonomous physical therapist practice.* American Physical Therapy Association. https://www.apta.org/apta-and-you/leadership-and-governance/policies/autonomous-pt-practice.

Barrett, C. M. (2021). *Dreeben-Irimia's introduction to physical therapist practice for physical therapist assistants* (4th ed.). Jones & Bartlett Learning.

Barrimore, S. E., Cameron, A. E., Young, A. M., Hickman, I. J., & Campbell, K. L. (2020). Translating research into practice: How confident are allied health clinicians? *Journal of Allied Health, 49*(4), 258–262.

Bauer, M. S., Damschroder, L., Hagedorn, H., Smith, J., & Kilbourne, A. M. (2015). An introduction to implementation science for the non-specialist. *BioMed Central Psychology, 3*(32), 1–12.

Bebeau, M. J., & Monson, V. E. (2012). Professional identity formation and transformation across the life span. In A. Mc Kee & M. Eraut (Eds.), *Learning trajectories, innovation and identity for professional development* (pp. 135–162). Springer Netherlands.

Become a Board-Certified Specialist. (2022). *APTA Specialist Certification - Governed by ABPTS.* https://specialization.apta.org/become-a-specialist.

Becoming a physical therapist. (2021). American Physical Therapy Association. https://www.apta.org/your-career/careers-in-physical-therapy/becoming-a-pt

Bennett, S., Laver, K., & Clemson, L. (2018). Progressing knowledge translation in occupational therapy. *Australian Occupational Therapy Journal, 65*(2), 156–160.

Best practice in mentoring in physical therapy. (2018, August 30). APTA. https://www.apta.org/apta-and-you/leadership-and-governance/policies/best-practice-in-mentoring-in-physical-therapy.

Bing, R. K. (1981). Eleanor Clarke Slagle Lectureship–1981. Occupational therapy revisited: A paraphrastic journey. *The American Journal of Occupational Therapy: Official Publication of the American Occupational Therapy Association, 35*(8), 499–518.

Bloom's Taxonomy. (n.d.). *What is Bloom's Taxonomy?* https://bloomstaxonomy.net/.

Brown, C. (2017). *The evidence-based practitioner: Applying research to meet client needs.* FA Davis.

Burgess, A., van Diggele, C., & Mellis, C. (2018). Mentorship in the health professions: A review. *The Clinical Teacher, 15*(3), 197–202.

Chisholm, D. & Schell, B. A. B. (2019). Overview of the occupational therapy process and outcomes. In B. A. B. Schell & G. Gillen (Eds.). *Willard and Spackman's occupational therapy* (13th ed., pp. 352–368). Wolters Kluwer.

CINHAL. (2022). *CINAHL Database.* https://www.ebsco.com/products/research-databases/cinahl-database.

Cochrane. (2022). *Cochrane.* www.cochrane.org.

Covey, S. R. (2013). *The 7 habits of highly effective people: Powerful lessons in personal change (25th anniversary edition).* Simon & Schuster.

Crable, J., Farrar, M. E., & Patmon, F. (2020). Evidence-based practice knowledge, attitudes, practices, and barriers: A nurse survey. *Nursing Critical Care, 15*(5). 24–32.

Ditwiler, R., Wagner, B., Swisher, L., & Anderson, S. (2021). *DPT student professional behaviors in academic and clinical settings: Introducing a novel tool (RISE)*. APTA CSM, Virtual.

Dunton, W. R. (1918). The principles of occupational therapy. *Public Health Nurse, 18*, 316–321.

Eames, S., Bennett, S., Whitehead, M., Fleming, J., Low, S. O., Mickan, S., & Caldwell, E. (2018). A pre-post evaluation of a knowledge translation capacity-building intervention. *Australian Occupational Therapy Journal, 65*(6). 479–493.

Edwards, H. & Dirette, D. (2010). The relationship between professional identity and burnout among occupational therapists. *Occupational Therapy in Health Care, 24*(2), 119–129.

ERIC. (n.d.). *FAQ Home*. https://eric.ed.gov/?faq.

Federation of State Boards of Physical Therapy. (2009). *Ethics remediation*. https://www.fsbpt.org/Secondary-Pages/Licensees/Ethical-Conduct/Ethics-Remediation.

Fetters, L., & Tilson, J. (2012). *Evidence based physical therapy*. F. A. Davis Company.

Foronda, C., Baptiste, D. L., Reinholdt, M. M., & Ousman, K. (2016). Cultural humility: A concept analysis. *Journal of Transcultural Nursing: Official Journal of the Transcultural Nursing Society, 27*(3), 210–217.

Fritz, J., & Flynn, T. W. (2005). Autonomy in physical therapy: Less is more. *The Journal of Orthopaedic and Sports Physical Therapy, 35*(11), 696–698.

Fulton, J. (2013). Mentorship: Excellence in the mundane. *British Journal of Healthcare Assistants, 7*, 142–145.

Gillette, N., & Kielhofner, G. (1979). The impact of specialization on the professionalization and survival of occupational therapy. *American Journal of Occupational Therapy, 33*, 21–28.

Godges, J. J. (2004). Mentorship in physical therapy practice. *Journal of Orthopaedic & Sports Physical Therapy, 34*(1), 1–3.

Granger, B. B. (2020). Life after PICOT: Taking the next step in a clinical inquiry project. *AACN Advanced Critical Care, 31*(1), 92–97.

Greathouse, D. G., Young, B. A., & Shaffer, S. W. (2021). US military physical therapy: 1970–2020. *Physical Therapy, 101*(3), pzab087.

Hachtel, Y., & Plummer, T. (2015). Leadership in academic settings. In S. B. Dunbar & K. Winston (Eds.), *An occupational perspective on leadership: Theoretical and practical dimensions*. (2nd ed., pp. 149–165). SLACK.

Halle, M. C., Bussières, A., Asseraf-Pasin, L., Storr, C., Mak, S., Root, K., & Thomas, A. (2021). Building evidence-based practice competencies among rehabilitation students: A qualitative exploration of faculty and preceptors' perspectives. *Advances in Health Sciences Education, 26*, 1311–1338.

Harvard Second Generation Study. (2015). *Harvardstudy*. https://www.adultdevelopmentstudy.org.

Harvey-Krefting, L. (1985). The concept of work in occupational therapy: A historical review. *The American Journal of Occupational Therapy, 39*(5), 301–307.

Health Insurance Association of America. (1984). Health Insurance Association of America: Update on occupational therapy. *American Journal of Occupational Therapy, 38*, 341–343.

Hirsch, J. L., & Clark, M. S. (2019). Multiple paths to belonging that we should study together. *Perspectives on Psychological Science, 14*(2), 238–255.

Hissong, A. N., Lape, J. E., & Bailey, D. M. (2015). *Research for the health professional* (3rd ed.). F. A. Davis Company.

Holden, M., Buck, E., Clark, M., Szauter, K., & Trumble, J. (2012). Professional identity formation in medical education: The convergence of multiple domains. *HEC forum: An Interdisciplinary Journal on Hospitals' Ethical And Legal Issues, 24*(4), 245–255.

Holm, M. B. (2000). Our mandate for the new millennium: Evidence-based practice, 2000 Eleanor Clarke Slagle lecture. *American Journal of Occupational Therapy, 54*, 575–585.

Holt-Lunstad, J., Smith, T. B., & Layton, J. B. (2010). Social relationships and mortality risk: A meta-analytic review. *PLoS Medicine, 7*(7), e1000316.

Howick, J., Chalmers, I., Glasziou, P., Greenhalgh, T., Heneghan, C., Liberati, A., Moschetti, I., Phillips, B., & Thornton, H. *The 2011 Oxford CEBM Evidence Levels of Evidence (Introductory Document)*. Oxford Centre for Evidence-Based Medicine. https://www.cebm.ox.ac.uk/resources/levels-of-evidence/levels-of-evidence-introductory-document.

Jensen, G. M. (2011). 42nd Mary McMillan Lecture: Learning: What matters most. *Journal of the American Physical Therapy Association, 91*(11), 1674–1689.

Johnson, J. A. (1975). Nationally speaking: Res.400-74 on licensure. *American Journal of Occupational Therapy, 29*, 73.

Johnson, S. G., Titlestad, K. B., Larun, L., Ciliska, D., & Olsen, N. R. (2021). Experiences with using a mobile application for learning evidence-based practice in health and social care education: An interpretive descriptive study. *PLoS One, 16*(7), e0254272.

Johnson, M. P., & Abrams, S. L. (2005). Historical perspectives of autonomy within the medical profession: Considerations for 21st century physical therapy practice. *The Journal of Orthopaedic and Sports Physical Therapy, 35*(10), 628–636.

Juckett, L. A., Robinson, M. L., Malloy, J., & Oliver, H. V. (2021). Health policy perspectives—Translating knowledge to optimize value-based occupational therapy: Strategies for educators, practitioners, and researchers. *American Journal of Occupational Therapy, 75*, 7506090020.

Kalet, A., Buckvar-Keltz, L., Monson, V., Harnik, V., Hubbard, S., Crowe, R., Ark, T., Song, H., Tewksbury, L., & Yingling, S. (2018). Professional identity formation in medical school: One measure reflects changes during pre-clerkship training. *MedEdPublish, 7*, 41. https://doi.org/10.15694/mep.2018.0000041.1.

Kegan, R. (1982). *The evolving self: Problem and process in human development* (Reprint edition). Harvard University Press.

Kilgallon, K., & Thompson, J. (2012). *Mentoring in nursing and healthcare: A practical approach*. Wiley-Blackwell.

Klavins, R. (1972). Work-play behavior: Cultural influences. *American Journal of Occupational Therapy, 26*(4), 176–179.

Krueger, R. B., Sweetman, M. A., Martin, M., & Cappaert, T. A. (2020a). Occupational therapists' implementation of evidence-based practice: A cross sectional survey. *Occupational Therapy in Health Care, 34*(3), 253–276.

Krueger, R. B., Sweetman, A. M., Martin, M., & Cappaert, T. A. (2020b). Self-reflection as a support to evidence-based practice: A grounded theory exploration. *Occupational Therapy in Health Care, 34*(4), 320–350.

Law, M., & MacDermid, J. (2014). *Evidence-based rehabilitation: A guide to practice* (3rd ed.). SLACK.

Lawrence, C., Mhlaba, T., Stewart, K. A., Moletsane, R., Gaede, B., & Moshabela, M. (2018). The hidden curricula of medical education: A scoping review. *Academic Medicine: Journal of the Association of American Medical Colleges, 93*(4), 648–656.

Le, B. M., Impett, E. A., Lemay, E. P., Muise, A., & Tskhay, K. O. (2018). Communal motivation and well-being in interpersonal relationships: An integrative review and meta-analysis. *Psychological Bulletin, 144*(1), 1–25.

Leahy, E., Chipchase, L., & Blackstock, F. (2017). Which learning activities enhance physiotherapy practice? A systematic review protocol of quantitative and qualitative studies. *Systematic Reviews, 6*(1), 83.

Lecours, A., Baril, N., & Drolet, M. J. (2021). What is professionalism in occupational therapy? A concept analysis. [Qu'est-ce que le professionnalisme en ergothérapie? Analyse de ce concept.] *Canadian*

Journal of Occupational Therapy [Revue Canadienne D'ergotherapie], *88*(2), 117–130.

Li, S. A., Jeffs, L., Barwick, M., & Stevens, B. (2018). Organizational contextual features that influence the implementation of evidence-based practices across healthcare settings: A systematic integrative review. *Systematic Reviews, 7*(72), 1–19.

MacDonald, G. (2012). Individual differences in self-esteem. In M. R. Leary (Ed.), *Handbook of self and identity* (2nd ed., pp. 354–377). The Guilford Press.

Mann, A. (2018, January 15). *Why we need best friends at work.* Gallup.Com. https://www.gallup.com/workplace/236213/why-need-best-friends-work.aspx.

Matheson, L. N., Dempster Ogden, L., & Violette, K. (1985). Work hardening: Occupational therapy in industrial rehabilitation. *The American Journal of Occupational Therapy, 39*, 314–321.

Maurer, P. (1971). Antecedents of work behavior. *The American journal of occupational therapy: official publication of the American Occupational Therapy Association, 25*(6), 295–297.

Maxwell, J. D., & Maxwell, M. P. (1984). Inner fraternity and outer sorority: Social structure and the professionalization of occupational therapy. In A. Wipper (Ed.), *The sociology of work: Papers in honour of Oswald Hall* (pp. 330–358). Ottawa, Ontario, Canada: Carleton University Press.

McLoughlin Gray, J. (1998). Putting occupation into practice: Occupation as ends, occupation as means. *The American Journal of Occupational Therapy, 52*, 354–364.

MEDLINE. (2022). *MEDLINE: Overview.* https://www.nlm.nih.gov/medline/medline_overview.html.

Melnyk, B. M., Tan, A., Hsieh, A. P., & Gallagher-Ford, L. (2021). Evidence-based practice culture and mentorship predict EBP implementation, nurse job satisfaction, and intent to stay: Support for the ARCC© Model. *Worldviews on Evidence-Based Nursing, 18*(4), 272–281.

Merriam, S. B., Caffarella, R. S., & Baumgartner, L. (2007). *Learning in adulthood: A comprehensive guide.* San Francisco: Jossey-Bass.

Moffat, M. (2003). The history of physical therapy practice in the United States. *Journal of Physical Therapy Education, 17*(3), 15–25.

Moorhead, L. (1969). The occupational history. *The American Journal of Occupational Therapy: Official Publication of the American Occupational Therapy Association, 23*(4), 329–334.

Murphy, M. (2018). *Neuroscience explains why you need to write down your goals if you actually want to achieve them.* Forbes. https://www.forbes.com/sites/markmurphy/2018/04/15/neuroscience-explains-why-you-need-to-write-down-your-goals-if-you-actually-want-to-achieve-them/.

Musolino, G. M., & Jensen, G. M. (2020). *Clinical reasoning and decision-making in physical therapy: Facilitation, assessment, and implementation.* SLACK.

Nelson, D. L. (1997). Why the profession of occupational therapy will flourish in the 21st century. The 1996 Eleanor Clarke Slagle Lecture. *The American Journal of Occupational Therapy, 51*(1), 11–24.

Occupational therapy profession-continuing competence requirements. (2022). https://www.aota.org/-/media/corporate/files/advocacy/licensure/stateregs/contcomp/continuing-competence-chart-summary.pdf.

O'Neil, C. A., Fisher, C. A., Newbold, S. K., & Newbold, S. K. (2009). *Developing online learning environments in nursing education* (2nd ed.). New York: Springer.

OTSeeker. (n.d.). *Welcome to OTseeker.* http://www.otseeker.com/.

Ovid. (2022). *Ovid.* https://www.wolterskluwer.com/en/solutions/ovid.

PEDro. (2022). *Welcome to PEDro.* https://pedro.org.au/.

Peterson, S., Weible, K., Halpert, B., & Rhon, D. I. (2022). Continuing education courses for orthopedic and sports physical therapists in the United States often lack supporting evidence: A review of available intervention courses. *Physical Therapy, 102*(6), pzac031.

PsycINFO. (2022). *APA PsycInfo.* https://www.apa.org/pubs/databases/psycinfo.

PubMed. (n.d.). *PubMed overview.* https://pubmed.ncbi.nlm.nih.gov/about/.

Questionable Conferences. (2021). University of Indianapolis Library. UIndy. https://libguides.uindy.edu/c.php?g=981357&p=7095715.

Quiroga, V. A. (1995). *Occupational therapy: The first thirty years.* AOTA Press.

Reed, K. L., & Peters, C. O. (2010). Values and Beliefs: Part V 1986-2000: Is this really occupational therapy? *OT Practice, 15*(6), 15–18.

Reiter, K., Helgeson, L., & Lee, S. (2018). Enhancing professionalism among OT students: The culture of professionalism. *Journal of Occupational Therapy Education, 2*(3). https://doi.org/10.26681/jote.2018.020308.

Rothstein, J. M. (2002). Autonomy and dependency. *Physical Therapy, 82*(8), 750–751.

Rothstein, J. M. (2003). Autonomy or professionalism? *Physical Therapy, 83*(3), 206–207.

Sandstrom, R. W. (2007). The meanings of autonomy for physical therapy. *Physical Therapy, 87*(1), 98–106.

Schwartz, K. B. (2009). Reclaiming our heritage: Connecting the founding vision to the centennial vision. *The American Journal of Occupational Therapy, 63*(6), 681–690.

Seligman, M. E. P. (2011). *Flourish: A visionary new understanding of happiness and well-being* (pp. xii, 349). Free Press.

Shanafelt, T. D., Dyrbye, L. N., & West, C. P. (2017). Addressing physician burnout: The way forward. *JAMA, 317*(9), 901–902.

Shulman, L. S. (1986). Those who understand: Knowledge growth in teaching. *Educational Researcher, 15*(2), 4–14.

Skaletski, E. (2021). Start Here: A Straightforward Guide to Searching for Evidence. https://www.aota.org/publications/ot-practice/ot-practice-issues/2021/searching-for-evidence.

Slagle, E. C. (1927). To organize an "OT" department. *Occupational Therapy & Rehabilitation*, (6),2, 125–130.

Staffileno, B., Heitschmidt, M., & Tucker, S. (2022). Using a generous leadership model to promote evidence-based practice. *American Journal of Nursing, 122*(3), 57–62.

Swisher, L. L., & Page, C. G. (2005). *Professionalism in physical therapy: History, practice & development.* Elsevier Saunders.

Tenbrunsel, A. E., & Messick, D. M. (2004). Ethical fading: The role of self-deception in unethical behavior. *Social Justice Research, 17*(2), 223–236.

Tipton, D. J. (2017). *Personal and professional growth for health care professionals.* Jones & Bartlett Learning.

Trombly, C. A. (1995). Occupation: Purposefulness and meaningfulness as therapeutic mechanisms. 1995 Eleanor Clarke Slagle Lecture. *The American Journal of Occupational Therapy, 49*(10), 960–972.

Tucker, S., McNett, M., Melnyk, B. M., Hanrahan, K., Hunter, S. C., Kim, B., Cullen, L., & Kitson, A. (2021). Implementation science: Application of evidence-based practice models to improve healthcare quality. *Worldviews on Evidence-Based Nursing, 18*(2), 272–281.

Vingerhoets, C., Hay-Smith, J., & Graham, F. (2020). Intersection of the elements of evidence-based practice in interdisciplinary stroke rehabilitation: A qualitative study. *New Zealand Journal of Physiotherapy, 48*(3), 148–154.

Yerxa, E. (1979). The philosophical base of OT. In *Occupational therapy: 2001 AD* (pp. 26–30). Rockville, MD: American Occupational Therapy Association.

Yerxa, E. J. (1998). Occupation: The keystone of a curriculum for a self-defined profession. *American Journal of Occupational Therapy, 53*, 365–372.

7

Interprofessionalism

PATRICIA A. MEYERS, OTD, OTR/L; and MICHELE FAVOLISE, PT, DPT, CFE

LEARNING OBJECTIVES

By the end of this chapter, the reader will be able to:

- Define interprofessionalism
- Explain how interprofessionalism is fostered in practice
- Articulate leadership approaches for developing effective interprofessional teams, work culture, and collaborative practice

- Understand the effect and impact of interprofessionalism on clinical practice
- Articulate the value of interprofessional education for future clinical practice

CHAPTER OUTLINE

Introduction

Interprofessional collaboration in healthcare is integral to optimal patient outcomes and cost-efficient care. In the face of patient safety concerns, ineffective and inefficient care, excessive costs of providing complex care, which are compounded by staffing shortages, collaborative care is recognized globally as the best means to optimize patient outcomes (Arth et al., 2018; Bainbridge et al., 2010; Reeves et al., 2018; Weiss et al., 2018, Wood et al., 2020.). Increased communication and collaboration among healthcare providers decreases medical errors, coordinates treatment, improves staff retention, enhances patient satisfaction and increases effective patient-centered care.

Interprofessionalism in Healthcare

Interprofessionalism describes how professionals from different disciplines collaborate to provide an integrated and cohesive approach to patient care (Légaré et al., 2011; Wei et al., 2020). This collaboration is characterized by communication, teamwork, mutual respect, and a team approach with decisions made in the patient's best interest (Fig. 7.1). The team shares responsibility and decision-making between themselves and the patient, reducing medical errors and improving patient care while containing health costs. Interprofessionalism is based on a team approach that values and emphasizes collaboration.

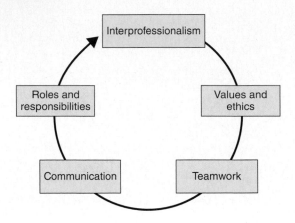

• **Fig. 7.1** Interprofessionalism is important for client-centered care and optimal outcomes.

TABLE 7.1	SHARE Approach to Patient Care
Step 1	**S**eek your patient's participation.
Step 2	**H**elp your patient explore and compare treatment options.
Step 3	**A**ssess your patient's values and preferences.
Step 4	**R**each a decision with your patient.
Step 5	**E**valuate your patient's decision.

Agency for Healthcare Research and Quality. The SHARE approach: A model for shared decisionmaking - fact sheet. (Content last reviewed September 2020). Agency for Healthcare Research and Quality, Rockville, MD. https://www.ahrq.gov/health-literacy/professional-training/shared-decision/tools/factsheet.html

Creating this positive culture fosters increased collaboration between members, with greater feelings of self-efficacy. Each team member feels their expertise is trusted and their contributions are valued and welcomed. Professionals are accountable for their input and each opinion is respected. Group expectations for each member are delineated, with a focus on the best interest of the patient. Such teams have high standards, flexibility, individual and group responsibility, clarity, and team commitment for the patient's benefit (Weiss et al., 2018).

Shared Decision-Making

Shared decision-making between the healthcare team and the patient led to the development of the Shared Decision Making Model and an appreciation for establishing and building interprofessional relationships in the fluid healthcare environment (Hall et al., 2013). The Shared Decision Making Model emphasizes decisions regarding patient care made between the practitioner and the patient through an evidence-based approach that considers the patient's perspective and values. This model values patient input and collaboration with the patient as the focus (Baca-Dietz et al., 2020; Elwyn et al., 2012; Légaré et al., 2011, Shakhman et al. 2019). It proposed an interprofessional approach to shared decision-making involving the interprofessional team working with the patient. The Shared Decision Making Model, or SHARE approach to patient care, as outlined in Table 7.1, has yielded improvements in quality of care, including better professional relationships between the healthcare practitioner and the patient, decreased costs as patients make informed decisions regarding their care, improved patient satisfaction and patient adherence to care recommendations (AHRQ.gov. 2020).

Clarification of professional time commitments, roles, and responsibilities assists with shared decision-making. Positive dialogue and discussion between members who are open to innovative ideas and creative approaches tend to be more productive and have positive outcomes. (Dogba et al., 2020; Hall et al., 2013; Weiss et al., 2018). Creating this

positive culture fosters improved collaboration between members, with greater feelings of self-efficacy. Individual members feel their contributions are welcomed, capabilities are trusted, opinions are respected, and team members feel valued. Each member is accountable for their input. Personal values, which include honesty and transparency regarding goals and errors, discipline to complete responsibilities autonomously, creative problem-solving, and humility to value the knowledge and expertise of others, contribute to an effective interprofessional team. Expectations for each member are clear, with a focus on the best interest of the patient. These teams have exacting standards, high flexibility, individual and group responsibility, clarity, and team commitment (Weiss et al., 2018).

Collaboration

Successful interprofessionalism and interprofessional practice emphasize a collaborative approach (Fig. 7.2). It is critical for clinicians to note potential institutional challenges and to enact an approach that is flexible and patient-centered. As noted by Matt Vorensky, "The key is to ask and adapt" (Loria 2022, p. 36). Ask and adapt entails conferring with team members to coordinate rehabilitation efforts and goals to provide the plan of care that best addresses the patient's needs. For example, scheduling treatment sessions and family education after traditional working hours to accommodate a caregiver's schedule. A care plan may require more complex tasks and incorporate strategies from different disciplines to address the patient's needs for returning home and going back to work. For example, the physical therapist may use communication strategies provided by the speech-language pathologist or cognitive strategies recommended by the occupational therapist to optimize the patient's performance and plan of care. This collaboration helps ensure the carryover of the strategies and interventions to maximize patient outcomes. According to Arth et al. (2018), "Collaborative Practice is when multiple health workers from different professional backgrounds provide comprehensive services by working with

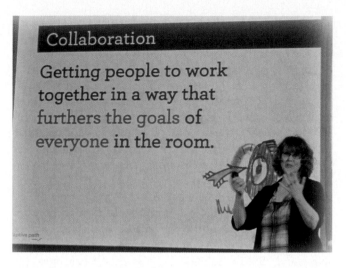

Collaboration

Getting people to work together in a way that furthers the goals of everyone in the room.

• **Fig. 7.2** How would you define collaboration? (From https://www.flickr.com/photos/36947317@N02/5629405358).

patients to deliver the highest quality of care across settings. Healthcare teams improve professional communication, reduce medical errors, improve patient experience and outcomes, increase the efficiency of health services and create a collaborative workforce" (p. 227).

"As clinicians aim to promote self-management, rehabilitation often takes team management. Identifying current and potential team members with the patient in other areas of healthcare and in the community is a fundamental interpersonal strategy," remarked Matt Vorensky (Loria 2022, p. 36.). Collaborative teamwork requires time and value for role clarification, resolving interprofessional conflict, sharing leadership, and understanding and appreciating team dynamics (Dogba et al., 2020). Each member is valued for their role on the team and mutual respect is given to each contribution. Recognizing the value of human connections and the importance of cultivating these relationships forged

by interprofessionalism positively impacts interprofessional collaborative practice (Wei et al., 2020).

Regardless of the team structure, there is shared leadership (Table 7.2). Team dynamics focuses on fulfilling realistic patient wishes and meeting the patient's and family's needs. The success of interprofessional teams is guided by the organization's culture, where the healthcare professionals feel supported. Team members share a sense of belonging when clarifying roles and responsibilities and cultivating trust. Essential elements for team success include role clarity, trust, confidence, ability to overcome adversity, personal differences, and collective leadership (Bosch & Mansell, 2015; Chamberlain-Salaun et al., 2013; Choi & Pak, 2006, Wei et al., 2022).

Role Clarity

Role clarity defines the function of each member of the interprofessional team. Each discipline has a unique role inherent in its specialty, though there is discipline overlap based on practice setting, expertise, and experience. Traditionally, examples include physical therapist and mobility, occupational therapist and self-care, nursing and medical care, speech-language pathologist and communication, social worker and discharge disposition, physician and medical care, dietician and nutrition, clergy and faith and support. Depending on the practice setting, each discipline's role may encompass all or some aspects of patient care. The team's primary focus is the best possible patient care and outcomes that value their wishes. Each member serves and executes unique functions; however, they may step outside their traditional roles and often overlap with other team members. This overlap of skills provides different perspectives.

Traditionally in the medical model, the physician assumes the leadership role, which may change as determined by the most pertinent or presenting problems. Within their roles, each member must recognize their professional strengths and

TABLE 7.2	Types of Healthcare Teams	
Interprofessional[a]	Collaboration among a team of professionals from different professions.
Intraprofessional[a]	Collaboration among a team of professionals from the same profession.
Interdisciplinary[b]	Analyzes, synthesizes, and harmonizes links between disciplines into a coordinated and coherent whole.
Transdisciplinary[b]	Integrates the natural, social, and health sciences in a humanities context and transcends their traditional boundaries.
Multidisciplinary[b]	Knowledge from different disciplines but remaining within their boundaries.

[a]Professional is the preferred terminology in healthcare.
[b]Disciplines are described as individual sciences that study different subjects independently of each other to develop theories as a means of scientifically understanding the world.
From Chamberlain-Salaun J, Mills J, & Usher K. (2013). Terminology used to describe health care teams: An integrative review of the literature. *Journal of Multidisciplinary Healthcare* 6, 65–74;
Choi BCK, & Pak AWP. (2006). Multidisciplinarity, interdisciplinarity and transdisciplinarity in health research, services, education and policy: 1. Definitions, objectives, and evidence of effectiveness. *Clinical and Investigative Medicine. Medecine Clininique et Experimentale* 29(6), 351–364.

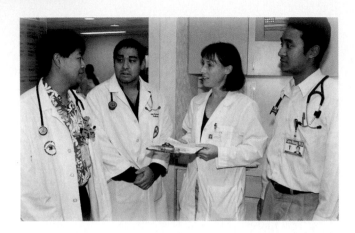

• **Fig. 7.3** A prerequisite to trust includes opportunities for team members to learn about each other. (From https://www.flickr.com/photos/52167074@N07/8362721478).

limitations and when to defer or consult, as necessary. Knowing when to defer to the expertise of others is a valuable trait for leaders and members of interprofessional healthcare teams. High-performing teams are goal-focused and encourage collaboration and innovation and appreciate the complimentary skills of team members (Ulrich & Crider, 2017). The team's strength lies in its ability to leverage the skills of multiple disciplines toward the common goal of client-centered care. Collaboration facilitates mutual respect and improves relationships amongst the team.

Trust and Confidence

Interprofessionalism considers the importance of trust between each professional on the team to address conflict and different perspectives while being supportive of others' expertise and autonomy. While trust and confidence in each other's skills and judgment develop with interaction and time spent together, a prerequisite to trust includes opportunities for team members to learn about each other (Fig. 7.3). Through experience, role clarification, expectations, and regular interaction with various disciplines, members develop confidence and comfort specific to the individual team members and their expected roles and responsibilities. Education and training focused on the discipline's purpose, parameters, and limitations are integral to the continued interactions. Professional identity and self-confidence, guided partly by professional competence, contribute to mutual interprofessional respect and trust. Trust improves working relationships as role identity is clarified and mutual respect is developed, encouraging innovative practice while improving job satisfaction and morale (Jones & Jones, 2011; Sifaki-Pistolla et al., 2020; Ulrich & Crider 2017; Wei et al., 2022).

Challenges to Interprofessional Practice

Comprehensive medical care involves the knowledge and expertise of professionals from various disciplines working together to address the complexity of patient care. It is important to recognize that each brings personal and professional perspectives (Irvine et al., 2004). The desire of all healthcare providers for effective, efficient, and safe treatment can serve as the reference point for interaction and collaboration. This reference point is also influenced by the challenges of healthcare policies and regulation that considers effective and efficient care to address cost. This focus, cost-cutting measures, and staff shortages have greater significance to interprofessional collaboration between medical professionals, including occupational and physical therapists (Bainbridge et al., 2010).

The healthcare team will often face adversity such as inadequate staffing, conflicting professional wishes, equipment needs, scheduling, logistical issues, financial hardships, and lack of support. Despite these challenges, the team must be dedicated to the best outcome for the patient. In these scenarios, the overlap of skills acts as checks and balances and can assist in compromised situations. The team may experience conflict due to differences in professional opinion, feelings of territorialism, or personal reasons. Perceived power imbalances and inequalities between professionals are significant barriers to relationships and effective interprofessional working. (Boland et al., 2019; Laurenson & Brocklehurst, 2011, p. 188.) The patient's needs are paramount and supersede any personal differences. Egos and personal differences are set aside, and the benefit to the patient is placed first. Through collective leadership, there is a team-based approach to patient care. While the medical director is often a physician, the patient's needs drive the team's decision-making. A patient-centered process allows the team to be creative problem-solvers who address the patient's medical care challenges and provide a safe discharge disposition.

Influence of Leadership on Interprofessional Practice

Strong relationships between healthcare providers and healthcare organizations facilitate change to improve the value of care for patients. By assuming a leadership role, healthcare providers direct the healthcare system to improve value and sustainability (Trastek et al., 2014). Leadership is the ability to guide, persuade or motivate others. Effective leadership is influenced by both an intrinsic and extrinsic perspective. Specific personality traits are associated with leadership and include enthusiasm, charisma, extraversion, and passion. Successful leadership may be driven by the desire for professional advancement or motivation to create change and leadership skills may be learned and developed.

Leadership Styles

Organizational culture may influence and be influenced by leadership styles (Chapter 10). Definitions of leadership provide a collective understanding and limit confusion, inferences, and assumptions. Healthcare leadership with an understanding of ethics and processes to shape the various disciplines on the team reinforces a hierarchical leadership perspective. Team leaders provide clear expectations and methods for communication for team members and are ultimately responsible for the work of the team (Ulrich & Crider, 2017). Definitions of leadership that lack detailed and accurate descriptions impact role clarity and challenge methods to measure the effectiveness and impact of team outcomes (Willgerodt et al., 2020).

A plethora of research focuses on effective leadership, which traditionally has had a hierarchical focus. Transformational and transactional leadership are prominent styles of leadership. Transactional leadership focuses on self-interest and the basic exchange between leaders and team members when working toward an established goal. Transformational leadership moves beyond self-interest while focusing on the team by building on shared vision, purpose, and values, which inspires cohesiveness and commitment (Bass, 1999). Thus transformational leadership is associated with greater process quality and is better suited for interprofessional practice (Samarakoon, 2019; Sfantou et al., 2017).

Shared or democratic leadership involves allocating leadership responsibilities to team members whose skill, knowledge, and experience best support established outcomes. This leadership style moves from the traditionally hierarchal perspective toward the recognition and value of team member leadership, accountability, and active engagement. "Other styles, such as quantum, authentic and servant, while more aligned with interprofessional practice in healthcare settings, require sophisticated self-awareness, reflective skills, and high levels of emotional intelligence" (Brewer et al., 2016, p.412). The servant leadership style encourages creativity that is responsive to the needs of the individuals and the whole team. This approach allows more efficient medical procedures, innovative medical equipment technology, and new treatments, resulting in increased safety, improved patient outcomes, service, and greater efficiency within the healthcare system (Trastek et al., 2014). Understanding leadership styles within the interprofessional team may guide the team in a more effective approach.

Leading Teams

Teamwork supports engagement while advancing patient safety and quality performance. Teamwork moves beyond a group where individuals primarily interact to achieve a common goal. A team works together and encompasses shared leadership, collective responsibility, and performance toward reaching the desired goal. Interdisciplinary teams in healthcare invoke the team's makeup, which involves professionals from different disciplines intentionally coordinating and communicating to contribute to the patient care plan. An effective team demonstrates a shared vision and goals, collective leadership, and accountability, recognizing that the team process is fluid with learning, growth, and feedback opportunities (Braveman 2016, p. 218).

To be effective, leaders of an interprofessional team must understand the roles and responsibilities of each healthcare professional to recognize emerging roles and responsibilities

that will occur as part of an interprofessional team. Although the overarching goal of healthcare teams is effective, safe, and efficient patient care, successful interprofessional leadership recognizes the differences between teams and that a one-size approach will not fit all. The work culture and environment negatively or positively impact the interprofessional team; therefore, communication, coordination, and distinctive training specific to role responsibilities are imperative.

Leaders create the culture of the team and must demonstrate support for each healthcare professional on the team by initially developing an environment of trust where the team will thrive and succeed. Leaders and team members willing to self-examine and acknowledge that their roles and responsibilities are influenced by the team strengthen interprofessionalism. When the leadership role is not clarified, it results in decreased team interaction, which impacts communication and information sharing (Folkman et al., 2019; Ulrich & Crider, 2017). As interprofessionalism in healthcare continues to develop with the successes in cost reduction, improved patient mortality, and improved safety, the value of interprofessional teams, is the expectation rather than the exception. Although leadership is considered crucial to the successful outcomes of the interprofessional team, it has not traditionally been the focus of research. In the realm of interprofessional practice, leadership styles most aligned with interprofessional practice embrace a collective approach with terms including collaborative or shared. While these styles are appreciated in theory, the challenge is apparent in practice when medicine has traditionally been viewed from a hierarchical lens that reinforces competition and individual achievement (Fig. 7.4).

Building an Effective Team

Interprofessional leaders must intentionally address the conditions that negatively impact effective teams, including lack of training, support, and alignment between incentives and interdependent functions of team members to address common goals. Leaders should create an organizational culture that values teamwork by incorporating opportunities for team members to get to know each other to build trust (Ulrich & Crider, 2017), team training and meetings for direct patient care needs and methods for recognition and reimbursement for all team members. This reinforces and supports interprofessional collaboration. Team cultures that value and actively seek each member's contribution inspire collaboration, commitment, and active engagement in achieving common goals (Weiss, et al., 2018), ideally, to achieve the best outcome for the patient.

Creating an effective interprofessional culture involves evaluating policies and procedures that support leadership delegation and workflow clarification. Leaders can facilitate this positive collaborative culture. By welcoming each team member's input while offering their own, there is an exchange of information and knowledge guided by the best interest of the patient. When senior members adopt a culture of positive regard for all, this attitude will positively

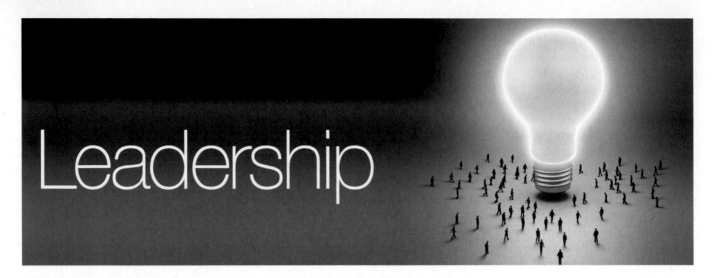

• **Fig. 7.4** Leadership in healthcare must move away from the traditional hierarchical lens that reinforces competition and individual achievement. (From https://commons.wikimedia.org/w/index.php?curid=32407807).

impact the rest of the staff, facilitating reflection and inquiry amongst the team and the process. When respect and trust are fostered by leadership and translated to the team members, it creates an environment of mutual respect and allows for progress where all members are equal. Effective interprofessional teams and leadership positively influence the culture and create a culture of safety (Taplin et al., 2013).

Leaders and members who use inclusionary practices such as soliciting input from all stakeholders in the healthcare process, recognizing successful practices, and consistently facilitating positive communication create psychological safety, encouraging participation and engagement in collaborative healthcare practices. Mindful attention to relationship building mitigates the tensions accompanying interdependence, resulting in safe, effective, and high-quality patient-centered care (Weiss et al., 2018).

Interprofessional Leadership Models

Interprofessional leadership models require a systematic approach that is multifaceted. While there is consensus and core belief in the value of interprofessional teams in healthcare as an effective approach to patient care, the move from the traditional hierarchical view and the implementation of this approach is less clear. Thus it requires leaders who champion implementation and ongoing support of interprofessionalism. Leadership theories have traditionally addressed leadership development; however, intentional focus on individuals' awareness of their behavior and how it influences the team is less developed.

Leadership models have contributed to interprofessionalism, including the Relational Model of Organizational Change, which considers the organizational process to improve team function. The Institute of Medicine Interprofessional Learning Continuum Model considers the formal and informal learning from teams, while the theoretical framework for Integrated Teamwork training tool addresses interprofessionalism in conjunction with shared decision-making. An interprofessional leadership council model tailored to the practice setting focuses on best practices for implementing sustainable interprofessional collaboration (Allen, 2021; Smith et al., 2020; Willgerodt et al., 2020).

Interprofessional Culture, Collaboration, and Communication

The practice settings for occupational therapists and physical therapists are vast and varied. The healthcare professionals within these settings are equally diverse, with complex roles and responsibilities that change and influence the organization's culture. Factors that positively influence and promote interprofessionalism include communication in an environment that encourages and appreciates sharing knowledge, collaboration, and ethics. Irvine et al. (2004) describe the common desire for safe, efficient, and effective treatment as the reference point for healthcare collaboration. Dialogic ethics refers to the opportunity and exchange between two or more different professionals to express their views and opinions (Weiss et al., 2018). Regardless of the care setting, the most successful healthcare teams possess mutual respect, nonhierarchical team structures, clear communication, and shared decision-making. As noted by Farrell (2016, pp. 889–890), "it is the foundation of shared ethics and values that collectively creates a vision for a more collaborative, communicative and inclusive clinical culture."

Interprofessional healthcare teams are complex. The length and focus of the education degree guided by discipline-specific accreditation and license or certificate requirements contribute to this complexity. When considering allied health disciplines, a commonality is the role of professionalism, which consistently includes discipline-specific knowledge and technical skills and the value of peer relationships. Factors that support collaboration and collective focus include shared purpose, critical reflection intervention, and leadership (Sims et al., 2015; Wagner et al., 2007).

Effective Professional Relationships

When building effective professional relationships, teams work together to provide optimum care and solve patient care problems. According to Weiss et al. (2018), healthcare teams that are empowered and enabled to learn about each other as individuals, work together in their respective roles, and address group dynamics and procedures, are better equipped to identify and solve problems. As members work alongside each other, learning more in-depth about the scope of each other's practice, the team can learn to anticipate each other's concerns and find solutions to the myriad of problems that arise. With patient care as the focal point for all members, each member can express viewpoints to maximize the patient's status. The goals are medical management, patient safety, optimizing patient status, aiding, and discharge planning while honoring patient and family wishes. Each team member possesses a unique perspective on managing the patient's needs. There is frequent dialogue, both formal and informal, amongst team members. Formal discussion occurs during patient care rounds or meetings, with the interprofessional team present, each contributing to report patient status and goals. Informally, discussions occur between two or more healthcare team members to discuss current care or to progress findings. Regardless of the method, the view of each member is given respect and value, with the patient wishes and desires at the forefront of consideration. Each team member's input is needed to develop the plan of care and discharge, with recommendations based on their unique perspective. Discharge planning requires coordination between all disciplines and the need for a complex array of services highlights the interdependence of all the stakeholders in the healthcare arena (Weiss et al., 2018).

Communication

Open communication creates a collaborative community among disciplines, increasing the value of each member and mutual respect. Also, it fosters interdisciplinary professionalism, confidence, and trust, which transcends beyond immediate healthcare team members. Communication is paramount in the healthcare environment, particularly for effective interprofessional collaboration to ensure safe, effective treatment, to reduce medical errors, to avoid duplication of services, and to manage medical costs, focusing on patient-centered care.

Interprofessional teams incorporate informal and formal communication. Informal communication may occur as an impromptu conversation between team members regarding patient information needed for appropriate care; for example, a physical therapist or occupational therapist may discuss the patient's general status with the nurse prior to the therapy evaluation, and between therapists to plan interventions or to correlate the functional status seen with each discipline and nursing. Formal communication occurs when healthcare team members contribute their clinical assessment to direct patient care during healthcare team rounds, patient care conferences, and medical record documentation. Formal team meetings and rounds involve discussion about updated patient status, with each member contributing and making recommendations for the patient. The team reaches a consensus, proposing solutions and addressing concerns to the patient and family to allow for informed consent and decision-making. Thus each member contributes to executing these established plans by fulfilling their unique roles.

Electronic Medical Record

Technology affords the healthcare team or student learning environments with ease of use, real-time access to patient care information, and collaboration, therefore minimizing logistical barriers (Weiss et al., 2018). The electronic medical record and other shared documents allow the healthcare team directly involved with the patient's care to access information regarding the medical status and overall wellbeing, which are essential for safe and proper patient care. It also makes available a secure, centralized location for the patient's information, permitting various team members simultaneously to document their clinical impressions and to view those of other disciplines. This centralized location affords a more efficient system of communicating the patient's medical history and current status, including the prevalent issues impacting prognosis and progress. The use of technology allows information exchange and collaboration between team members, enabling higher-order thinking, clinical reasoning, and informed clinical decision-making (Fig. 7.5).

Interprofessional Education

The World Health Organization (2010) defines interprofessional education (IPE) as follows: "when students of two or more professions learn about, from, and with each other to enable effective collaboration and improve health outcomes." IPE, globally recognized and endorsed by educators, focuses on collaborative practice, whereby students who learn together create a knowledge-rich environment

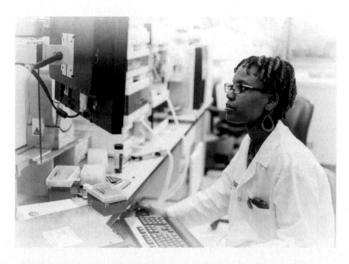

• **Fig. 7.5** Electronic medical records can acquire, process, store, and secure patient information. (From https://www.flickr.com/photos/64860478@N05/10424826743/in/photostream/).

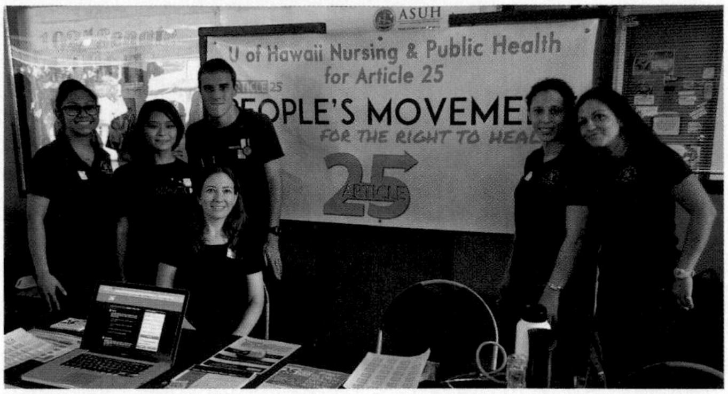

• **Fig. 7.6** When students from multiple health professions are educated together, they enter the workforce with respect and a willingness to collaborate. (From https://commons.wikimedia.org/w/index.php?curid=40235917).

that shares characteristics of community practice (Arth et al., 2018; Lôbo de Carvalho et al., 2018; Weiss et al., 2018). This concept is fueled by the belief that when students from multiple health professions are educated together, they will enter the workforce with respect and a willingness to collaborate. The evidence supports students will function better in cooperative healthcare teams to address complex issues and improve patient outcomes (Fig. 7.6). Arth et al., (2018) noted that initially, the roles and responsibilities of the other disciplines were not well understood by students; however, learning, competency, autonomy, teamwork, collaboration, communication, and readiness to learn all improved and were positive regardless of the IPE methodology. Understanding roles and responsibilities, communication, and positive professional identity development improve with IPE activities. Conversely, results included students who had negative perceptions of the other disciplines after the IPE experience were acknowledged. Implementing IPE early on and throughout the curriculum may combat stereotyping and negative perceptions while fostering greater respect and understanding of the other disciplines. IPE may also provide future healthcare professionals with an intrinsic value for collaboration as well as the foundational knowledge to address institutional structures and policies that negatively impact interprofessional collaboration (Ansa et al., 2020; Laurenson & Brocklehurst, 2011; Lôbo de Carvalho et al., 2018.).

Competencies

Competencies are skills or abilities required to perform essential job functions and duties. Interprofessional competence prepares healthcare students to work in teams and is dependent on the depth and breadth of opportunities for education and practice involving other disciplines (Bainbridge et al., 2010; Keshmiri & Mehrparvar, 2021; Wood et al., 2009). Interprofessional healthcare collaboration reduces medical costs and improves patient outcomes and care. Recognizing the value of interprofessionalism, the Interprofessional Education Collaboration (IPEC) Expert Panel, formed in 2009 to advance interprofessional learning experiences, identified core competencies which were published in 2011 and updated in 2016. The initial goal of this health profession collaboration was and continues to be "to help prepare future health professionals for enhanced team-based care of patients and improved population health outcomes" (IPEC, 2016, p.1). Four core competencies with related subcompetencies provide detailed information and are listed for interprofessional collaborative practice. The four topical areas fall under the single domain of Interprofessional Collaboration, in which four core competencies exist (Table 7.3).

The practice setting partly influences competencies from an interprofessional perspective. Individual competencies are discipline-specific but may overlap between different disciplines within the interprofessional team. One or more professions may share common competencies. In collaborative competencies, when individual disciplines work together, learners and practitioners form partnerships with the healthcare team and the patient (Braveman, 2016). Individuals understand their roles and responsibilities and those of the various members of the interdisciplinary team. Members are valued for their input and contribution to the collaborative decision-making process. Communication, team dynamics, and leadership are appreciated as the team seeks solutions to problems and provides optimal patient care.

Strategies and Implementation

The strategies and implementation of interprofessional education vary, as do the outcome measures among the different curricula. The teaching methodology of IPE includes didactic (lecture or presentations, group discussion), simulations (scenarios to fulfill objectives), and a mix of different methods (two or more methods). Educational methods include workshops, didactic lectures, subject modules, in-classroom learning, clinical scenarios, competencies and case studies. Outcome measures also vary between standardized measures or informal means. Validated and standardized measures include the Interdisciplinary Education Perception Scale (IEPS), Readiness for Interprofessional Learning Scale

TABLE 7.3	The Four Core Competencies of Interprofessional Collaboration	
Topic	**Core Competency**	**Competency Description**
Values/ethics for interprofessional practice	Competency 1	Work with individuals of other professions to maintain a climate of mutual respect and shared values.
Roles/responsibilities	Competency 2	Use the knowledge of one's role and those of other professions to appropriately assess and address the healthcare needs of patients and promote and advance the health of populations.
Interprofessional communication	Competency 3	Communicate with patients, families, communities, and professionals in health and other fields responsively and responsibly that supports a team approach to promoting and maintaining health and preventing and treating disease.
Teams and teamwork	Competency 4	Apply relationship-building values and the principles of team dynamics to perform effectively in different team roles to plan, deliver, and evaluate patient/population-centered care and population health programs and policies that are safe, timely, efficient, effective, and equitable.

Adapted from Interprofessional Education Collaborative. (2016). *Core competencies for interprofessional collaborative practice: 2016 update*. Washington, DC: Interprofessional Education Collaborative.

(RIPLS), Attitude Towards Health Care Teams Scale (ATHCTS), Teams Skills Scale (TSS), Health Professional Collaboration Scale (HPCS), IPEC Competency Self-Assessment Tool and Communication and Teamwork Scale of the West of England (CTS). Informal assessments include journals, reflections, and objective-specific tools (Arth, 2018, Roberts et al., 2018.). Various methods of implementation and assessment, with outcomes clarified, should be used throughout the curriculum to show the efficacy of IPE in both short-term or immediately postactivity as well as long-term or postgraduation effects (Arth et al., 2018).

Barriers to IPE implementation usually involve competing schedules and the various course demands of each discipline (Shakhman et al., 2019; Weiss et al.; 2018). Although each discipline must meet the demands of its profession and accreditation by covering specific content, where and when content is covered is program-specific, making coordination difficult. The differing course structure and educational levels among disciplines increase the difficulty of coordinating educational activities and determining where the programs align to implement experiences can be challenging. Finally, faculty bias in interprofessional healthcare can and often does influence the curriculum and student perceptions. Although some faculty members are knowledgeable and experienced in interprofessional teamwork, others may practice in silos (Wood et al., 2020). This solitary clinical practice where interaction with other disciplines of the healthcare team is limited can diminish the importance of a collaborative team approach. This experience shapes the clinician's viewpoint and influences their teaching, which may result in decreased support of IPE or seeing little value in its implementation.

There are various methods of instruction in which IPE can be implemented. In didactic learning, students from multiple disciplines share common foundational topics in which they may all be taught together. Topics such as professionalism, ethics, patient confidentiality, leadership, research, and empathy are central to all healthcare members (Shakhman et al., 2019). Face-to-face lectures, small group discussions, or presentations allow for sharing of perspectives and values. Community-based learning is employed when faculty and students from two or more disciplines attend a clinical facility or community function to perform healthcare tasks and provide services and education. This setting allows students to practice skills and work cohesively as a team as they gain professional exposure under faculty supervision.

Interprofessional interactions where students work together in a case scenario to achieve an objective or patient outcome are, in effect, simulations. These experiential sessions mimic real-life clinical situations and allow students to role-play and make clinical decisions in a safe, controlled environment (Fig. 7.7). Each simulation, followed by a

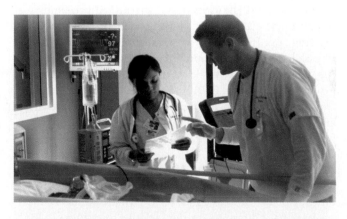

• **Fig. 7.7** Simulations can facilitate students working together in a case scenario that mimics real-life clinical situations to make clinical decisions in a safe, supervised, and controlled environment. (From https://www.flickr.com/photos/41431665@N07/8637884629).

debriefing session, enables students and instructors to analyze and reflect on the simulation and its outcomes, often finding ways to improve future performance. Other IPE delivery methods include journal clubs, debates, class or online discussions, and competency-based assessments. Most interprofessional curricula employ a mixed methodology in graduate and undergraduate healthcare programs to prepare students for collaborative clinical practice.

To succeed, IPE requires the administration's support to champion the initiative. Interprofessional programmatic infrastructure is needed to provide financial, logistical, communication, and coordination resources for activities to accommodate various program specialties. Faculty facilitating IPE should be dedicated and experienced in collaborative practice and readily promote integrated interprofessional opportunities with training and mentorship to disseminate and advance the implementation of interdisciplinary activities. It is crucial that faculty model the essential skills and core values of interprofessional collaboration for learners." (AOTA, 2022, p.11). Educational programming and resources may be needed to ensure that everyone understands the objectives of this educational component. This may be accomplished through internal programs, committees, and external interprofessional education organizations, conferences, and workshops (AOTA, 2022). Lastly, student participation and efforts should be acknowledged as they navigate their way through shared decision-making, shared leadership, collaborative and cooperative engagement, and conflicts. Through these learning opportunities, students may learn to value the communication between the team members and the roles, functions, and responsibilities of each discipline, including their own.

Practice Standards in Healthcare Education

Interprofessional education and collaborative practice are outlined in the Framework for Action on Interprofessional Education and Collaborative Practice (WHO, 2010). From a world perspective, this framework details the value and implementation of interprofessional collaboration in clinical practice and the classroom. The accrediting bodies of physical and occupational therapists include standards addressing IPE. In 2016, the Commission on Accreditation in Physical Therapy Education (CAPTE) included IPE into the standards for entry-level physical therapist education programs (CAPTE, 2020) in support of the core competencies of the American Physical Therapy Association (APTA) and the American Council on Academic Physical Therapy (ACAPT). To further support IPE in 2019, The Health Professions Accreditors Collaborative (Health Professions Accreditors Collaborative, 2019) and the National Center for Interprofessional Practice and Education collaborated on the document "Guidance on Developing Quality Interprofessional Education for the Health Professions."

Upon release of the initial IPEC report in 2011, AOTA signed on as a supporting organization and, in 2016, became professionally represented as an institutional member.

IPE aligns with the core values of occupational therapy and interprofessionalism, as an essential skill for practitioners, and has been reinforced through AOTA supported continuing education (Johnson, 2017; McLaughlin Gray et al. 2015). The Accreditation Council for Occupational Therapy Education (ACOTE) Standards were updated in 2018. Within this update, Standard B.4.25: Principles of Interprofessional Team Dynamics states that occupational therapy students will demonstrate knowledge of the principles of interprofessional team dynamics to perform effectively in different team roles (ACOTE, 2018).

Code of Ethics

Each healthcare profession is guided by its code of conduct and ethics to safeguard patient care and establish standards of professional behavior (Chapter 5; APTA, 2020a). The Code of Ethics for the Physical Therapist is built upon the five roles of the physical therapist, the core values of the physical therapy profession, and the realms of ethical action. Effective in 2010, this revised document defines the foundational principles that govern the behavior and the mandatory ethical obligations of practicing physical therapists as determined by the House of Delegates of the APTA. For example, Code of Ethics Principle number 3 declares that physical therapists shall be accountable for making sound professional judgments that incorporate interprofessionalism. In Principle 3C, physical therapists shall make judgments within their scope of practice and expertise and communicate with, collaborate with, or refer to peers or other healthcare professionals when necessary (APTA, 2020b). This principle demands that the physical therapist communicates with other healthcare team members to coordinate services and care efforts in the patient's best interest.

The Occupational Therapy Code of Ethics, updated in 2020, defines core values and ethical principles to guide professional decision-making and enforceable Standards of Conduct to AOTA members. (AOTA, 2020, p.1), These core values of altruism, equality, freedom, justice, dignity, truth, and prudence guide occupational therapy personnel in their interaction and collaboration on interprofessional teams. Specific to interprofessionalism and interprofessional practice, it is the ethical principle of fidelity that states that "occupational therapy personnel shall treat clients (persons, groups, or populations) colleagues and other professionals with respect, fairness, discretion and integrity" (AOTA, 2020, p.4).

Interprofessionalism Resources

For further information on interprofessionalism and interprofessional education, consult your professional organization for practice standards and requirements. Additional resources and organizations are listed below.
- World Health Organization (WHO) https://www.who.int/
- Interprofessional Education Collaborative (IPEC) https://ipecollaborative.org

- The National Center for Interprofessional Practice and Education https://nexusipe.org
- American Physical Therapy Association (APTA) https://www.apta.org/
- American Occupational Therapy Association (AOTA) https://www.aota.org/
- American Association of Colleges of Nursing (AACN) https://www.aacnnursing.org/
- Journal of Interprofessional Care http://informahealthcare.com/journal/jic
- Journal of Research in Interprofessional Practice and Education http://www.jripe.org/index.php/journal
- American Association of Medical Colleges https://www.mededportal.org/interprofessional-education

References

Accreditation Council for Occupational Therapy Education (ACOTE). (2018). Standards and interpretive guide (effective July 31, 2020). *American Journal of Occupational Therapy, 72*(Suppl. 2), 7212410005p1–7212410005p83.

Agency for Healthcare Research and Quality. (2020). *The SHARE approach: A model for shared decision making.* https://www.ahrq.gov/sites/default/files/publications/files/share-approach_factsheet.pdf.

Allen, D. (2021). Interdisciplinary leadership council: A model for excellence in improving interprofessional collaboration. *Nursing Management (Springhouse), 52*(10), 51–54.

Ansa, B. E., Zechariah, S., Gates, A. M., Johnson, S. W., Heboyan, V., & De Leo, G. (2020). Attitudes and behavior towards interprofessional collaboration among healthcare professionals in a large academic medical center. *Healthcare (Basel, Switzerland), 8*(3), 323.

American Occupational Therapy Association. (2020). AOTA 2020 occupational therapy code of ethics. *American Journal of Occupational Therapy, 74*(Suppl. 3), 7413410005.

American Occupational Therapy Association. (2022). Importance of interprofessional education for occupational therapy. *American Journal of Occupational Therapy, 76*(Suppl. 3), 7613410250. https://doi.org/ 10.5014/ajot.2022.76S3007.

American Physical Therapy Association (APTA). (2020a). *APTA Guide for professional conduct.* https://www.apta.org/your-practice/ethics-and-professionalism/apta-guide-for-professional-conduct.

American Physical Therapy Association (APTA). (2020b). *Code of ethics for the physical therapist.* https://www.apta.org/apta-and-you/leadership-and-governance/policies/code-of-ethics-for-the-physical-therapist.

Arth, K., Shumaker, E., Bergman, A., Nolan, A., Ritzline, P., & Paz, J. (2018). Physical therapist student outcomes of Interprofessional Education in Professional (Entry-level) Physical therapist education programs: A systematic review. *Journal of Physical Therapy Education, 32*(3), 226–239.

Baca-Dietz, D., Wojnar, D. M., & Espina, C. R. (2020). The shared decision-making model: Providers' and patients' knowledge and understanding in clinical practice. *Journal of the American Association of Nurse Practitioners, 33*(7), 529–536.

Bainbridge, L., Nasmith, L., Orchard, C., & Wood, V. (2010). Competencies for interprofessional collaboration. *Journal of Physical Therapy Education (American Physical Therapy Association, Education Section), 24*(1), 6–11.

Bass, B. M. (1999). Current developments in transformational leadership: Research and applications. *The Psychologist-Manager Journal, 3*(1), 5–21.

Boland, L., Graham, I. D., Légaré, F., Lewis, K., Jull, J., Shephard, A., Lawson, M. L., Davis, A., Yameogo, A., & Stacey, D. (2019). Barriers and facilitators of pediatric shared decision-making: A systematic review. *Implementation Science, 14*, 7.

Bosch, B., & Mansell, H. (2015). Interprofessional collaboration in Health care: Lessons to be learned from competitive sports. *CPJ/RPC, 148*, 176–179.

Braveman, B. (2016). *Leading & managing occupational therapy services: An evidence-based approach* (2nd ed.). F.A. Davis Company.

Brewer, M. L., Flavell, H. L., Trede, F., & Smith, M. (2016). A scoping review to understand "leadership" in interprofessional education and practice. *Journal of Interprofessional Care, 30*(4), 408–415.

Chamberlain-Salaun, J., Mills, J., & Usher, K. (2013). Terminology used to describe health care teams: An integrative review of the literature. *Journal of Multidisciplinary Healthcare, 6*, 65–74.

Choi, B. C. K., & Pak, A. W. P. (2006). Multidisciplinarity, interdisciplinarity and transdisciplinarity in health research, services, education and policy: 1. Definitions, objectives, and evidence of effectiveness. *Clinical & Investigative Medicine, 29*(6), 351–364.

Commission on Accreditation in Physical Therapy Education. (2020). *Standards and required elements for accreditation of physical therapist education programs.* CAPTE Accreditation Handbook. https://www.capteonline.org/globalassets/capte-docs/capte-pta-standards-required-elements.pdf.

Dogba, M. J., Menear, M., Brière, N., Freitas, A., Emond, J., Stacey, D., & Légaré, F. (2020). Enhancing interprofessionalism in shared decision-making training within homecare settings: a short report. *Journal of Interprofessional Care, 34*(1), 143–146.

Elwyn, G., Frosch, D., Thomson, R., Joseph-Williams, N., Lloyd, A., Kinnersley, P., Cording, E., Tomson, D., Dodd, C., Rollnick, S., Edwards, A., & Barry, M. (2012). Shared decision making: A model for clinical practice. *Journal of General Internal Medicine, 27*(10), 1361–1367.

Farrell, C. (2016). The Ethics and Value of True Interprofessionalism. *American Medical Association Journal of Ethics, 18*(9), 887–890.

Folkman, A. K., Tveit, B., & Sverdrup, S. (2019). Leadership in interprofessional collaboration in health care. *Journal of Multidisciplinary Healthcare, 12*, 97–107.

Hall, P., Weaver, L., & Grassau, P. A. (2013). Theories, relationships and interprofessionalism: Learning to weave. *Journal of Interprofessional Care, 27*(1), 73–80.

Health Professions Accreditors Collaborative. (2019). *Guidance on developing quality interprofessional education for the health professions.* Chicago, IL: Health Professions Accreditors Collaborative. https://healthprofessionsaccreditors.org/wp-content/uploads/2019/02/HPACGuidance02-01-19.pdf.

Interprofessional Education Collaborative. (2016). *Core competencies for interprofessional collaborative practice: 2016 update.* Washington, DC: Interprofessional Education Collaborative.

Irvine, R., Kerridge, I., & McPhee, J. (2004). Towards a dialogical ethics of interprofessionalism. *Journal of Postgraduate Medicine, 50*(4), 278–280.

Jones, A., & Jones, D. (2011). Improving teamwork, trust and safety: An ethnographic study of an interprofessional initiative. *Journal of Interprofessional Care, 25*(3), 175–181.

Johnson, C. (2017). Understanding interprofessional collaboration: An essential skill for all practitioners. *OT Practice, 22*(11), CE1–CE7. https://www.aota.org/~/media/Corporate/Files/Publications/CE-Articles/CE-Article-June-2017.pdf.

Keshmiri, F., & Mehrparvar, A. H. (2021). Developing a competency framework of interprofessional occupational health team: A first step to interprofessional education in occupational health field.

Journal of Occupational and Environmental Medicine, 63(11), e765–e773.

Laurenson, M., & Brocklehurst, H. (2011). Interprofessionalism, personalization and care provision. *British Journal of Community Nursing, 16*(4), 184–190.

Légaré, F., Stacey, D., Pouliot, S., Gauvin, F. P., Desroches, S., Kryworuchko, J., Dunn, S., Elwyn, G., Frosh, D., Gagnon, M. P., Harrison, M., Pluye, P., & Graham, I. (2011). Interprofessionalism and shared decision-making in primary care: a stepwise approach towards a new model. *Journal of Interprofessional Care, 25*(1), 18–25.

Lôbo de Carvalho, V., Tôrres Tomaz, J. M., & Falcão Tavares, C. H. (2018). Interprofessionalism and interdisciplinarity in academic formation: The perception of graduates in physiotherapy. *Journal of Nursing UFPE/Revista de Enfermagem UFPE, 12*(4), 908–915.

Loria, K. (2022). Using fundamental interventions to address social determinants of health. *APTA Magazine, 14*(2), 30–42. https://www.apta.org/apta-magazine/2022/03/01/interventions-to-address-social-determinants-health.

McLaughlin Gray, J., Coker-Bolt, P., Gupta, J., Hissong, A., Hartmann, K. D., & Kern, S. B. (2015). Importance of interprofessional education in occupational therapy curricula. *American Journal of Occupational Therapy, 69*, 1–14.

Reeves, S., Pelone, F., Harrison, R., Goldman, J., & Zwarenstein, M. (2018). Interprofessional collaboration to improve professional practice and healthcare outcomes. *The Cochrane Database of Systematic Reviews, 6*(6), CD000072.

Roberts, S. D., Lindsey, P., & Limon, J. (2018). Assessing students' and health professionals' competency learning from interprofessional education collaborative workshops. *Journal of Interprofessional Care, 33*(1), 38–46.

Samarakoon, K. B. (2019). Leadership styles for healthcare. *International Journal of Scientific and Research Publications, 9*(9), ISSN2250–ISSN3153.

Sfantou, D. F., Laliotis, A., Patelarou, A. E., Sifaki-Pistolla, D., Matalliotakis, M., & Patelarou, E. (2017). Importance of leadership style towards quality of care measures in healthcare settings: A systematic review. *Healthcare (Basel, Switzerland), 5*(4), 73.

Shakhman, L. M., Al Omari, O., Arulappan, J., & Wynaden, D. (2019). Interprofessional education and collaboration: Strategies for implementation. *Oman Medical Journal, 35*(4), e160.

Sifaki-Pistolla, D., Melidoniotis, E., Dey, N., & Chatzea, V. E. (2020). How trust affects performance of interprofessional healthcare teams. *Journal of Interprofessional Care, 34*(2), 218–224.

Sims, S., Hewitt, G., & Harris, R. (2015). Evidence of a shared purpose, critical reflection, innovation and leadership in interprofessional healthcare teams: A realist synthesis. *Journal of Interprofessional Care, 29*(3), 209–215.

Smith, T., Fowler Davis, S., Nancarrow, S., Ariss, S., & Enderby, P. (2020). Towards a theoretical framework for Integrated Team Leadership (IgTL). *Journal of Interprofessional Care, 34*(6), 726–736.

Taplin, S. H., Foster, M. K., & Shortell, S. M. (2013). Organizational leadership for building effective health care teams. *Annals of Family Medicine, 11*(3), 279–281.

Trastek, V. F., Hamilton, N. W., & Niles, E. E. (2014). Leadership models in health care—A case for servant leadership. *Mayo Clinic Proceedings, 89*(3), 374–381.

Ulrich, B., & Crider, N. M. (2017). Using teams to improve outcomes and performance. *Nephrology Nursing Journal, 44*(2), 141–152.

Wagner, P., Hendrich, J., Moseley, G., & Hudson, V. (2007). Defining medical professionalism: A qualitative study. *Medical Education, 41*(3), 288–294.

Wei, H., Horns, P., Sears, S. F., Huang, K., Smith, C. M., & Wei, T. L. (2022). A systematic meta-review of systematic reviews about interprofessional collaboration: Facilitators, barriers, and outcomes. *Journal of Interprofessional Care, 36*, 735–749. doi:10.1080/13561820.2021.1973975.

Wei, H., Corbett, R. W., Ray, J., & Wei, T. L. (2020). A culture of caring: The essence of healthcare interprofessional collaboration. *Journal of Interprofessional Care, 34*(3), 324–331.

Weiss, D., Tilin, F., & Morgan, M. (2018). *The interprofessional health care team*. Massachusetts: Jones and Bartlett Learning.

Willgerodt, M. A., Abu-Rish Blakeney, E., Summerside, N., Vogel, M. T., Liner, D. A., & Zierler, B. (2020). Impact of leadership development workshops in facilitating team-based practice transformation. *Journal of Interprofessional Care, 34*(1), 76–86.

Wood, A. J., Grudzinskas, K., Ross, J. A., Bailey, S., Gordon, G. E., Burton, C., & Wishart, L. R. (2020) Strengthening teamwork capability in allied health: Implementation of a team development program in a metropolitan health service. *Australian Health Review, 44*, 443–450.

Wood, V., Flavell, A., Vanstolk, D., Bainbridge, L., & Nasmith, L. (2009). The road to collaboration: Developing an interprofessional competency framework. *Journal of Interprofessional Care, 23*(6), 621–629.

World Health Organization. (2010). *Framework for action on interprofessional education & collaborative practice*. Geneva, Switzerland: Health Professions Network Nursing and Midwifery Office, Department of Human Resources for Health. http://www.who.int/hrh/nursing_midwifery/en/.

8

Diversity, Equity, and Inclusion

THERESA RHETT-DAVIS, EdD, OTR/L; and SARAH CORCORAN, OTD, OTR/L

LEARNING OBJECTIVES

After completion of this chapter, learners will be able to:

- Define key terms related to diversity, equity, inclusion (DEI), and belonging.
- Relate diversity, equity, and inclusion to macro-, meso-, and micro-systems levels.
- Describe the history of the PT and OT professions through to current times, using the lens of DEI.
- Give an example of how legal and ethical contexts transact with DEI across systems levels.

- Discuss how social capital affects the healthcare workforce and clients.
- Provide a plan for how PT and OT students and practitioners can build the capacity of the professions related to DEI.

Related ACOTE Standards: B.1.2, B.3.1, B.5.1, B.5.2, B.5.4, B.7.1, B.7.2

Related to CAPTE Standards: 7D4, 7D5, 7D8, 7D13, 7D14

CHAPTER OUTLINE

Introduction

Greater diversity, equity, and inclusion (DEI) in the healthcare workforce are essential for improving healthcare delivery and outcomes in an increasingly diverse population. All health professions, including occupational therapy (OT) and physical therapy (PT), must be prepared to address the needs of the changing population demographics. This chapter will facilitate conversation and continued dialogue addressing DEI issues and solutions within our professions related to leadership and management in healthcare. DEI is dynamic, multifaceted, and complex; therefore it is impossible to cover this topic's breadth and depth in one chapter. While this chapter aims to be inclusive, content and examples may be

related more closely to one or more aspects of an individual's identity for synthesis and application.

This chapter utilizes a three-legged approach to examine DEI at macro-, meso-, and micro-levels. These three system levels comprise the cornerstone upon which DEI is supported or rejected. This chapter focuses on DEI related to leadership and management in healthcare professions, including OT and PT. Examples of macro-, meso-, and micro-levels illustrate essential concepts. People in many disciplines, from sociology to engineering to healthcare, use these terms to describe different, interrelated system levels. Analysis and action at each level are critical to whether DEI is supported or rejected. All system levels are essential and interdependent. The authors offer definitions (see Fig. 8.1)

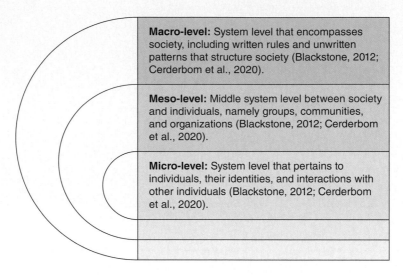

• **Fig. 8.1** Macro-, Meso- and Micro-Level Definitions

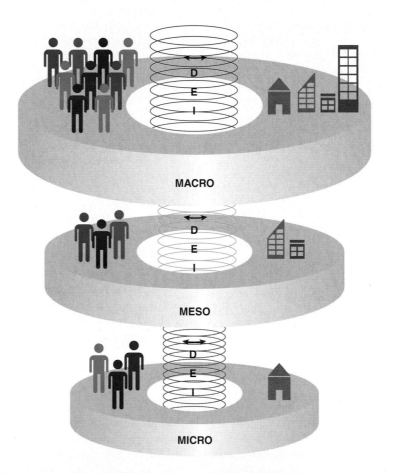

• **Fig. 8.2** Diversity, Equity, and Inclusion (DEI) Flow Through Systems Levels. (Original graphic designed by Theresa Rhett-Davis, Sarah Corcoran, and artist Marie Lyani Nicandro.)

of the system levels to help you understand each level and how they relate to DEI (Fig. 8.2).

- **Macro-level** encompasses society, including written rules and unwritten patterns that structure society (Blackstone, 2012; Cerderbom et al., 2020). Kendi (2019), who wrote *How to Be an Antiracist,* explains that this level of systems, such as legal and social systems, directs the experience of groups.

- **Meso-level** refers to the middle system between society and individuals, namely groups, communities, and organizations (Blackstone, 2012; Cerderbom et al., 2020). At the meso-level, practitioners engage with professional teams and organizations.

- **Micro-level** pertains to individuals, their identities, and interactions with other individuals (Blackstone, 2012;

Cerderbom et al., 2020). We may be most aware of the micro-level in our daily routines when directly engaging with clients and colleagues.

When DEI is supported across all system levels, written laws are equitable, organizational culture is fair and impartial, and cultural humility is standard practice. *Cultural humility* has been defined as the commitment to lifelong learning, self-reflection, and repair of power imbalances to build relationships and communities (Tervalon & Murray-Garcia, 1998). When DEI is rejected at any system level, anti-discrimination laws are not followed or enforced, discriminatory practices are standard in organizational culture, and individuals operate out of bias and prejudices in existing power dynamics. Many people have witnessed the fragmented connections between the system levels concerning DEI. These broken connections create barriers and perpetuate policies, practices, and procedures that work against individuals and collectives of people. Because DEI touches all facets of life, individuals, groups, and communities are impacted when DEI is not valued and actively promoted. One example is how the COVID-19 pandemic demonstrated the lack of health access and quality healthcare for African Americans (Chowkwanyun & Reed, 2020; Lavizzo-Mourey et al., 2021). DEI can help support individuals' and communities' healthcare needs by eliminating healthcare disparities. Healthcare professionals, including OT and PT practitioners, must understand their role in supporting or hindering DEI at all system levels.

Diversity, Equity, and Inclusion Defined

It is important to know the definitions of essential terms used in this chapter, starting with diversity, equity, inclusion, and belonging. The concept of diversity is forever changing. *Diversity* is the quantitative representation of unique aspects of identity present within a person, a group, or a population, such as healthcare professionals, students, and clients (Race Forward, n.d.; Togioka et al., 2021). These internal and external aspects of identity include and are not limited to race, ethnicity, gender, gender identity, ability, age, religion, social class, socioeconomic status, sexual orientation, primary spoken language, education, geographic origin, values, and beliefs (American Occupational Therapy Association [AOTA], 2020a; American Physical Therapy Association [APTA], 2019; Taff & Blash, 2017; Togioka et al., 2021). Diversity among people in the workplace promotes diversity of ideas, engagement, retention of employees, and business success (Rosenkranz et al., 2021). Based on social conditions and political, legal, and economic systems of power, the aspects that make persons unique from one another also create advantages and barriers to participation in society (AOTA, 2020a; Peterson et al., 2021; World Health Organization, 2022).

The World Health Organization (2022) defines *equity* as "the absence of unfair, avoidable, or remediable differences among groups of people, whether those groups are defined socially, economically, demographically, or geographically or by other dimensions of inequality (e.g., sex, gender, ethnicity, disability, or sexual orientation)" (para. 1). The concept of equity differs from equality, which implies the sameness of treatment or resources for everyone. Instead, equity entails recognizing and correcting the advantages and barriers that individuals, groups, and populations experience due to social conditions, institutions, and systems (AOTA, 2020a). OT and PT practitioners can promote equity for themselves, clients, colleagues, teams, groups, communities, and populations.

Inclusion is the act of fostering an environment in which differences are not only accepted but continuously invited and embraced so that all people can participate as their authentic selves (Bailey et al., 2020). While diversity is quantitative representation or presence, "inclusion is a qualitative measure of representation and participation" (Race Forward, n.d.). Inclusion can be viewed as an active "function of connection" (Ross, 2011, p. 38). Teams, communities, classrooms, and organizations are inclusive when all the people feel valued and connected, share power, and have a say in decisions. Inclusion emphasizes the value, respect, and support of individuals' and groups' unique qualities, characteristics, and experiences to facilitate belonging.

Belonging is the personal experience of feeling valued and perceiving a good fit between our identity and environment, including social systems and work organizations (Hagerty et al., 1992). Although contextual factors influence a person's sense of belongingness, only each person can assess whether or not they feel like they belong. Consider belongingness the sweet spot reached when diversity, equity, and inclusion are at their best.

As you read this chapter, you may want to refer to this resource that provides additional definitions of terms related to DEI: https://www.edi.nih.gov/blog/communities/understanding-racial-terms-and-differences

Throughout this chapter, we offer examples to help you apply what is learned about DEI and belonging in the context of leadership and management. Opportunities for application are found in the case of vignette boxes at the end of each section. The following case vignettes introduce Bryan, the practitioner, and Meera, the student.

CASE VIGNETTE

Meet Bryan the Practitioner

Bryan has 15 years of experience working as an occupational therapist. He currently works in an outpatient therapy clinic at a hospital. Bryan's career history includes work in the school system and a skilled nursing facility. Bryan actively engages in professional associations and regularly serves as a fieldwork educator with OT students. Bryan is 40 years old, identifies as male, and uses he/him pronouns. He is Black and Hispanic. Bryan and his partner, Diego, have been married for 5 years and have two school-aged children. They live together in the southwest region of the United States.

Consider how Bryan's identities and roles may relate to diversity, equity, and inclusion at macro-, meso-, and micro-levels.

Meet Meera the Student

Meera is the first person to attend college in her family. Meera attended public schools from kindergarten through 12th grade and is a current student in an entry-level physical therapy program at a predominantly White institution in a city in the Northeast region of the United States. Meera is 21 years old, identifies as a cisgender, heterosexual female, and uses she/her pronouns. Meera is a first-generation American, the daughter of parents who emigrated from India to the United States. Meera and her family practice the Islamic religion. Meera speaks English as a second language.

Consider how Meera's identities and roles may relate to diversity, equity, and inclusion at macro-, meso-, and micro-levels.

Historical Overview

The long history of social injustices, such as systemic racism in the United States, must be addressed to become an egalitarian society. Systemic racism involves any structure, organization, or society that embeds any form of racism in its laws or regulations. It is deeply rooted in discriminatory practices in healthcare, education, law, criminal justice, employment, housing, and politics (Braveman et al., 2022). Racism is considered a public health crisis, and the health of the members of a society is connected to the health of its democracy (Pollock et al., 2022). Therefore systemic racism directly affects all members of society.

The United States' founding document, the Declaration of Independence, states that all people are "created equal." The words "created equal" are written to establish an egalitarian society. However, centuries later, since the document was written, widespread social injustice still occurs based on race, gender, class, religion, disability, sexual orientation, and other identity factors and crosses all industries. It is undeniable that some progress has been made toward becoming an egalitarian society. However, it must not be denied that there is still improvement to be made to actualize a genuinely egalitarian society practicing social justice in all areas. The healthcare industry in the United States is one of these areas that will be discussed regarding DEI.

According to the United States Census Bureau's County Business Patterns (CBP), the healthcare industry has the highest employment of any other industry in the United States (United States Census Bureau, 2022). Organizations provide healthcare in the United States and these organizations or healthcare systems employ many people. Healthcare organizations are usually supported by federal, state, and local funding and secure additional financial support via charitable contributions. Healthcare systems include the client, the healthcare professional, the setting in which it takes place, the agencies that regulate healthcare, and the channels that provide financial support. A segregated workforce for OT and PT is evident in these healthcare systems. OT is a majority white profession (Salvant et al.,

2021; Sterman & Njelesani, 2021), as is PT (Matthews et al., 2021; Vazir et al., 2019). An understanding of the history of OT and PT is essential for practitioners to diminish individual and systemic racism today and in the future (Matthews et al., 2021; Sterman & Njelesani, 2021).

Marginalization results from isolation, which can occur when working in a segregated work environment where DEI is absent. Healthcare organizations should make DEI intentional by incorporating DEI in their mission, vision, value statement, strategic plan, policies, and procedures. Healthcare organizations that embrace and vividly declare DEI as an integral part of their organization enable the organization to adapt to the needs of all stakeholders. Any workplace discrimination and lack of support for workers to address discrimination can potentially damage the work and the workplace overall.

There is no time like the present to do an evaluation of race in the disciplines of OT and PT. Since the inception of the fields of OT and PT, the professions have struggled to address racial disparities among their students, practitioners, and educators (Matthews et al., 2021; Salvant et al., 2021; Sterman & Njelesani, 2021). Thus change must occur. Most recently, AOTA established a Diversity, Equity, and Inclusion Task Force and obligated this task force to focus on DEI related to governance, strategic planning, and the development of a DEI roadmap revealing a plan of action (Salvant et al., 2021). Additionally, in the summer of 2020, AOTA hosted four virtual Be Heard We're Listening sessions with Black Indigenous People of Color (BIPOC) students, practitioners, and educators (Salvant et al., 2021). BIPOC students, practitioners, and educators shared their experiences related to patterns of covert and overt forms of racism faced by BIPOC OT students, practitioners, and educators. These sessions reveal three primary themes as a starting point to address disparities within the OT profession: (1) limited diversity and BIPOC representation at all levels within the profession; (2) the experience of racialized trauma, stress, and fatigue; and (3) anti-racism" (Salvant et al., 2021 p. 3). Likewise, APTA has established the Office of Minority Affairs and the Minority scholarship Fund to address the diversity issues in the profession (Matthews et al., 2021). However, according to Mathews et al. (2021), professional physical therapy organizations must develop comprehensive standards and practical strategies to work toward a profession where DEI is embedded as core values.

BIPOC practitioners have been excluded from better-paid, secure, and more desirable jobs in OT and PT through systemic practices in the workforce and other areas such as the educational system. These systemic practices can reinforce and sustain the long-standing hegemonic ideas contradictory to DEI concepts and ideas in the workplace. Therefore according to Sterman and Njelesani (2021), OT practitioners should address racism in the workplace occurring at the micro- and meso-system levels. Case vignettes explore the situation of Bryan and Meera from a societal, historical perspective related to DEI.

CASE VIGNETTE

Bryan the Practitioner

Bryan feels safe identifying as a gay man in the workplace; however, his colleague confided in him that at work, he identifies as Tim, and in private, she is Tracey, a trans woman. Tracey has not openly come out at work as a trans woman for fear of not feeling safe in the work environment to self-identify as a member of the Lesbian, Gay, Bisexual, Transgender, Queer/Questioning, Intersex, Asexual (LGBTQIA+) Community. She worries about not being accepted as a trans woman and being terminated. Both Bryan and Tracey discuss the still lingering gaps between equality and the reality for LGBTQIA+ workers. One issue that is of genuine concern is the use of a safe restroom in the workplace. Access to a public bathroom is necessary for activities of daily living (ADLs) participation in the workplace and a ban on the use of bathroom access for transgender persons is a reality. It is no secret about controversial and legal discussions about transgender women having access to the women's bathroom in public places. Tracey would like to avoid embarrassment, trauma, or humiliation if she were to come out as a trans woman in the workplace and not be allowed to use the bathroom according to her identity. They both agree that clearer, more explicit laws and regulations that are effective need to be established to protect transgender persons in the use of public bathrooms. Likewise, both concur that their current workplace must adopt policies and procedures that focus on DEI so that every employee receives fair and equitable treatment and has a sense of belonging.

CASE VIGNETTE

Meera the Student

Meera has learned through experience that her intersecting identities of being an Indian American woman and Muslim in the United States are often met with discrimination and prejudice. However, Meera believes her darker skin is the cause of discrimination more so than being an Indian woman or Muslim. Meera knows in reality, lighter skin is preferred in the United States and India. She understands that skin color is linked to Black slavery and systemic racism. Meera knows that all her intersecting identities matter; she also recognizes that color matters. She knows she cannot hide her skin color and has come to live with the reality that she may be evaluated by individuals with skin tone bias who will judge her based on her skin color and not by her ability, intellect, or skills. During one of her fieldwork experiences, Meera was placed in a hospital in a predominately white community. During this fieldwork experience, she overheard her fieldwork educator comment to her colleague about her skin color. She remembers the words most vividly "She is rather dark and some of the older white patients might refuse to work with her." She contacted the fieldwork educator at her school to let her know what she overheard and to request reassignment to another fieldwork placement. She explained that she was uncomfortable remaining in this setting. The school's fieldwork educator used this situation as a teaching opportunity for Meera and the fieldwork site. The fieldwork educator contacted the fieldwork site coordinator to discuss the situation and to offer educational training to her staff on colorism in the workplace, unconscious bias and strategies to interrupt bias in the workplace. The fieldwork coordinator at the site agreed and welcomed the staff training. Meera was encouraged and empowered to help develop and participate in the staff training to help decrease racial inequity and barriers to equal opportunities for people with darker skin tones.

Law and Ethics

Law and ethics, in different ways, structure society, groups, and individuals. This section focuses on DEI, considering legal and ethical contexts that influence OT and PT practice, management, and leadership at all system levels. With the importance of representation, values, and decision-making, it should be understood that all legal and ethical matters connect to DEI. This chapter intends not to provide a comprehensive list of laws and ethical codes but to help you understand the relationship between law and ethics and DEI. The Cambridge Dictionary (Cambridge University Press, n.d.) defines "law" as "a rule, usually made by a government that is used to order how a society behaves." Ethics is "a set of standards for behavior that helps us decide how we ought to act in a range of situations" (Brown University, 2022). Law and ethics differ in their goals and sanctions, but both affect how people live their lives, including professional aspects.

First, consider the legal context and DEI. While the nature of law is to provide justice and order, there are many experiences of inequity and lack of access due to discrimination in American society, including health inequities evidenced by COVID-19. Due to long-standing social conditions and hegemonic practices, laws and policies can serve as structures that sustain systemic discrimination, including racism (Braveman, 2022). OT and PT practitioners have a professional responsibility to understand the relationship of laws to DEI and advocate for actively eliminating or changing policies that work against DEI to support equitable opportunities in an inclusive society.

At a macro-level, in the United States, laws are made at federal, state, and local levels based on constitutions, statutes, administrative agencies, and decisions made through the court system (National Paralegal College, 2022). As healthcare practitioners, we recognize that laws aim to define and protect the rights of our workforce and the populations we serve. For example, state practice acts structure the scope of services for the OT and PT professions. Another example of macro-level law is the Civil Rights Act. In 1964, the Civil Rights Act disallowed segregation in public places and employment discrimination based on race, religion, national origin, and gender. This law created the Equal Employment Opportunity Commission, whose mission is to "prevent and remedy unlawful employment discrimination and advance equal opportunity for all in the workplace" (United States Equal Employment Opportunity Commission, n.d.). The Voting Rights Act of 1965 and the Fair Housing Act of 1968 expanded the prohibition of discrimination to voting and housing sale, rental, and financing (History.com Editors, 2022). Later, in 1990, the Americans with Disabilities Act (ADA) was instituted to protect the civil rights of people with disabilities to participate in the same opportunities as all Americans, including access to employment, government programs, and public and commercial buildings (ADA.gov, n.d.). These laws assure the rights of all Americans, including healthcare workers and consumers. They affect our collective and individual experiences, opportunities, decisions, and consequences in all facets of our lives.

A couple of examples of macro-level legislation are the Equality Act (H.R.5) and the Allied Health Workforce Diversity Act (H.R. 3320/S.1679). The Equality Act, awaiting next steps in Congress at the time of this chapter's writing, prohibits discrimination based on sex, sexual orientation, and gender identity in public places, education, federal funding, employment, housing, credit, and the jury system (Congress.gov, n.d). The Allied Health Workforce Diversity Act, signed into law on December 29, 2022, provides financial support to education programs to recruit students from underrepresented backgrounds to OT, PT, speech-language pathology, respiratory therapy, and audiology (Congress.gov, n.d.). This legislation is supported by the American Occupational Therapy Association and the American Physical Therapy Association (AOTA, 2021a; APTA, 2021a). More information can be found on advocacy and other federal and state laws that affect OT and PT practitioners and clients through your professional associations.

At the meso-level, policies structure how specific organizations, institutions, communities, and groups work. For example, a hospital often has policies guiding PT and OT service delivery. The organization uses these policies to form job descriptions and balance workload among team members. These policies are informed by macro-level practice acts and the organization's needs and resources. Guidelines from professional associations, while not laws, may be considered in developing policies that affect the routines and roles of students and practitioners. Likewise, the institutions where healthcare practitioners learn and work have policies and procedures related to admission and hiring. These meso-level rules can support diversity, equity, and inclusion. For instance, institutional policies regarding holistic admissions in healthcare education programs, including OT and PT, have supported increased diversity in healthcare professions (Brotherton et al., 2021; Coleman-Salgado, 2021; Glazer et al., 2014). Holistic review is a process that balances consideration of student applicants' experiences, attributes, and traditional academic metrics like grades and test scores as criteria for admission to an educational program (Glazer et al., 2014). Holistic hiring practices emphasize candidates' demonstrated skills and competencies over qualifications and work history (Fuller et al., 2022).

Laws and policies affect all aspects of life. Macro-level rules and norms influence whether and how individuals participate in society. Meso-level policies depend on macro-level rules and affect each person on a micro-level. Additionally, individuals, particularly people in positions of power, influence decisions about laws and policies at the macro-level and meso-level. For example, consider the role of elected officials in creating and adopting laws in the United States or the role of an administrator with authority to make final decisions about workplace policies.

Recognizing the transactions between system levels invites us to consider how OT and PT practitioners contribute to meso- and macro-level change from the micro-level and how ethics guide our responses and actions. Although ethical decision-making can occur at all system levels, ethics has personal and interpersonal components. Our decisions at the micro-level affect groups, organizations, communities, and society. Respective professional and organizational codes of ethics should be consulted to guide our decisions and actions. The OT and PT Codes of Ethics organize core values, principles, and standards that members of each profession should share and follow. In the *Code of Ethics for the Physical Therapist,* APTA (2020) recognizes the core values of integrity and social responsibility, specifying behaviors that show respect for all people and advocacy to reduce inequities. In the *AOTA 2020, Occupational Therapy Code of Ethics,* AOTA (2020b) includes justice as a core value and principle to guide practitioners in promoting equity and inclusion, with standards addressing inequities and reporting discriminatory policies. With knowledge about the historical and current legal contexts and ethical decisions guided by shared core values, practitioners can work toward DEI at the macro-, meso-, and micro-levels in all professional roles. Examples of law and ethics impacting DEI are provided in Fig. 8.3. Refer to following case vignettes 8.6 for applying law and ethics related to DEI.

CASE VIGNETTE

Bryan the Practitioner

While attending a meeting for his state OT association, Bryan listened to a call for members to support the Allied Health Workforce Diversity Act, legislation to increase diverse representation in professional healthcare education programs and workforce, including OT. Bryan reflected on his path to becoming an OT. As a Black and Hispanic man among mostly White women in his OT program, Bryan often felt alone. He rarely saw practitioners with similar racial and ethnic identities portrayed in textbook images and as authors of professional resources. Bryan did not meet a male OT practitioner from a similar racial and ethnic background until he had been working for 3 years. Bryan also reflects on his experiences as a member of the LGBTQIA+ community in the healthcare profession. While Bryan's employer insured his own spouse and children before Bryan's marriage to Diego, Bryan was not offered insurance coverage for his life partner. As a fieldwork educator, Bryan has supervised students from underrepresented backgrounds. He enjoys this role and recognizes the benefits students from diverse backgrounds bring to the OT workforce and clients. Bryan appreciates the resources students tell him about from their universities, including student organizations promoting diversity and inclusion. However, he has also listened to students describe challenges in their educational programs and workforce interactions that include microaggressions by educators, classmates, and clients. Bryan relates to these experiences and can quickly think of examples in his education and day-to-day work in which he has been affected by implicit biases and discrimination on a micro-, meso-, and macro-level. With all this on his mind, Bryan joined advocacy efforts for the Allied Health Workforce Diversity Act through his state and national professional organizations. He has visited legislators and OT programs to encourage awareness and action regarding support for this legislation. Bryan also finds opportunities for everyday advocacy within his team and throughout his workplace.

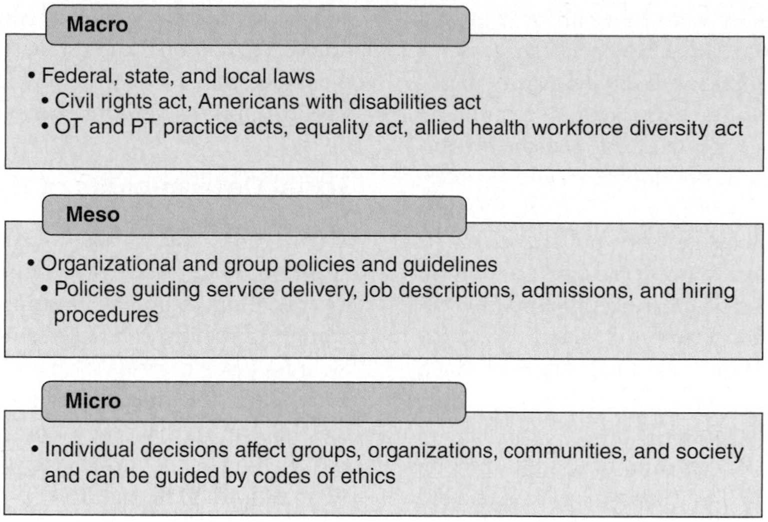

Macro

- Federal, state, and local laws
  - Civil rights act, Americans with disabilities act
  - OT and PT practice acts, equality act, allied health workforce diversity act

Meso

- Organizational and group policies and guidelines
  - Policies guiding service delivery, job descriptions, admissions, and hiring procedures

Micro

- Individual decisions affect groups, organizations, communities, and society and can be guided by codes of ethics

• **Fig. 8.3** Laws and Ethics Impacting Diversity, Equity, and Inclusion

CASE VIGNETTE

Meera the Student

Meera loves being a student in the DPT program. During her admissions interview, Meera felt welcomed and listened to as she shared her experiences as a first-generation college student. This feeling was important in Meera's decision about where to attend PT school. This predominantly White institution is committed to efforts to increase diversity among students and faculty. Meera's experience as a student has not been without challenges. As one of a few minority-status students in the program, Meera sometimes feels pressure to speak on behalf of underrepresented groups and communities during class conversations. Meera works diligently and has high expectations for herself regarding academic performance but sometimes struggles with writing assignments and finds limited support at the writing center. Despite these challenges, Meera generally feels a sense of community with peers and faculty in this program. Meera learned about the Allied Health Workforce Diversity Act during a professional rights and responsibilities class. Meera's instructor is involved in advocacy efforts within the PT profession, including those focused on this legislation. Meera was inspired by her professor's passion and advocacy for DEI and asked how she could become involved. With support from this faculty member, Meera offered an educational presentation and coordinated student advocacy efforts through the PT student organization at her school. The organization joined efforts with healthcare students from nearby schools for advocacy action with legislators and political action committees. When it was time for Meera's capstone course, Meera suggested an opportunity to work with her professor in examining the use of holistic review in admissions practices across DPT programs.

Social Capital

Social capital has increased prominence across multiple domains, such as healthcare and education. Leaders in healthcare and education are interested in how social capital can positively or negatively impact healthcare and education.

Many definitions in the literature define social capital, and Pierre Bourdieu's description differs from the current conceptual definitions of social capital (Claridge, 2020; Xu et al., 2020). Bourdieu's definition of social capital is linked to his theory of social stratification and is attached to the reproduction of class and status through power relations (Bourdieu, 1984, 1986; Claridge, 2015). According to Bourdieu, social capital stems from social, economic, and cultural structures that create differential power and status for specific individuals while reinforcing the social stratification of others based on race, class, and gender (Bourdieu, 1984, 1986; Claridge, 2015). It is essential to mention that the stigmatization of social identities reinforces social stratification and creates systems of oppression and dominance by maintaining hegemony (Davis, 2015).

Consequently, Robert Putnam defines social capital as the social networks, norms of reciprocity, and social trust in social organizations that facilitate coordination and cooperation towards shared goals (Putnam, 1993, 2000). Since the inception and popularization of Bourdieu's and Putnam's concepts of social capital, various social capital theories have emerged, been adapted, and expanded across different disciplines (Claridge, 2015, 2020; Xu et al., 2020), including healthcare. Therefore it is important to understand how social capital is formed and operates within the OT and PT health professions.

Many practitioners and scholars have discussed social capital implications related to the lack of DEI in the current OT and PT workforce and the overall educational and healthcare system. Healthcare organizations and professional organizations can use social capital as an asset to mobilize action for DEI integration in the workforce. At the micro-level, social capital supports social interactions among diverse workers, workers' rights to belong socially, and opportunities for social mobility. An example of this would be a healthcare worker's refusal to engage in employee social isolation by inviting all employees to be a part of the social group where they are valued. This effort creates a sense of belonging to the social group. Social capital at the meso-level impacts the integration of inclusive systems reinforcing collaboration between healthcare workers, focusing on employee conditions, training and development, and developing networking systems. For example, at this level, a healthcare system can integrate inclusive work policies for all its employees. Social capital can support resource allocation and funding at the macro level, creating pipelines for minority populations' social and economic mobility. An example is the Allied Health Workforce Diversity Act, which focuses on increasing racial diversity in education and the health professions such as OT and PT.

Diversity in healthcare is vital as minorities shift to represent the majority of the United States population. Table 8.1 presents the changing demographics of race and ethnicity in the United States. However, as race and ethnicity demographics in the United States change, occupational and physical therapy professions need to shift to reflect a more diverse

pool of therapists for the workforce. Therefore a representation of occupational and physical therapists will better reflect the population changes. Table 8.2 provides a snapshot of the respective profession's race and ethnicity demographics.

Social Determinants of Health

Many health threats are linked to social determinants of health (SDOH). Social determinants include access to quality education, affordable housing in a safe community, jobs, economic stability, and access to quality healthcare. It also includes other negative social determinants such as discrimination, bias, prejudices, violence, and racism (Healthy People 2030, n.d.) that "significantly correlates with the health and well-being of those who experience them" (Lucas & Washington, 2020, p. CE-4).

Individuals belonging to minority groups are more often affected by healthcare disparities. Some individuals in this group may be less likely to have health insurance or a routine source of healthcare. For example, regarding SDOH, the

TABLE 8.1 Race and Ethnicity Demographics in the United States

| Characteristics | Population Percentages | | | Population Change Percentages |
	2016	2030	2060	2016 to 2060
White	76.9	74.2	68.0	10.7
Non-Hispanic White	61.3	55.8	44.3	-9.5
Black or African American	13.3	13.8	15.0	41.1
American Indian and Alaska Native	1.3	1.3	1.4	37.7
Asian	5.7	6.9	9.1	101.0
Native Hawaiian and Other Pacific Islander	0.2	0.3	0.3	45.9
Two or more races	2.6	3.6	6.2	197.8
Hispanic	17.8	21.1	27.5	93.5

Vespa, J., Medina, L., & Armstrong, D.M. (2020). *Demographic turning points for the United States: Population projections for 2020 to 2060 (P25-1144).* United States Census Bureau. https://www.census.gov/content/dam/Census/library/publications/2020/demo/p25-1144.pdf

TABLE 8.2 Practitioner Race Demographics

| Profession | Percentage of Race Representation in the Profession | | | | | | |
	White	Black or African American	Asian	Hispanic or Latino	Pacific Islander	American Indian	Other
Occupational Therapist	83.3	3.0	5.8	4.0	Percentage reported with Asian Population	Not reported	Not reported
Physical Therapist	84.3	2.5	6.9	3.5	Not reported	0.4	2.4

PT statistics are from American Physical Therapy Association. (2020). *APTA physical therapy workforce analysis.* https://www.apta.org/your-career/careers-in-physical-therapy/workforce-data/apta-physical-therapy-workforce-analysis.
OT statistics are from American Occupational Therapy Association. (2020). *AOTA 2019 workforce and salary survey.*

Native American population's geographical isolation and income may be factors regarding receiving adequate healthcare. Other SDOH factors, such as living conditions related to inadequate water supply and proper disposal of waste and sewage stemming from a lack of access to indoor plumbing, may lead to infectious diseases (Ehrenpreis & Ehrenpreis, 2022). Likewise, some individuals in the LGBTQIA+ community may be less likely to seek healthcare due to fear of stigmatization and discrimination (McKay, 2011). Persons of the LBGTQIA+ community are more likely to be bullied, injured, raped, and victimized (Kassing et al., 2021; McKay et al., 2019). It is critical for the OT and PT practitioner to have awareness and understanding of managing the healthcare needs of diverse populations. Creating a nonjudgmental environment and practicing cultural humility when caring for diverse patients can influence positive health outcomes. OT and PT practitioners must be aware that their personal bias can cause them to ignore SDOH factors.

Health Equity and Health Disparities

Many definitions of health equity are present in the literature. Healthy People 2030 (n.d.) describes health equity as providing every individual fair and just opportunity to achieve the highest level of health and well-being by eliminating health and healthcare disparities for everyone. In comparison, Braveman (2013) asserts that health equity is the goal that drives efforts to remove health disparities for groups of people who are socially and economically disadvantaged than groups of people who are not.

Some vulnerable groups at risk of health disparities include minority groups, homeless individuals or people living in poverty, individuals with chronic health problems and disabilities, refugees, immigrants, limited English proficiency, members of the LBGTQIA+ community, and individuals who are incarcerated. These vulnerable groups experience more significant risk factors, lack of access to care, and increased mortality and morbidity compared with the general populations in healthcare

(Wesson & Kitzman, 2018). The healthcare professional's self-awareness of their values, beliefs, culture, ethics, and communication style helps to foster optimal health outcomes for patients of diverse populations. Healthcare professionals who recognize their biases and practice cultural humility toward all people can affect care satisfaction. The potential impacts of social capital on DEI are represented in Fig. 8.4. Refer to case vignettes for applying the information about social capital.

CASE VIGNETTE

Bryan the Practitioner

Bryan is an expert OT practitioner. He has been in practice for 15 years and has acquired a wealth of experience, allowing him to view situations holistically and process and integrate information efficiently. He can make decisions using an advanced level of intuition, analytical ability, and skill. Bryan currently serves as a quality improvement committee representative. He helps develop policies and procedures, collects information and data on staff adherence to established policies and procedures, helps create budgets to implement new policies and procedures, and assists with education and training to improve staff performance. The rehabilitation director informed the staff that he would retire at the year's end. Bryan is considering applying for the position as his career goal is to transition to an administrative role within his organization. He has all the qualifications required to apply for the rehabilitation director position.

Bryan recognizes that there is little diversity in upper management positions and has a strong desire to change the status quo of homogeny in upper management in his organization. During his interview for the rehabilitation director position, Bryan advocated for himself based on his accomplishments at the organization, national, state, and local levels. He discussed DEI and how diversity in the workplace at all levels can benefit the organization, employees, and clients. Likewise, Bryan's peers and colleagues advocated for Bryan to be promoted to the position. This is an example of the positive impact of social capital, illustrating social networking, norms of reciprocity, and social trust between Bryan, his peers, and colleagues.

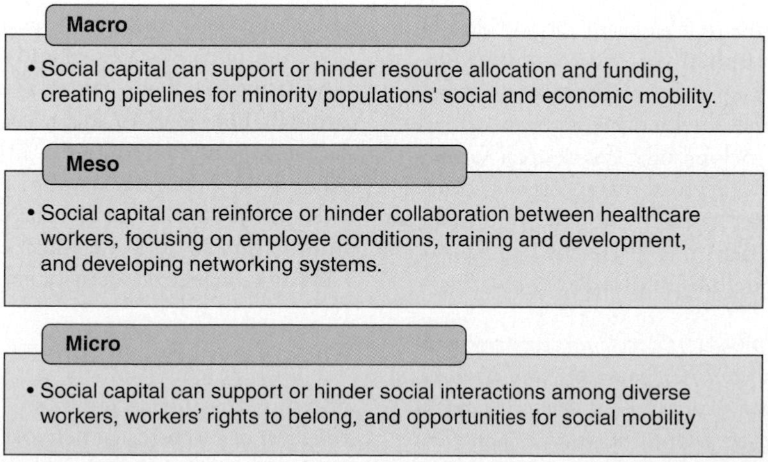

Macro

- Social capital can support or hinder resource allocation and funding, creating pipelines for minority populations' social and economic mobility.

Meso

- Social capital can reinforce or hinder collaboration between healthcare workers, focusing on employee conditions, training and development, and developing networking systems.

Micro

- Social capital can support or hinder social interactions among diverse workers, workers' rights to belong, and opportunities for social mobility

• **Fig. 8.4** Social Capital Impacting Diversity, Equity, and Inclusion

Meera the Student

Meera's parents migrated to the United States for a better life. Her parents are considered working class based on their education level, occupation, and income. Meera remembers her parents barely covering rent, utilities, food, clothing, transportation, and healthcare expenses. Meera moved around as a child because her parents needed to secure employment or housing. Her parents frequently experienced difficulty navigating the structural barriers of the social and political environments in the United States and also adapting to cultural norms. Meera spoke her native language when at home and she did not know any English when she entered the school for the first time. Meera was placed in an ESL (English as a Second Language) class to learn language skills and speak English. As Meera became proficient in English, she became an interpreter for her parents, who spoke little English. Her parents worked hard and wanted a better life for Meera, mandating that Meera would attend college after graduating from high school. Her parents instilled in her to work hard and get good grades to attend college. Meera also wanted to attend college because she saw how hard her parents worked and wanted a better social and financial life for herself. One of Meera's teachers told her, "If you want to get out of poverty, you must get an education." Meera has etched this statement in her mind and it is her mantra to keep pushing forward to the finish line-DPT degree. Meera's educational journey has not always been easy. It was challenging for her. She often felt she was not considered a good student or capable of attending college by some of her teachers even though she earned good grades. Meera reflects on a time when she met with her guidance counselor to find out her options for attending college. She was interested in going to college for physical therapy. Meera became aware of the PT profession when a physical therapist came to her school to talk about a career in physical therapy. Meera thought this was something she would like to do as a career. Her counselor responded, "I thought you would get a job like your parents after graduating." This is an example of the negative impact of social capital, illustrating social stratification based on race, class, and gender stigmatization.

Professional Engagement and Building Capacity

It is easy for everyone to agree that we want the world to be better. Perhaps this vision inspired you to choose your professional field. From the perspective of DEI, we can consider a better world to be one in which every person experiences a continual sense of belonging. This section focuses on building the capacity of ourselves, teams, organizations, professions, communities, and society through professional engagement and DEI. To orient this discussion, we refer to the United Nations' (n.d.) definition of *capacity-building*:

Capacity building is the process of developing and strengthening the skills, instincts, abilities, processes, and resources that organizations and communities need to survive, adapt and thrive in a fast-changing world. An essential ingredient in capacity-building is transformation that is generated and sustained over time from within; transformation of this

kind goes beyond performing tasks to changing mindsets and attitudes. (para. 1)

We propose that, while this process is often discussed from the perspective of organizations, it is helpful to consider how capacity is built through all system levels. How do we transform what we think and do to actualize our vision for our best possible selves, teams, organizations, professions, communities, and society? Inherent in answering this question is our need to connect. Consider the role of connection as you plan to engage in capacity building at each system level.

Macro-Level Engagement

Professional engagement at the macro-level is essential to building society's capacity for DEI. We engage at the macro-level by learning about systems, including social, political, economic, and legal systems, and how power operates within these contexts. When we know about structures that support or reject DEI in the United States, we can decide how to create, vote, and advocate for policies that contribute to DEI at the macro-level. Outcomes at this level traverse all system levels. For example, by understanding structures that codify education stratification and their effect on enrollment and graduation rates in OT and PT education, we can make informed decisions for ourselves and groups to advocate for laws and policies that facilitate equitable educational access and diversity in the OT and PT workforce.

Advocacy is an important skill and action for all members of the OT and PT communities to facilitate change related to DEI in society. Kirsh (2015) described advocacy as a "professional imperative" that pulls together all system levels for change (p. 213). Kirsh (2015) suggests that practitioners move beyond helping individual clients face challenges to understand and "chip away" at the structures and systems that create these challenges (p. 217). According to Kirsh (2015), strategies involved with advocacy can include identifying the causes of inequity, generating relationships for a supportive community, planning for change, crafting and communicating your message to stakeholders, and facilitating public awareness and engagement. To get started advocating for change within systems and institutions, practitioners may refer to the advocacy efforts of their professional associations. APTA (2021b) offers a position paper to guide PT practitioners toward priority public policies that affect the profession and its clients. AOTA (2021b) provides information to help guide advocacy efforts on aota.org, including guidance for decisions related to everyday advocacy.

Meso-Level Engagement

Societal transformation also requires collaboration at the level of professional networks and organizations. At the meso-level, OT and PT practitioners in all roles extend the visions of their professions through teams, communities,

TABLE 8.3 Professional Organization Vision and DEI Statements

Statement	Occupational Therapy	Physical Therapy
Vision	As an inclusive profession, occupational therapy maximizes health, well-being, and quality of life for all people, populations, and communities through effective solutions that facilitate participation in everyday living (AOTA, 2019).	Transforming society by optimizing movement to improve the human experience (APTA, 2022)
DEI Statement	AOTA affirms the inalienable right of every individual to feel welcomed, valued, a sense of belonging, and respected while accessing and participating in society, regardless of the internal or external factors that make every individual unique (AOTA, 2020).	APTA is committed to increasing diversity, equity, and inclusion in the association, profession, and society (APTA, 2022).

American Occupational Therapy Association. (2019). AOTA board expands Vision 2025. *The American Journal of Occupational Therapy, 73*(3), 7303420010p1-7303420010p1.

American Occupational Therapy Association. (2020). Occupational therapy's commitment to diversity, equity, and inclusion. *American Journal of Occupational Therapy, 74*(Suppl. 3), 7413410030.

American Physical Therapy Association (APTA). (2022). *APTA strategic plan 2022-2025.* https://www.apta.org/contentassets/14be4b91c1b94da8a92dfb76fe041b99/apta-strategic-plan-2022-2025.pdf

schools, and workplaces. The AOTA and APTA set an intentional course for DEI through their vision and DEI commitment statements (See Table 8.3). Active engagement within professional associations provides opportunities to make a difference by taking an honest look at how we fulfill the mission of our profession, how we recruit and educate future professionals, and how we advocate for changes that sustain positive outcomes for all people in the contexts of healthcare, legislation, politics, economy, and education. Lucas and Washington (2020) recommend that OT educators, students, and practitioners reflect on historical and current hegemonic policies and the frameworks of systemic racism to work toward occupational justice, considered an essential outcome of occupational therapy.

Practitioners can support DEI by offering input on standards of education and practice. Academic communities can assess curriculum, policies, and procedures, including those related to admission, to promote inclusion and belonging among all faculty, staff, and students. OT and PT practitioners can build capacity for DEI through continuing professional development opportunities, including AOTA (aota.org) and APTA (apta.org) educational series and resources. In addition to formal offerings, practitioners build the profession's capacity for DEI by volunteering on committees, engaging in mentorship, and dialoguing with fellow practitioners, community members, and organizational leaders. Interprofessional collaborations provide opportunities to foster DEI on a broad platform. For example, a group of PT, OT, and nursing members of the National Academies of Practice (NAP) came together to organize a workshop about DEI priorities across professions and develop an action plan for anti-racist interprofessional healthcare organizations (Bishop et al., 2022).

Students can also contribute toward DEI at the level of their future profession by joining groups of committed students and community members, for example, a profession-based student organization that hosts a series of DEI discussions and learning events at a university or an informal learning community that shares resources and perspectives to deepen understanding of DEI topics. In OT, a group of practitioners started the Coalition of Occupational Therapy Advocates for Diversity (COTAD) in 2014 to promote justice, equity, diversity, inclusion, and antiracism in the OT profession (COTAD, n.d.). At the time of this chapter's writing, there are 118 student chapters of this organization. Physical therapy practitioners have created groups such as PT Proud, the LGBTQIA+ Committee of the Health Policy and Administration Section of the APTA, which advocates for equity among LGBTQIA+ practitioners and clients (PT Proud, n.d.), and the National Association of Black Physical Therapists, which includes 23 established or developing chapters throughout the United States (NABPT, 2020).

At the meso-level, OT and PT practitioners can focus efforts on DEI through organizational engagement. Examples may range from critically examining hiring policies at a small outpatient clinic for sources of inequity to mindfully developing partnerships between extensive healthcare and community organizations to developing and implementing DEI training for work teams. The American Hospital Association Institute for Diversity and Health Equity (2020) proposes that healthcare settings continuously monitor and report how they work toward DEI, specifically in data collection, training opportunities, leadership, and community partnerships. Diverse representation at all levels of an organization is a starting point for moving toward inclusion and the experience of belonging for everyone in the organization. Emphasis on diversity and inclusion where decisions are made, for example, among organizational leadership teams and governing boards, moves the organization toward a culture of representation, inclusion, and quality (Bass, 2020). DEI committees at the organizational level can also yield progress. Lingras et al. (2023) offer a framework for health centers to get started with dedicated committees for DEI, *A Model for Developing a Departmental Diversity, Equity, Inclusion (DEI) Committee.* Fig. 8.5 represents the steps of this model.

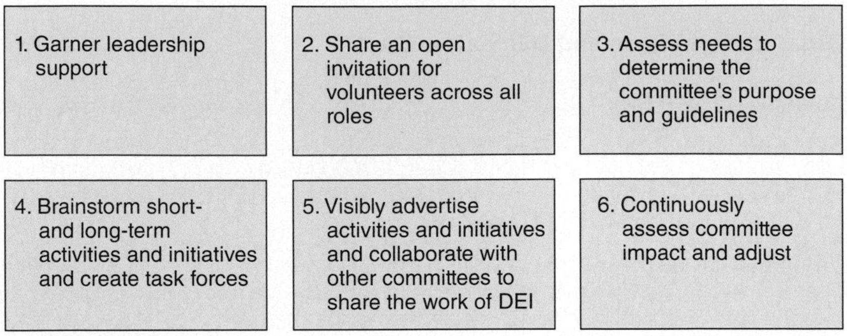

• **Fig. 8.5** A model for developing a departmental diversity, equity, inclusion (DEI) committee. (From Lingras, K. A., Alexander, M. E., & Vrieze, D. M. (2023). Diversity, Equity, and Inclusion Efforts at a Departmental Level: Building a Committee as a Vehicle for Advancing Progress. *Journal of clinical psychology in medical settings*, 30(2), 356–379. https://doi.org/10.1007/s10880-021-09809-w.

Micro-Level Engagement

Throughout this chapter, we have noted the interconnectedness of systems levels. The larger societal level affects the organizational and team levels, affecting individuals and interpersonal dynamics. It is also necessary to understand the influence of the micro-level on the meso- and macro-levels. Individuals live, work, lead, and make decisions at all system levels. OT and PT practitioners, like all members of society, must intentionally work toward DEI for transformation to occur. This work involves learning and critically reflecting on ourselves, others, and the power between us, mindfully interacting with each other, and taking action. Such work is aligned with the Social Change Model of Leadership (Komives & Wagner, 2016), a holistic model that everyone, regardless of position, can use to work towards being socially responsible. Please refer to the Chapter 10 in this book for more about this model.

Those who practice cultural humility are curious about how they and the people they interact with think and act. Agner (2020) broadly discusses culture as consisting of all aspects of identity we continuously learn about through interpersonal interactions rather than aspects we can assume and know for sure. This approach requires authentic dialogue, not a checklist. With this in mind, Agner also acknowledges that bias is human and encourages practitioners and educators to investigate the nature and sources of bias to promote inclusion. Lastly, Agner summarizes the reality that many researchers, social leaders, and advocates have confirmed—power is in play, and knowing how it works based on our social conditions and how it is used matters profoundly in the support or rejection of DEI.

At the micro-level, we think, dialogue, and act with one another. DEI at the micro-level requires consideration of the spaces that we create with each other and how they promote or limit the capacity for change and belonging. Researchers have described these spaces as safe and brave (Arao & Clemens, 2013). Safe spaces may imply physical, emotional, psychological, and social protection, trust, and even comfort for all people in the space.

People may associate safety with a lack of fear. For example, in a class group, you may agree to ground rules

regarding the space being a "judgment-free zone" for all to feel free to speak their mind. This zone can be beneficial, especially as we begin conversations about DEI in our homes, workplaces, classrooms, and communities. Experts such as Arao and Clemens (2013) recognize that spaces may more effectively promote DEI, belonging, and justice when accountability is present and when we dare to take a risk for positive change. See Table 8.4 for Arao and Clemens' comparison of the "rules" often related to safe spaces and the "challenges" invited in brave spaces.

Tulshyan (2022) emphasizes the value of an inclusion mindset for leaders and shares the BRIDGE framework (see Fig. 8.6). To leverage personal and interpersonal impact on DEI at meso- and macro-levels, we can use this framework to lead ourselves and others from fear to growth, a critical path for change related to DEI. With cultural humility, brave spaces, and the BRIDGE Framework, we have resources to add to professionally based supports for micro-level

TABLE 8.4 Characteristics of Safe and Brave Spaces

Typical ground rules for safe spaces	Challenges invited in brave spaces
"Agree to disagree"	"Controversy with civility"
"Don't take it personally"	Own your intentions and impact.
Choose your challenge	Reflect on how and why we choose to challenge or not challenge.
Respect	Be mindful of the different ways we each define and show respect.
Do not attack	Recognize that discomfort can lead to defense and explore why we defend.

Source Arao, B., & Clemens, K. (2013). From safe spaces to brave spaces: A new way to frame dialogue around diversity and social justice. In L. M. Landreman (Ed.), *The art of effective facilitation: Reflections from social justice educators* (1st ed.; pp. 135–150). Stylus Publishing, LLC.

Bridge framework

1. Be uncomfortable
2. Reflect (on what you don't know)
3. Invite feedback
4. Defensiveness doesn't help
5. Grow from your mistakes
6. Expect that change takes time

• **Fig. 8.6** BRIDGE Framework. (Tulshyan, Ruchika. Foreword by Ijeoma Oluo, Inclusion on Purpose, Table: Bridge Framework, © 2022 Ruchika Tulshyan, by permission of The MIT Press.)

engagement and capacity building related to DEI. Suggestions for professional engagement and building capacity related to DEI at each system level are provided in Fig. 8.7. Refer to case vignettes to apply this information.

CASE VIGNETTE

Bryan the Practitioner

During his career, Bryan has grappled with how best to help clients who experience health concerns related to social determinants of health. He has advocated for many clients who experience medical issues and make decisions about their health and healthcare based on transportation availability, access to nutritious food choices, and the need for income. Bryan sees the impact of systemic racism and homophobia on clients, families, and communities. Through Bryan's professional association and civic engagement, he has connected with national and regional advocacy efforts that support progress toward health equity. Since accepting the administrative role at the health system, Bryan has engaged with people on his team and throughout the organization in DEI work. Bryan regularly uses resources from AOTA and APTA to coordinate staff training opportunities and inform policy and administrative decisions based on data. Bryan frequently implements and shares the BRIDGE Framework to build an inclusive mindset amid his work pressures and busy days (Tulshyan, 2022). With humility, Bryan invites feedback, often asking staff and administrators questions about things that can be difficult to discuss. Bryan is committed to building trust while taking risks that promote the growth of his team and the organization and the care they provide to clients.

How do you think Bryan engages at each system level? Which skills and resources support Bryan in promoting DEI at these levels?

CASE VIGNETTE

Meera the Student

Meera and some classmates meet informally to share perspectives and experiences in their education and a passion for DEI at all levels. Their time together may be spent listening to a classmate's experience of microaggression, checking out news and resources from APTA, or introducing new friends with common interests in PT and DEI. Meera values these interpersonal connections and feels drawn to organize a more formal group inclusive of all students at the university and even neighboring schools who want to learn more and advocate for DEI. Meera engages her friends in a discussion about this and petitions to initiate a new student organization called Building Belonging in the Health Professions. So far, in the organization's first year, the group has connected with similar organizations at two other higher education institutions in their region to host educational networking events and provided a space for students and faculty from across professional programs to listen and share stories and experiences related to DEI.

How does Meera's experience highlight engagement toward DEI related to her education and future profession? How might this influence how Meera contributes to DEI as a practitioner?

Macro

• Learn how power operates in social, political, economic, and legal systems to make informed decisions on how to create, vote, and advocate for policies that contribute to diversity, equity, and inclusion (DEI).

Meso

• Extend the visions of the professions through teams, communities, schools and workplaces through formal training, working for organizational policies that support DEI, and volunteering.

Micro

• Critically reflect on ourselves, others, and the power between us, mindfully interacting with each other and taking action for DEI; supports include cultural humility, brave spaces, and the BRIDGE framework.

• **Fig. 8.7** Professional Engagement and Building Capacity Impacting Diversity, Equity, and Inclusion

Conclusion

Diversity, equity, inclusion, and belonging are supported or rejected at macro-, meso-, and micro-levels. These systems levels are interconnected and dependent on one another. Members of the OT and PT professional communities must understand their roles in supporting or hindering DEI at each system level. Critical reflection on the history of society, healthcare, and the OT and PT professions provides a necessary starting point for moving toward DEI. Practitioners, guided by the ethics and core values of their professions, have a responsibility to know and advocate for laws, policies, and procedures that support DEI at all levels. OTs and PTs must also learn the effect of social capital on clients, the workforce, and society to work toward health equity. When practitioners engage at the macro-, meso-, and micro levels, the capacity of the professions to support DEI and belonging is built and actualized.

DEI Resource List

As resources related to DEI and belonging in education, healthcare, and the workforce become available, we encourage you to engage with all you can to learn, connect, advocate and be a part of the change that matters to you. We offer some resources to help you get started. We look forward to the future resources that will help us all build the capacity of the PT and OT professions and communities for DEI and belonging.

Governmental Resources

- The White House Executive order on Diversity, equity, inclusion, and accessibility in the federal workforce (https://www.whitehouse.gov/briefing-room/presidential-actions/2021/06/25/executive-order-on-diversity-equity-inclusion-and-accessibility-in-the-federal-workforce/)

Educational Resources

- Journal article about DEI textbook inventory
  Dillard-Wright, J., Gazaway, S. (2021). Drafting a diversity, equity, and inclusion textbook inventory: Assumptions, concepts, conceptual framework. *Teaching and Learning in Nursing, 16* (3), 247-253. https://doi.org/10.1016/j.teln.2021.02.001
- TED Talk about gender equity:
  Singh, L. (2021). "A seat at the table" isn't the solution for gender equity [video]. YouTube. https://youtu.be/9EBkS2kE7uk
- Fitzhugh Mullan Institute for Health Workforce Equity. Health Workforce Diversity Tracker. Washington, DC: George Washington University, 2021. https://www.gwhwi.org/workforce-trackers.html
- American Hospital Association's Health Equity, Diversity & Inclusion Measures for Hospitals and Health System Dashboards https://ifdhe.aha.org/health-equity-diversity-inclusion-measures-hospitals-and-health-system-dashboards

Professional Organization Resources

- AOTA DEI Resource Library https://www.aota.org/practice/practice-essentials/dei/diversity-equity-inclusion-toolkit-resource-library
- AOTA DEI Framework https://www.aota.org/media/Corporate/Files/AboutOT/DEI/DEI-Framework.pdf
- APTA Diversity, Equity, Inclusion Activity Report Form https://www.apta.org/apta-and-you/diversity-equity-and-inclusion/diversity-equity-and-inclusion-activity-report-form
- 2021 Lynda D. Woodruff Lecture by Charlene Portee, PT, Ph.D., "The Road to Success: Are We Ready to Change Direction?" https://youtu.be/FePjgK8Agm8

Organizations and Advocacy Group Resources

- AORTA: Anti-Oppression Resource and Training Alliance https://aorta.coop/
- ACLU webpage on LGBTQ Rights: https://www.aclu.org/know-your-rights/lgbtq-rights
- Coalition of Occupational Therapy Advocates for Diversity https://www.cotad.org/
- National Association of Black Physical Therapists, Inc. https://nabpt.org/

References

ADA.gov. (n.d.). *Introduction to the ADA.* https://www.ada.gov/ada_intro.htm.

Agner, J. (2020). Moving from cultural competence to cultural humility in occupational therapy: A paradigm shift. *American Journal of Occupational Therapy, 74*(4), 7404347010-7404347010p7.

American Hospital Association Institute for Diversity and Health Equity. (2020). *Health equity, diversity & inclusion measures for hospitals and health system dashboards.* American Hospital Association. https://ifdhe.aha.org/system/files/media/file/2020/12/ifdhe_inclusion_dashboard.pdf.

Table 8.3 American Occupational Therapy Association. (2020a). Occupational therapy's commitment to diversity, equity, and inclusion. *American Journal of Occupational Therapy, 74*(Suppl. 3), 7413410030.

American Occupational Therapy Association. (2020b). AOTA 2020 occupational therapy code of ethics. *American Journal of Occupational Therapy, 74*(Suppl. 3), 7413410005.

American Occupational Therapy Association. (2021a). *Our nation is facing a health workforce diversity crisis.* https://www.aota.org/-/media/corporate/files/advocacy/ahwd-2021-supporting-data-one-pager.pdf.

American Occupational Therapy Association. (2021b). *Everyday advocacy decision guide.* https://www.aota.org/-/media/corporate/files/advocacy/everyday-advocacy-decision-guide.pdf.

American Physical Therapy Association (APTA). (2019). *APTA diversity and inclusion strategic plan.* APTA.

American Physical Therapy Association (APTA). (2020). *Code of ethics for the physical therapist.* https://www.apta.org/siteassets/pdfs/policies/codeofethicshods06-20-28-25.pdf.

American Physical Therapy Association (APTA). (2021a). *Position paper: The Allied Health Work Diversity Act (H.R. 3320/S. 1679).*

https://www.apta.org/advocacy/issues/education-and-workforce-legislation/allied-health-workforce-diversity.

American Physical Therapy Association (APTA). (2021b). *APTA public policy priorities 2021-2022* [Position Paper]. APTA. https://www.apta.org/advocacy/issues/apta-public-policy-priorities.

Arao, B., & Clemens, K. (2013). From safe spaces to brave spaces: A new way to frame dialogue around diversity and social justice. In L. M. Landreman (Ed.), *The art of effective facilitation: Reflections from social justice educators* (1st ed., pp. 135–150). Stylus Publishing, LLC.

Bailey, E., Lipton, A., Miller, J., & Moll, S. (2020). *The three A's of inclusion: Awareness, authenticity, and accountability.* Harvard Business Publishing Corporate Learning. https://www.harvardbusiness.org/insight/the-three-as-of-inclusion-awareness-authenticity-and-accountability/.

Bass, K. H. (2020). *Recruiting for a diverse health care board: Practices and processes to better reflect community diversity.* American Hospital Association. https://trustees.aha.org/recruiting-diverse-health-care-board.

Bishop, K. L., Abbruzzese, L. P., Adeniran, R., Dunleavy, K., Maxwell, B., Oluwole-Sangoseni, O., Simon, P., Smith, S. S., & Thurston, L. (2022). Becoming an anti-racist interprofessional healthcare organization: Our journey. *Journal of Interprofessional Education & Practice, 27,* 100509.

Blackstone, A. (2012). *Principles of sociological inquiry: Qualitative and quantitative methods.* Saylor Foundation. https://saylordotorg.github.io/text_principles-of-sociological-inquiry-qualitative-and-quantitative-methods/.

Bourdieu, P. (1984). *Distinction: A social critique of the judgement of taste.* Harvard University Press.

Bourdieu, P. (1986). The forms of capital. In J. G. Richardson (Ed.), *Handbook of theory and research for the sociology of education* (pp. 241–258). New York: Greenwood Press.

Braveman, P. (2013). What is health equity: And how does a life-course approach take us further toward it? *Maternal and Child Health Journal, 18*(2), 366–372.

Braveman, P. A., Arkin, E., Proctor, D., Kauh, T., & Holm, N. (2022). Systemic and structural racism: definitions, examples, health damages, and approaches to dismantling. *Health Affairs, 41*(2), 171–178.

Brotherton, S., Smith, C. R., Boissonneault, G., Wager, K. A., Velozo, C., & de Arellano, M. (2021). Holistic admissions: Strategies for increasing student diversity in occupational therapy, physical therapy, and physician assistant studies programs. *Journal of Allied Health, 50*(3), 91E–97E. https://www.ingentaconnect.com/content/asahp/jah/2021/00000050/00000003/art00014.

Brown University. (2022). *A framework for making ethical decisions.* https://www.brown.edu/academics/science-and-technology-studies/framework-making-ethical-decisions.

Cambridge University Press. (n.d.). *Cambridge dictionary.* Retrieved from February 2, 2022. https://dictionary.cambridge.org/us/dictionary/english/law.

Cerderbom, S., Bjerk, M., & Bergland, A. (2020). The tensions between micro-, meso- and macro-levels: Physiotherapists' views of their role towards fall prevention in the community – a qualitative study. *BMC Health Services Research, 20*(1), 97.

Chowkwanyun, M., & Reed, A. L. (2020). Racial health disparities and Covid-19 — Caution and context. *The New England Journal of Medicine, 383*(3), 201–203. https://www.nejm.org/doi/10.1056/NEJMp2012910.

Claridge, T. (2015). *Bourdieu on social capital: Theory of capital.* Institute for Social Capital. https://www.socialcapitalresearch.com/bourdieu-on-social-capital-theory-of-capital/.

Claridge, T. (2020). *Current definitions of social capital: Academic definitions in 2019.* Institute for Social Capital. https://www.socialcapitalresearch.com/current-definitions-of-social-capital/.

Coalition of Occupational Therapy Advocates for Diversity. (n.d.). *Our Mission—COTAD National.* https://www.cotad.org/about.

Coleman-Salgado, B. (2021). Admissions holistic review of socioeconomic factors fosters diversity in a doctor of physical therapy program. *Journal of Physical Therapy Education, 35*(3), 182–194.

Congress.gov. (n.d.). *H.R.5—117th Congress (2021-2022): Equality Act.* https://www.congress.gov/bill/117th-congress/house-bill/5/text.

Congress.gov. (n.d.). *S.1679—117th Congress (2021-2022): Allied Health Workforce Diversity Act of 2021.* https://www.congress.gov/bill/117th-congress/senate-bill/1679/actions?r=56&s=1.

Davis, J. B. (2015). Stratification economics and identity economics. *Cambridge Journal of Economics, 39*(5), 1215–1229. https://doi.org/10.1093/cje/beu071.

Ehrenpreis, J. A., & Ehrenpreis, E. D. (2022). A historical perspective of healthcare disparity and infectious disease in the Native American Population. *The American Journal of the Medical Sciences, 363*(4), 288–294.

Fuller, J., Langer, C., & Sigelman, M. (2022, February 11). *Skills-based hiring is on the rise.* Harvard Business Review. https://hbr.org/2022/02/skills-based-hiring-is-on-the-rise.

Glazer, G., Danek, J., Michaels, J., Bankston, K., Fair, M., Johnson, S. & Nivet, M. (2014). *Holistic admissions in the health professions: Findings from a national survey.* Washington, DC: Urban Universities for HEALTH.

Hagerty, B. M. K., Lynch-Sauer, J., Patusky, K. L., Bouwsema, M., & Collier, P. (1992). Sense of belonging: A vital mental health concept. *Archives of Psychiatric Nursing, 6*(3), 172–177.

Healthy People 2030. (n.d.). *Social determinants of health.* U.S. Department of Health and Human Services, Office of Disease Prevention and Health Promotion. Retrieved from February 9, 2022. https://health.gov/healthypeople/priority-areas/social-determinants-health.

History.com Editors. (2022, January 20). *Civil Rights Act of 1964—Definition, summary & significance.* https://www.history.com/topics/black-history/civil-rights-act.

Kassing, F., Casanova, T., Griffin, J. A., Wood, E., & Stepleman, L. M. (2021). The effects of polyvictimization on mental and physical health outcomes in an LGBTQ sample. *Journal of Traumatic Stress, 34*(1), 161–171. https://doi.org/10.1002/jts.22579.

Kendi, I. X. (2019). *How to be an antiracist* (1st ed.). One World.

Kirsh, B. H. (2015). Transforming values into action: Advocacy as a professional imperative. *Canadian Journal of Occupational Therapy, 82*(4), 212–223.

Komives, S. R., & Wagner, W. (Eds.). (2016). *Leadership for a better world: Understanding the social change model of leadership development* (2nd ed.). Jossey-Bass.

Lavizzo-Mourey, R. J., Besser, R. E., & Williams, D. R. (2021). Understanding and mitigating health inequities — past, current, and future directions. *The New England Journal of Medicine, 384*(18), 1681–1684.

Lingras, K. A., Alexander, M. E., & Vrieze, D. M. (2023). Diversity, equity, and inclusion efforts at a departmental level: Building a committee as a vehicle for advancing progress. *Journal of Clinical Psychology in Medical Settings, 30*(2), 356–379. https://doi.org/10.1007/s10880-021-09809-w.

Lucas, C., & Washington, S. (2020). *Understanding systemic racism in the United States: Educating our students and ourselves.* AOTA Continuing Education.

Matthews, N. D., Rowley, K. M., Dusing, S. C., Krause, L., Yamaguchi, N., & Gordon, J. (2021). Beyond a statement of support: Changing the culture of equity, diversity, and inclusion in physical therapy. *Physical Therapy, 101*(12), pzab212.

McKay, B. (2011). Lesbian, gay, bisexual, and transgender health issues, disparities, and information resources. *Medical Reference Services Quarterly, 30*(4), 393–401.

McKay, T., Lindquist, C. H., & Misra, S. (2019). Understanding (and acting on) 20 years of research on violence and LGBTQ + communities. *Trauma Violence & Abuse, 20*(5), 665–678. https://doi.org/10.1177/1524838017728708.

NABPT. (2020). *National Association of Black Physical Therapists, Inc.* https://nabpt.org/about/.

National Paralegal College. (2022). *Sources of law in the United States.* https://lawshelf.com/shortvideoscontentview/sources-of-law-in-the-united-states.

Peterson, A., Charles, V., Yeung, D., & Coyle, K. (2021). The health equity framework: A science- and justice-based model for public health researchers and practitioners. *Health Promotion Practice, 22*(6), 741–746.

Pollock, E. A., Givens, M. L., & Johnson, S. P. (2022). *Voting and civic engagement rights are eroding: What does it mean for health and equity?* Health Affairs Forefront.

PT Proud. (n.d.). *Home [Facebook page].* Facebook. Retrieved from March 12, 2022. https://www.facebook.com/PTProud/.

Putnam, R. (1993). The prosperous community: Social capital and public life. *The American Prospect, 13*, 35–42.

Putnam, R. (2000). *Bowling alone: The collapse and revival of American community.* New York: Simon and Schuster.

Race Forward. (n.d.). *What is Racial Equity?* https://www.raceforward.org/about/what-is-racial-equity-key-concepts#diversity-inclusion.

Rosenkranz, K. M., Arora, T. K., Termuhlen, P. M., Stain, S. C., Misra, S., Dent, D., & Nfonsam, V. (2021). Diversity, equity and inclusion in medicine: Why it matters and how do we achieve it? *Journal of Surgical Education, 78*(4), 1058–1065.

Ross, H. J. (2011). *Reinventing diversity transforming organizational community to strengthen people, purpose, and performance.* Rowman & Littlefield Publishers.

Salvant, S., Kleine, E. A., & Gibbs, V. D. (2021). The issue is...Be heard-we're listening: Emerging issues and potential solutions from the voices of BIPOC occupational therapy students, practitioners, and educators. *American Journal of Occupational Therapy, 75*, 7506347010.

Sterman, J., & Njelesani, J. (2021). Becoming anti-racist occupational therapy practitioners: A scoping study. *OTJR, 41*(4), 232–242.

Taff, S. D., & Blash, D. (2017). Diversity and inclusion in occupational therapy: Where we are, where we must go. *Occupational Therapy in Health Care, 31*(1), 72–83.

Tervalon, M., & Murray-Garcia, J. (1998). Cultural humility versus cultural competence: A critical distinction in defining physician training outcomes in multicultural education. *Journal of Health Care for the Poor and Underserved, 9*(2), 117–125.

Togioka, B. M., Duvivier, D., & Young, E. (2021). Diversity and discrimination in healthcare. In *StatPearls.* StatPearls Publishing. http://www.ncbi.nlm.nih.gov/books/NBK568721/.

Tulshyan, R. (2022). *Inclusion on purpose: An intersectional approach to creating a culture of belonging at work.* The MIT Press.

United Nations. (n.d.). *Capacity-building.* United Nations: Academic impact. https://www.un.org/en/academic-impact/capacity-building.

United States Census Bureau. (2022). 2020 *County business patterns first look.* https://www.census.gov/data/tables/2020/econ/cbp/2020-first-look.html.

U.S. Equal Employment Opportunity Commission. (n.d.). *Overview.* https://www.eeoc.gov/overview.

Vazir, S., Newman, K., Kispal, L., Morin, A. E., Mu, Y. (Yusuf), Smith, M., & Nixon, S. (2019). Perspectives of racialized physiotherapists in Canada on their experiences with racism in the physiotherapy profession. *Physiotherapy Canada, 71*(4), 335–345.

Wesson, D. & Kitzman, H. (2018). How academic health systems can achieve population health in vulnerable populations through value-based care: The critical importance of establishing trusted agency. *Academic Medicine, 93*(6), 839–842.

World Health Organization. (2022). *Health equity.* https://www.who.int/health-topics/health-equity#tab=tab_1.

Xu, J., Kunaviktikul, W., Akkadechanunt, T., Nantsupawat, A., & Stark, A. T. (2020). A contemporary understanding of nurses' workplace social capital: A response to the rapid changes in the nursing workforce. *Journal of Nursing Management, 28*(2), 247–258.

9

Communication With Clients and Providers

MATTHEW B. GARBER, PT, DSc, OCS, FAAOMPT;
and JULIA HAWKINS-POKABLA, OTD, OTR/L

LEARNING OBJECTIVES

After completion of this chapter, learners will be able to:

- The student will identify five ways to use effective communication with clients.
- The student will define health literacy.
- The student will list three evidence-based strategies that support quality interviewing skills.

- The student will list one strategy to improve communication in three different practice settings.
- The student will give three examples of different types of communication in a therapy setting.

CHAPTER OUTLINE

An Overview of Communication With Clients

Considerable research has revealed the positive impact and importance of effective communication in improved health outcomes over the past 40 years. Clients working with rehabilitation professionals value positive communication characteristics expressed during client-physician encounters. Bialosky and colleagues (2010) noted that clients were more satisfied with their care and had better recall and understanding of provided information with quality communication. Beattie and colleagues (2002) reported a strong association between client satisfaction and the perceived quality of client-provider interactions. In particular, providers spending adequate time with the client, exhibiting strong listening and communication skills, and offering clear explanations of treatments were desirable qualities (Fig. 9.1).

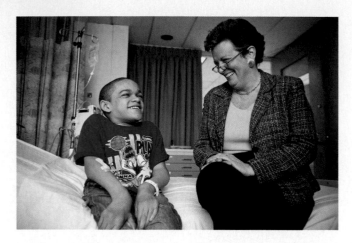

• **Fig. 9.1** Avoiding interruptions and confusing terminology improves the quality of pertinent data gained through the interview. (From https://www.flickr.com/photos/64860478@N05/7139600519).

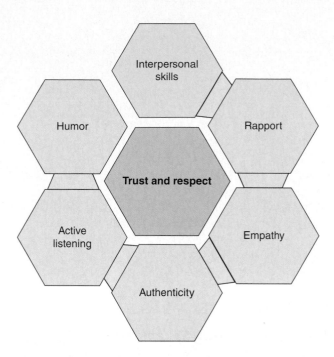

• **Fig. 9.2** These interpersonal and communication skills profoundly influence client-therapist interactions.

Despite the evidence showing the importance of strong communication skills in healthcare settings, many providers struggle to integrate effective communication during client encounters. It is common for providers to interrupt clients early and often during a visit, hindering effective care. Physicians have been shown to take control of the interview after interrupting the client and use more closed-ended questions for the remainder of the interview (Beckman & Frankel, 1984). After being interrupted, clients may not volunteer their primary concerns, hindering the amount and quality of pertinent data gained through the interview (Phillips & Ospina, 2017; Realini et al., 1995; Rosenstein & O'Daniel, 2005). Therapists spend twice as much time talking during a visit than clients (Roberts & Bucksey, 2007).

Appropriate medical terminology, including clarifying clients' understanding of terms, is critical to successful communication. Wright & Hopkins (1978) found that physicians, therapists, and clients commonly disagree about the definition of commonly used medical terms. Physicians and clients showed poor agreement on more than 40% of the words in a questionnaire. Therapists and clients showed poor agreement for *numbness, ligaments, lumbar, back,* and *sciatic nerve.* Even more alarming is that physicians and therapists could not agree on 30% of these commonly used medical terms. Among words with fair to poor agreement were *arthritis, back, arm weakness, joint swelling,* and *sciatic nerve* .

A recent systematic review by O'Keeffe et al. (2016) found that the therapist's interpersonal and communication skills profoundly influence client-therapist interactions in the outpatient setting. The communication elements associated with these positive interactions were active listening, empathy, friendliness, confidence, and encouragement. Therapists who listen help their clients feel understood and valued, strengthening the client-provider relationship. Clients also want their therapist to be empathetic and understand how their condition impacts their life. Effective therapists who have developed strong interpersonal skills foster a positive client-provider relationship that improves client outcomes. Clients with confidence in their therapist, resulting from a trusting and respectful relationship, are also more likely to adhere to treatment plans (O'Keefe et al., 2016).

Therapists who are relaxed and incorporate humor, develop a stronger bond with their clients. Therapists who offer emotional support and encouragement are more likely to motivate their clients to adhere to treatment recommendations. Finally, clients who feel confident in their therapist are more likely to trust and respect their opinions and recommendations (Fig. 9.2). Physical therapists who have mastered these interpersonal skills foster a positive client-therapist relationship, leading to better results (O'Keeffe et al., 2016). Occupational therapists with more training in the *therapeutic use of self* (i.e., conscious use of personality and knowledge to improve interactions with clients) were more likely to feel positive regard and genuine concern for their clients (Taylor et al., 2009). These findings suggest that more attention and training on the therapeutic relationship and the therapeutic use of self may be warranted. Families who trust a therapeutic relationship and view healthcare professionals as collaborative and cooperative may also be more faithful to recommendations (Dimatteo, 2004).

Clients also notice when providers try to adjust treatment when difficulties are encountered. Healthcare providers that consider the clients' points of view and opinions result in more active client engagement in the rehabilitation process and more positive interactions between clients and their providers (O'Keeffe et al., 2016). The Institute of Medicine's report supports that client satisfaction is linked to shared decision-making between providers and clients (Alston et al., 2012).

While it is important to understand the positive association between effective communication and health outcomes, negative outcomes, such as poor health literacy (Chapter 4), cultural differences, and patient beliefs about treatment efficacy are also associated with poor communication. Most complaints about healthcare providers are associated with ineffective communication, not clinical skills (Richards, 1990; Shapiro et al., 1989). Most malpractice allegations against physicians arise from communication problems (Roter et al., 1997). Clients and families are more likely to sue if they think the healthcare provider is not caring or compassionate (Levin & Riley, 1984). Beckman et al. (1994) found that 70% of malpractice depositions were attributed to communication problems between the client and the physician. Primary care physicians who use active listening and facilitate client input have been found to have fewer malpractice claims than other physicians (Levinson et al., 1997). A 2015 report examining over 23,000 malpractice claims in obstetrics, nursing, surgery, and general medicine found that 30% of all malpractice complaints involve some communication error, with the vast majority of these provider-to-provider miscommunications, not provider to client (Blackstone & Pressman, 2016).

Healthcare professionals can sometimes undervalue or forget the potency of quality communication skills (May, 1994). Limiting communication with clients because of administrative burdens, regulatory requirements, payment policies, practices, or other workplace pressures can lead to longer recovery times and poor client outcomes due to gaps or errors in collecting pertinent client data (May, 1994). Becoming a skilled communicator with clients, physicians, and insurers, among others, should be a high priority for any rehabilitation professional. This chapter will provide recommendations and guidance to assist occupational and physical therapists in providing evidence-based communication strategies to key stakeholders in various healthcare settings.

Quality Communication With Clients

Building Rapport

Building rapport is a soft skill that therapists should focus on early on in their professional journey so that a connection can be made with clients and trust can guide the therapeutic process. Building rapport is connecting with someone so that communication channels are open and effective, which helps create a relationship and supports collaboration regarding an end goal in therapy. "Developing a therapeutic client-therapist relationship is believed to be critical to facilitating the occupational therapy process and ensuring positive client outcomes" (Cole & McLean, 2003; Palmadottir, 2006; Taylor et al., 2009). Effective therapeutic relationships include authentic and respectful interpersonal communication with clients (Cole & McLean, 2003; Palmadottir, 2006; Punwar et al., 2000; Taylor, 2020). *The Intentional Relationship Model* (IRM) guides therapists using six communication modes based on the therapist's personality and needs, and preferences (Fan et al., 2022). The modes are advocating, collaborating, empathizing, encouraging, instructing, and problem-solving so that the client can remain engaged, supported, and dedicated to their progress (Fig. 9.3).

Client-Centered Interviews

The client-centered interview is a method that incorporates biopsychosocial concepts. A biopsychosocial approach is "a

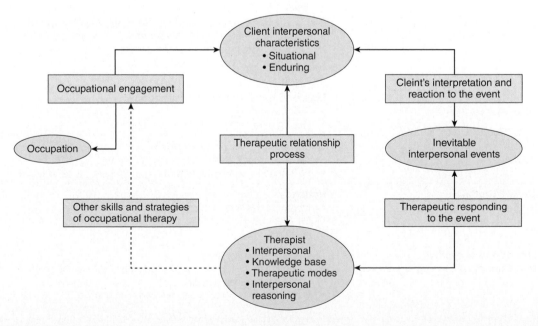

• **Fig. 9.3** The intentional relationship model. (Taylor, R. R. [2020]. *The Intentional Relationship: Occupational Therapy and Use of Self.* [2nd ed.]. Philadelphia: FA Davis.)

way of understanding the patient's subjective experience as an essential contributor to accurate diagnosis, health outcomes, and humane care" (Wittink & Oosterhaven, 2018). The biopsychosocial approach when interviewing a client encourages more client participation during the medical encounter and diagnosing and treating their disorder (Epstein, 2000). The client-centered interview allows the therapist to develop a more effective relationship with clients and ensure that clients are understood and valued (Platt et al., 2001).

The client-centered interview consists of six interactive components: (1) exploration of both the client's disease/diagnosis and its impact on their life; (2) understanding the whole person; (3) finding common ground regarding intervention or management; (4) prevention and health promotion; (5) enhancement of the client-provider relationship; and (6) realistic expectations (Evans et al., 1991).

Understanding the importance of communication is the foundation for the client interview. The goals of completing the client interview and obtaining the client's history include establishing rapport, identifying any barriers to communication, identifying the client's preferred learning style, and establishing the client's goals for treatment. Table 9.1 lists common barriers to communication and possible solutions (Ali, 2017, Button & Rossera, 1990).

Furthermore, the client history that the therapist gathers enables the therapist to establish an early hypothesis about the source of the client's symptoms. Then the therapist can plan an appropriate physical exam, establish a "baseline" of symptoms and determine a functional level to measure changes after any interventions. The client interview should be conducted in a room with as little noise and distraction as possible. Rooms with bright lights and clutter can inhibit good eye contact and should be avoided.

An Effective Occupational Profile

The most valuable step in the evaluation portion of the therapeutic process is the occupational profile, where communication skills are vital to gathering the information that leads to a client-centered plan of care. The occupational profile is a conversation, an interview, with the client and relevant caregivers where strengths and barriers in the client's routine are discussed and prioritized. The occupational profile is the client's story and drives the therapeutic process. Therapists must listen to and value the client's wants and needs to develop an effective treatment plan. Current procedural terminology codes established in 2017 require the inclusion of an occupational profile for occupational therapists in initial evaluation documentation (American Occupational Therapy Association, 2021).

Once the occupational profile is established through effective communication skills between the therapist and the client/caregivers, a plan of care can be established (AOTA Occupational Profile Template, 2017). Goals are

TABLE 9.1	Barriers and Solutions to Communication
Barriers to Communication	**Possible Solutions**
Physical and environmental • Time, place, space, climate, and noise • Choice of medium	**Ask the client questions about preferences:** • Scheduling • Treatment area (e.g., private room) • Email? Text? Phone call?
Wrong choice of medium • Frequent therapy no-shows/cancelations • Noncompliance • Distractions • Language Barriers	**Discuss what's working and not working with the client:** • "Do you have time to check your email?" "Do you prefer to hang a home program worksheet on your refrigerator?" • "Do you check your text messages frequently?"
Semantic Varied connotative meanings	**Listen to the client's use of language** • Ask if everything is clear • Return demonstration/discussion summary
Cultural Diversity of cultures	**Complete an occupational profile** • Asks questions about cultural preferences • Follow up for feedback from the client regarding satisfaction
Psychological/Attitudinal Moods, attitudes, and relationships	**Patience** • Involve caregivers in communication • Be client-centered: "What do you want to work on?" "You're doing good; let's also..."
Varying perceptions of reality Levels of understanding and comprehension	**Ask about reading level** • Ask preference for medium (read to them, email, interpretive services): • Review evaluation results • Review plan of care, goals, progress, discharge

From Ali, M. (2017) Communication skills 2: Overcoming barriers to effective communication. *Nursing Times, 114,* 1, 40–42; Button, K., & Rossera, F. (1990). Barriers to communication. *The Annals of Regional Science, 24*(4), 337–357.

created with client and caregiver input so that all individuals that are part of the therapy team can contribute to the goals laid out and are invested in the steps needed to produce positive outcomes for the client. Clear communication lines will not be open if therapists do not start conversations, ask questions, or repeat ideas and goals to create an open dialogue between all therapy team partners. The plan of care should be shared in a conversation between the therapist, client, and primary caregivers so that changes and revisions can be made as therapy moves forward. Interventions are chosen based on the plan of care conversation and can be revised through further communication so that all parties involved are invested in the client's positive outcome. If the therapist establishes a plan of care, only their investment in it is represented. Like a business meeting, everyone involved in the client's care should know the steps and goals. A written copy or electronic summary of the plan of care, including medication management and client goals, should be provided to the family by the therapist to be a resource for ongoing and necessary communication (Dimatteo, 2004).

Strategies for Effective Verbal Communication

Effective verbal communication skills are critical during the client interview. Open-ended questions allow the client to elaborate on details surrounding their condition, while closed-ended questions provide limited information. It is best to start with open-ended questions and then "funnel" to closed-ended questions that require a "yes" or "no" response to clarify information. It is also important not to use biased questions that lead the client to provide the answer the therapist wants to hear. Other effective verbal communication strategies include asking only one question, speaking slowly and deliberately, and keeping questions brief. These strategies prevent the client from getting confused and help the client answer questions more accurately. Simple sentences free of medical jargon are also helpful in preventing client confusion. Using the client's own words whenever possible is also an effective strategy to improve communication and rapport with the client. Using the client's line of thought, or paralleling the client's mental processes, may also be helpful. The therapist is more likely to get an accurate picture of the client's symptoms and their impact on daily activities. Assumptions should be avoided and any misunderstanding should focus first on the therapist's inability to communicate effectively. Physicians have been found to often attribute communication problems to the client rather than their limitations (Levinson et al., 1993). Attributing frustration to client characteristics alone may interfere with building a trusting relationship necessary for an optimal client-provider relationship (Levinson et al., 1993). These moments of misunderstanding and clarification allow the therapist to self-evaluate and reflect on ways to improve communication skills. Periodic self-assessment of the entire examination, including the interview, and using videotapes and audiotapes are useful tools to reflect on communication skills.

Motivational Interviewing

A technique that has gained popularity in rehabilitation settings to assist behavior modification is motivational interviewing. Motivational interviewing is a counseling method that evolved from Carl Rogers' person-centered approach to therapy that helps people resolve insecurities and feelings to find the internal motivation necessary to make life changes (Hettema et al., 2005). It is a practical and short-term process that helps therapists show empathy while considering the difficulties of behavior change. The interviewer focuses on listening and reflecting on the client's thoughts to hear their reasons and motivations expressed back to them (Clifford & Curtis, 2016; Hettema et al., 2005).

Motivational interviewing involves four communication skills that support and strengthen the therapist-client relationship, commonly referred to as OARS (Souders, 2019). Box 9.1 provides motivational interviewing strategies and sample questions:

1. **Open-ended questions** allow the client to provide more information about their perspective and ideas for change.

• BOX 9.1 Motivational Interviewing Strategies and Questions

1. **Ask open-ended questions:** "What has worked well for you in the past?"
2. **Express empathy:** "I understand that it has been difficult for you to exercise in the past. Many of my clients find this to be difficult. I think it is still important for us to try to find ways for you to work on this."
3. **Provide positive feedback:** "You have been working hard and it is paying off with good results."
4. **Elicit intrinsic motivation** (don't just tell the client what they *should* do) "What are the most important things for you?; "If you decided to change, what might your options be?"; "How can I help you succeed?"
5. **Reflect back thoughts and feelings:** "Watching less TV and exercising more is one thing you'd like to change."
6. **Have the client connect the dots:** "So you said you want to live long enough to see your grandchildren. What are the key points we discussed about how you might make that happen?"
7. **Roll with resistance:** If the client says, "I just always go back to my previous habits of watching TV and not exercising," the therapist could say, "That is a common problem. What would make you more confident about making these changes stick?"
8. **Make it personal:** Personal relationships are the basis for change. Rather than offering generic advice, specifically link action steps to the client's needs. "You said it was important for you to be outside more often so you can be more active. How do you think that would work for you?"

Adapted from Miller, M. (2021, May 3). *Motivational interviewing: 8 questions to ask clients to motivate change. 6 seconds: the emotional intelligence network.* https://www.6seconds.org/2021/05/03/motivational-interviewing-change/ © Six Seconds, used by permission.

2. **Affirming:** recognizing and commenting on the client's strengths and abilities.
3. **Reflective listening:** repeating what the client has said in our own words.
4. **Summarizing:** allows the therapist and client to identify key elements of the client's story.

Other behavior change models that may be useful in working with clients include the transtheoretical model (Prochaska & Velicer, 1997) and social cognitive theory (Bandura, 1995). The transtheoretical model (TTM) proposes that health behavior change progresses through six stages: precontemplation, contemplation, preparation, action, maintenance, and termination (see Box 9.2). TTM has been shown to improve the physical activity levels of college-aged students, supporting the idea that individuals' stages of change affect their self-efficacy level, or the ability to make positive and negative decisions impacting performance (Liu et al., 2018). A key component of social cognitive theory is self-efficacy, which is the belief in one's capability to complete a course of action, such as exercise (Bandura, 1995). Building self-efficacy involves experiencing success, seeing others similar to them, having positive experiences and successfully applying those strategies, receiving encouragement from others, and experiencing enjoyment or positive mood states (see Box 9.3; Bandura, 1995).

Carefully chosen words and phrases have been identified that help build empathy, allowing the provider to enhance their relationship with the client (Coulehan et al., 2001). Alternatively, other words and phrases can increase client anxiety or poor outcomes (see Box 9.4). Sloan and Walsh (2010) found that clients with chronic low back pain were exposed to degenerative terms from clinicians, such as "disc space loss," "wear and tear," and "deterioration," commonly found on radiology reports associated with a poor prognosis. Using these degenerative terms may not be helpful for clients

---

• BOX 9.3 How to Build Self Efficacy

1. **Mastery experiences** = experiencing success yourself
2. **Vicarious experiences** = seeing others who are similar to you having positive experiences and successful application of strategies (clients observing others in the clinic succeed)
3. **Verbal persuasion** = encouragement from others (including healthcare providers)
4. **Physiological feedback** = enjoyment, positive mood states

Adapted from Bandura, A. (1995). Exercise of personal and collective efficacy in changing societies. In A. Bandura (Ed.), *Self-efficacy in changing societies.* Cambridge: Cambridge University Press.

• BOX 9.4 Words That Harm

Provocative Terms (increase fear and anxiety)

1. Disc degeneration
2. Wear and tear
3. Disc space loss
4. Crumbling
5. Instability
6. Collapsing
7. Bone on bone

Adapted from Sloan, T.I. & Walsh, D.A. (2010). Explanatory and diagnostic labels and perceived prognosis in chronic low back pain. *Spine, 35,* 21, E1120-E1125.

---

and the authors suggest that clinicians use caution when reviewing radiology reports with clients. Explaining radiology findings to clients presents an opportunity to challenge unhelpful or misinformed beliefs about the diagnosis and prognosis and advocate for active treatment strategies (Sloan & Walsh, 2010). Using medical jargon, technical terms, and frightening metaphors can lead to client misunderstanding and create fear (Bedell et al., 2004). Clinicians should be mindful of their words' power and choose them wisely so they do not evoke fear and anxiety in the client (Stewart and Loftus, 2018). Healing language (see Box 9.5) avoids words that intensify these emotions and adapts and responds to the client's experience (Bedell et al., 2004; Stewart and Loftus, 2018). Healing language involves collaborative decision-making between the client and the clinician and provides information about treatment options while incorporating client preferences related to these choices (Bedell et al., 2004). Language should assist in healing by supporting the client's strengths, validating their perspective, and teaching them how to be more independent (Coulehan et al., 2001). The language therapists use should be strength-based, positive, and client-centered.

Communication in Different Practice Settings

Therapists should consider the entire context of the practice setting and use communication styles accordingly. Communication styles can differ between individuals and

---

• BOX 9.2 Transtheoretical Model of Change

1. **Precontemplation:** I don't see how my lack of exercise is a concern, but I hope that by agreeing to talk about it, my wife will feel reassured.
2. **Contemplation:** I can picture how exercising could improve my self-esteem, but I can't imagine exercising on a regular basis.
3. **Preparation:** I'm feeling good about setting a start date and joining a gym, but I'm wondering if I have the courage to follow through.
4. **Action:** Exercising for the past 3 weeks really makes me feel good, but part of me wants to celebrate by taking some days off and eating a pizza.
5. **Maintenance:** These recent months of exercise have made me feel that I'm progressing toward goals, but I'm still wondering whether exercising this much is really necessary.
6. **Termination:** Behaviors are well established and part of the person's new identity.

Adapted from Prochaska, J. O., & Velicer, W. F. (1997). The transtheoretical model of health behavior change. *American Journal of Health Promotion 12*(1), 38–48.

• BOX 9.5   Say This Not That: Words to Avoid and Alternatives When Discussing Client Conditions

Say This
- Normal age changes
- Narrowing; Tightening
- Condition
- It may persist, but you can overcome it
- You may have to make adjustments
- Reparable harm
- Everything will be OK
- The normal curve in your back
- Needs more strength and control

Avoid This
- Degenerative changes; arthritis; wear and tear
- Bone on bone
- Disease
- Chronic
- You are going to have to live with it
- Damage
- Don't worry
- Kyphosis; lordosis
- Instability

Adapted from Stewart, M. & Loftus, S. (2018). Sticks and stones: the impact of language in musculoskeletal rehabilitation. *Journal of Orthopaedic & Sports Physical Therapy, 48*(7), 519–522.

---

developmental levels of people. Institutions may even portray diversity in how they communicate with their clients. Therapists should consider the entire context they practice and use communication styles accordingly.

Outpatient

Communication in an outpatient setting should be clear and applicable to the client's routine outside of a hospital or clinic setting. Therapists should address daily routines that the client values in the plan of care as the client engages at home and in the community. Understanding client preferences supports client-centeredness and client-practitioner relationships and is recommended as an evidence-based technique to improve client commitment in an outpatient setting (Valdes & Campbell, 2017). Therapists in an outpatient setting should create plans of care and home programs that can be applied in the context of the clients improving skills, expanding roles, and growing independence. According to one study, clients prefer video copies of home programs in outpatient settings (Valdes & Campbell, 2017). *A Family Centered Training Program (FCTP)* is a method of caregiver education that can effectively provide knowledge to caregivers of people with dementia to assist with ADL independence if clients require more support at home (DiZazzo-Miller et al., 2017).

Acute Care

Hemsley and Balandin (2014) recommended strategies to improve communication between clients and providers in the acute care setting. First, healthcare facilities must develop systems, services, and policies supporting improved communication. In addition, devoting time to communicating and having access to appropriate communication devices is critical. Lastly, and perhaps most importantly, focusing on improving provider competence in effective communication strategies and collaborating with caregivers, family members, and clients' spouses is critical to good outcomes. Critical care clients, especially those receiving mechanical ventilation, frequently experience frustration and anxiety over their limited communication ability. Subsequently, using a communication board for critically ill clients has decreased client anxiety

and frustration while improving communication with healthcare providers (Patak et al., 2006). During ICU rounds, Choi and Tate (2021) recommend that clinicians be able to address: (1) whether the client can communicate effectively and by what mechanism; (2) posting a sign in the room indicating communication difficulty; (3) whether a speech-language pathologist has been consulted; and (4) whether there has been a change in the client's condition that could affect their ability to communicate. They also suggest posting a communication plan at the bedside listing how the client can convey thoughts, needs, and symptoms and whether the client can understand what care providers are communicating, including their need for hearing aids, glasses, or other assistive communication devices (Choi & Tate, 2021).

Skilled Nursing

Majerovitz et al. (2009) conducted two studies to examine the sources of conflict and miscommunication between skilled nursing facility staff and family members of residents. Institutional barriers included understaffing, frequent staff turnover, poor training, policies based on a medical model, and poor communication between staff. Psychosocial factors that hindered family communication included guilt, unrealistic expectations, cultural differences, and conflicting responsibilities. Families identified communication problems, including using guilt to alter thoughts or behaviors, criticism of their involvement, limited information, changes made in care without consultation, high staff turnover, and poor communication between staff members. Nursing personnel expressed similar concerns and stated they valued trusting, respectful relationships with supervisors and families, consultation prior to changes in care plans, support addressing racist or abusive comments, appropriate staffing, and teamwork. Certified nursing assistants expressed concern that family members are quick to complain but seldom praised care provided and those family members rarely recognize their considerable familiarity with the resident's functional status. Educational programs like *"Partners in Caregiving"* (Pillemer et al., 1998) can be used by therapists. *"Partners in Caregiving"* provides communication technique training to nursing staff and family members of residents to improve cooperation and communication of nursing facility staff and family members. Researchers reported positive outcomes in family and nursing staff who completed the training. In particular, family members of residents with dementia reported less conflict with nursing staff, while staff reported a lower likelihood of resigning (Pillemer et al., 1998).

Pediatrics

Therapists in pediatric settings should prioritize mindful connections with the entire family unit for communication to be impactful. An emphasis on rapport building with the child and the child's caregivers is integral. Home activities, safety education, developmental milestone resources, and supporting success are important when working with the diverse issues and families seen with children and youth. Dimatteo (2004) reports that the sicker the family believes their child is, the less likely the family is to follow recommendations from healthcare providers (Dimatteo, 2004). The therapist's communication skills and styles vary as it is necessary to connect with a child and educate the caregiver. Healthcare providers can become a normative influence in pediatric care when caregivers participate in direct and effective communication (Dimatteo, 2004). Sensitive questioning should be used to explore cultural differences and to fully understand the influence of others in the family's life (Dimatteo, 2004). The tone of voice, use of language, organizing ideas, and follow-up of education are all components of effective communication in a pediatric setting that should be considered. Even when caregivers believe care is family-centered, some gaps limit the partnership and effectiveness of interventions, further supporting the need to communicate clearly and often with children and their caregivers (Gafni-Lachter et al., 2021). Cultural humility is important during family communication and can be achieved by understanding bias, asking questions, and recognizing power dynamics in healthcare (Agner, 2020). Clinicians should consider the child's developmental level and communicate with them directly during intervention education while considering the accuracy of resources youth might find when using technology to explore their condition (Dimatteo, 2004).

Written Communication

While documentation is extremely important for client care, documenting during an episode of care can have negative consequences. In an analysis of 113 client physical therapy interactions, Schoeb and Hiller (2018) found that documentation during the episode led to pauses in communication, decreased eye contact, and restricted client participation, hindering client-centered communication. These findings were consistent with other healthcare settings (Jones, 2009; Toerien, 2013). Thus Schoeb and Hiller (2018) recommend increasing awareness regarding the impact of documentation on impaired communication and self-reflection to consider personal practices regarding documentation that could impact effective communication. Adjusting the clinical practice environment to avoid pauses

or interruptions by including all appropriate forms for clients to access during the visit is also recommended (Schoeb & Hiller, 2018). Literature supports that 59%–62% of clients believe they should be able to add comments to a doctor's note and one out of three clients believe they should approve contents in a note (Delbanco et al., 2012).

HIPAA

Communicating health information requires discretion. The Health Insurance Portability and Accountability Act of 1996 (HIPAA) is "a federal law that required the creation of national standards to protect sensitive patient health information from being disclosed without the patient's consent or knowledge" (HIPAA, 2016). The HIPAA Privacy Rule was first enacted by the U.S. Department of Health and Human Services in 2002 to protect the confidentiality of clients and their healthcare information while allowing pertinent client healthcare information to flow to other parties when necessary. Also known as the "Standards for Privacy of Individually Identifiable Health Information," the HIPAA Privacy Rule "regulates who can have access to protected health information (PHI), the circumstances in which it can be used, and who it can be disclosed to" (*HIPAA Privacy Rule*, 2016).

Different organizations and individuals are protected by the Privacy Rule and are considered "covered entities." These include:

- **Healthcare providers:** Any healthcare provider who electronically transmits health information (e.g., claims, benefit eligibility inquiries, referral authorization requests).
- **Health plans:** Entities that provide or pay the cost of medical care (e.g., HMOs, Medicare, Medicaid, government and church-sponsored health plans).
- **Healthcare clearinghouses:** Entities that process nonstandard information they receive from another entity into a standard.
- **Business associates:** A person or organization (other than a member of a covered entity's workforce) using or disclosing individually identifiable health information to perform or provide functions, activities, or services for a covered entity (e.g., billing, utilization review, claims processing, data analysis).

The Privacy Rule protects all identifiable health information, including social security numbers, medical record numbers, insurance beneficiary numbers, names, addresses, and other unique identifiers (see Box 9.6). There are limited circumstances when PHI can be disclosed, such as for treatment, payment, or organizational activities, including fraud and abuse detection, quality improvement measures, and competency assessment. For payment and organizational activities, the "minimum necessary standard" applies, which states that "protected health information should not be used or disclosed when it is not necessary to satisfy a particular purpose or carry out a function." (U.S. Department of Health and Humans Services, Health Information Privacy, 2013).

BOX 9.6 HIPAA Privacy Rule

Protected Health Information

https://www.hhs.gov/hipaagor-professionas/privacy/laws-regulations/index.html

Protected Health Information (PHI)

- Name
- Address (smaller than state)
- Date
- Phone no
- Fax no
- Email address
- Social security no
- Medical record no
- Health insurance beneficiary no
- Account no
- Certificate/license no
- Driver's license or license plate no
- Device ID and serial no
- Web URL
- IP address
- Finger print
- Full face photo
- Any other unique ID no or characteristic that could reasonably be associated with the individual

BOX 9.7 HIPAA Security Rule

Reasonable and Appropriate Safeguards
Specific to electronic protected hearth information (e-PHI)
https://www.hhs.gov/hipaa/for-professionals/security/index.html
Reasonable and Appropriate Safeguards (for e-PHI)
- **Administrative Safeguards**
  - Policies and procedures, security officer, training, privacy notices, discipline
- **Physical Safeguards**
  - Lock and key, security, cameras
  - Data backup, removal, and disposal
- **Technical Safeguards**
  - Moving workspaces to private areas
  - Logging out
  - Never sharing passwords
  - Never emailing sensitive information
  - Technology security, encrypting hard drives

The HIPAA Security Rule was established to protect a subset of information covered by the Privacy Rule (HIPAA, 2016). This subset is "all individually identifiable health information a covered entity creates, receives, maintains, or transmits in electronic form" and is called "electronically protected health information" (e-PHI). The Security Rule only applies to e-PHI, not PHI transmitted orally or in writing (HIPAA, 2016). Healthcare organizations and providers must maintain reasonable and appropriate safeguards, including administrative (e.g., policies and procedures, training, privacy notices), physical (e.g., security, data backup), and technical (e.g., logging out, encryption, password security) measures to prevent the unauthorized release of PHI (see Box 9.7) (U.S. Department of Health and Humans Services, Health Information Privacy, 2020).

The HIPAA Breach Notification Rule requires HIPAA-covered entities and their business associates to provide notification following a breach of unsecured PHI. There are three types of breaches (U.S. Department of Health and Humans Services, Health Information Privacy, 2013):

1. **Incidental:** an unavoidable occurrence that happens during an otherwise compliant activity. For example, conversations overheard in a hospital or information displayed on a whiteboard at the nurse's station. These are not considered true breaches and do not need to be reported.
2. **Accidental:** mistakenly providing PHI, for example, sending an email or fax to the wrong person. This breach must be reported to the privacy officer. Providers should assist in helping to correct the breach and learn from these unintended breaches.
3. **Intentional:** carelessly or deliberately using or disclosing PHI. Violators are subject to criminal and civil charges. This breach must be reported to the privacy officer. Within 60 days of any known breach, the organization must notify the U.S. Department of Health and Human Services, the clients involved, and, if greater than 500 individuals were involved, the media.

When engaged in client care, healthcare providers must maintain awareness of these laws, regulations, and policies. Most facilities require regular refresher training on HIPAA. Rehabilitation professionals are advised to consult HIPAA resources to ensure they abide by appropriate privacy standards. Protecting patient privacy and optimal communication between providers for safety and patient outcomes is a synergistic goal that all healthcare providers should strive to achieve.

Modes of Therapeutic Communication

Telehealth

Telehealth has become increasingly utilized in healthcare as an information and communication technology (ICT). According to Dahl-Popolizio et al. (2020), AOTA defines the term telehealth as "inclusive of evaluation, intervention, consultation, supervision, and remote monitoring provided by OTPs (Occupational Therapy Practitioners) across practice settings" (p. 77). With technological advances and the COVID-19 pandemic, telehealth is emerging and becoming more common in practice. However, relevant internationally recognized guidelines about terminology were not available pre-pandemic, which has caused terms such as teletherapy, telehealth, and telerehabilitation to be used interchangeably, creating confusion (Leochico et al., 2021). Research suggests that it may be just as effective in certain populations as face-to-face interventions (Nobakht et al., 2018). "Occupational therapy outcomes aligned with telehealth include the facilitation of occupational performance, adaptation, health and wellness, prevention, and quality of life" (AOTA, 2013, p. 1–2).

Telehealth is used with underserved clients to help develop skills, incorporate assistive technology and adaptive techniques, modify work/home or school environments and support health promotion (*Telehealth in Occupational*

Therapy, 2018). Occupation-based coaching via telehealth (or teletherapy) effectively improves parent efficacy and participation among families of children with autism spectrum disorder (Little et al., 2018). Overall, telehealth can lead to improved access to therapy for clients for various reasons, including transportation challenges and staffing shortages. Therapists should refer to their state practice acts to be aware of policies and procedures for the use and reimbursement of telehealth services. Telephone-based treatment can be effective when paired with traditional rehabilitation programs (Little et al., 2018). Telehealth can be chosen as a service delivery model on a case-by-case basis and requires strong clinical judgment to ensure best practices for effective evaluation, communication, and client outcomes.

Unless therapists use telephone-based treatment that can be effective when paired with traditional rehabilitation programs (Little et al., 2018), a good video connection is important when using synchronous or asynchronous telehealth services. Reliable technology connections can be a challenge to effective communication using ICT. Secure video chat platforms are often used in telehealth services. There can be a lag in video or audio connection when using telehealth platforms, so it is important to summarize the session at the end to ensure important content is not missed. Confidentiality and HIPAA compliance are integral when using telehealth services with clients to ensure information is not passed to outside parties. Chat functions can send links to resources or written instructions for clients and caregivers. Most software platforms can record the "meeting" so that clients can watch it again to clarify information or practice techniques learned in the session. Therapists should carefully consider if they want the session recorded because it becomes a saved documentary of everything said and done in the treatment session. Overall, therapists should consider the evidence that supports the increased rates of client satisfaction with telehealth services in clients in rural areas (Patterson et al., 2021). It is important to note that virtual therapy settings, such as telehealth, can limit hands-on interaction and provide emotional support for individuals like frail older adults (Little et al., 2018). Telehealth access greatly varies by the demographics and location of clients and requires digital literacy (Proffitt et al., 2021). Thus clinicians should ask the questions of reimbursement, access, and preference for face-to-face versus telehealth to best serve clients.

Electronic Medical Records

Electronic medical records (EMRs) allow electronic messaging in healthcare and have become more widespread since ICT has expanded. Most electronic medical records have the ability for healthcare providers to send an electronic message, such as email, from within the medical system software. This efficient communication allows for sharing content such as client status, prescription of services, updates in plans of care, discharge instructions, and home program directions to be stored and passed between providers and

---

> ### • BOX 9.8 Situation-Background-Assessment-Recommendation (SBAR)
>
> **SBAR Example**
> - **Situation:** "My client is a 57-year-old male complaining of shortness of breath and chest pain."
> - **Background:** "He had a knee replacement 2 weeks ago and has not been able to ambulate as much as usual. His calf is warm and swollen, his BP is 140/90, and his heart rate is 115."
> - **Assessment:** "I am concerned he may be having a pulmonary embolism or cardiac event."
> - **Recommendation:** "I recommend we activate EMS and continue monitoring vitals and retrieve the AED and be prepared to begin CPR."
>
> From Institute for Healthcare Communication. (2011). *Impact of Communication in Healthcare*. https://healthcarecomm.org/about-us/impact-of-communication-in-healthcare/; Institute for Healthcare improvement. *SBAR tool: situation-background-assessment-recommendation*. http://www.ihi.org/resources/Pages/Tools/SBARToolkit.aspx

---

provided to clients electronically. Communication can be fast, concise, and organized when using an EMR. Clients can access accurate information from the EMR when a release is signed and the information is sent securely via email, within the software messaging system, or printed out from the EMR. The client then has access to accurate communication directly from the chart. It also "enables improved communication and collaboration between hospitals and municipal healthcare services" (Melby, 2015).

Transferring information about a client to another healthcare teammate is a critical skill that requires attention and practice. Many errors in client care are due to poor communication (Blackstone & Pressman, 2016) and several frameworks have therefore been developed to assist in effective client handoffs and collaborative care. One of the more commonly used communication frameworks in healthcare settings, especially hospitals, is the Situation-Background-Assessment-Recommendation (SBAR) (Institute for Healthcare Communication, 2011). The SBAR (see Box 9.8) provides a simple and concise format to relay important client information to another healthcare provider. The guideline and template can be downloaded for free from http://www.ihi.org/resources/Pages/Tools/SBARToolkit.aspx.

Another useful tool to assist in communication leading to improved client safety is Team Strategies and Tools to Enhance Performance and Patient Safety (TeamSTEPPS), developed by the Department of Defense and the Agency for Healthcare Research and Quality (*About TeamSTEPPS*, 2019). TeamSTEPPS is an evidence-based system to improve teamwork and communication skills between healthcare professionals. With over 20 years of research, TeamSTEPPS has been shown to improve information sharing and resolve conflicts resulting in improved client quality and safety (*About TeamSTEPPS*, 2019). Training materials, including an app and a downloadable pocket guide, are available for free through the AHRQ website at https://www.ahrq.gov/teamstepps/index.html.

Health Literacy

A client's perspective of their healing process, from their awareness of symptoms to diagnosis to their acceptance of a diagnosis, is a process. Health literacy is involved in the transfer and communication of information with clients, and personal health literacy is defined by *Healthy People* (2030) as "the degree to which individuals can find, understand, and use information and services to inform health-related decisions and actions for themselves and others." (U.S. Department of Health and Human Services, 2022). An estimated 90 million Americans have low health literacy; many with lower socioeconomic status or education, older adults with low English proficiency, or those receiving publicly financed health coverage or socioeconomic assistance (Institute of Medicine Committee on Health Literacy, 2004). Allied healthcare providers should consider preparing materials at a sixth- to eighth-grade reading level to target most individuals' reading capabilities (Rooney et al., 2021). All healthcare providers need to gather information while considering health literacy status and communicate at the individual level of each client when sharing and receiving information.

A biopsychosocial approach helps to ensure the therapist and client have a mutual understanding of the client's skills required to understand their healthcare process. This approach considers the complex interactions of the biological elements of illness and disease and the client's important psychological and social factors that impact their health. The biopsychosocial approach is apparent when clinicians interview a client so that facts can be collected and the client's perspective is understood (Diener et al., 2016). Therapists can best communicate with clients when they understand the multitude of factors that define their client's perspective of their health needs.

Therapists need to open an ongoing dialogue with clients and caregivers to know their perspectives and level of health literacy, only then can the therapist carry out the most effective treatment. Sometimes clients may appear to be listening; however, information processing may be difficult, and the client may not remember or understand what is being said to them. Repetition is key in communicating information to families, especially when clients have a cognitive or language difference. The teach-back method is one approach that can be applied during treatment sessions to reinforce understanding of intervention education, and evidence shows its effectiveness when used with individuals with chronic disease (Wittink & Oosterhaven, 2018). Therapists ask clients to repeat key instruction points so both parties can ensure that education is understood and clear. Follow the link to learn more about this communication method: https://www.ahrq.gov/patient-safety/reports/engage/interventions/teachback-mod.html.

Clear communication in client educational materials is a crucial first step to providing the best client-centered care. Poor health literacy has negatively impacted health outcomes

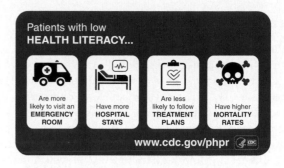

• **Fig. 9.4** Communication between healthcare providers and their clients is essential to achieving optimal health outcomes. (From https://www.cdc.gov/cpr/infographics/healthliteracy.htm)

and medical self-management (Fig. 9.4). "Nearly 9 out of 10 adults have difficulty using the everyday health information that is routinely available in our healthcare facilities, retail outlets, media, and communities" (U.S. Department of Health and Human Services, 2010). One basic tool for supporting clients with low health literacy is clear written communication (Dignan & Hunter, 2015). People with physical disabilities (PWPDs) are at higher risk of health disparities and challenges with health literacy. Therapists can help PWPDs to access equitable healthcare related to their needs for accommodation, rights to care, and ability to request accommodations (VanPuymbrouck et al., 2021). In pediatric therapy services, health literacy is complicated by the therapist's ability to communicate during play with a child and the therapist's skill in passing information to families about evaluation and treatment. Therapists can optimize family participation by increasing the accessibility to written materials, limiting jargon, and providing materials in the family's preferred language. Health literacy can also be supported by improving system accessibility, providers' communication skills, and accessibility of materials. These health literacy components can influence child health outcomes, especially in caring for newborns and young children with special healthcare needs (Blair & Raver, 2015). Addressing the components of health literacy is important in therapy practice to ensure that clients understand the information provided to them by their therapists and other healthcare professionals they encounter (Smith et al., 2010).

Health literacy also encompasses the use of the internet for health information. According to the Centers for Disease Control and Prevention, 80% of adults use the internet as the primary mode of learning about health (Runyen & Benner, 2020). However, PWPDs may have multiple limitations related to independently accessing information or using the devices that allow them to access their medical record (computers, cell phones, tablets). If a client cannot understand how to navigate their medical record, an OT can create a goal and treatment strategies to improve the client's health literacy skills to increase the independence needed to navigate the healthcare arena. For more information on health literacy, refer to Chapter 4.

Interpretive Services

The United States is composed of diverse individuals who are entitled to healthcare services. Not all Americans speak English as their primary language, so interpretive or translation services may be required for clients to understand their medical and therapeutic services best. National standards for culturally and linguistically appropriate services are spearheaded by the U.S. Department of Health and Human Services, Office of Minority Health (2022), which seeks to "provide effective, equitable, understandable, and respectful quality care and services." The federal government requires those agencies that serve individuals and receive federal financial assistance to develop a system and issue guidance to recipients so that people with limited English proficiency can meaningfully access services (U.S. Department of Justice, Executive Order 13166, August 11, 2000). In the United States, patients with limited English proficiency (LEP) have a right to access healthcare in their preferred language (Basu et al., 2017) and it is integral that clinicians work within each practice setting to access these services for their clients (Fig. 9.5). Literature supports that interpretation services help overcome communication barriers and improve client satisfaction, equity, and healthcare quality (Hadziabdic & Hjelm, 2014). The Certification Commission for Healthcare Interpreters (CCHI) was formed to create a national, valid, credible, and vendor-neutral certification program in the United States (Youdelman, 2013). A therapist may know some words in the client's native language that can be used during treatment or play with a toddler to build rapport, but an interpreter should be used during an interview, discussion of evaluation results, or communication of information related to the plan of care. Discharge is also important when interpretation services can help clients and families transition successfully. Some facilities hire interpreters for face-to-face evaluation or ongoing treatment sessions; at other times, an interpreter can enter the session on the phone through video-conferencing to translate.

Interpretive services help to provide clear communication to clients. Best practice includes the use of a competent professional interpreter. Untrained interpreters, including family or minors, are more likely to make errors and cause poor outcomes, including violating confidentiality (Juckett & Unger, 2014). Clinicians should address the client directly and position the interpreter next to or slightly behind the client (Juckett & Unger, 2014). Printed resources in the client's preferred language are important for home programming. Telephone conferencing is an option, while video conferencing was a preference of clients with LEP during the COVID-19 pandemic and may be the preferred option in the future (Rajiv et al., 2021). Video conference interpretation can support positive communication lines as being able to view the team can build trust amongst stakeholders. Follow the link to learn more about client rights about language access: https://www.lawhelp.org/files/1814550B-B14C-5F28-66B9-295AF39C97B1/attachments/A97E4DE9-2530-48D0-A25B-418E68C2F660/basic-info-language-access-law.pdf.

Communicating With Caregivers

A client may be cognitively, emotionally, or physically challenged when a disease process or disability leads them to need therapy services. It is important that caregivers and individuals offering support be identified to assist the client in their journey to health, wellness, and potential independence. The caregiver can be vital to the client's success as they navigate information provided by therapists and are found to provide over 80% of the care for clients with diagnoses such as dementia and chronic illness (Parmar et al., 2020). The results of these interactions therapists have

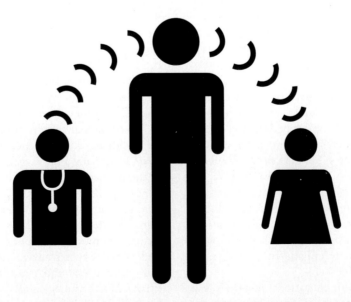

• **Fig. 9.5** For legal and ethical reasons, United States therapists must use certified medical interpreters and translation services for clients with limited English proficiency. (From https://commons.wikimedia.org/wiki/File:Medical_Interpreter_-_The_Noun_Project.svg).

with caregivers are variable. Coaching is a common intervention strategy in pediatric practice when the therapist verbally guides the caregiver to learn and demonstrate intervention strategies. The therapist should ask the family what barriers they might have when coaching them, so that the carryover of intervention strategies is successful. Caregivers may not follow through with strategies in the daily routine because of poor understanding of therapeutic techniques, limited time in the family routine, or decreased caregiver motivation. Collaborative decision-making and shared power are prevalent needs in pediatric practice regarding communication between therapists and caregivers. Home programs and conversations are common avenues to communicate with caregivers about pediatric clients (Riley & Lane, 2016). Hands-on training and return demonstration of techniques by caregivers are important ways to communicate and practice interventions with caregivers across the lifespan. Family Caregiver Training Programs (FCTPs) are used with caregivers of clients with dementia, and common dementia caregiving tasks include activities of daily living (ADLs), instrumental activities of daily living (IADLs), and behavioral management (DiZazzo-Miller et al., 2017).

As the aging population continues and is predicted to grow, therapists must explore age-friendly care. Therapists can pull from evidence-based strategies that help with *age-friendly* care like the 4 Ms (Table 9.2). The 4 Ms framework can reduce the cognitive load of caregivers when working with older adult clients and improve communication (Mate et al., 2021). Connecting with caregivers who take on a strong support role for our clients is important. Evaluation of the caregiver can foster effective communication and result in better client outcomes. The Family Caregiver Communication Tool (FCCT) is a caregiver assessment tool that can provide information about caregiver needs (Wittenberg et al., 2017). It is a 10-item Likert scale tool that measures family conversation and conformity. These age-friendly healthcare approaches that involve attention to the communication styles of caregivers and simplify the healthcare system can ensure that older adults receive high-quality care from their therapists.

TABLE 9.2	**Age Friendly Care: the 4 Ms**	
What **M**atters	Prioritize outcomes specific to the client in context
Medication	Be mindful of medication choice impact
Mentation	Pay attention to mood and memory
Mobility	Move safely every day in function

Data from Institute for Healthcare Improvement. (2020). *Age-friendly health systems: Guide to using the 4Ms in the care of older adults.* Age-Friendly Health Systems. Available at: https://www.ihi.org/Engage/Initiatives/Age-Friendly-Health-Systems/Pages/default.aspx.

At Initial Evaluation

Therapist communication of the therapeutic process begins with data gathering at the initial evaluation, and evaluation results should be provided promptly to the client and primary caregiver in a private, face-to-face environment if possible. Therapists should be clear, concise, and as positive as possible when highlighting pertinent evaluation results related to the client's plan of care. Therapy goals should be presented to the client and caregiver and the therapist should confirm if the goals are client-centered and allow open dialogue to modify the goals per the family's wishes. Evidence shows that caregivers welcome support in communicating with children and youth about treatment goals (Santer et al., 2014). Engaging the parent in the plan of care includes connecting, listening, explaining, demonstrating, discussing, valuing input, and collaborating (D'Arrigo et al., 2020). Discussing the frequency and duration of treatment should also be agreed upon between all parties. The therapist should continue the dialogue as treatment commences with a summary to the client and caregiver after each treatment session, including straightforward statements about the progress, continued areas of improvement, and home activity training. The plan of care can be communicated verbally and with a written handout or electronically per the family's preference. The use of specific tools can be helpful for clients so that they can guide their own healthcare decisions. One example is the Speak Up tool which helps with advanced care planning for clients in outpatient settings (Howard et al., 2021). Therapists should be aware of the importance of reviewing and modifying home activities as the plan of care evolves by discussing specific changes with the family and requiring a return demonstration of any changes.

Discharge Planning

Preparing the client and caregivers for discharge is important to ensure success with sustaining treatment outcomes and the emotional well-being of the treatment team, especially in pediatrics. In pediatric acute rehabilitative settings, caregiver readiness for discharge should occur through assessment at admission and prior to discharge (Ragni et al., 2021). Home activities should be reviewed at the end of each session and solidified in the second to last session so that caregivers can ask questions about carryover at the last treatment session. Therapists can help families overcome the burden of treatment expectations for children with long-term conditions that are resistant by minimizing the impact on family life (Santer et al., 2014). Pediatric teams tend to bond over the developmental milestone attainment of the child and caregiving interactions and clear professional boundaries are therefore important to set at the beginning of treatment for best practice and should be maintained with professional communication styles. The pediatric therapeutic triad includes the parent-child, child-practitioner, and parent-practitioner, making discharge planning complex (Hines et al., 2020). Discharge planning may need to be discussed earlier than 2 weeks before the discharge date for some complex cases to support the discharge transition with caregivers or clients more emotionally tied to their therapists. Well-designed IT solutions may help improve communication in hospital settings regarding the discharge plan (Newnham et al., 2017). Some families may fear negative changes after discharge without therapists present to communicate feedback. Therefore ongoing dialogue about the discharge transition can ease the inevitable change for clients and families.

Communication With Other Providers

Physical and occupational therapists do not address all healthcare practice areas; therefore interprofessional consultation can help provide high-quality care to our clients. Therapists may need to consult with experts in a therapy specialty area of practice. Alternatively, therapists may move outside the therapy realm to consult with other healthcare professionals who can best meet the client's needs. Following up with a referring physician to ask clarifying questions should be a priority and the first step. Psychologists, nurses, case managers, social workers, speech-language pathologists, and dieticians are just some other professionals physical and occupational therapists may need to communicate with to pass on information or gather information related to a client. Face-to-face discussions, phone calls, encrypted emails, and providing and reviewing written documentation in a client's file are all ways therapists can reach out to consult with other healthcare providers. Identifying our lack of knowledge and understanding other professionals' scope of practice is integral in consulting about a client. Physical and occupational therapists may also be asked to consult with these providers and screen or request a formal prescription be written to evaluate the client as needed.

Collaboration and Consultation

Collaboration is an active process that requires clear, respectful, and inquisitive communication practices by all individuals involved in a client's care. Most professionals find their time valuable; thus being concise with communication skills and style is important. In some cases, encrypted email communication and written documentation of a client's information may serve as the only information needed to collaborate. In other circumstances, more formal team meetings or rounds may be structured in the workday where therapists must take turns and provide clear and beneficial information in these open dialogues. These meetings require the therapist to come prepared with documentation or specific notes to add to the collaborative process for the client. Preparation, evidence or outcome sharing, and collaboration are paramount when working with other providers, whether with conversation or written communication.

Collaboration and consultation also occur inter- and intraprofessionally between therapists and therapy assistants. However, each state has supervision regulations for therapy assistants that may vary slightly. Therefore clinicians should consult their state practice act regarding the specific requirements related to supervision and communication.

It is both the responsibility of the therapists and therapy assistants to communicate their role to the client and family. This delineation of responsibilities does not need to be lengthy when speaking with the family but should be provided by the evaluating therapist and any other therapy assistant involved in the client's care. The therapy team should introduce themselves at the initial evaluation and delineate their roles to the client and family for transparency and clarity. The client should know that the therapy assistant and supervising therapist work together to provide optimal care. Therapy assistants should always be honest when reporting progress to therapists, leaving out any bias related to how their competence impacted the client's progress or not. Therapists and therapy assistants should meet before discharge to clarify discharge and home activity plans to support a positive transition out of treatment for the client and family.

Conclusion

Communication is a vital skill for all health professionals. The positive impact of effective communication skills on health outcomes cannot be overlooked. Like any other clinical skill, developing effective verbal and nonverbal communication skills requires patience, intentional practice, and ongoing professional reflection. Incorporating evidence-based communication strategies can enhance a fulfilling clinical practice and make a difference in the lives of those therapists are entrusted to serve.

Acknowledgments

The authors would like to thank Anna Miller, SPT and Carlos Bautista, SPT, Alexandra Hotz, OTS, Miranda MacWhirter, OTS, Elizabeth Maurer, OTS, and Katelyn Miles, OTS for their assistance in preparing this chapter.

References

About TeamSTEPPS. (2019). https://www.ahrq.gov/teamstepps/about-teamstepps/index.html

Ali, M. (2017). Communication skills 2: Overcoming barriers to effective communication. Nursing Times, 114(1), 40–42.

Agner, J. (2020). Moving From cultural competence to cultural humility in occupational therapy: A paradigm shift. The American Journal of Occupational Therapy, 74(4), 7404347010p1–7404347010p7.

Alston, C., Paget, L., Halvorson, G. C., Novelli, B., Guest, J., McCabe, P., Hoffman, K., Koepke, C., Simon, M., Sutton, S., Okun, S., Wicks, P., Undem, T., Rohrbach, V., Von Kohorn, I., Informed Medical Decisions Foundation, Permanente, K., Georgetown University, ... Institute of Medicine. (2012). Communicating with patients on health care evidence. NAM Perspectives, 2(9), 1–17.

American Occupational Therapy Association. (2021). Improve your documentation and quality of care with AOTA's updated Occupational

Profile Template. *The American Journal of Occupational Therapy, 75,* 7502420010p1–7502420010p3.

AOTA Occupational Profile Template. (2017). *The American Journal of Occupational Therapy, 71*(Suppl. 2), 7412410010p1–7412410010p87.

Bandura, A. (1995). Exercise of personal and collective efficacy in changing societies. In A. Bandura (Ed.), *Self-efficacy in changing societies.* Cambridge University Press.

Basu, G., Costa, V. P., & Jain, P. (2017). Clinicians' obligations to use qualified medical interpreters when Caring for Patients with Limited English Proficiency. *AMA Journal of Ethics, 19*(3), 245–252.

Beattie, P. F., Pinto, M. B., Nelson, M. K., & Nelson, R. (2002). Patient satisfaction with outpatient physical therapy: Instrument validation. *Physical Therapy, 82*(6), 557–565.

Beckman, H. B., & Frankel, R. M. (1984). The effect of physician behavior on the collection of data. *Annals of Internal Medicine, 101*(5), 692–696.

Beckman, H. B., Markakis, K. M., Suchman, A. L., & Frankel, R. M. (1994). The doctor-patient relationship and malpractice. Lessons from plaintiff depositions. *Archives of Internal Medicine, 154*(12), 1365–1370.

Bedell, S. E., Graboys, T. B., Bedell, E., & Lown, B. (2004). Words that harm, words that heal. *Archives of Internal Medicine, 164*(13), 1365–1368.

Bialosky, J. E., Bishop, M. D., & Cleland, J. A. (2010). Individual expectation: An overlooked, but pertinent, factor in the treatment of individuals experiencing musculoskeletal pain. *Physical Therapy, 90*(9), 1345–1355.

Blackstone, S. W., & Pressman, H. (2016). Patient communication in health care settings: New opportunities for augmentative and alternative communication. *Augmentative and Alternative Communication, 32*(1), 69–79.

Blair, C., & Raver, C. C. (2015). School readiness and self-regulation: A developmental psychobiological approach. *Annual Review of Psychology, 66*, 711–731.

Button, K., & Rossera, F. (1990). Barriers to communication. *The Annals of Regional Science, 24*(4), 337–357.

Choi, J., & Tate, J. A. (2021). Evidence-based communication with critically ill older adults. *Critical Care Nursing Clinics of North America, 33*(4), 441–457.

Clifford, D., & Curtis, L. (2016). *Motivational interviewing in nutrition and fitness.* New York: Guilford Publications.

Cole, M. B., & McLean, V. (2003). Therapeutic relationships re-defined. *Occupational Therapy in Mental Health, 19*(2), 33–56.

Coulehan, J. L., Platt, F. W., Egener, B., Frankel, R., Lin, C. T., Lown, B., & Salazar, W. H. (2001). "Let me see if i have this right ...": Words that help build empathy. *Annals of Internal Medicine, 135*(3), 221–227.

Dahl-Popolizio, S., Carpenter, H., Coronado, M., Popolizio, N. J., & Swanson, C. (2020). Telehealth for the provision of occupational therapy: Reflections on experiences in COVID-19 pandemic. *International Journal of Telerehabilitation, 12*(2), 77–92.

D'Arrigo, R. G., Copley, J. A., Poulsen, A. A., & Ziviani, J. (2020). Strategies occupational therapists use to engage children and parents in therapy sessions. *Australian Occupational Therapy Journal, 67*(6), 537–549.

Delbanco, T., Walker, J., Bell, S. K., Darer, J. D., Elmore, J. G., Farag, N., Feldman, J. J., Mejilla, R., Ngo, L., Ralston, J. D., Ross, S. E., Trivedi, N., Vodicka, E., & Levelle, S. G. (2012). Inviting patients to read their doctors' notes: A quasi-experimental study and a look ahead. *Annals of Internal Medicine, 157*(7), 461–470.

Diener, I., Kargela, M., & Louw, A. (2016). Listening is therapy: Patient interviewing from a pain science perspective. *Physiotherapy Theory and Practice, 32*(5), 356–367.

Dignan, E., & Hunter, E. (2015). Assessing and adapting patient educational materials: addressing low health literacy in an inpatient rehabilitation setting. *The American Journal of Occupational Therapy, 69*(Suppl. 1), 6911515150–6911515150p1.

Dimatteo, M. R. (2004). The role of effective communication with children and their families in fostering adherence to pediatric regimens. *Patient Education and Counseling, 55*(3), 339–344.

DiZazzo-Miller, R., Winston, K., Winkler, S. L., & Donovan, M. L. (2017). Family caregiver training program (FCTP): A randomized controlled trial. *The American Journal of Occupational Therapy, 71*(5), 1–10.

Epstein, R. M. (2000). The science of patient-centered care [Review of *The science of patient-centered care*]. *The Journal of Family Practice, 49*(9), 805–807.

Evans, B. J., Stanley, R. O., Mestrovic, R., & Rose, L. (1991). Effects of communication skills training on students' diagnostic efficiency. *Medical Education, 25*(6), 517–526.

Fan, C. W., Hazlett, J. N., & Taylor, R. R. (2022). Perceiving therapeutic communication: Client–therapist discrepancies. *The American Journal of Occupational Therapy: Official Publication of the American Occupational Therapy Association, 76*(3), 7603345010. https://doi.org/10.5014/ajot.2022.047670.

Gafni-Lachter, L., Ben-Sasson, A., & Alsaaed, S. (2021). Gaps between parent and therapist perspectives on family-centered care as a factor of service setting. *The American Journal of Occupational Therapy, 75*(Suppl. 2), 7512510272p1.

Hadziabdic, E., & Hjelm, K. (2014). Arabic-speaking migrants' experiences of the use of interpreters in healthcare: A qualitative explorative study. *International Journal for Equity in Health, 13*, 49.

Health Insurance Portability and Accountability Act of 1996 (HIPAA). (2016, February 21). https://www.cdc.gov/phlp/publications/topic/hipaa.html.

Hemsley, B., & Balandin, S. (2014). A metasynthesis of patient-provider communication in hospital for patients with severe communication disabilities: Informing new translational research. *Augmentative and Alternative Communication, 30*(4), 329–343.

Hettema, J., Steele, J., & Miller, W. R. (2005). Motivational interviewing. *Annual Review of Clinical Psychology, 1*, 91–111.

Hines, D., York, K., & Kaul, E. (2020). Optimizing compliance with home programming through neuroplasticity education among parents of children receiving outpatient OT. *The American Journal of Occupational Therapy: Official Publication of the American Occupational Therapy Association, 74*(4_Supplement_1), 7411505129p1–p7411505129p1.

HIPAA Privacy Rule. (2016, April 1). HIPAA Journal. https://www.hipaajournal.com/hipaa-privacy-rule/.

Howard, M., Robinson, C. A., McKenzie, M., Fyles, G., Hanvey, L., Barwich, D., Bernard, C., Elston, D., Tan, A., Yeung, L., & Heyland, D. K. (2021). Effect of "Speak Up" educational tools to engage patients in advance care planning in outpatient healthcare settings: A prospective before-after study. *Patient Education and Counseling, 104*(4), 709–714.

Institute for Healthcare Communication. (2011). *Impact of communication in healthcare.* https://healthcarecomm.org/about-us/impact-of-communication-in-healthcare/.

Institute of Medicine (US) Committee on Health Literacy. (2004). *Health literacy: A prescription to end confusion.* In L. Nielsen-Bohlman, A. M. Panzer, & D. A. Kindig (Eds.). National Academies Press (US). https://nap.nationalacademies.org/catalog/10883/health-literacy-a-prescription-to-end-confusion.

Jones, A. (2009). Creating history: Documents and patient participation in nurse-patient interviews. *Sociology of Health & Illness, 31*(6), 907–923.

Juckett, G., & Unger, K. (2014). Appropriate use of medical interpreters. *American Family Physician, 90*(7), 476–480.

Leochico, C. F. D., Austria, E. M. V., & Espiritu, A. I. (2021). Global online interest in telehealth, telemedicine, telerehabilitation, and related search terms amid the COVID-19 pandemic: An infodemiological study. *Acta Medica Philippina, 56*(11). doi:10.47895/amp.vi0.3037.

Levin, M. F., & Riley, E. J. (1984). Effectiveness of teaching interviewing and communication skills to physiotherapy students. *Physiotherapy Canada. Physiotherapie Canada, 36*(4), 190–194.

Levinson, W., Roter, D. L., Mullooly, J. P., Dull, V. T., & Frankel, R. M. (1997). Physician-patient communication. The relationship with malpractice claims among primary care physicians and surgeons. *JAMA, 277*(7), 553–559.

Levinson, W., Stiles, W. B., Inui, T. S., & Engle, R. (1993). Physician frustration in communicating with patients. *Medical Care, 31*(4), 285–295.

Little, L. M., Pope, E., Wallisch, A., & Dunn, W. (2018). Occupation-based coaching by means of telehealth for families of young children with autism spectrum disorder. *The American Journal of Occupational Therapy, 72*(2), 7202205020p1–7202205020p7.

Liu, K. T., Kueh, Y. C., Arifin, W. N., Kim, Y., & Kuan, G. (2018). Application of transtheoretical model on behavioral changes, and amount of physical activity among university's atudents. *Frontiers in Psychology. 9*, 2402.

Majerovitz, S. D., Mollott, R. J., & Rudder, C. (2009). We're on the same side: Improving communication between nursing home and family. *Health Communication, 24*(1), 12–20.

Mate, K., Fulmer, T., Pelton, L., Berman, A., Bonner, A., Huang, W., & Zhang, J. (2021). Evidence for the 4Ms: Interactions and outcomes across the care continuum. *Journal of Aging and Health, 33*(7-8), 469–481.

May, W. F. (1994). Listening carefully [Review of *Listening carefully*]. *Second Opinion, 20*(1), 47–49. europepmc.org.

Melby, L. (2015). You've got an e-message! Improving healthcare professionals' communication and collaboration across the Norwegian healthcare sector. *International Journal of Integrated Care, 15*(5), 1–2.

Newnham, H., Barker, A., Ritchie, E., Hitchcock, K., Gibbs, H., & Holton, S. (2017). Discharge communication practices and healthcare provider and patient preferences, satisfaction and comprehension: A systematic review. *International Journal for Quality in Health Care, 29*(6), 752–768.

Nobakht, Z., Rassafiani, M., & Hosseini, S. A. (2018). A web-based caring training for caregivers of children with cerebral palsy: Development and evaluation. *Iranian Journal of Child Neurology, 12*(4), 65–84.

O'Keeffe, M., Cullinane, P., Hurley, J., Leahy, I., Bunzli, S., O'Sullivan, P. B., & O'Sullivan, K. (2016). What influences patient-therapist interactions in musculoskeletal physical therapy? Qualitative systematic review and meta-synthesis. *Physical Therapy, 96*(5), 609–622.

Palmadottir, G. (2006). Client-therapist relationships: Experiences of occupational therapy clients in rehabilitation. *The British Journal of Occupational Therapy, 69*(9), 394–401.

Parmar, J., Poole, L., Anderson, S., Cheryl, P., Duggleby, W., Charles, L., Brémault-Phillips, S., & Holyroyd-Leduc, J. (2020). Co-Designing Caregiver-Centered Care: Training the health workforce to support family caregivers. *Innovation in Aging, 4*(Supplement_1), 15–16.

Patak, L., Gawlinski, A., Fung, N. I., Doering, L., Berg, J., & Henneman, E. A. (2006). Communication boards in critical care: Patients' views. *Applied Nursing Research: ANR, 19*(4), 182–190.

Patterson, A., Harkey, L., Jung, S., & Newton, E. (2021). Patient satisfaction with telehealth in rural settings: A systematic review. *The American Journal of Occupational Therapy, 75*(Supplement_2), 1.

Phillips, K. A., & Ospina, N. S. (2017). Physicians interrupting patients. *JAMA, 318*(1), 93–94.

Pillemer, K., Hegeman, C. R., Albright, B., & Henderson, C. (1998). Building bridges between families and nursing home staff: The Partners in Caregiving Program. *The Gerontologist, 38*(4), 499–503.

Platt, F. W., Gaspar, D. L., Coulehan, J. L., Fox, L., Adler, A. J., Weston, W. W., Smith, R. C., & Stewart, M. (2001). "Tell me about yourself": The patient-centered interview. *Annals of Internal Medicine, 134*(11), 1079–1085.

Prochaska, J. O., & Velicer, W. F. (1997). The transtheoretical model of health behavior change. *American Journal of Health Promotion, 12*(1), 38–48.

Proffitt, R., Cason, J., Little, L., & Pickett, K. A. (2021). Stimulating research to advance evidence-based applications of telehealth in occupational therapy. *OTJR: Occupation Participation and Health, 41*(3), 153–162.

Punwar, J. A., & Peloquin, M. S. (2000). *Occupational therapy: Principles and practice.* Lippincott Williams & Wilkins.

Ragni, L. B., Velasco, C., Fitzsimons, T., & Shniderman, K. (2021). Pediatric Readiness for Hospital Discharge Scale (PedsRHDS): Use in interdisciplinary caregiver training program in acute inpatient rehabilitation. *The American Journal of Occupational Therapy, 75*(Supplement_2), 1.

Rajiv, P., Riggs, E., Brown, S., Szwarc, J., & Yelland, J. (2021). Communication interventions to support people with limited English proficiency in healthcare: A systematic review. *Journal of Communication in Healthcare, 14*(2), 176–187.

Realini, T., Kalet, A., & Sparling, J. (1995). Interruption in the medical interaction. *Archives of Family Medicine, 4*(12), 1028–1033.

Richards, T. (1990). Chasms in communication. *BMJ, 301*(6766), 1407–1408.

Riley, B., & Lane, S. J. (2016). Feasibility of engaging caregivers during pediatric occupational therapy services: A mixed-methods study. *The American Journal of Occupational Therapy, 70*(4_Supplement_1), 7011520294p1.

Roberts, L., & Bucksey, S. J. (2007). Communicating with patients: What happens in practice? *Physical Therapy, 87*(5), 586–594.

Rooney, M. K., Santiago, G., & Pernie, S. (2021). Readability of patient education materials from high-impact medical journals: A 20-year analysis. *Journal of Patient Experience, 8*, 1–9.

Rosenstein, A. H., & O'Daniel, M. (2005). Disruptive behavior and clinical outcomes: Perceptions of nurses and physicians. *The American Journal of Nursing, 105*(1), 54–64; quiz 64–65.

Roter, D. L., Stewart, M., Putnam, S. M., Lipkin, M., Jr., Stiles, W., & Inui, T. S. (1997). Communication patterns of primary care physicians. *JAMA, 277*(4), 350–356.

Runyen, M., & Benner, M. (2020). Enhancing health management by adapting technology and addressing electronic health literacy. *American Journal of Occupational Therapy, 74* (Supplement _1), 7411505174p1.

Santer, M., Ring, N., Yardley, L., Geraghty, A. W. A., & Wyke, S. (2014). Treatment non-adherence in pediatric long-term medical conditions: Systematic review and synthesis of qualitative studies of caregivers' views. *BMC Pediatrics, 14*, 63.

Schoeb, V., & Hiller, A. (2018). The impact of documentation on communication during patient-physiotherapist interactions: A qualitative observational study. *Physiotherapy Theory and Practice, 34*(11), 861–871.

Shapiro, R. S., Simpson, D. E., Lawrence, S. L., Talsky, A. M., Sobocinski, K. A., & Schiedermayer, D. L. (1989). A survey of sued and nonsued physicians and suing patients. *Archives of Internal Medicine, 149*(10), 2190–2196.

Sloan, T. J., & Walsh, D. A. (2010). Explanatory and diagnostic labels and perceived prognosis in chronic low back pain. *Spine, 35*(21), E1120–E1125.

Smith, D. L., Hedrick, W., Earhart, H., Galloway, H., & Arndt, A. (2010). Evaluating two health care facilities' ability to meet health literacy needs: A role for occupational therapy. *Occupational Therapy in Health Care, 24*(4), 348–359.

Souders, B. *17 Motivational interviewing questions and skills.* November 5, 2019. https://positivepsychology.com/motivational-interviewing/.

Stewart, M., & Loftus, S. (2018). Sticks and stones: The impact of language in musculoskeletal rehabilitation. *The Journal of Orthopaedic and Sports Physical Therapy, 48*(7), 519–522.

Taylor, R. R. (2020). *The intentional relationship: Occupational therapy and use of self.* F.A. Davis.

Taylor, R. R., Lee, S. W., Kielhofner, G., & Ketkar, M. (2009). Therapeutic use of self: A nationwide survey of practitioners' attitudes and experiences. *The American Journal of Occupational Therapy, 63*(2), 198–207.

Telehealth in Occupational Therapy. (2018). *The American Journal of Occupational Therapy, 72*(Supplement_2), 7212410059p1–7212410059p18.

Toerien, M. (2013). Using electronic patient records in practice: A focused review of the evidence of risks to the clinical interaction. *Seizure: The Journal of the British Epilepsy Association, 22*(8), 601–603.

U.S. Department of Health and Humans Services, Health Information Privacy. (2013 and 2020). *Minimum necessary requirement.* https://www.hhs.gov/hipaa/for-professionals/privacy/guidance/minimum-necessary-requirement/index.html.

U.S. Department of Health and Humans Services. (2020). *The security rule.* https://www.hhs.gov/hipaa/for-professionals/security/index.html.

U.S. Department of Health and Humans Services. (2013). *Breach notification rule.* https://www.hhs.gov/hipaa/for-professionals/breach-notification/index.html.

U.S. Department of Health and Human Services, Office of Disease Prevention and Health Promotion. (2010). *National action plan to improve health literacy.* Washington, DC.

U.S. Department of Health and Human Services. (2022, May 26). *Health literacy in healthy People 2030.* Office of Disease Prevention and Health Promotion. https://health.gov/healthypeople/priority-areas/health-literacy-healthy-people-2030.

U.S. Department of Health and Human Services, Office of Minority Health. (2022). *National Standards for Culturally and Linguistically Appropriate Services (CLAS) in health and health care.* Washington, DC.

U.S. Depart of Justice, Civil Rights Division. *Executive Order 13166, August 11, 2000.* https://www.justice.gov/crt/executive-order-13166. Accessed June 20, 2023.

Valdes, K., & Campbell, A. (2017). Patient preferences for home exercise program provision: A patient survey. *The American Journal of Occupational Therapy, 71*(4_Supplement_1), 7111510186p1.

VanPuymbrouck, L., Carey, J., Draper, A., & Follansbee, L. (2021). Recognizing inequity: A critical step of health literacy for people with disability. *The American Journal of Occupational Therapy, 75*(4). 1–10.

Wittenberg, E., Buller, H., Ferrell, B., Koczywas, M., & Borneman, T. (2017). Understanding family caregiver communication to provide family-centered cancer care. *Seminars in Oncology Nursing, 33*(5), 507–516.

Wittink, H., & Oosterhaven, J. (2018). Patient education and health literacy. *Musculoskeletal Science & Practice, 38*, 120–127.

Wright, V., & Hopkins, R. (1978). What the patient means. A study from rheumatology. *Physiotherapy, 64*(5), 146–147.

Youdelman, M. (2013). The development of certification for healthcare interpreters in the United States. *Translation and Interpreting, 5*(1), 1–13.

10

Leadership

SARAH CORCORAN, OTD, OTR/L; TRACEY E. RECIGNO, OTD, OTR/L;
and WILLIAM R. VANWYE, PT, DPT, PhD

LEARNING OBJECTIVES

By the end of this chapter, the reader will be able to:

1. Define leadership in the context of the occupational and physical therapy professions.
2. Describe evidence-informed supports for building personal leadership capacity.
3. Discuss the key aspects of leadership approaches and theories across four phases.
4. Identify opportunities to develop and contribute to leadership at local, state, national, and global professional levels.

CHAPTER OUTLINE

Introduction

Although change is often difficult, it is inevitable. Throughout human existence, adapting to change has been essential for survival. The uniqueness of today's change is that the *rate* is more rapid than ever, undoubtedly mainly due to the acceleration of technology (Fig. 10.1). In these times of hyperchange, it is no longer enough to be effective; to thrive in today's workforce, we must be highly effective (Covey, 2004; Hinojosa, 2007). Covey (2004) explained that people have adapted to change by evolving from hunter-gathers to farmers to industrial workers and, currently, to the knowledge workers. Drucker (2000) noted that emergence of knowledge workers is leading to an unprecedented change in the human condition. Workers must identify their strengths, find space to be effective, and, most importantly, learn to

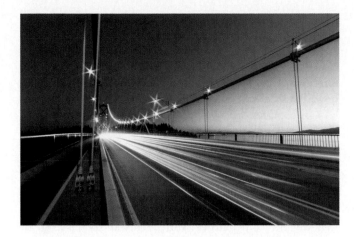

• **Fig. 10.1** We live in a period of hyper-change. Thus it is no longer enough to be effective; to thrive in today's workforce, we must be highly effective. (From https://www.flickr.com/photos/75472177@N08/9353095333).

manage themselves. Covey (2004) refers to this as finding one's voice.

While finding our voices sounds like a natural process, Drucker (2000) notes that society is unprepared for the challenge. According to Covey (2004), many older management techniques no longer work today. After all, these techniques seek to treat people like things instead of individuals, inhibiting many from finding their voice. Everyone's voice is unique and personal, consisting of talents, passions, needs, and conscience. Overall, finding this voice deals directly with the importance of leadership (Covey, 2004).

The varying levels of success throughout society often expose leadership's presence or absence. Thus a common question emerges; why is there such a lack of leadership? The issue may be that it is challenging to measure leadership. What are the standards? Is it the ability to inspire, to organize followers, and to set goals, or is it all about results? Are we looking for leadership in the wrong place or the wrong individuals? It is common for us to look at the highest levels of government, schools, and businesses for leadership, only to be disappointed. However, leaders can be found at all levels around the globe.

In this chapter, we explore the concept that everyone is responsible for leading at some point in life. As healthcare providers, we are called upon to be citizen or servant leaders because our true north principle is to serve others (Burns, 1995a; Couto, 1995a; Gardner, 1995; Greenleaf, 1995). Thus we have organized this chapter to focus on your capacity to lead and leadership contexts. We share leadership definitions, fundamental theories, skills, and resources relevant to the occupational therapy (OT) and physical therapy (PT) professions. Also, we explore actionable strategies for leadership spotlighted in the *Living Leadership* boxes, including examples of a developing leader named Carmen. In addition, we provide a *Capacity Building Resource List* at the end of the chapter to support your learning about leadership. See Box 10.1 to begin learning Carmen's story with leadership.

• **BOX 10.1   Living Leadership: Meet Carmen**

Carmen is an OT student currently completing fieldwork experience in a community hospital. Carmen uses "they/them" pronouns. Carmen is working hard to be an OT practitioner, both in their coursework and a part-time job as an aide in a skilled nursing facility. When Carmen has time, they like to engage in activities with other students, including those offered through their university's student OT association. As the first person to go to college, and the first soon-to-be OT, among their family and friends, Carmen has welcomed and valued opportunities to get to know OT practitioners, including professors, coworkers, clinical supervisors, and professionals from different fields. Carmen views many of these people as leaders and wonders how people develop into leaders, particularly in their profession.

What Is Leadership?

> *"Leadership is not about titles, positions or flowcharts. It's about one life influencing another."*
>
> **JOHN C. MAXWELL**

While a standard, operational definition of leadership is difficult to pinpoint in the overall body of literature, we share a few perspectives with you. Northouse (2022) defines leadership as "a process whereby an individual influences a group of individuals to achieve a common goal" (p. 5). Covey (2004) suggested that leadership is "communicating to people their worth and potential so clearly that they come to see it in themselves" (p. 98). According to Bass (1995), leadership is group-focused, a matter of personality, associated with direction, persuasion, power-related, an instrument to achieve goals, interaction, a role, and a structure. Kotter (1996) noted that "leadership defines what the future should look like, aligns people with that vision, and inspires them to make it happen despite the obstacles" (p. 28).

Kouzes and Posner (2017) note that "leadership is an observable pattern of practices and behaviors, and a definable set of skills and abilities" (p. 302). These behaviors are highlighted in their five leadership practices (see Capacity Building Resource List at the end of the chapter) (Kouzes & Posner, 2017). In addition, in their attempt to integrate the varied definitions of leadership, Winston and Patterson (2006) offered this integrated definition of leadership: "A leader is one or more people who selects, equips, trains, and influences one or more follower(s) who have diverse gifts, abilities, and skills and focuses the follower(s) to the organization's mission and objectives causing the follower(s) to willingly and enthusiastically expend spiritual, emotional, and physical energy in a concerted coordinated effort to achieve the organizational mission and objectives" (p. 7).

There is no official definition of leadership within OT and PT. A definition needs to consider the broad contexts in which therapists practice, including communities and systems. OT Dr. Brent Braveman (2022) defines leadership as "a process of creating structural change wherein the values, vision, and ethics of individuals are integrated into the culture of a community as a means of achieving sustainable change" (p. 6). In Braveman's definition, leadership is more than a person; it is an adaptable process that empowers lasting positive change.

We appreciate the salient aspects of leadership from these experts' perspectives. Also, we recognize that the collective understanding of leadership is always evolving. Thus we propose this definition as a guide to apply leadership in the context of PT and OT:

Leadership is the ethical, mindful application of a person's identity, strengths, and values, guided by critical reflection and emotional intelligence, to engage followers in transformation within a context, such as a workplace, community, or society.

Building Your Capacity for Leadership

"I believe that heartfelt leadership is a journey that begins with a clear picture of oneself and extends that heightened self-awareness to a deep awareness of others, and ultimately to organizations."

VIRGINIA C. STOFFEL

It is easy to believe that leadership is separate, even distant, from ourselves. How do we authentically connect to the concept of leadership? How do we begin to feel like leaders? Former Navy SEAL Jeff Boss emphasizes that leadership capacity building occurs around courage, clarity, and curiosity (Boss, 2017). If we consider capacity as possible when we are at our best, we can apply this to ourselves, our teams, communities, organizations, and professions. Leadership capacity is possible when we continuously maximize our strengths and skills to lead others.

Leadership is not a static outcome for healthcare professionals. Personal capacity building requires you to consistently reflect on your current skills and knowledge and then identify strategies and resources to advance those capabilities (Moyers, 2007). Capacity building can also be done at community, organizational, and professional levels. The ongoing process of leadership capacity building requires attention and action. This section includes how you can connect to your best leadership. Recognizing that you will develop your unique leadership capacity, we present evidence from leadership literature to help you get started. Specific evidence-based supports are organized using Boss' reflection on the essential concepts of courage, clarity, and curiosity.

Courage

We translate Boss' (2017) concept of courage to the ideas of leader identity and strengths, values, and ethical and moral leadership. Therapy practitioners' leadership skills are critical to negotiating successful outcomes in difficult situations. Courage is about using your strengths to face challenges. Courage is not easy, but it is a necessary attribute of leadership that drives change and upholds ethical decision-making. Leadership identity and courage are interrelated, and those

who identify themselves as leaders have more confidence in their skills (Clapp-Smith et al., 2019).

Leadership Identity & Personal Strengths

Often students and new healthcare practitioners question how their identity connects to leadership. You may feel a lack of experience and knowledge needed to be a leader, despite having many life experiences that may support you in this role. Doubting your abilities and feeling incompetent to fulfill the role of "leader" despite having the necessary skills is referred to as *imposter syndrome* (Lazarus, 2021). Leadership identity is not rooted in a supervisor or a manager position. Instead, leadership identity is understanding the contributions you can make to the team by leveraging your distinctive perspectives, experiences, and knowledge.

Using tools such as The CliftonStrengths Assessment or completing the VIA survey (see Capacity Building Resource List section) can provide helpful insights into personality traits and intrinsic qualities useful in leadership. Tapping into or strengthening these characteristics can further support a leadership identity. Visioning your capacity building into the future requires self-reflection and articulating your fundamental beliefs (Scott & Webber, 2008). Therefore it is also necessary that leaders clearly understand their values.

Values

*"Values should be what you do,
not just what you say they are."*

JAMIE EDWARDS

Values are the fundamental beliefs that guide or motivate attitudes and actions and help us determine our priorities. We often develop values early on in life to connect with the world. Johnson (2021) emphasizes, "we are more likely to act with courage, demonstrate grit, control our impulses, be just and compassionate, and remain true to ourselves if we have a clear sense of direction and identify a set of guiding principles for our lives" (p. 93). Exploration of values provide an understanding of intrinsic traits that influence how we see the world and act upon it. In essence, values frame our mindsets as people and practitioners.

Closely linked to leadership identities is the concept of leadership mindsets. When thinking about building leadership capacity, Jeanes (2021) frames it this way: "The alternative to leadership as ways of 'doing' (leadership skills and actions), 'behaving' (behavioral and style approaches to leadership) and being ('traits'), is how we 'see' the world – the frames that are described as mindsets." Values influence leadership mindsets. Healthcare professions have inherent and explicit values that guide practitioner decision-making, behaviors, and actions (Thomas et al., 2019). Chapter 5 provides more information on the core values and ethics of OT and PT. We invite you to reflect on how these professional values align and interact with your own. Evaluating personal values allows a better understanding of mindsets and adjust to promote growth and ethical behaviors.

Ultimately, values play a crucial role when leaders make ethical decisions.

Ethical and Moral Leadership

"The most important thing is not what you do, it's who you are...
you need to define who you are"

DANIEL GILBERT

Ethics is core to leadership and leadership is essential to ethical environments. Most healthcare professionals will probably encounter challenging ethical dilemmas or moral distress. Moral distress is an ethical problem when practitioners know the right thing but cannot act on it because of external barriers or concerns about the outcome. Ethical dilemmas are complex and often require making choices that conflict between values and moral principles (Chapter 5).

A closer examination of ethical leadership reveals that we must possess a solid moral compass to be considered leaders. One of the first steps in moral action when making ethical decisions is recognizing ethical behaviors. Recognizing ethical behaviors requires critical thinking skills, the "head and heart" to identify a course of action, and reflection (Johnson, 2021). Later in this chapter, we will explore how reflection impacts the reciprocal influence of the leader, the organization, and professional values that can play a role in ethical actions and behaviors. A good starting point for developing ethical behaviors as a professional is seeking guidance from your profession's code of ethics.

Overall, leaders must follow ethical principles. Without a moral compass, one cannot be labeled a leader. Consider notorious figures in our world's history and contemporary times who used their power for self-gain and fell into the dark side of leadership (Box 10.2).

Clarity

Another essential concept to building leadership capacity is clarity. Many hold leaders in high esteem when they simultaneously inspire others toward a future-oriented vision and thoughtfully navigate relationships and challenges in the present. We can think of a leader carrying a light bright enough to see what is possible ahead and what is happening now. We can develop this kind of light, or clarity, through mindfulness and emotional intelligence.

Mindfulness

Kabat-Zinn (Mindful Staff, 2017) defines mindfulness as awareness cultivated by intentional attention and presence. Many people use the term mindfulness in their everyday vocabulary and already incorporate mindfulness into their routines. Mindfulness can help us slow down and better understand ourselves and our world. As individuals, we can find a quiet space to calm our minds and detach from our thoughts. People who use mindfulness consistently train their minds, like athletes train their bodies, to maintain mental calm amidst difficult situations (Levey & Levey, 2019).

While we may think of training our minds as a personal experience, mindfulness also has the potential to build leadership capacity and professional relationships. We can be fully present in our interactions with others by listening with our whole body, and responding with thoughtful intention, even when chaos and challenges seem abundant. Mindfulness can provide clarity on how to best connect with colleagues, partners, employees, supervisors, clients, and customers through mindfulness. Mindfulness practice has improved healthcare workers' emotional intelligence, another critical leadership support (Jiménez-Picón et al., 2021). When we connect to the people on our teams, communities, and organizations, our work together can be highly effective. Evidence supports the value of mindfulness in professional leadership (see Capacity Building Resource List section).

Mindful leadership does not mean only to leave space and time to practice mindfulness independently. Instead, this leadership imbibes mindfulness throughout the organizational culture, procedures, and decision-making processes. Mindful leaders intentionally influence clarity among followers, benefiting all who have a stake in the organization (Levey & Levey, 2019). Literature supports that mindfulness is typically developed in organizations through skills-based training programs or systems approaches to build mindfulness into workplace culture (Levey & Levey, 2019; Rupprecht et al., 2019). While skills-based mindfulness training programs produce positive personal and short-term organizational outcomes (Johnson et al., 2020), systems-based mindfulness facilitates more profound, more sustainable change within workplace cultures (Levey & Levey, 2019). As a leader, when you choose a systems approach, you routinely include mindfulness in all practices, procedures, and policies (Box 10.3).

Emotional Intelligence

We recognize emotional intelligence as another support for clarity in leadership. Emotional intelligence is the ability to perceive and understand our own and others' emotions and use this information to guide our decisions and behaviors

---

> ## • BOX 10.2 The Dark Side of Leadership
>
> Leaders must first have integrity or character, or as Covey (1990) states, a leader must be principle-centered. Without moral behavior, leaders can become destructive or toxic. Toxic leaders are often charming but lack integrity. They search for followers who are conformers (i.e., lack confidence) or colluders (i.e., share the leader's views). Toxic leaders also seek a conducive environment; unstable, lacking checks and balances, or in crisis (Bass, 1999; Northouse, 2022; Padilla & Kaiser, 2007).
>
> Bass, B. M. (1999). Two decades of research and development in transformational leadership. *European Journal of Work and Organizational Psychology, 8*(1), 9–32.
> Covey, S. R. (1990). *Principle-centered leadership.* New York: Simon and Schuster.
> Northouse, P. G. (2022). *Leadership: Theory and practice* (9th ed.). SAGE.
> Padilla, A., Hogan, R., & Kaiser, R. B. (2007). The toxic triangle: Destructive leaders, susceptible followers, and conducive environments. *The Leadership Quarterly, 18*(3), 176–194.

Before heading out to the hospital today, Carmen had started the day with a 5-minute meditation for clarity through a mindfulness app on their phone. Later, at the hospital, Anju, the chief quality improvement officer, introduced a tool called the *Minding Safety Checklist* to all employees who worked in the rehabilitation unit. The tool was developed after a root-cause analysis identified a series of minor, avoidable errors or oversights made unintentionally by multiple staff members during a busy shift, contributing to a patient fall with severe injury. Carmen observed that Anju first acknowledged the stress that staff members experience and their shared value for safety. Then, Anju explained why and how this tool should be used and invited staff to share their questions and feelings about this checklist freely. The list would be used by each staff member during a shift and included keywords that staff members would use to remind each other to pause, assess identified physical areas of the unit, ask for help, and invite questions from each other, regardless of hierarchical position or rank. During the several weeks that followed, Carmen had opportunities to use the checklist with staff on the unit and recognized that use of the checklist was becoming part of shared work routines. Carmen admired how Anju led the team to adopt this tool through support, understanding, emphasis on shared goals, and gratitude for their contribution to the unit's culture of safety and teamwork.

(Salovey & Mayer, 1990). When you have emotional intelligence, you tend to see yourself and others more clearly. Emotional intelligence is an essential skill of healthcare leaders (Weiszbrod, 2020). Most healthcare providers value connections with people. Many may naturally possess a high emotional intelligence to serve therapeutic relationships with clients. This section emphasizes leveraging emotional intelligence to flourish as a leader.

Daniel Goleman (1995) popularized the importance of emotional intelligence in the workplace through the book *Emotional Intelligence: Why It Can Matter More Than IQ*. More recently, Goleman et al. (2017) compiled a set of competencies to develop skills necessary for four essential emotional intelligence components: self-awareness, self-management, social awareness, and relationship management. Since these capabilities rely on specific skills, emotional intelligence can be developed, unlike IQ and personality (Bradberry, 2017). Evidence supports connections between emotional intelligence and positive workplace outcomes, including improved leadership and managerial practices, team performance, collaboration, satisfaction, retention, perceived health, and burnout protection (Gransberry, 2021; Jiménez-Picón et al., 2021; Zhang et al., 2018). Researchers have suggested that organizations provide emotional intelligence training and competencies to foster employee effectiveness (Gorgens-Ekermans & Roux, 2021).

Scholars and industry leaders have also touted emotional intelligence qualities as integral to effective leadership. Especially in the current social, cultural, political, health, and economic contexts, demonstrations of humanity can spark change. The popular work of researcher and educator Brené Brown (2018) has reframed vulnerability from a perceived weakness to a powerful leadership strength. Knowing and sharing one's whole self and staying curious about what works and does not work in teams may be particularly helpful as we lead during times of hyperchange (Couris, 2020).

Like vulnerability, kindness is a modest but powerful leadership strategy. Leaders positively influence workplace culture by humbly and explicitly acknowledging mistakes, asking for help, and encouraging meaningful discourse among groups (Johnson, 2021). Groyberg and Seligson (2020) recognize kindness, emotional intelligence, and empathy as the most essential "soft skills" for leadership. Perhaps, these soft skills provide the infrastructure for working together as leaders and followers. Angie Vuyst (2021) points out that every leader is at some point a follower and encourages a perspective that honors the fundamental interconnectedness with others, like trees in a forest. Researchers have proposed that leaders and followers can be best understood by recognizing the social identity of their collective groups (e.g., workplaces, teams, organizations, communities) rather than viewing leadership as a solo operation (Haslam et al., 2017). Although being a follower often has a negative undertone, it would be impossible to have leaders without followers; one cannot exist without the other. Followership will be discussed later in the chapter. See Box 10.4 for an example of emotional intelligence in leadership development.

Curiosity

To achieve clarity, it is important to respect uncertainty and question assumptions that come from life experiences. Understanding experiences and contexts is essential to understanding ourselves as leaders. When you think of leadership, what or who comes to mind? Maybe it was a coach from high school or a leader of your Scout troop. It might

Carmen considers many leaders they have met in their professional training to be advisors. Carmen recognizes common characteristics in these mentors: they make time for other people, invite all perspectives and ideas, and give honest feedback. One leader with high emotional intelligence is Jada, Carmen's fieldwork educator. Jada serves on many committees at work; her voice is valued. Although Jada is not a supervisor or manager, Carmen sees that colleagues often look to Jada for advice about treating clients or working with teams. Jada mentors many new practitioners and students, like Carmen. People feel good about themselves and their work when they interact with Jada. Recently, Jada was awarded by the state professional association for a significant contribution to the profession through fieldwork education. Carmen recognizes that their mentorship with Jada does not emphasize power or feel hierarchical. While Carmen has learned much from Jada in a clinical sense, they also feel comfortable sharing their perspectives with Jada, which helps Carmen feel connected to Jada and the OT profession. Jada's words and actions consistently show self-awareness and understanding of the emotions of others. Jada's leadership is rooted in humility and kindness.

be the president of the United States or a CEO of a large corporation. We support leadership development when we commit to a natural curiosity about ourselves, what and whom we observe, and our assumptions. This section highlights two skills that require and support the role of curiosity in leadership development: lifelong learning and critical reflection.

Lifelong Learning and Critical Reflection

Learning is critical in leadership development to keep up with evolving global perspectives and needs (Torrez & Rocco, 2015). Curiosity involves the desire to learn and the willingness to challenge what has been learned. It invites us to check whether assumptions make sense based on new observations, information, and contexts. This essential component of leadership is critical reflection, the cognitive process that supports transformative learning (Torrez & Rocco, 2015). Transformative learning harmonizes assumptions with what is happening to produce change beyond the surface (Mezirow, 2003). Critical reflection involves understanding past and present situations to derive next steps into the future (The Institute of Leadership and Management, 2022). Since many people attribute the ability to facilitate change as the mark of a good leader, critical reflection is a valuable skill to promote new perspectives and lead to creative solutions instead of how things have always been done (Torrez & Rocco, 2015). A simple way of describing critical reflection may be to add what we have already discussed about mindfulness to the adage of "learn from your mistakes."

Critical reflection extends beyond the self to teams, organizations, and professional communities. When a problem requires questioning underlying beliefs and reasons for choices, a critical reflection on our thoughts, behaviors, and interactions with persons, teams, communities, organizations, and society can assist with clarification. We can practice critical reflection by recognizing and challenging assumptions that influence perceptions of leadership (Dugan, 2018).

Leadership is more than just a skill set of an individual. Leadership development entails a social process influenced by the transactive relationship between the leader and the environment, and *implicit leadership theory* is essential to understanding the social constructs of leadership (Schyns et al., 2011). Implicit leadership theory calls for critical reflection to examine preconceived ideas of what it means to be a leader, where these ideas come from, and how these assumptions guide thoughts and actions. Staying curious is one way to step outside long-held, societally-shaped beliefs about leadership to activate effective leadership and create environments that encourage people to reflect, learn, and grow. Learning is never finished and is a necessary process throughout your career (Chapter 6). See Box 10.5 for an application of critical reflection to leadership.

Leadership Approaches and Theories

There are numerous ways of conceptualizing leadership. Theoretical principles guide our actions and decisions as

---

• BOX 10.5 Living Leadership: Carmen and Critical Reflection

Carmen took a course called Leadership in the Health Professions with instructor Dr. Mack, a PT with expertise in leadership development. Carmen found one class activity particularly transformative concerning their concept of a leader. Dr. Mack instructed students working in groups to draw a picture of a leader. When each group reached an agreement about their "leader" picture, they presented it to the whole class. Carmen's group recognized that they thought differently about what a leader is. Some students acknowledged that they tended to think of a leader as a male with conservative but "fancy" clothing, like a suit and tie, denoting power and prestige. Some classmates suggested that they thought of a leader as a woman who wears their hair naturally and their "heart on their sleeve." A couple of group members depicted a "loud" leader who "takes charge," while some students included oversized ears in their picture because they admired leaders who quietly listened to followers' voices and ideas. Carmen considered the varied views on what a leader looks like and asked meaningful questions about the origin of team members' assumptions. The class activity prompted consideration of the influence of societal and cultural factors and life experiences on the concept of a leader. Dr. Mack helped Carmen and their classmates deepen reflective discussions, consider new perspectives, and reconcile differences between old and current ways of thinking. Since this class, Carmen intentionally reflects on and welcomes perspectives that challenge their assumptions about leadership.

Adapted from Schyns, B., Kiefer, T., Kerschreiter, R., & Tymon, A. (2011). Teaching implicit leadership theories to develop leaders and leadership: How and why it can make a difference. *Academy of Management Learning & Education, 10*(3), 397–408.

---

leaders, just as theories guide our therapy practice. There are many leadership theories, each focusing on a unique aspect of leadership and how it is applied and perceived. The continuum ranges from a focus on intrinsic leadership characteristics to societal leadership systems. Since leadership identity may be closely connected to the most observed approaches, it is helpful to see the breadth of leadership perspectives.

Leadership theories and models can be divided into three main phases: trait, behavioral, and situational/contingency (Ledlow & Stephens, 2018). The trait and behavioral phases focus on the leader by identifying a person's characteristics, skills, behaviors, or styles. Later research focused on the situational/contingency phase by examining leaders in the context of work situations and environments and the ability to adapt (Ledlow & Stephens, 2018). We propose a fourth phase termed the socially responsive phase, in which theories focus on the leader as a change maker. This section highlights some of the major approaches and ideas that emerged during each phase. Table 10.1 provides an overview of commonly cited leadership theories and approaches.

Leader as Self: Trait and Behavioral Phases

"Leaders are not born or made—they are self-made."

STEPHEN R. COVEY

TABLE 10.1	Common Leadership Approaches and Theories			
Phase	**Leadership Theory/Approach**	**Primary Theorist(s)**	**Focus**	**Key Words**
Trait	Trait	• Kurt Lewin • Ronald Lippitt • Ralph White • Ralph Stogdill	• Unique characteristics of effective leaders	• Personality • Big five • Strengths leadership
Behavioral	Skills	• Robert Katz • Michael Mumford	• Skills required for effective leadership	• Technical, human, and conceptual skills • Competencies, individual attributes, leadership outcomes, career experiences, environmental influences
	Style	• Ralph Stogdill • Alvin Coons • Robert Blake • Jane Mouton	• What leaders do and their behaviors	• Bandura's social learning theory • McGregor's theory X and theory Y • Autocratic, directive, and task-oriented • Democratic, collaborative, and relationship-oriented • Managerial / leadership grid®
Situational/ Contingency	Contingency	• Fred Fiedler	• Using context to match a leader's style to the setting	• Context • Task/goal-motivated • Relationship/people-motivated
	Situational	• Paul Hersey • Kenneth Blanchard	• Changing one's style or behavior to fit the situation	• Directing • Coaching • Supporting • Delegating
	Transformational	• James Burns • Bernard Bass	• How relationship-motivated leaders empower followers to create positive change	• Transactional • Transforming • Followership • Charisma • Idealized influence • Inspirational motivation • Intellectual stimulation • Individualized consideration
	Authentic	• Bill George	• Effective leaders are genuine and stay true to their values	• Self-awareness • Balanced processing • Internalized moral perspective • Relational transparency
	Servant	• Robert Greenleaf	• Leaders place the needs of the followers before their own	• Stewardship • Obligation • Partnership • Emotional healing • Elevating purpose
	Adaptive	• Ronald Heifetz • Marty Linsky	• Leaders help followers adapt and manage change	• Technical challenges • Adaptive challenges
	Followership	• Abraham Zaleznik • Robert Kelley • Ira Chaleff • Barbara Kellerman	• Individuals who are engaged, committed, and take the initiative. They are independent thinkers who are active in the leadership process, even leading when needed	• Motivation • Engagement

TABLE 10.1 Common Leadership Approaches and Theories—cont'd

Phase	Leadership Theory/Approach	Primary Theorist(s)	Focus	Key Words
Socially Responsive	Social Change Model	• Susan Komives • Wendy Wagner • Higher Education Research Institute (HERI) of UCLA	• Leadership is a process, not a position • Collaborative vision of community leadership • Values-driven • Emphasis on the 7 "C's" of leadership	• Consciousness of self • Congruence • Commitment • Collaboration • Common purpose • Controversy with civility • Citizenship • Change
	Transformative	• William Foster • Richard Quantz, Judy Rogers, Michael Dantley • Carolyn Shields	• Leaders affect deep and equitable change with critical reflection and moral action to dismantle hegemonic structures and promote the common good	• Moral activism • Social justice • Equity and inclusion • Balancing critique and promise

Sources Johnson, C. (2021). *Meeting the ethical challenges of leadership: Casting light or shadow* (7th ed.). SAGE Publications; Komives, S. R., & Wagner, W. (Eds.). (2016). *Leadership for a better world: Understanding the social change model of leadership development* (2nd ed.). Jossey-Bass; Ledlow, G. R., & Stephens, J. H. (2018). *Leadership for health professionals: Theory, skills, and applications* (3rd ed.). Jones & Bartlett Learning; Northouse, P. G. (2013). Leadership: Theory and practice (6th ed.). SAGE Publications; Northouse, P. G. (2022). *Leadership: Theory and practice* (9th ed.). SAGE Publications; Shields, C. M. (2020). Transformative leadership. In C. M. Shields, *Oxford Research Encyclopedia of Education*. Oxford University Press.

Early leadership research focused on how leaders somehow seemed different from their subordinates. Thus researchers sought to identify the unique characteristics associated with leadership; although some common characteristics were identified, traits alone could not identify what led to a leader's success. The limitations of the trait phase led to the emergence of the behavioral phase, which focused on leadership skills and styles. What emerged from both phases is that there is no universal set of leadership traits or behaviors; however, these phases were the foundation for the leadership theories of today. Refer to Table 10.2 for an overview of common traits, skills, and styles of effective leaders. Interestingly, these traits, skills, and styles are common in expert therapists (Embrey et al., 1996; Gilliland & Wainwright, 2017; Huhn et al., 2019; Jensen et al., 1990, 1992, 2000; Musolino & Jensen, 2020).

Trait Phase

The *trait approach* or *great man theory* was one of the earliest ways of considering leadership. The assumption was that leaders were born with certain traits leading to their exceptional abilities. Early history writers focused on the importance of leaders demonstrating courage and physical strength, primarily for conquest. Around 1530, Machiavelli (1914) described the traits of a successful leader: be clever—choose being feared over loved but avoid cruelty—show mercy and generosity, but judiciously—be honest, but lie if needed to maintain power—trust advisors, but do not be naïve. In the 1800s, theorists identified great leaders based

TABLE 10.2 Traits, Skills, and Styles of Leaders and Expert Therapists

Traits	Skills	Styles
• Integrity • Confidence • Intelligence • Sociability • Determination • Compassion • Altruistic • Responsibility • Motivation	• Communication • Efficiency • Time-management • Problem-solving • Flexibility • Intuition • Vision • Reflection	• Relationship-oriented • Biopsycho-social • Person-centered • Team leadership

From Embrey, D. G., Guthrie, M. R., White, O. R., & Dietz, J. (1996). Clinical decision making by experienced and inexperienced pediatric physical therapists for children with diplegic cerebral palsy. *Physical Therapy*, 76(1), 20–33; Gilliland, S., & Wainwright, S. F. (2017). Patterns of clinical reasoning in physical therapist students. *Physical Therapy*, 97(5), 499–511; Huhn, K., Gilliland, S. J., Black, L. L., Wainwright, S. F., & Christensen, N. (2019). Clinical reasoning in physical therapy: A concept analysis. *Physical Therapy*, 99(4), 440–456; Jensen, G. M., Shepard, K., & Hack, L. (1990). The novice versus the experienced clinician: Insights into the work of the physical therapist. *Physical Therapy*, 70, 314–32; Jensen, G. M., Shepard, K. F., Gwyer, J., & Hack, L. M. (1992). Attribute dimensions that distinguish master and novice physical therapy clinicians in orthopedic settings. *Physical Therapy*, 72(10), 711–722; Jensen, G. M., Gwyer, J., Shepard, K. F., & Hack, L. M. (2000). Expert practice in physical therapy. *Physical Therapy*, 80(1), 28–43; Musolino, G. M., & Jensen, G. M. (2020). *Clinical reasoning and decision-making in physical therapy: Facilitation, assessment, and implementation*. SLACK.; Northouse, P. G. (2022). *Leadership: Theory and practice* (9th ed.). SAGE.

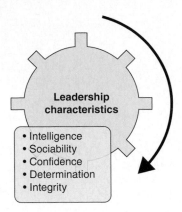

• **Fig. 10.2** Common Leadership Characteristics

on their affluence and throughout the 1900s, researchers focused on identifying specific characteristics that distinguished leaders from followers (Ledlow & Stephens, 2018).

Although it was ultimately established that there is no universal set of traits, there are characteristics that consistently emerge from the research (Fig. 10.2) (Northouse, 2022). In addition, trait approach research produced the Big Five personality factors associated with strong leadership. In order of importance, these factors are extraversion, conscientiousness, openness, low neuroticism, and agreeableness. A metaanalysis demonstrated a strong correlation between these five traits and leadership, confirming that certain traits are associated with leadership (Judge et al., 2002).

Behavioral Phase

Since traits alone could not fully explain leaders' success, researchers transitioned to identifying behaviors, such as skills and styles. The *skills approach* focuses on the leader's capabilities and knowledge (Ledlow & Stephens, 2018; Northouse, 2022). Overall, leaders need to possess technical, human, administrative, and conceptual skills. Technical skills require competence and proficiency in work. Human (i.e., people or interpersonal) skills include listening and understanding others' feelings and motivations. Human skills focus on people, whereas technical skills address things. Administrative skills involve managerial functions, including hiring, budgeting, planning, organizing, delegating, and mentoring. Lastly, conceptual skills relate to ideas and, thus are most important at the top management levels. Leaders with conceptual skills can put the organization's goals, vision, and strategic plan into words.

The behavioral phase also includes the *style approach*, emphasizing that a leader's style or behavior is crucial (Ledlow & Stephens, 2018; Northouse, 2022). The style approach is associated with Bandura's social learning theory, which describes human behavior as a continuous reciprocal interaction where individuals observe, imitate, and model behavior. Thus the style approach ushered in an important revelation; *leadership could be learned*. The style approach

classifies leaders as more goal/task-oriented versus employee/relationship-oriented.

The task-oriented versus relationship-oriented distinction is consistent with McGregor's Theory X and Theory Y (Ledlow & Stephens, 2018). Theory X involves managers and leaders assuming that their followers are indifferent, extrinsically motivated, undisciplined, and uncooperative. On the other hand, Theory Y views followers as responsible, intrinsically motivated, energetic, bright, and collaborative. Based on the leader's viewpoint of their follower, they will utilize different styles. For example, a Theory X leader would use autocratic and directive styles (i.e., task-oriented), whereas a Theory Y leader would utilize democratic and collaborative styles (relationship-oriented). Thus the concept that leaders must alter their style to fit the demands of the situation emerged.

Leader as a Team Member: Situational/Contingency Phase

The situational/contingency phase emerged after researchers identified that leadership effectiveness depends on the context. This phase identified the notion that leaders must change their style to fit the demands of the situation and that organizations may need to change leaders based on current needs. Successful organizations and leaders diagnose the situation, account for context, and adapt to followers' needs.

Contingency Theory and Situational Leadership Approach

Contingency theory contends that a leader's effectiveness is contingent on matching the leader's style to the situation (Ledlow & Stephens, 2018; Northouse, 2013). Thus leaders can be effective in certain contexts, but not all. Leaders are either task-motivated or relationship-motivated based on the context of the situation. For example, a sports team with experienced veteran leadership may replace a disciplinarian coach (i.e., task-motivated) with a players' coach (i.e., relationship-motivated). While the trait and behavioral phases focus on a leader's characteristics, skills, or styles, contingency theory matches the leader to the situation. Contingency theory is distinct in that it recognizes that leaders should not be expected to lead in every situation and must be optimally placed for success.

Although the situational leadership approach and contingency theory sound similar on the surface, there is a distinction. *Situational leadership* involves changing one's leadership style to fit the situation (Ledlow & Stephens, 2018; Northouse, 2022). Contingency theory promotes finding the best leader for the situation. Thus in contingency theory, the leader's style is relatively fixed, whereas, in situational leadership, the style is dynamic. Situational leadership requires that the leader change or adapt their style based on how much support and direction the follower needs. Situational leaders select a style based on the development level of

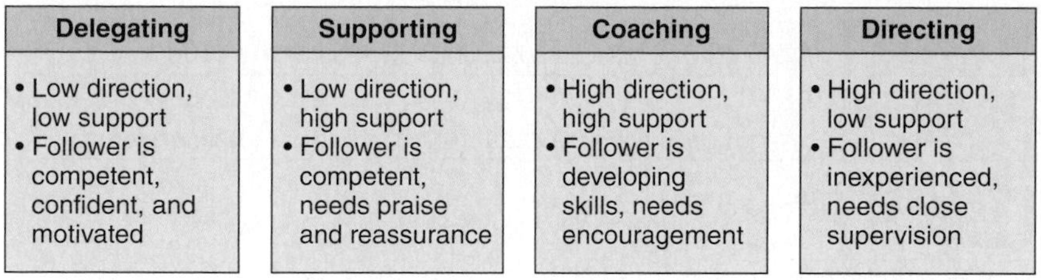

Delegating	Supporting	Coaching	Directing
• Low direction, low support • Follower is competent, confident, and motivated	• Low direction, high support • Follower is competent, needs praise and reassurance	• High direction, high support • Follower is developing skills, needs encouragement	• High direction, low support • Follower is inexperienced, needs close supervision

• **Fig. 10.3** Situational Leadership Styles. (From: Northouse, P. G. [2022]. *Leadership: Theory and practice* [9th ed.]. SAGE.)

• BOX 10.6   Situational Leadership for OTs and PTs

- What situational leadership style might be most common among OTs and PTs?
- What situational leadership style might be most effective for the following individuals?
  - A 67-year-old patient who is 1-week status post rotator cuff repair
  - A 25-year-old experienced weightlifter with acute low back pain but cannot afford more than two sessions

---

the followers, specifically their competence and commitment to accomplishing the goal. The four leadership styles are *directing, coaching, supporting,* and *delegating* (Fig. 10.3).

Since some patients need more support and direction than others, OTs and PTs commonly adapt their behavior to create an ideal patient-therapist interaction. During patient-therapist interaction, therapists commonly use a coaching style (Box 10.6) (Northouse, 2013; Rasmussen-Barr et al., 2019).

Transforming and Transformational Leadership

Transformational leadership is an evolution of transforming leadership, initially introduced by Burns (1978). When describing transforming leadership, Burns contrasted it with transactional leadership. Transactional leadership is task-motivated and concerned with extrinsic rewards and equal exchanges. In contrast, transforming leadership is relationship-motivated. The leader engages followers' intrinsic motivation to work toward a common purpose. Transforming leadership has moral and ethical aspirations. The leader-follower interaction rises above self-interest, transforming the leader and followers into a united front with like-minded values (Burns, 1995b; Couto, 1995b).

Over time there has been a blending of Burns' (1978) transforming leadership with what Bass (1985) refers to as transformational leadership. Transformational leadership is a radical departure from the traditional management approach, which focuses on maintaining order and productivity. In contrast, transformational leadership focuses on elevating the performance of followers. The factors involved in helping followers achieve their full potential include the "four I's" of transformational leadership (Table 10.3) (Lee, 2014; Northouse, 2022).

TABLE 10.3   The Four I's of Transformational Leadership

Inspirational Motivation	Transformational leaders use enthusiasm, encouragement, and pep talks to facilitate necessary change
Intellectual Stimulation	Transformational leaders encourage followers to identify and solve problems via innovation and critical thinking
Individual Consideration	Transformational leaders establish a supportive environment for advisement and coaching
Idealized Influence	Transformational leaders possess confidence, vision, and charisma

From Bass, B. M. (1999). Two decades of research and development in transformational leadership. *European Journal of Work and Organizational Psychology, 8*(1), 9–32; Couto, R. A. (1995b). The transformation of transforming leadership. In J. T. Wren (Ed.), *Leaders companion: Insights on leadership through the ages* (pp. 102–107). Free Press; Lee, M. (2014). Transformational leadership: Is it time for a recall? *International Journal of Management and Applied Research, 1*(1), 17–29; Northouse, P. G. (2022). *Leadership: Theory and practice* (9th ed.). SAGE.

Transformational leaders have vision and charisma (Bass, 1999; Couto, 1995b; Lee, 2014; Northouse, 2022). However, Bass (1999) prefers the term idealized influence because charisma has become notorious figures throughout history who have used their charisma to accomplish unspeakable atrocities. Thus many people are skeptical of anyone labeled charismatic, which could extend to transformational leadership (Lee, 2014; Northouse, 2022). Beyond using idealized influence over charism, Bass (1999) addressed the potential for the dark side of leadership or what he referred to as pseudo-transformational leadership. Pseudo-transformational leaders are immature and self-aggrandizing charismatics. They appear uplifting and responsible but lack an ethical or moral foundation. In addition to being immoral, pseudo-transformational leaders are self-consumed, exploitive, and power-hungry.

Authentic Leadership

Authentic leadership focuses on being real or genuine. Thacker (2016), the author of the book, *The Art of Authenticity,* notes that "We think of authentic leadership as being the real us, the real deal. The problem is that there is no one

Self-awareness	An internal reflection of your unique traits and perceptions
Balanced processing	Being open-minded and fact-focused when receiving information
Internalized moral perspective	Using intrinsic values to drive behaviors and actions
Relational transparency	Sharing thoughts and feelings openly and respectfully

• **Fig. 10.4** Components of Authentic Leadership (From Johnson, C. [2021]. *Meeting the ethical challenges of leadership: Casting light or shadow* (7th ed.). SAGE; Thacker, K. [2016]. *The art of authenticity: Tools to become an authentic leader and your best self.* Wiley.)

real deal. There is no one single version of any of us to behold. We show different sides of ourselves in different contexts all the time" (p. 73). It is important to be pragmatic and realistic about the human condition. Authentic leadership requires you to be a more skilled version of yourself (Thacker, 2016). There are four key components of authentic leadership (Fig. 10.4).

Authentic leaders do not compromise on their values, even during challenging times (Northouse, 2022). Challenging times strengthen their values. They also know how to build strong relationships with followers because of their firmly held beliefs. Their steadfastness creates a connection between them and their followers.

There is a strong relationship between authenticity and ethical leadership. Authentic leaders are self-aware, consistent, emotionally balanced, transparent, and moral (Northouse, 2022; Thacker, 2016). They remain cool, calm, and objective in emotional times. They avoid favoritism and biased decisions. Authentic leaders are transparent and because they possess integrity, they have no fear of exposure. They are an open book and beyond reproach. Transparency, however, is not an all-or-nothing proposition; it needs to be intentional. Within authentic leadership lies a paradox; while an individual may feel authentic, authenticity is ultimately a perception of others (Thacker, 2016).

Servant Leadership

Developed by Robert Greenleaf, *servant leadership theory* fits well with the core philosophies of health professions by emphasizing service to others and the betterment of society (Greenleaf, 2002; Northouse, 2022). This leadership approach emphasizes empowering the follower and developing a sense of community, focusing on wellbeing and ethics (Eva et al., 2019). Servant leadership theory emphasizes social justice principles and collaborative environments within healthcare and human service fields (Eva et al., 2019; Fields et al., 2015; Garber et al., 2009). Servant leadership theory offers a holistic perspective on the attributes and characteristics integral to an effective therapist. Servant leadership acknowledges the human side of people and moves beyond typical transactional leadership approaches to empower others.

Servant leaders position themselves in the background and act as a conduit to strengthen the community around

them. Like transformational leadership, servant leadership empowers others to transform yet differs by fostering independence in followers rather than creating a dependent relationship (Johnson, 2021). Johnson (2021) emphasizes that a servant leader acts as a partner and does not treat followers as subordinates. This mutual respect promotes more positive interactions and self-efficacy.

Johnson (2021) notes that servant leaders put followers and their needs at the forefront of their approach, practice "humble inquiry over telling," and effectively promote follower growth (p. 249). Introversion is a strength in this leadership style, and research is starting to validate the efficacy of servant leadership (Spark & O'Connor, 2017). Servant leadership and self-awareness are inherently linked and individuals who choose this leadership style need to have insight into their nature. Mindfulness and spirituality play a substantial role in this type of leadership and being present for followers through open body language, active listening, compassion, leader self-care, and understanding connection to a higher purpose contribute to successful outcomes (Bunting, 2016; Johnson, 2021).

Adaptive Leadership

The goal of *adaptive leadership* is to help followers adapt and manage change (Northouse, 2022). Adaptive leadership takes a process approach, accounting for the complexities between leaders, followers, and situations. Leaders must have a holistic perspective, acknowledging the followers' logistical and psychological needs. Adaptive leadership is used when there is no current system or practice to help the team navigate challenges, problems, or changes (Northouse, 2022).

Adaptive leadership is prescriptive because the process gives leaders the tools to help organize followers to facilitate change (Northouse, 2022). The leader surveys the current situation, identifies the challenge, creates structure, monitors for distress, encourages followers to focus on the challenge, and finally gives the work back to the people. Another critical aspect of adaptive leadership is acknowledging diverse viewpoints to gain an inclusive perspective. In this way, adaptive leadership is follower-focused. It moves away from the top-down approach and allows leaders to engage followers close to the problem and most familiar with day-to-day operations.

- How might you use adaptive leadership to encourage an individual with heart disease risk factors to begin exercising?
- How might you use adaptive leadership to integrate occupational therapy and Speech Language Pathology (SLP) into your school's already established physical therapy pro bono clinic?

Collaboration is essential because it acknowledges that the leader does not have all the answers. Adaptive leaders are not directors; they are facilitators who allow followers to implement solutions for a successful change. This theory is unique and directs authority to help followers deal with conflicting values in changing organizational environments and social contexts. Leaders offer followers transparency by discussing what must change, why it is needed, how it will occur, and the data behind the innovative approach. Adaptive leadership fosters resiliency through cohesion, creating a shared vision, and facilitating ownership (Box 10.7). There is a focus on the bigger picture and fluidity in meeting goals (Ramalingam et al., 2020).

Followership

Being labeled a follower often has a negative connotation. However, it would be impossible to have leaders without followers, and thus followers are just as important as leaders. Followership is the active process of an individual accepting influence from another, typically to achieve a common goal (Northouse, 2022). Both followers and leaders must be engaged in the process; one cannot take place without active participation from the other.

There are various classifications to describe followers (Table 10.4). Kelly (1988) focused on follower motivation. Followers range from unmotivated and dependent to motivated and independent. Kellerman (2007) focused on follower engagement and noted that regardless of context, the follower's degree of involvement determines the nature of the leader-follower relationship. Follower engagement ranges from feeling and doing nothing to extreme devotion.

As with leaders, certain characteristics and behaviors make a successful follower (Northouse, 2022). Successful followers are credible, competent, motivated, and independent thinkers who manage themselves. Followers are committed to meeting the mission and have shared values with the leader. They support and learn from their leader and challenge them honestly and respectfully (Box 10.8).

Leader as Change-Maker: Socially Responsive Phase

Leadership can be understood through theories that go beyond self and team to include a change at the societal level. National and global OT and PT professional associations call practitioners to change that supports equity and inclusion. The strategic plans of both the American Occupational Therapy Association (AOTA) and the American Physical Therapy Association (APTA) focus on inclusive and transformative efforts connected to the value system of each profession (American Occupational Therapy Association, 2021; American Physical Therapy Association, 2022a). This section introduces two leadership theories that can help you respond to the call for leaders to facilitate profound societal change: the *social change*

TABLE 10.4   Types of Followers

Kelley's Types of Followers				
Passive (Sheep)	**Alienated** (Cynics)	**Pragmatics** (Survivors)	**Conformists** (Yes-people)	**Exemplary** (Stars)
• Not motivated • Dependent • Requires constant supervision	• Not motivated • Independent • Critical and negative, but does not actively participate	• Motivated • Independent • Prefers the status quo	• Motivated • Dependent • Content to take orders; defers to leader	• Motivated • Independent • Actively engaged and takes initiative

Kellerman's Types of Followers				
Isolates	**Bystanders**	**Participants**	**Activists**	**Diehards**
• Not engaged • Unaware • Lacks commitment • Prefers the status quo	• Not engaged • Aware • Lacks commitment • Prefers the status quo	• Engaged • Supports or opposes the leader depending on whether they agree	• Highly engaged • Works on behalf of the leader or challenges the leader	• Extremely engaged • Devoted to supporting or opposing the leader • Would die for the cause

Kelley, R. (1988, November 1). In praise of followers. *Harvard Business Review.* https://hbr.org/1988/11/in-praise-of-followers; Kellerman, B. (2007, December 1). What every leader needs to know about followers. *Harvard Business Review.* https://hbr.org/2007/12/what-every-leader-needs-to-know-about-followers; Northouse, P. G. (2022). *Leadership: Theory and practice* (9th ed.). SAGE.

Carmen attends a departmental meeting during one of their clinical rotations. One of the therapists working in the department approaches Carmen and Jada and remarks, "these meetings are a waste of time." Carmen observes that some individuals are uninvolved during the meeting, playing on their phones or documenting on their computers. Jada actively participated, asking questions, and seeking solutions to problems within the department. After the meeting, Carmen hears a therapist ask questions about the new practice guidelines announced during the meeting. Each question was covered moments ago, in detail, during the meeting. Carmen considers the importance of being an engaged follower and how it might impact patient care.

model of leadership development and *transformative leadership theory*.

Social Change Model of Leadership

Developed initially with students in mind, the social change leadership model takes a collaborative approach to promote social change through leadership. Socially responsible leadership considers the transaction between the individual, group, and community values (Dugan, 2015; Komives & Wagner, 2016). This model is based on the following assumptions (Komives & Wagner, 2016) (p. xv):

- Leadership is concerned with effecting change on behalf of others and society.
- Leadership is collaborative.
- Leadership is a process rather than a position.
- Leadership should be value-based.
- All students (not just those who hold formal leadership positions) are potential leaders.
- Service is a powerful vehicle for developing students' leadership skills.

This holistic perspective emphasizes that leadership is accessible to all persons and does not require a management position but rather the commitment to learning and growing

as a person and a team. Komives and Wagner (2016) offer seven values within three leadership domains to use as a mechanism to work toward social change, also known as the 7 Cs (Fig. 10.5).

Using the social change model of leadership enables health professionals to address the needs of diverse clients that encompass individuals, groups, and communities (Liotta-Kleinfeld et al., 2018). This model can be used both as a process model guiding individuals and teams toward social change or can also be used as a development model, identifying areas in which students can advance their skills and behaviors (Dugan, 2015). Experiential learning, such as clinical rotations or service-learning requirements in coursework, provides an excellent opportunity to use the tenets of the social change leadership model. You are encouraged to explore these values during your experiences and reflect on these elements. The take-home message of this model is to remind you that despite inexperience or position within your field, you are still well-positioned to be a catalyst for societal change.

Transformative Leadership Theory

Rooted in Burns' concept of transforming leadership (1978), *transformative leadership theory* has explicit connections with equity, inclusion, and social justice (Shields, 2020). Transformative leadership originated with theorists critically examining power in the reform of the educational system (Foster, 1986; Quantz et al., 1991). According to this theory, leaders facilitate change for the greatest good. This theory relies on the leadership essentials connected to courage, clarity, and curiosity, particularly critical reflection. It recognizes that a path to the greatest good is achieved through equity and inclusion, requiring dismantling what has been done for a long time. Shields (2020) shares eight guiding tenets for transformative leadership theory:

- mandate for deep and equitable change
- need to deconstruct knowledge frameworks that perpetuate injustice
- need to address inequitable distribution of power

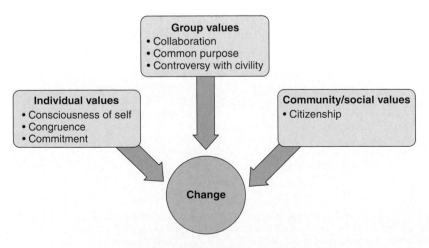

• **Fig. 10.5** 7 C's of Social Change

- emphasis on private (individual) and public (collective) good
- focus on emancipation, democracy, equity, and justice
- emphasis on interdependence, interconnectedness, and global awareness
- need to balance critique with promise
- call to exhibit moral courage

Transformative leaders move beyond the ability to create positive change toward actions that cause change within societal contexts. Shields (2020) proposes that such actions involve questioning, discourse, and relationships to understand and begin to deconstruct hegemonic structures. As OT and PT professions address inequities related to the workforce and clients, therapists can reaffirm professional core values, including equity and inclusion. Knowing and acting from these values requires courage. We can challenge bias and discrimination by questioning our learned assumptions. In other words, we can apply continuous curiosity about how power is at play in our relationships, communities, professions, and organizations. Recognizing inequities is a prerequisite to equity. We can build relationships and engage in active discourse with tension and difficulties around us. Considering the nature of this theory, a discussion that leads to change will inherently challenge us to act and to take risks.

Leadership in Action: Building Capacity of the Professions

Now that you have read the sections of this chapter related to defining leadership, building your capacity to lead, and understanding leadership theories, we invite you to consider the reciprocal relationship between you and your profession. Healthcare leaders emphasize that future leaders require fundamental skills in creating professional relationships (Heard, 2014; Stoffel, 2013). When you take an active role and connect with members of your professional community, you contribute to the capacity of your profession to meet society's rapidly changing, complex needs. The OT and PT professions regard leadership as critical to the profession's sustainability, as evidenced by the emphasis on leadership in the national associations' strategic plans (American Occupational Therapy Association, 2021; American Physical Therapy Association, 2022a). This section of the chapter highlights opportunities for developing leadership in the contexts of your local, state, national, and global communities while contributing to your profession's mission, vision, and goals in tandem.

Local – Academic Program/University and Workplace

Locally, students and practitioners develop and apply leadership within school and work contexts. Opportunities for the development of leadership capacity at these local levels abound. Examples include formal education and training, informal interactions with classmates, faculty, and colleagues, volunteering, engaged membership, mentorship, and advocacy.

First, consider the context of your professional program at school. You likely receive formal training related to leadership in your coursework and field experiences. Developing competency in leadership among students builds outstanding clinician-leaders (Blumenthal et al., 2012; Sebelski et al., 2020) and the capacity of our broader profession to transform systems like healthcare (Onyura et al., 2019). As a student, you may engage with leadership training through leadership development programs, course content, field experiences, interprofessional learning opportunities, and advanced projects, like a capstone. Students in an OT program perceived improved leadership after participating in their doctoral capstone experience (Recigno et al., 2020). Everyday student experiences also contribute to leadership behaviors. Engaging in profession-based student organizations invites opportunities to develop leadership that directly connects to your career (Lebrón et al., 2017). Your student organization may be a local chapter of a larger professional organization or an original group based on the specific needs of your school. Student organizations foster professional communities while inviting students to explore their leadership identity by holding officer positions, through events and initiatives related to mentorship, professional networks, community outreach, and advocacy efforts.

Similar to leadership training opportunities at a university, there are opportunities for leadership development within work settings. Workplace opportunities can build our capacity to lead while also offering ways for us to contribute to an organization's mission and vision. We can learn about leadership and lead from any role within an organization, beginning with mindful everyday interactions with colleagues, staff members, and clients or customers. For example, you may foster interprofessional collaboration during client care, engage in mentorship, advocate for your client, or host activities to promote awareness of your profession at your place of employment. Practitioners share unique perspectives by volunteering on committees. Guided by professional values, PT and OT professionals facilitate change for organizations, employees, colleagues, and clients. For example, a PT invested in client-centered care and frustrated by the limitations of note templates in an electronic medical record can lead a task group to bring evidence-informed suggestions to administrators and the documentation system vendor. This leadership can yield change that promotes accurate documentation of client-centered PT services. There are also formal ways to learn about leadership in the workplace. Examples include traditional mentorship programs and professional development sessions related to communication and teamwork. These structured opportunities may be provided, or even required, by the organization.

State

State-level professional associations provide another context for leadership development and application with your state professional community members. Students and practitioners contribute to the capacity of professions at the state level when they become a part of the state's professional association. This membership offers access to resources about state advocacy efforts, licensure, and practice issues. Like a school's profession-based organization, state-level membership offers opportunities to develop and apply leadership skills to directly support the profession while expanding your professional network beyond your work setting. Such options include volunteering at a sponsored event to promote awareness of OT or PT among community members, attending professional development events and conferences, serving in an elected board position, and lobbying for legislation, such as the decision to join an interstate licensure compact.

National

National-level initiatives invite you to engage with members of your professional community from around the country as you develop your leadership identity. Many opportunities are coordinated through the AOTA and APTA. This national context offers ways to build your capacity and contribute to your profession through formal and informal opportunities requiring varied commitment and time. Such opportunities include micro-volunteering, which entails sharing a limited amount of time and specific talents to work on smaller tasks that contribute to larger projects and meaningful change (AOTA, 2022). For example, members may volunteer at the annual conference or review manuscripts for professional magazines and journals. You may also consider an elected position within your national association. While a formal position is not necessary to lead, you may find that this provides a dedicated way to utilize your knowledge, skills, and vision for the profession's future. Another way to lead in the national context, engaging in national advocacy efforts, closely aligns with the societal lens of leadership. Opportunities for lifelong learning, such as leadership training programs, fellowships, and communities of practice, produce outcomes for individual learners and support the future advancement of professions (Alsop & Lloyd, 2002). One example of a specialized leadership learning opportunity is the APTA's LAMP Institute of Leadership Certificate in Healthcare Leadership, a program for healthcare professionals to grow their personal and professional leadership (American Physical Therapy Association, 2022b). Fellowships are advanced educational experiences that can help prepare individuals for leadership roles (McGowan & K. Stokes, 2015). Both the AOTA and APTA coordinate fellowships with sponsoring organizations in focused practice areas. Lastly, communities of practice are groups of professionals who meet regularly to learn together and share resources about a common interest related to practice, including leadership (Wenger-Trayner & Wenger-Trayner, 2015). These social networks may be created organically by members and formally recognized by organizations, such as the AOTA. To learn about specific opportunities to get involved in your national professional context, visit the APTA and AOTA websites (apta.org and aota.org).

Global

Similar to engagement at a national level, leadership opportunities on a global level are often facilitated through professional organizations such as the World Federation of Occupational Therapy or World Physiotherapy (aka World Confederation for Physical Therapy) (World Federation of Occupational Therapists, 2022; World Physiotherapy, 2022). These international organizations have elected delegates representing members from each country and can be a way for involvement on this global level. If there is interest in leadership opportunities outside of the delegate role, individuals are encouraged to reach out to their national delegates to match current initiatives. Projects often involve partnerships with international organizations such as the World Health Organization (WHO) or the International Society for Prosthetics and Orthotics (ISPO). You can also be involved in global leadership through participation in World PT Day or World Occupational Therapy Day advocacy and service activities. The world organizations provide information on their websites on participating and supporting these events.

Leadership Development Planning

Perhaps you have read this chapter so far and still question how to lead. This section offers you information to help guide your leadership development. Plotting the course for leadership is a continuous process. It begins now and may not have an endpoint. To start writing a leadership development plan or map, start where you are. There may be a natural tendency to wait until you learn more and can do more; however, engaging in leadership is often the best way to learn more and do more.

It is important to take the time to reflect upon what is important to you and what drives you to lead. One helpful strategy is to craft a personal mission and vision statement. Mission statements are a guiding force and serve as a reminder of your values, purpose, and who you are. Vision statements are forward-thinking and communicate the goal of where you want to go and how you want to be known in the future. These two statements then serve as a foundation for direct activities and actions that support your leadership development.

The University of Nebraska Office of Graduate Studies (2022) offers advice on creating a professional development plan. This advice may also contribute to your leadership development. First, mark where you are in your leadership development by reflecting on your current roles and responsibilities. Think about what has motivated and supported you to arrive at this point. You may reflect on how these roles and responsibilities connect or do not connect to your identities. Do not hesitate to approach doubts and vulnerabilities with curiosity. Consider your current knowledge and skills

Throughout the examples in this chapter, Carmen has had many encounters with leaders and leadership. Thinking about leadership identity, Carmen reflects on their leadership journey and goals and decides to plan leadership intentionally. See this example below for Carmen's leadership development plan.

- Mission Statement: To be an ethical leader in my everyday actions, live a balanced and mindful life, and make a difference.
- Vision Statement: To be a socially responsive leader who leverages connections and skills for the promotion of an inclusive profession capable of change
- Leadership Goal 1: Develop or join a committee that focuses on diversity, equity, and inclusion (DEI) initiatives in the workplace and community
  - Timeline: 2 years
  - Enabling Objectives:
    - Take a continuing education course on best practices in DEI
    - Discuss with supervisor interest in DEI work
    - Start or join a DEI centered journal or book club
- Leadership Goal 2: Serve in a supervisory/advanced practice role within my clinical setting
  - Timeline: 5 years
  - Enabling Objectives:
    - Apply for a leadership fellowship
    - Join a leadership community of practice
    - Connect with Jada to enter a formal mentoring relationship
    - Mentor and supervise students on clinicals/fieldwork
- Leadership Goal 3: Attain a leadership position within the state or national association
  - Timeline: 10 years
  - Enabling Objectives:
    - Volunteer for a lead role in the student association
    - Be an active member in a state and national association
    - Participate in state or national committees, taskforce, or ad hoc group

and those you would like to improve. Next, formulate meaningful goals with timelines that make sense to you. Determine feasible actions to facilitate your progress toward each goal. Document leadership planning and keep this a resource that you can readily and routinely access (Box 10.9).

Leading into the Future

Leadership is the ethical, mindful application of a person's identity, strengths, and values, guided by critical reflection and emotional intelligence, to engage followers in transformation within a context, such as a workplace, community, or society. The emergence of the knowledge worker has brought about a time of hyperchange, in which leadership is necessary for all. Leadership is not a static outcome; it is a continuous process. As an OT or PT who will be called to lead, intentional leadership development is critical. Building the capacity to lead requires courage, clarity, and curiosity.

Leadership has been studied from multiple angles, emphasizing traits, behaviors, situational variables, to social change responsibility. What is known now is that no single theory or approach can completely describe effective leadership. Pairing

components from theoretical approaches with your own leadership identity facilitates your capacity to lead in your profession.

There is an effort to build capacity for leadership within the OT and PT professions. There are opportunities at the local, state, national, and global levels—also opportunities via volunteering, elective positions, advocacy, leadership training programs, fellowships, and communities of practice. Students and practitioners who want to plot their leadership development journey can start with a leadership development plan that evolves as they build leadership capacity.

Capacity Building Resource List

Selected resources to learn more about the information in the chapter.

What Is Leadership

- Covey, S. R. (2013). The 7 habits of highly effective people: Powerful lessons in personal change (25th anniversary edition). Simon & Schuster.
- Kouzes, J. M., & Posner, B. Z. (2017). The leadership challenge (6th ed.). John Wiley & Sons.

Building Your Capacity for Leadership

- Brown, B. (2018). Dare to lead: Brave work, tough conversations, whole hearts. Vermilion.
- VIA Institute on Character. (2023). https://www.viacharacter.org/
- Gallup, Inc. (2023). The CliftonStrengths® Assessment: Find the report that's right for you. https://www.gallup.com/cliftonstrengths/en/253868/popular-cliftonstrengths-assessment-products.aspx
- Grenny, J., Patterson, K., McMillan, R., Switzler, A., & Gregory, E. (2021). Crucial Conversations: Tools for Talking When Stakes are High, Third Edition (3rd edition). McGraw Hill.
- Institute for Mindful Leadership. (2022). Institute for Mindful Leadership. https://instituteformindfulleadership.org/
- Johnson, C. (2021). Meeting the ethical challenges of leadership: Casting light or shadow (7th ed.). SAGE.

Leadership Approaches and Theories

- Northouse, P. G. (2022). Leadership: Theory and practice (9th ed.). SAGE.

Leadership In Action: Building Capacity of the Professions

- American Physical Therapy Association. (2022). APTA. https://www.apta.org/
- Join AOTA to Fuel Your Passion | AOTA. (2022). https://www.aota.org/

Leadership Development and Planning

- The Regents of the University of California. (2023). UC learning center: Professional development guide. https://training.ucsf.edu/professional-development-guide

References

Alsop, A., & Lloyd, C. (2002). The purpose and practicalities of postgraduate education. *British Journal of Occupational Therapy*, *65*(5), 245–251. https://doi.org/10.1177/030802260206500512.

American Occupational Therapy Association. (2021). *AOTA strategic framework*. https://www.aota.org/-/media/Corporate/Files/About AOTA/BOD/2021%20AOTA%20Strategic%20Framework.pdf.

American Occupational Therapy Association. (2022). *Get involved at AOTA*. https://www.aota.org/community/get-involved.

American Physical Therapy Association. (2022a). *APTA strategic plan 2022-2025*. https://www.apta.org/contentassets/14be4b91c1b94 da8a92dfb76fe041b99/apta-strategic-plan-2022-2025.pdf.

American Physical Therapy Association. (2022b). *LAMP leadership institute—HPA The catalyst*. https://www.aptahpa.org/page/LAMP.

Bass, B. M. (1985). *Leadership and performance beyond expectations*. Free Press.

Bass, B. M. (1995). The meaning of leadership. In J. T. Wren (Ed.), *Leaders companion: Insights on leadership through the ages* (pp. 37–38). Free Press.

Bass, B. M. (1999). Two decades of research and development in transformational leadership. *European Journal of Work and Organizational Psychology*, *8*(1), 9–32.

Blumenthal, D. M., Bernard, K., Bohnen, J., & Bohmer, R. (2012). Addressing the leadership gap in medicine: Residents' need for systematic leadership development training. *Academic Medicine: Journal of the Association of American Medical Colleges*, *87*(4), 513–522.

Boss, J. (2017). *How to build your leadership capacity*. Forbes. https://www.forbes.com/sites/jeffboss/2017/09/08/how-to-build-your-leadership-capacity/.

Bradberry, T. (2017, February 13). *Emotional intelligence: What it is and why you need it*. World Economic Forum. https://www.weforum.org/agenda/2017/02/why-you-need-emotional-intelligence/.

Braveman, B. (2022). *Leading & managing occupational therapy services: An evidence-based approach* (3rd ed.). F. A. Davis Company.

Brown, B. (2018). *Dare to lead: Brave work, tough conversations, whole hearts*. Vermilion.

Bunting, M. (2016). *The mindful leader: 7 practices for transforming your leadership, your organisation and your life* (1st ed.). Wiley.

Burns, J. M. (1978). *Leadership*. Harper & Row.

Burns, J. M. (1995a). The crisis of leadership. In J. T. Wren (Ed.), *Leaders companion: Insights on leadership through the ages* (pp. 8–10). Free Press.

Burns, J. M. (1995b). Transactional and transforming leadership. In J. T. Wren (Ed.), *Leaders companion: Insights on leadership through the ages* (pp. 100–101). Free Press.

Clapp-Smith, R., Hammond, M. M., Lester, G. V., & Palanski, M. (2019). Promoting identity development in leadership education: A multidomain approach to developing the whole leader. *Journal of Management Education*, *43*(1), 10–34.

Couris, J. D. (2020). Vulnerability: The secret to authentic leadership through the pandemic. *Journal of Healthcare Management*, *65*(4), 248–251. ABI/INFORM Collection; Research Library.

Couto, R. A. (1995a). Defining the citizen leader. In J. T. Wren (Ed.), *Leaders companion: Insights on leadership through the ages* (pp. 11–17). Free Press.

Couto, R. A. (1995b). The transformation of transforming leadership. In J. T. Wren (Ed.), *Leaders companion: Insights on leadership through the ages* (pp. 102–107). Free Press.

Covey, S. R. (2004). *The 8th habit: From effectiveness to greatness*. Free Press.

Drucker, P. (2000). *Managing knowledge means managing oneself* (No. 16; pp. 8–10). Leader to Leader.

Dugan, J. P. (2015). The measurement of socially responsible leadership: Considerations in establishing psychometric rigor. *ECPS - Educational Cultural and Psychological Studies*, *12*, 23–42.

Dugan, J. P. (2018). Critical perspectives on capacity-building for international leadership. *New Directions for Student Leadership*, *2018*(160), 31–39.

Embrey, D. G., Guthrie, M. R., White, O. R., & Dietz, J. (1996). Clinical decision making by experienced and inexperienced pediatric physical therapists for children with diplegic cerebral palsy. *Physical Therapy*, *76*(1), 20–33.

Eva, N., Robin, M., Sendjaya, S., van Dierendonck, D., & Liden, R. C. (2019). Servant leadership: A systematic review and call for future research. *The Leadership Quarterly*, *30*(1), 111–132.

Fields, J., Thompson, K., & Hawkins, J. (2015). Servant leadership: Teaching the helping professional. *The Journal of Leadership Education*, *14*(4), 92–105.

Foster, W. (1986). *Paradigms and promises: New approaches to educational administration*. Prometheus Books.

Garber, J. S., Madigan, E. A., Click, E. R., & Fitzpatrick, J. J. (2009). Attitudes towards collaboration and servant leadership among nurses, physicians and residents. *Journal of Interprofessional Care*, *23*(4), 331–340.

Gardner, J. W. (1995). The cry for leadership. In J. T. Wren (Ed.), *Leaders companion: Insights on leadership through the ages* (pp. 3–7). Free Press.

Gilliland, S., & Wainwright, S. F. (2017). Patterns of clinical reasoning in physical therapist students. *Physical Therapy*, *97*(5), 499–511.

Goleman, D. (1995). *Emotional intelligence: Why it can matter more than IQ*. Bantam Books.

Goleman, D., Boyatzis, R., Druskat, V., Davidson, R. J., Kohlrieser, G., McKee, A., Boell, M. M., Pitagorsky, G., Nevarez, M., Lippincott, M., Petry, A. F., Senge, P., Taylor, M., Gallo, A., & Fernandez-Araoz, C. (2017). *Building blocks of emotional intelligence: 12 leadership competency primers*. Key Step Media. https://www.keystepmedia.com/shop/12-leadership-competency-primers/#.YiDwBujMKUk.

Gorgens-Ekermans, G., & Roux, C. (2021). Revisiting the emotional intelligence and transformational leadership debate: Does emotional intelligence matter to effective leadership? *SA Journal of Human Resource Management*, *19*(2), e1–e13.

Gransberry, C. K. (2021). How emotional intelligence promotes leadership and management practices. *Public Organization Review*, *22*(4), 935–948.

Greenleaf, R. K. (1995). Servant leadership. In J. T. Wren (Ed.), *Leaders companion: Insights on leadership through the ages* (pp. 18–23). Free Press.

Greenleaf, R. K. (2002). *Servant leadership: A journey into the nature of legitimate power and greatness 25th anniversary edition* (3rd ed.). Paulist Press.

Groyberg, B., & Seligson, S. (2020, November 1). *Good leadership is an act of kindness—HBS working knowledge*. Working Knowledge: Business Research for Business Leaders. https://hbswk.hbs.edu/item/good-leadership-is-an-act-of-kindness.

Haslam, S. A., Steffens, N. K., Peters, K., Boyce, R. A., Mallett, C. J., & Fransen, K. (2017). A social identity approach to leadership development: The 5R program. *Journal of Personnel Psychology*, *16*(3), 113–124.

Heard, C. P. (2014). Choosing the path of leadership in occupational therapy. *The Open Journal of Occupational Therapy*, *2*(1). https://doi.org/10.15453/2168-6408.1055.

Hinojosa, J. (2007). Becoming innovators in an era of hyperchange. *American Journal of Occupational Therapy*, *61*(6), 629–637.

Huhn, K., Gilliland, S. J., Black, L. L., Wainwright, S. F., & Christensen, N. (2019). Clinical reasoning in physical therapy: A concept analysis. *Physical Therapy*, *99*(4), 440–456.

Jeanes, E. (2021). A meeting of mind(sets). Integrating the pedagogy and andragogy of mindsets for leadership development. *Thinking Skills and Creativity*, *39*, 100758.

Jensen, G. M., Gwyer, J., Shepard, K. F., & Hack, L. M. (2000). Expert practice in physical therapy. *Physical Therapy*, *80*(1), 28–43.

Jensen, G. M., Shepard, K. F., Gwyer, J., & Hack, L. M. (1992). Attribute dimensions that distinguish master and novice physical therapy clinicians in orthopedic settings. *Physical Therapy*, *72*(10), 711–722.

Jensen, G. M., Shepard, K., & Hack, L. (1990). The novice versus the experienced clinician: Insights into the work of the physical therapist. *Physical Therapy*, *70*, 314–323.

Jiménez-Picón, N., Romero-Martín, M., Ponce-Blandón, J. A., Ramirez-Baena, L., Palomo-Lara, J. C., & Gómez-Salgado, J. (2021). The relationship between mindfulness and emotional intelligence as a protective factor for healthcare professionals: Systematic review. *International Journal of Environmental Research and Public Health*, *18*(10), 5491.

Johnson, C. (2021). *Meeting the ethical challenges of leadership: Casting light or shadow* (7th ed.). SAGE.

Johnson, K. R., Park, S., & Chaudhuri, S. (2020). Mindfulness training in the workplace: Exploring its scope and outcomes. *European Journal of Training and Development*, *44*(4/5), 341–354.

Judge, T. A., Bono, J. E., Ilies, R., & Gerhardt, M. W. (2002). Personality and leadership: A qualitative and quantitative review. *Journal of Applied Psychology*, *87*(4), 765–780.

Kellerman, B. (2007, December 1). *What every leader needs to know about followers*. Harvard Business Review. https://hbr.org/2007/12/what-every-leader-needs-to-know-about-followers.

Kelley, R. (1988, November 1). *In praise of followers*. Harvard Business Review. https://hbr.org/1988/11/in-praise-of-followers.

Komives, S. R., & Wagner, W. (Eds.). (2016). *Leadership for a better world: Understanding the social change model of leadership development* (2nd ed.). Jossey-Bass.

Kotter, J. (1996). *Leading change*. Harvard Business Press.

Kouzes, J. M., & Posner, B. Z. (2017). *The leadership challenge* (6th ed.). John Wiley & Sons.

Lazarus, A. (2021). Impact of imposter syndrome on physicians' practice and leadership development. *The Journal of Medical Practice Management*, *37*(1), 367–372.

Lebrón, M. J., Stanley, C. L., Kim, A. J., & Thomas, K. H. (2017). The empowering role of profession-based student organizations in developing student leadership capacity. *New Directions for Student Leadership*, *2017*(155), 83–94.

Ledlow, G. R., & Stephens, J. H. (2018). *Leadership for health professionals: Theory, skills, and applications* (3rd ed.). Jones & Bartlett Learning.

Lee, M. (2014). Transformational leadership: Is it time for a recall? *International Journal of Management and Applied Research*, *1*(1), 17–29.

Levey, J., & Levey, M. (2019). Mindful leadership for personal and organisational resilience. *Clinical Radiology*, *74*(10), 739–745.

Liotta-Kleinfeld, L., Gibbs, D., Hachtel, Y., & Plummer, T. (2018). Applying the social change model of leadership to an entry-level occupational therapy doctorate program. *Journal of Occupational Therapy Education*, *2*(1). doi:10.26681/jote.2018.020107.

Machiavelli, N. (1914). Instructions on how to rule wisely. In *The Prince: Vol. XXXVI, Part 1*. P.F. Collier & Son. https://www.bartleby.com/36/1/.

McGowan, E., & K. Stokes, E. (2015). Leadership in the profession of physical therapy. *Physical Therapy Reviews*, *20*(2), 122–131.

Mezirow, J. (2003). Transformative learning as discourse. *Journal of Transformative Education*, *1*(1), 58–63.

Mindful Staff. (2017, January 11). *Jon Kabat-Zinn: Defining mindfulness—Mindful*. Mindful: Healthy Mind, Healthy Life. https://www.mindful.org/jon-kabat-zinn-defining-mindfulness/.

Moyers, P. A. (2007). A legacy of leadership: Achieving our centennial vision. *American Journal of Occupational Therapy*, *61*(6), 622–628.

Musolino, G. M., & Jensen, G. M. (2020). *Clinical reasoning and decision-making in physical therapy: Facilitation, assessment, and implementation*. SLACK.

Northouse, P. G. (2013). *Leadership: Theory and practice* (6th ed.). SAGE.

Northouse, P. G. (2022). *Leadership: Theory and practice* (9th ed.). SAGE.

Onyura, B., Crann, S., Tannenbaum, D., Whittaker, M. K., Murdoch, S., & Freeman, R. (2019). Is postgraduate leadership education a match for the wicked problems of health systems leadership? A critical systematic review. *Perspectives on Medical Education*, *8*(3), 133–142.

Padilla, A., Hogan, R., & Kaiser, R. B. (2007). The toxic triangle: Destructive leaders, susceptible followers, and conducive environments. *The Leadership Quarterly*, *18*(3), 176–194.

Quantz, R. A., Rogers, J., & Dantley, M. (1991). Rethinking transformative leadership: Toward democratic reform of schools. *Journal of Education*, *173*(3), 96–118.

Ramalingam, B., Nabarro, D., Oqubay, A., Carnall, D. R., & Wild, L. (2020, September 11). *5 principles to guide adaptive leadership*. Harvard Business Review. https://hbr.org/2020/09/5-principles-to-guide-adaptive-leadership.

Rasmussen-Barr, E., Savage, M., & Von Knorring, M. (2019). How does leadership manifest in the patient-therapist interaction among physiotherapists in primary health care? A qualitative study. *Physiotherapy Theory and Practice*, *35*(12), 1194–1201.

Recigno, T., Benham, S., & Breen-Franklin, A. (2020). Exploration of self-perceived leadership practices of entry-level doctoral students during the doctoral capstone experience. *Journal of Occupational Therapy Education (JOTE)*, *4*(1). https://doi.org/10.26681/jote.2020.040113.

Rupprecht, S., Falke, P., Kohls, N., Tamdjidi, C., Wittmann, M., & Kersemaekers, W. M. (2019). Mindful leader development: How leaders experience the effects of mindfulness training on leader capabilities. *Frontiers in Psychology*, *10*, 1081–1081.

Salovey, P., & Mayer, J. D. (1990). Emotional intelligence. *Imagination, Cognition and Personality*, *9*(3), 185–211.

Schyns, B., Kiefer, T., Kerschreiter, R., & Tymon, A. (2011). Teaching implicit leadership theories to develop leaders and leadership: How and why it can make a difference. *Academy of Management Learning & Education*, *10*(3), 397–408.

Scott, S., & Webber, C. F. (2008). Evidence-based leadership development: The 4L framework. *Journal of Educational Administration*, *46*(6), 762–776.

Sebelski, C. A., Green-Wilson, J., Zeigler, S., Clark, D., & Tschoepe, B. (2020). Leadership competencies for physical therapists: A Delphi determination. *Journal of Physical Therapy Education*, *34*(2), 96–104.

Shields, C. M. (2020). Transformative leadership. In C. M. Shields (Ed.), *Oxford research encyclopedia of education*. Oxford University Press.

Spark, A., & O'Connor, P. (2017, September 25). *Introverts think they won't like being leaders but they are capable*. The Conversation. http://theconversation.com/introverts-think-they-wont-like-being-leaders-but-they-are-capable-84371.

Stoffel, V. C. (2013). From heartfelt leadership to compassionate care. *American Journal of Occupational Therapy, 67*(6), 633–640.

Thacker, K. (2016). *The art of authenticity: Tools to become an authentic leader and your best self*. Wiley.

The Institute of Leadership and Management. (2022). *Leadership essentials: Critical reflection*. https://www.institutelm.com/learning/leadership-framework/ownership/critical-reflection/leadership-essentials-critical-reflection.html.

Thomas, Y., Seedhouse, D., Peutherer, V., & Loughlin, M. (2019). An empirical investigation into the role of values in occupational therapy decision-making. *The British Journal of Occupational Therapy, 82*(6), 357–366.

Torrez, M. A., & Rocco, M. L. (2015). Building critical capacities for leadership learning. *New Directions for Student Leadership, 2015*(145), 19–34.

University of Nebraska Office of Graduate Studies. (2022). *The individual professional development plan (IPDP): A career management tool*. Graduate Connections. https://www.unl.edu/gradstudies/connections/individual-professional-development-plan-ipdp-career-management-tool.

Vuyst, A. (2021, September 13). *Reframing the way we think about following the leader. Be like a tree*. Leadership PSYCH 485 Blog. https://sites.psu.edu/leadership/2021/09/13/reframing-the-way-we-think-about-following-the-leader-be-like-a-tree/.

Weiszbrod, T. (2020). Health care leader competencies and the relevance of emotional intelligence. *The Health Care Manager, 39*(4), 190–196.

Wenger-Trayner, E., & Wenger-Trayner, B. (2015). *Communities of practice a brief introduction*. https://wenger-trayner.com/wp-content/uploads/2015/04/07-Brief-introduction-to-communities-of-practice.pdf.

Winston, B. E., & Patterson, K. (2006). An integrative definition of leadership. *International Journal of Leadership Studies, 1*, 6–66.

World Federation of Occupational Therapists. (2022, May 17). WFOT. https://wfot.org.

World Physiotherapy. (2022). Home | World Physiotherapy. https://world.physio/node/232.

Zhang, L., Cao, T., & Wang, Y. (2018). The mediation role of leadership styles in integrated project collaboration: An emotional intelligence perspective. *International Journal of Project Management, 36*(2), 317–330.

11

Healthcare Management and Administration

SCOTT TRUSKOWSKI, PhD, OTR/L, ACUE;
and WILLIAM R. VANWYE, PT, DPT, PhD

LEARNING OBJECTIVES

After reading this chapter, you should be able to:

1. Describe the internal and external factors that influence the provision of therapy services.
2. Differentiate between the technical, people, and conceptual skills necessary to manage in a healthcare setting.
3. Explain the connections between an organization's strategic, budget, and marketing plans.
4. Refine each step in your organization's hiring processes, from job descriptions through orientation.
5. Apply the steps inherent to the therapy process to align personal and organizational goals.
6. Design a clear and consistent performance evaluation process.

CHAPTER OUTLINE

Introduction

Managing personnel in today's healthcare environment is challenging. Therapists who hold a managerial role are often expected to balance their time, energy, and resources to ensure appropriate staffing levels; meeting unit level expectations related to service provision; monthly and yearly budgeting; provision of quality services; as well as supervising other therapists (Koverman & Braveman, 2016a; Fisher, 2011). These management roles are commonly listed as planning, organizing, directing, and controlling (Braveman, 2016c). When describing each of these functions, it is important to consider the context in which each will be carried out. For example, organizing and directing a team of therapists will look vastly different and require more time when a manager oversees all pediatric therapy services in a large regional hospital system than when a private therapy clinic owner carries these responsibilities. The functions themselves will be similar, but the scope will be different by necessity.

Management has been described as the art and process of getting things done through and with people (Braveman, 2016c). Management can be construed as focused on outcomes. Supervision, a related element of management, is more process-driven and aligns with the directing function of management. Supervision (i.e., directing the work of others) includes training new employees, establishing agreed-upon professional goals, and assessing employee performance (Braveman, 2016c). It is relevant for allied health professionals who hold managerial or supervisory positions to recognize that occupational therapists (OTs), occupational therapy assistants, physical therapists (PTs), physical therapy assistants, and speech/language pathologists are independently licensed professionals. The goal is to align the therapist's personal and professional aims with the organization. In short, effective healthcare management strives to meet the goals and objectives of the organization as well as the personal and professional goals of the staff being managed. The remainder of this chapter will describe how each of the four management functions allows effective management of the professional staff in a healthcare organization, which is the most important and most expensive resource to be managed.

Factors That Influence Organizations

For clinicians to transition effectively into administrative positions, it is essential for therapy managers to broaden their focus toward an ongoing awareness and assessment of external and internal factors that influence the organization (Ledlow & Stephens, 2018).

External Environment

The external environment includes local, state, and national elements that must be monitored and assessed. Managers who understand the potential effects of various external factors are positioned to ensure the healthcare organization fulfills its mission while being nimble enough to respond to a changing environment and remain viable over time (Braveman & Phipps, 2016; Ledlow & Stephens, 2018).

Legislation

Federal and state legislation can profoundly influence service provision, billing, and reimbursement of therapy services and disciplinary scopes of practice. State practice acts include oversight and supervision requirements for occupational and physical therapy assistants and rehabilitation technicians. Managers must remain abreast of the frequency and types of supervision required to schedule the most cost-efficient staffing mix (Koverman & Braveman, 2016; Page, 2015). State regulatory boards routinely update the requirements for licensure. For example, in Michigan, initial and relicensure requirements for human trafficking, pain management, and implicit bias training have been added since 2017. Therapy managers can utilize these requirements to inform budgetary decisions regarding hosting training for therapy staff or providing continuing education funds to offset the cost of off-site training.

Finance Changes

Economic and healthcare finance changes are closely related to legislative effects on service provision. At the federal level, the Centers for Medicare and Medicaid Services (CMS) shifted from a volume-based focus to a more value-based model in post-acute care settings. Under the previous volume-based model, healthcare organizations were incentivized to employ more skilled practitioners, maximize the staff's productivity, and document/bill for as much patient care time as possible (American Occupational Therapy Association [AOTA], 2018). Skilled nursing facilities have shifted from providing and tracking minutes of service under Resource Utilization Groups (RUGs) to the Patient-Driven Payment Model (PDPM), which focuses on each patient's individualized needs, goals, and characteristics to determine the number of services required as well as the reimbursement for those services (CMS, 2021b). Home health organizations faced a similar shift with the patient-driven groupings model, which eliminates therapy use thresholds and redirects the service provision and reimbursement on patient characteristics (CMS, 2022). State legislation can have a similar, drastic effect. For example, in 2019, Michigan passed a major reform to the existing auto no-fault insurance law. This new legislation restricts the amount medical providers can charge insurance companies. After 1 year of being in effect, the Brain Injury Association of Michigan (BIAMI) has reported that over 1500 individuals with brain and spinal cord injuries were discharged by healthcare providers based on hitting the newly imposed reimbursement cap rather than by meeting therapy goals. The same survey estimates that over 3000 jobs have been eliminated, due to these discharges, as healthcare providers have had to adapt their staffing plans to remain solvent (BIAMI, 2021). These examples are provided to discuss briefly the ramifications of federal and state-level changes to the reimbursement policy.

Geographic Location

The healthcare organization's geographic location is a third distinct portion of the external environment. Managers can utilize information related to the city/county/regional: population density, socioeconomic status, and racial and ethnic mix to determine service priorities and marketing strategies. A second important element of the local geography is the presence or absence of other organizations that may compete for the same client base. Managers can assess the market saturation in a given area to determine if a planned location provides sufficient access to potential patients. In urban population centers, the local population is likely to support multiple providers of similar services. In more rural areas, a single outpatient therapy clinic may serve an entire county or grouping of counties.

Internal Environment

The internal environment of an organization includes the organization's physical plant, guiding documents, and workplace culture. These factors combine to influence day-to-day operations.

Physical Plant

The physical plant of an organization refers to the available infrastructure in which healthcare services are provided. These areas include treatment and storage spaces, the number and types of equipment available, décor, accessibility, and parking. The setup of the treatment spaces has two profound influences on therapy provision. First, the types of therapy sessions that can be planned are dictated by the physical environment. For example, an outpatient pediatric therapy clinic equipped with sensory equipment and a large play area designed to provide "heavy work" to young children may not be equipped to accept a referral of a 19-year-old transitioning from school-based therapy to learning rudimentary vocational skills. The second physical influence is on the number of clients scheduled at a given time. The number of mat tables, plinths, and private treatment rooms could limit the therapy schedule. Recently, the COVID-19 pandemic added to this limit through a combination of potential local spacing guidelines, added cleaning/sterilization procedures between clients, and apprehension of proximity and crowds on the part of some patients.

Guiding Documents: Mission, Vision, and Core Values

Another internal influence on everyday operations is the overall set of guiding documents specific to the organization. These documents include the organization's mission, vision, core values, and policies and procedures. Simply put, a company's mission statement describes the purpose for the organization exists; the mission serves as the *why* for a company. An organization's vision statement is more aspirational and addresses an ideal future for the clients or community the organization serves; the vision provides what is hoped to be accomplished (Braveman & Phipps, 2016). A

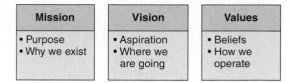

• **Fig. 11.1** Mission, Vision, and Core Values Overview

company's core values, or the guiding principles that guide behavior and decision-making, are closely related to the mission and vision. Core values articulate *how* an organization and its employees operate (Fig. 11.1).

Guiding Documents: Policies and Procedures

Administration refers to the use of systems for planning and organizing. Any business without systems is doomed to fail due to chaos, inconsistency, and confusion (Gerber, 2004). Systems are typically set up via policies and procedures. Policies and procedures serve numerous functions, including compliance, consistency, accountability, orientation, and safety (Page, 2015).

Policies and procedures are frequently housed together in a single policy and procedure manual. Like many other aspects of healthcare administration, the size and scope of a policy and procedure manual vary on the size and nature of the organization itself. A large, multi-site organization that maintains accreditation through The Joint Commission will have a much larger manual than an individually owned outpatient clinic. Policies can be thought of as the rules that frame expectations for employee actions; they provide information about what to do in a given situation (Braveman, 2016c; Page, 2015). Procedures provide the particular steps used to implement the related policy; procedures tell the employees how that action is carried out within the organization. Policy and procedure manuals should utilize consistent language across policies and be written so that the important details and steps are understandable. A policy and procedure manual has the most value and utility when it is: accessible to employees, updated, and focused on expectations rather than negative examples (Page, 2015). While there is no universal format for policies and procedures, the following headings are commonly included:

- Title or name of the policy
- Dates for implementation and revision
- Policy
  - Purpose: why the policy exists
  - Scope: why the policy applies within the organization
  - Definitions
- Procedures
  - Person(s) responsible
  - Materials needed
- Approvals: names or signatures

Other Administrative Documents

Additional documents that help with administrative processes include bylaws, clinical practice guidelines, and protocols.

Bylaws set up the legal framework of a business. Clinical practice guidelines, also known as pathways, help clinicians with *deciding*. In contrast, protocols are detailed plans about *doing* (Page, 2015).

Organizational Culture

The next element of the internal environment is the organizational culture. Although the policy and procedure manual provides written expectations, the organizational culture influences how things are carried out. According to Page, culture is "how we do things around here" (2015, p. 32). Workplace culture can be very nuanced and involves much more than an organization describing its culture as a family. An integral element of workplace culture is understanding where knowledge, power, or decision-making authority lies within an organization. For some scenarios, such as requesting reimbursement for a continuing education course, the decision-making authority may be laid out in a policy statement. At the same time, other situations have an unwritten go-to person that is always included in a discussion or decision. The second aspect of organizational culture is the layered social structure of the company, also referred to as office politics. A non-exhaustive list of some of the layers that make up the social fabric of an organization includes which groups eat lunch or take breaks together, who maintains a social relationship outside of the work setting, and forms of communication that exist between employees and those in administrative roles (Page, 2015). The third characteristic of an organization's culture is the level of acceptance of the change. Some organizations have existed and operated similarly for years; others strive to be at the forefront of service delivery and actively seek new opportunities. Each mindset can become hard-wired into the culture and ultimately shape individual and collective responses to external presses for change.

Organizational Structure

The overall organizational structure is the last element of the internal environment discussed here. The size and scope of the organization have a profound effect on the reporting relationships and whether the institution has flattened communication and decision making or if it functions with bureaucratic layers. The private practice would be more likely to have a single person functioning as the primary administrator while available to all employees. A large regional healthcare system that functions as a Level I trauma unit would be more apt to have different teams or units, each with its team lead or therapy supervisor, as well as additional levels of administration that have reporting relationships up the organizational chart that extend to the C-suite (e.g., CEO, CFO, COO) (Fig. 11.2). The scale of the organizational structure affects two primary elements—geography and availability. The geography relates to the physical plant and the organizational chart; the location of manager and supervisor offices may have those with decision-making authority far removed from day-to-day therapy provision. The availability piece is more about the management style a person uses. Availability can be directly observable in the form of regular and meaningful engagement with individual members of the team, having a clearly articulated open-door policy, and facilitating group discussions to share ideas and problem-solving situations.

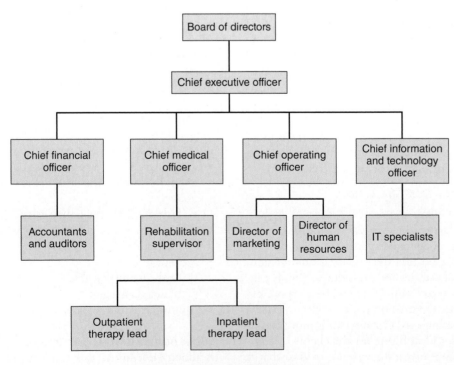

• **Fig. 11.2** Sample Organizational Chart

Becoming a Rehabilitation Manager

PTs and OTs are trained as clinicians and typically spend their initial years honing technical skills to treat clients better. This training is typically accomplished by participating in continuing education courses, acquiring specialist credentials, or understanding current evidence surrounding a particular treatment strategy. Initially, therapists may not anticipate taking on a management or supervisory role. However, there are considerable similarities between patient care management and healthcare management. Thus it is not uncommon for a successful clinician to be promoted into managerial and supervisory roles within the organization.

Common initial roles for clinicians include using their clinical degrees and experience to become program coordinators or frontline supervisors (Page, 2015). Often, these individuals work a dual role with management responsibilities while continuing patient care. Individuals may move into mid-level managerial roles and away from direct patient care. Lastly, therapists may move into executive positions. These higher-level positions may require more advanced training, such as an advanced degree (e.g., Master of Business Administration [MBA], Master of Healthcare [MHA]) or certification. Larger organizations often have in-house training, tuition deferment, and structured mentorship to encourage growth within the organization.

Managerial Skills

A manager's skills will vary based on their work setting and management category. Blanchard and Bowles (2001) described three basic skills that managers must possess: technical, human, and conceptual. These skills can be imagined on a sliding scale, with certain managers requiring higher levels of each.

Technical Skills

Technical skills include the specific abilities necessary to provide rehabilitation services. PTs and OTs acquire these skills through education, continuing education, reviewing current research or evidence, and treating clients. A rehabilitation professional then implements this skill with clients. The technical skill also includes understanding billing practices, development, execution of a plan of care, educating clients, and delegating appropriate tasks to support staff. Technical skill is effectively evaluating and treating a client to meet their needs.

Human Skills

Human or "soft" skills are concerned with the ability to interact effectively with other individuals (Fig. 11.3). PTs and OTs exhibit human skills when interacting with patients and colleagues by effectively communicating and

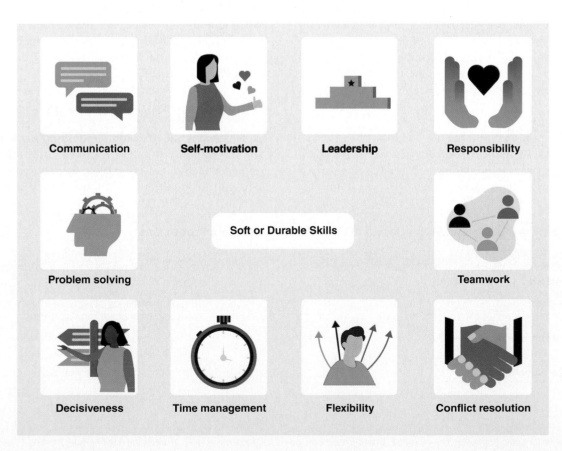

• **Fig. 11.3** Soft skills, now referred to as durable skills, are personal attributes that enable someone to interact effectively and harmoniously with others.

discussing client care. Managers utilize human skills when interacting with the employees they manage. Understanding what motivates employees and communicating job roles, responsibilities, and expectations are critical to the organization's success.

Conceptual Skills

Conceptual skills are considered higher-level skills required by managers. Understanding the goals of an organization, realizing growth opportunities, and carrying out necessary plans all require a conceptual framework of the organization and its landscape. Conceptual skill includes having a broader knowledge base about the bigger picture of the organization to meet the needs of their clients more effectively. Implementing a new program or offering a new service takes planning, knowledge, and consideration from all stakeholders. Success requires the conceptual skill of the manager.

Management Skills in Action

Generally, a higher-level manager requires more conceptual skills, less technical skills, and vice versa. For example, PT or OT team leads will work with clients, which requires a higher level of technical skill. Because a team lead position is not typically making large decisions about implementing a new service line to the organization, they do not require higher levels of conceptual skill. In contrast, a top-level manager is considering adding home care services to their organization. This manager must have more conceptual skills to implement this service effectively. Although they require some general understanding of providing home-care services (technical skills), this is less important. Higher-level managers rely on middle, or first-line managers to ensure the services are delivered effectively.

Managerial Styles

Over the years, many management styles have categorized different approaches to overseeing and guiding an organization or a team of individuals. A manager may utilize one style for all duties or different styles depending on their circumstances. Common management styles are charismatic, consultative, delegating, persuasive, transactional, and transformational (Northouse, 2022).

A charismatic manager utilizes their personality to inspire others. This type of manager requires excellent communication ability and interpersonal skills. A consultative manager readily receives input from employees before deciding. A delegating manager identifies employees' strengths and assigns tasks that fit their skill set. A persuasive manager uses their ability to convince employees that the predetermined course of action is the most appropriate. A transactional manager uses a reward system (i.e., quid pro quo). If an employee follows directions initiated by the manager, the manager may offer increased pay or a bonus. A transformational manager works to develop the culture of the business by focusing on staff/employee development, such as offering continuing education or opportunities for development.

Like leadership, there is not one style that fits each situation. There are pros and cons to each. In a situation where a quick decision must be made, a persuasive style may be more effective. In other situations, employees may value being part of the decision-making, such as in a consultative style. Other times employees are motivated by a reward system used by a transactional manager. Effective managers adjust styles accordingly. The Managerial Grid, known today as the Leadership Grid, is a manager or leadership behavior model with five styles based on the leader's concern for production and people (Ledlow & Stephens, 2018; Northouse, 2022). These five styles reveal that priorities guide behavior (Table 11.1). Lastly, it is important to recognize and avoid toxic managers (Table 11.2) (Northouse, 2022; Padilla et al., 2007).

Primary Functions of Managers

Understanding the roles and responsibilities of a rehabilitation manager and the skills necessary to be effective is essential. A manager is responsible for developing, carrying out, and accomplishing a healthcare organization's goals.

TABLE 11.1	The Five Managerial Styles Based on Concern for People and Production		
Style	**Concern for People**	**Concern for Production**	**Overview**
Impoverished	Low	Low	Apathetic, expecting minimum effort
Country-club	High	Low	People pleaser, creating a friendly environment with minimal concern for production
Middle of the road	Average	Average	Strikes a balance, seeking moderate results with satisfactory relationships
Authority-compliance	Low	High	Controlling, demanding, and lacking compassion
Team	High	High	Utilizes an optimal balance of developing relationships and achieving results

From Blake, R. R., & McCanse, A. A. (1991). *Leadership dilemmas—grid solutions*. Gulf Pub. Co; Blake, R. R., & Mouton, J. S. (1964). *The managerial grid: Key orientations for achieving production through people*. Gulf Pub. Co; Northouse, P. G. (2022). *Leadership: Theory and practice* (9th ed.). SAGE.

TABLE 11.2	**Characteristics and Behaviors of Toxic Managers**
Narcissistic or self-consumed	Lacking empathy, preoccupied with themselves
Power-hungry	Overly ambitious with a strong drive for power
Information hoarding	Ensuring all communication flows through them
Ambiguity	Creating an environment to maintain intellectual superiority via unclear expectations and instructions
Inconsistent or erratic behavior	Allowing behaviors in some instances but not others Allowing behaviors for certain subordinates but not for others
Indifferent or exploitive	Lacking concern for employees' problems or using their troubles against them
Lead by fear	Using positional power through threats and intimidation
Lack integrity	Untrustworthy, lack a moral compass

From Northouse, P. G. (2022). *Leadership: Theory and practice* (9th ed.). SAGE; Padilla, A., Hogan, R., & Kaiser, R. B. (2007). The toxic triangle: Destructive leaders, susceptible followers, and conducive environments. *The Leadership Quarterly, 18*(3), 176–194.

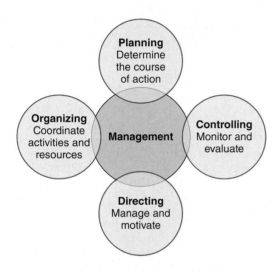

• **Fig. 11.4** Management Functions

Taking on the responsibility of a manager can be daunting. Keeping in mind the management skills discussed here, we can now shift attention to the more specific roles and responsibilities that a therapy manager holds. Management can include aspects of *planning, organizing, directing, and controlling*; the following section of this chapter will further explore each of these (Fig. 11.4).

Planning

Planning as an overarching management process includes identifying organizational aspirations and tangible goals, understanding the financial implications related to the healthcare organization, and developing strategies to market the business to potential clients and referral sources effectively.

Strategic Planning

Strategic planning is the intentional process undertaken by organizations to identify current operational capacity and envision a potential future (Page, 2015). This review is

of the current state with an eye on the future, allowing organizations to remain relevant to their stakeholders (Commission for the Accreditation of Rehabilitation Facilities [CARF], 2022). The strategic planning process has been incorporated into accreditation standards for clinical settings (CARF, 2022) and educational programs (Accreditation Council for Occupational Therapy Education [ACOTE], 2022; APTA, 2022).

An organization's strategic plan provides a series of connected stages that, when carried through to completion, can help the organization fulfill its stated mission. The stages of a fully articulated strategic plan include long-term goals, short-term objectives, tangible action steps directed to achieving the short and long-term goals, and a specific person responsible for each action step (Page, 2015). Multiple processes can be followed to facilitate the development of a strategic plan (Fig. 11.5). Two common healthcare organizations include a SWOT analysis (Fig. 11.6), which explores Strengths, Weaknesses, Opportunities, and Threats, and a

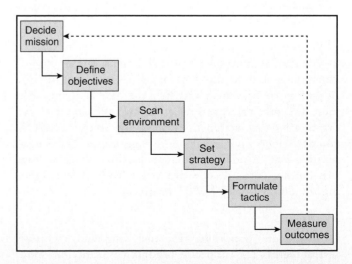

• **Fig. 11.5** Strategic Planning Example. (From https://upload.wikimedia.org/wikipedia/commons/2/2f/Strategic-Planning-Cycle.png)

Swot Analysis

Internal		External	
Strengths	Weaknesses	Opportunities	Threats

• **Fig. 11.6** A SWOT analysis can help managers understand their organization's advantages, disadvantages, struggles, and areas for improvement. (From https://commons.wikimedia.org/w/index.php?curid=31368987)

TABLE 11.3 Common Metrics

Capacity	Expected number of patients or units per day e.g., • 12 patients/clients per day • 25 units billed per day
Units/visit	Number billable units a therapist bills per patient visit
Cancel/no show rate	Number of scheduled patients that did not keep their appointments
Full-time equivalent (FTE)	Employees' scheduled hours divided by the hours they worked that week e.g., • Scheduled 40 hours, worked 40 hours = 1 FTE • Scheduled 40 hours, worked 20 hours = 0.5 FTE
Variance reports	Budget versus what was spent
Volume-related reports	Number of sales in a period
Benchmarking	Process of comparing business processes and performance metrics to others in the industry

SOAR analysis, which delves into Strengths, Opportunities, Aspirations, and Results (Braveman, 2016c; Page, 2015). According to Braveman (2016c), the SOAR approach is more strengths-based and seeks to build off aspects of the organization that are functioning at a high level; the SWOT approach offers a potentially more realistic view of the organization that includes areas that are lacking, as well as those that are not currently effective. See Chapter 14 for more information regarding SWOT analysis.

Financials

Managers are responsible for reviewing and reporting several metrics (e.g., capacity, productivity, cancel/no-show rates) (Table 11.3). These metrics are essential for numerous business matters, including hiring, employee performance,

and assessing marketing efforts. Financials assist with adjustments to meet strategic goals.

Billing practices and oversight of the rehabilitation services budget fluctuate based on the organization's size. Large organizations often employ professionals with specific skills in accounting and finance and possibly a legal team to ensure success in being financially stable. In these organizations, a top-level manager may need to review and manage a large budget, while a frontline manager may focus on billing practices and reimbursement for services rendered. An owner and manager of a private practice manager may be responsible for overseeing all financial aspects of the business. At a given point in time, an organization's financial stability contains *assets, liabilities,* and the determination of *net worth*. Financial statements such as pro forma, profit

<table>
<tr><td rowspan="1">TABLE 11.4</td><td>Financial Statements</td></tr>
</table>

Pro forma	• Used for projections, forecasting, predicting, and budgeting
Profit and loss	• Also known as Income Statement • Summarizes a company's revenues and expenses during a specific period (e.g., monthly, quarterly, and yearly)
Balance sheet	• Tracks profits and losses from the time the business started (or was bought) until the day it was sold • Reports overall assets, liabilities, and shareholders' equity

and loss statements, and balance sheets are essential for forecasting and monitoring financial stability (Table 11.4).

Assets

As a company grows, it will typically accumulate assets. Assets are items that have value. Purchased equipment or owned buildings are common examples of assets of a rehabilitation facility. Managers may need to decide on purchasing versus renting equipment and space, seeing that all assets depreciate as they age and purchased equipment requires maintenance and replacement. A cost-benefit analysis can be implemented when making this decision. Calculate the cost to purchase and maintain a piece of equipment minus the predicted depreciation and then add the predicted investment return. Comparing this figure to the cost-benefit of renting the equipment will provide a clearer answer.

Liabilities

Liabilities do not have value; they are outstanding expenses for items or equipment. Think of a company that purchases a large piece of state-of-the-art equipment. The upfront cost is, perhaps, $100,000. Imagine that the company must take out a loan to purchase this item. Therefore the new piece of equipment begins its shelf life as a liability of $100,000. Eventually, the equipment will result in increased revenue and be paid off. Despite depreciation, it will then become an asset. Liabilities can be thought of as outstanding debts.

Net Worth

Net worth is a simple way of looking at a company's financial position at one point in time. *Net worth* is total assets minus total liabilities. A manager may oversee the cost of conducting business in rehabilitation. How much does it cost to provide skilled rehabilitation services for clients? Before answering this question, we must also consider how much money is made by providing services, typically from reimbursement from insurance companies.

More specifically, for every patient that comes through the door, a manager should know how much money it costs to provide services while considering how much therapy revenue the client is likely to bring in. These figures will provide an idea of the cost per visit and the expected revenue per visit. When receiving reimbursement from insurance companies, the money received for services rendered cannot be determined solely by the business. A rehabilitation facility often develops a contract with an insurance company with a determined amount that they will receive for each Common Procedural Terminology (CPT) code. This process is typical for outpatient billing to private insurance companies. Federal insurance programs often set prices that are not negotiable. Each year, Medicare employs actuaries who review historical claims paid to companies to set what they believe is an appropriate amount of money to provide for rendering those services (i.e., fee-schedule). The specifics for each rehabilitation setting and type of insurance are beyond the scope of this chapter (see Chapters 13, 15–19).

Costs

There are two major categories of costs: *direct and indirect.* Direct costs are expenses that are directly related to providing services. Some examples are the salaries or wages of the personnel who provide care, equipment, and necessary supplies. There is a linear relationship between the number of clients and the necessary direct costs—the more clients are being treated, the more direct costs the business will incur. Indirect costs are expenses that are not directly related to providing care. Rent, utilities, maintenance of equipment, and clerical supplies are examples. Indirect costs do not vary based on the number of clients being served.

Costs can be further classified as being *fixed or variable.* A fixed cost such as rent does not change. A company will sign a lease for a specific amount over a determined period. In contrast, a variable cost such as clinic supplies fluctuates based on the number of clients. If more clients are coming into the facility, there will be a need for more supplies. Sometimes, a cost can be a combination of both (*semi-fixed*). Consider a wage paid to a physical or occupational therapy assistant. The hours and wages are probably fixed; however, if patient volume decreases, their hours could be decreased.

Revenue

Money coming into a business from services rendered or goods sold is known as revenue. Rehabilitation professionals provide a valuable service to their clients. Revenue typically comes from the services provided via reimbursement from insurance companies. In the outpatient setting, it is becoming more common for clinics to offer cash-based services without contracting with insurance companies. Clients will pay cash for the rehabilitation services that they receive. Additionally, a business may offer items for sale that generate additional revenue.

Close attention must be paid to the specific contracts that providers enter into with insurance companies. The variety of contracts and clients from each insurer is known as a *payor mix*. A manager should understand how many clients they serve from each insurance company and their contracted reimbursement to determine the revenue each client brings in.

Profit Margin

The goal of most businesses is to make a profit. Once cost and revenue is understood, a profit margin can be calculated. The profit margin is a ratio of a company's profit and is calculated by revenue minus expenses and then divided by the revenue.

Budget

A budget is an estimated projection of revenue and expenses over time. It is a way to monitor and predict the financial solvency of the organization and assists in making decisions. It can simply be a spreadsheet with revenue and all expenses that a business or department may incur. At the end of the fiscal or calendar year, a manager may review the revenue and expenses and, based on the results, develop a budget for the next year. If a company is very profitable, decisions can be made about investing in the organization, offering raises, buying additional equipment, and adding a service line. Conversely, if the company cannot make a profit, the manager may need to decrease expenses, adjust employee hours, or make other cuts in preparation for next year.

Marketing

Marketing is an important element of the managerial function of planning. Regardless of the size of the healthcare organization, therapy managers will have some level of responsibility for marketing their services. This section will address some of the more common marketing skills required of therapy managers. Chapter 14 of this book will delve more fully into specific marketing tasks.

Therapy managers must understand their organization's target market; those who benefit from or pay for therapy services (Braveman, 2016b). Effective managers explicitly attempt to determine what will satisfy their target market such as new lines of service, convenient scheduling options for patients and families, or patient outcomes reported in a particular format for third-party payers. Therapy managers also need to be aware of potential competitors within a geographic area in order to answer as many of the following questions as possible:

- What similar providers exist within a given city, county, or region of a state?
- Where are they located? Does the local population support multiple clinics providing similar services?
- What specific service lines do they offer?
- In what ways do their patient outcomes compare? What are their funding sources?

The third managerial marketing skill is benchmarking or comparing current internal processes and outcomes against identified best practices of similar companies (Page, 2015). Benchmarking can be done with direct local competitors or organizations offering similar services in a comparable geographic location. Therapy managers may also need to develop an active social media presence to share news, patient success stories, and clinic event details with those in the target market. Managers in large healthcare organizations may be assisted by a marketing team employed by the organization, while smaller clinic managers/owners may be solely responsible for this form of marketing.

Organizing

The managerial function of organizing is predicated on developing working relationships, reporting relationships, and lines of service that most efficiently meet the needs of those receiving skilled services (Braveman, 2016c). Depending on the organization's size, the role of the therapy manager can fluctuate widely. For example, a rehabilitation supervisor at a Level 1 trauma center may be responsible for staffing and scheduling therapy services across the intensive care unit (ICU), acute care floors, long-term acute care (LTAC), and inpatient rehabilitation units of the hospital system. Organizations like this probably include additional administrative roles and responsibilities within each unit, with the overall authority for organizing, or reorganizing, resting with higher-level management. Therapists who open their practice will find that, by necessity, they have a more hands-on role in organizing the staff mix and reporting relationships within the business.

Staffing

Staffing can be thought of as the intentional process of identifying that the right (and best) people are positioned to complete those tasks essential for the organization (Braveman, 2016c). Staffing is a process aimed at ensuring the fit among the people; the daily, weekly, and monthly tasks that need to be completed; and the workgroup or organization as a whole. Law et al. (1996) utilized similar terms of person, environment, and occupation in designing a model of practice (PEO) that allows therapists to account for and include all three areas throughout the therapy process.

Therapy managers and administrators can use the PEO mindset throughout the staffing process to best position the organization's human resources for success. Some may read the heading of this section and the preceding sentence and think, "that is HR's job," meaning the human resources department of an organization. HR will play a role in staffing within large healthcare organizations; however, all therapy managers and administrators should have a baseline knowledge of each area.

Human Resources

Organizing and staffing may be the most important function of human resource management. Across all industries, wage and salary costs accounted for nearly 70% of employer expenses as recently as 2021 (United States Department of Labor, 2022). While hoping to avoid a cliché, this financial outlay makes the people within an organization the most valuable resource. The aim is to identify who is the best fit for the organization, the daily/weekly/monthly tasks that need to be completed (staffing), how each position in the company fits within the organizational structure (organizing), and how each of these steps contributes to the fulfillment of the organization's strategic plan.

Staffing Plan

Therapy managers must clearly understand the organization's service provision, client base, referral sources, and anticipated patient volume to develop an effective staffing plan (Braveman, 2016c). Staffing plans act as a general guideline for managers that identifies a projected roster of therapists, therapy assistants, and aides that will enable the organization to meet the needs of its client base as well as the financial goals of the organization.

A staffing plan enables a therapy manager to determine the most cost-effective way of providing skilled therapy services. The skill mix, or the number of therapists, therapy assistants, and therapy aides, is ultimately determined by the therapy manager but can be influenced by several factors (Braveman, 2016c). State rules or practice acts may dictate the ratio of therapy assistants that an OT or a PT may supervise. Frequent reimbursement practices by third-party payor sources can play a critical role in hiring plans. Therapists who prefer a routine, hands-on role with patients on their caseload may mitigate the potential role of a therapy assistant (Page, 2015).

Large-scale shifts in healthcare can also change an organization's staffing plan. An example of this change would be the 2019 shift in skilled nursing facilities from RUG levels to the PDPM. This shift in practice from volume billing to a more value-based model that reimburses positive patient outcomes at a higher level. Two approaches to the PDPM shift could be: to reduce the number of therapy staff and provide the same type of care as in the past to reduce labor costs or to increase the number of therapists and therapy assistants with the intent to provide more individualized therapy that is not specifically tied to minutes of therapy in hopes of improving patient (and facility) outcomes.

By necessity, staffing plans are highly individualized to each practice setting. The staffing plan will probably be relatively stable in established practice settings such as an inpatient rehabilitation unit. There may be periodic fluctuations in therapy staffing needs based on patient census, but when viewed over time, there will be an anticipated turnover of individual staff members, but the number of therapy staff positions remains unchanged. Owners of private therapy clinics and managers of new areas of service provision are likely to find staffing plans to be more of a routine area of focus. These managers may begin as the sole clinical staff member and utilize outcomes such as the revenue generated and the volume of billable time as indicators that the staffing level needs to change. As the patient volume reaches a critical mass, the manager has to make calculated decisions about whom to add to the therapy team and when. Managers need to consider therapist wages/salary expectations, the cost of benefits associated with a position, and whether the hiring is being done to address the current volume of patients or with a projected eye on the future volume.

The most flexible hire would be to bring one or more contingent or "pro re nata" (PRN) therapists into the fold. These nonpermanent roles allow the manager to utilize them as needed without immediately adding a full salary and benefits package. There are downsides to utilizing PRN staff, including hourly wages that tend to be higher than full-time members of the organization and the likelihood that the PRN role is a second position, meaning the organization will be second priority to the person's more regular work role. Managers who opt for or require a more recurring type of position must decide between adding a half-time or full-time position. Half-time positions tend to either not offer or offer a reduced benefits package. Full-time positions will come with the increased costs associated with wages and benefits but also increased continuity and communication with staff and patients.

Job Descriptions

Once the organizational staffing plan is clarified, the next step is to develop or refine the job descriptions (Fig. 11.7) for each position within the staffing plan. Job descriptions:
- Identify the work tasks, responsibilities, and performance expectations.
- Include the qualifications aligned with each position. These can include education, certification(s), and licensure.
- Form the basis for performance evaluation (Koverman & Braveman, 2016; Page, 2015).

Similar to the therapy manager's input on organizing, the healthcare administrator's level of input on the content of job descriptions will vary based on the type of organization. The owner or operating manager of a small private practice will have a high degree of autonomy in determining each job description; by contrast, managers in large healthcare entities are likely to utilize more standardized job descriptions (Munoz et al., 2017). Regardless of their origins, thorough job descriptions will include the job title, Fair Labor Standards Act (FLSA) status, reporting relationship(s), an overview of the available position, essential functions such

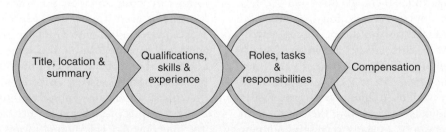

• **Fig. 11.7** Job Description Components. (Courtesy Bold Limited.)

as knowledge, skills, and abilities required for the position, and qualifications (Page, 2015).

A therapy manager may utilize the job description to identify experiences or certifications to help the organization meet the current or projected case-mix needs. For example, consider a manager who seeks to replace an OT with 15 years of pediatric experience. In addition to their experience, they held multiple specialty certifications, including Ayres Sensory Integration (ASI) and a Board Certification in Pediatrics (BC-P) through the American Occupational Therapy Association. Although it is unlikely that this administrator will successfully hire a single therapist with all the same experiences and expertise, the job description could be amended to include a statement that "Preference will be given for candidates with either an ASI certification or BC-P credential." In this example, the manager is seeking to replace a therapist (P) who was a good fit with the organization (E) and was competent in a wide range of therapy skills and tasks (O). During the hiring phase, managers must carefully review the candidate pool to determine who will best fit the organization—a therapist with experience and the desired certifications or one with less experience who is amenable to additional training.

Recruitment

Organizations with up-to-date staffing plans and job descriptions are positioned for recruitment success (Page, 2015). The clarity in these two areas helps therapy managers understand who will help the organization's PEO fit. The recruitment process has changed dramatically since the turn of the millennium; with four generations making up the healthcare workforce, effective and inclusive recruitment strategies are warranted to help organizations identify the best fit for their current staffing needs.

Managers and administrators entering the hiring process must balance the immediacy of filling the position with patience to find the right person to fit the organization. The recruitment process can be exciting, but it also can be expensive; every week or month that a position remains unfilled leads to the ongoing cost of advertising coupled with a reduction of reimbursement based on staffing shortages to meet patient needs. Posting a Help Wanted sign or a position announcement in the local newspaper's classified section are strategies of a bygone era. A variety of internet-based recruitment options are available to managers, including hiring websites such as Monster.com and Indeed.com; job postings through professional organizations such as the American Occupational Therapy Association (AOTA) or American Physical Therapy Association (APTA); local and regional news sites such as the author's home state of Michigan, would be Mlive.com; advertising on social media platforms; as well as an organization's website.

Depending on the candidate pool the organization is hoping to attract, various offline recruitment tactics can be employed simultaneously. Having the organization represented at job fairs can be a means to recruit both new employees and some experienced therapists who may have shifted away from full-time employment. Therapists who are members of the Baby Boomer generation may no longer want, or need, to work full-time but do want to maintain their role as a clinician. While staffing in all industries has been affected by the COVID-19 pandemic, healthcare staffing among Baby Boomer practitioners has been declining since 2010 (Corporate Screening, 2022). Additional offline recruitment strategies can include maintaining regular connections with local and regional programs that graduate new therapists yearly; most academic programs also have alum email lists or social media pages that allow job postings to reach a combination of new graduates and experienced therapists. More robust strategies to connect with potential candidates can include having members of the therapy team act as guest speakers or adjunct faculty for these academic programs, hosting groups of students for observation hours or as part of a structured lab, and routinely hosting student fieldwork or clinical education placements (Page, 2015).

Hiring

Once the organization has identified its optimal staffing plan, updated the relevant job descriptions, and formally recruited qualified candidates, the focus shifts to the hiring process. Assuming that the recruitment strategies have been effective, the first step in the hiring process is to screen applicants to ensure they meet the organization's posted criteria for the position.

The screening process can be valuable as each candidate brought in for an interview means time for the hiring manager and potentially for other team members to talk with the candidate. Some baseline criteria may include a candidate's licensure status or eligibility for state licensure; the requisite experience or entry-level degree that is posted for the position; and the ability to demonstrate any population-specific competencies (e.g., sensory integration training, proficiency with physical agent modalities, or training in the Mckenzie Method). The applicants who pass the screening process becomes eligible for the next phase of the hiring process—interviewing.

Depending on the number of candidates to interview, scheduling an initial phone or videoconference interview may be worthwhile to narrow the field before scheduling face-to-face interviews. A candidate's ability to navigate a virtual meeting can be a telling indicator of their flexibility and problem-solving and, in some practice settings their ability to conduct teletherapy sessions. With multiple platforms to choose from, such as Zoom, FaceTime, Google Meets, Microsoft Teams, or GoToMeeting, a hiring manager can meet in real time with potential candidates for little additional expense. During this stage of the hiring process, questions should focus on ensuring that the applicant can meet the position's essential functions (Page, 2015).

With the candidate pool sorted into several interviewees, the next step is preparation for the face-to-face interviews. The interview day is an initial means for the applicants to learn more about the organization from the hiring manager and the current staff. The extent of staff involvement in the interview process can range from brief introductions during a tour of the therapy space to scheduling a block of time for current staff members to meet with the candidates. Therapy managers should go into each interview to ensure the values and skills of the candidate are aligned with the organization's mission, vision, and values (Page, 2015) and that the candidate will be a good fit within the organizational culture (Braveman, 2016c).

These goals can seem daunting; however, with the right preparation, the interview process can simultaneously be objective and include input from multiple therapy team members. Page (2015) recommends that managers determine what qualities and skills they are looking for in new hires and plan to gather that information through the interview. This process includes asking the other therapy team members what they are looking for in the new hire and collating the responses into the list of interview questions. The interview questions should be open-ended or scenario-based to allow the manager to determine each candidate's attributes (Braveman, 2016c). This approach is similar to qualitative research interviews, where each candidate answers the same questions from the manager's interview guide, with follow-up inquiries tailored to the individual responses (Pedersen et al., 2016).

The questions that are not asked are equally as crucial as the questions posed to the candidates. The United States Equal Employment Opportunity Commission (EEOC) enforces employment laws that make it illegal to discriminate against someone based upon their race, color, religion, sex (inclusive of gender, gender identity, sexual orientation, and pregnancy status), national origin, age (40 years and older), disability status, or genetic information (United States EEOC, 2022). In larger healthcare institutions with a human resources department, an employment specialist can answer questions for new managers and those with experience during the hiring process. Managers in smaller practices, or those in private practices, are more likely to find this information for themselves. All therapy managers are recommended to familiarize themselves with the basics of federal employment law at a minimum and complete an internet search for questions and conversation topics to avoid during the interview process (Martin, 2021).

Final Hiring Steps

Once your organization has identified the candidate who best meets the position's requirements, a handful of steps remain before making the final, formal job offer. First, the therapy manager should obtain the results of a background check and required drug screens and verify professional credentials and licensure status. The therapy manager should focus on contacting the selected candidate's references as these checks are in process. The remaining aspect of this phase of the hiring process is negotiating the candidate's compensation package. Negotiation is not listed last to imply it is the last thing to address before hiring. The

negotiation process works best if it is handled more like an ongoing conversation than a one-time discussion with a set number of talking points (Braveman, 2016c; Page, 2015).

While the obvious starting point to this conversation is salary, the manager needs to convey the overall value of the compensation package. According to Fisher (2011), the total compensation package for a full-time salaried employee can be estimated to add the equivalent of one-third of the salary. Aspects of the compensation package can include salary; retirement plans or employer contribution matching; life, health, and disability insurance; continuing education; paid time off, holidays, and bereavement leave; and payment or reimbursement of licensure or professional society membership costs. For example, a PT accepts a position within a rehabilitation hospital with a starting salary of $80,000. When factoring in the retirement plan, health/vision/dental insurance, reimbursement of their state license and APTA dues, and a generous continuing education stipend, the overall compensation package is worth $106,400 ($80,000×33%=$26,400; then add this onto the starting salary $80,000 + $26,400= $106,400 for total compensation).

Orientation

Following the acceptance of the formal job offer, the therapy manager's responsibilities shift to onboarding the new hire. Once again, depending upon the organization's size, the new hire's orientation may span two or three workdays on the low end or it may last longer than a full workweek. Regardless of duration, effective orientation periods: share pertinent information related to policies and safety; highlight responsibilities, expectations, and processes (such as documentation systems); and strive to make the new hire feel welcome in the organization (Braveman, 2016c; Page, 2015).

Orientation will likely vary based on the experience level of the new hire; it is natural to assume that someone will need a longer acclimation period for their first therapy job than an OT or a PT with a decade of practice experience. Orientation items to build into the initial few days may include:

- A facility tour to ensure the therapist is familiar with the layout of treatment spaces, exits, restrooms, and break areas, and to complete documentation.
- Provide a schedule for the first week to allow sufficient time to review policies and procedures.
- Blocked time for the manager to meet the therapist to answer any questions.
- Meeting times with other members of the therapy team.
- Starting a personnel file to keep updated employment documents including, but not limited to, the therapist's license, background check and drug screen results, and eventually the therapist's performance review materials (Page, 2015).

Legal, Ethical, and Risk

Managers are responsible for maintaining ethical and legal compliance, including risk management. Risk management identifies potential threats that could severely damage or ruin an organization and takes action via systems and processes to detect, assess, mitigate, and prevent risks (Catalyst, 2018; Page, 2015). Managers must be proactive to protect patients and their organization's assets, accreditation, and community standing (Catalyst, 2018). Risk management is guided by ethics, legal awareness, and accreditation.

Ethical Considerations

The AOTA and APTA have established ethical practices for therapists (Chapter 5). Ethical practice begins with beneficence, nonmaleficence, justice, and autonomy, with additional principles such as patient-centered practice, respect for privacy, equity, honesty, transparency, and competence (Card, 2020). An example of ethics in risk management is informed consent, the process of educating a patient about the risks, benefits, and alternatives of a given procedure or intervention (Shah et al., 2022). Additional considerations for ethical practice include enforcing the code of ethics, encouraging employees to bring errors and problems forward, being transparent about mistakes, and disclosing any potential conflicts of interest.

Legal Considerations

Numerous entities regulate legal healthcare matters at the federal (e.g., Medicare, HIPAA) and state levels (e.g., Medicaid, Workers' Compensation, state practice acts, business licensing). In addition, the Occupational Safety and Health Administration (OSHA) ensures employees safe and healthy working conditions by identifying potential threats and taking steps to address them (Fig. 11.8) (OSHA, 2022a). OSHA provides safety data sheets (SDS, formerly MSDS), used to communicate the risks of hazardous chemical products (OSHA, 2022a; OSHA, 2022b). Additional regulations are set by accreditation bodies such as The Joint Commission (TJC), the Utilization Review Accreditation Commission (URAC), the Commission on Accreditation of Rehabilitation Facilities (CARF), the Accreditation Commission for Health Care (ACHC), and the Center for Improvement in Healthcare Quality (CIHQ) (CMS, 2022). Accreditation is not required for all settings; however, the Centers for Medicare and Medicaid Services requires hospitals to be accredited to receive Medicare reimbursement.

Types of Risk

Risks in healthcare settings include hazard, reputation, operations, market, or human capital (Table 11.5) (Page, 2015). Centers for Medicare and Medicaid Services requires plans to address the potential for hazards (e.g., tornados, hurricanes), which must include ongoing training and testing (CMS, 2021a; APTA, 2020). Operational hazards can be mitigated by equipment inspection, maintenance, and other measures that coincide with safety and compliance. Notoriety and reputation are critical in healthcare; thus managers must be vigilant to maintain awareness of market changes and factors affecting the organization's standing in the community. Last, avoiding human capital risks includes ensuring proper staffing, recruitment, and retention of skilled practitioners.

A common risk for all healthcare organizations is medical errors. Medical errors are preventable adverse events, regardless of harm (Carver et al., 2022). Most errors are caused by flawed systems, policies, procedures, or conditions instead of an individual's recklessness. Medical errors are commonly due to improper patient management and failure to supervise and monitor care (*Physical Therapy Professional Liability Exposure Claim Report*, 2021).

Negligence or gross negligence is when a medical error or breach of duty results in harm (i.e., tort) (Page, 2015). Negligence is a general term to describe any professional deviation from the standard of care (SOC), i.e., what a reasonable person with similar training would do in a particular set of circumstances. However, if the SOC is followed and an incident occurs, it is not negligence; it is a bad outcome. Determining negligence typically involves testimony from expert witnesses in the same field. For an incident to

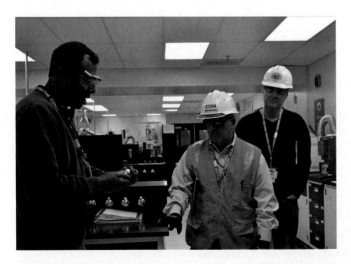

• **Fig. 11.8** OSHA Review. (From https://commons.wikimedia.org/w/index.php?curid=80268448)

TABLE 11.5	Types of Risk	
Risk	**Examples**
Hazard	Attacks, diseases, disasters
Market	Changes to insurance, referral source, target market, technology
Reputation	Poor patient outcomes, suspicious accounting, fraud, false advertising, unprofessional behavior, data breach
Operations	Equipment inspection and maintenance, injuries, safety, compliance, documentation
Human capital	Staffing, recruitment, retention, professional development, mentoring, terminations

From Page, C. G. (2015). *Management in physical therapy practices* (2nd ed.). F.A. Davis Company.

be labeled negligent, four essential elements are needed: (1) the professional owed a duty (i.e., a patient-provider relationship existed), (2) the professional breached this duty (i.e., did not follow the SOC), (3) the breach caused an injury, and (4) lastly, the individual suffered damages due to the breach (e.g., pain and suffering, medical bills, reduced quality of life).

Malpractice is a more specific term associated with professionals in healthcare (Bono et al., 2022; Page, 2015). Malpractice requires the same four elements of medical negligence; however, it comes with the added element; *intent*. It must be proved that the provider knew they should have done something different but failed to do so, knowing that failure could cause harm to the patient. Thus intent can mean that the provider planned to harm or knew there was a risk of harm and acted nonetheless (e.g., performing spinal manipulation on a patient with osteoporosis).

Risk Documentation

If an incident occurs, it must be reported and documented. Incident reports (Fig. 11.9) are internal documents detailing adverse events, errors, or near misses/close calls (Page, 2015). Sentinel and never events are incidents resulting in death or serious physical or psychological injury (*Never Events*, 2019; Patra & De Jesus, 2021).

Documentation on incidents includes the date, time, location, patient specifics, witness accounts, responses, treatments, and the preparer's signature. Do not offer a prognosis, speculation, assumptions, or opinion on how the event could have been prevented. Because incident reports are internal documents, they are not part of the medical record. Although the incident is documented in the patient's chart, there should be no reference to the *report* (Page, 2015). Incidents should be evaluated using a root cause analysis, which includes identifying the problem, gathering data, identifying the cause, finding the "root cause," and implementing solutions (Singh et al., 2022). A root cause analysis should focus on identifying faulty systems, not individual blame.

Directing

The direction of the therapy team has been described as "the process of providing guidance and oversight so that the work performed is goal-oriented and focuses on achieving desired departmental and organizational outcomes" (Braveman, 2016c, p. 175). This definition is appropriate in some industries but stops short of a collaborative approach that connects with the modern healthcare workforce. This description implies that the therapy team and the everyday tasks they complete are subservient to the organization. OTs and PTs and assistants in each field are highly educated, highly skilled, and independently licensed healthcare providers. Many unlicensed staff members (rehabilitation aides or techs) often take on these positions to accrue hands-on patient care experience with aspirations to become OTs or PTs. Directing a therapy team can be a collaborative process of guidance, growth, and oversight so that the work of each member of the therapy team is aligned to achieve outcomes that mutually benefit the team members, recipients of care, as well as the organization.

Meeting therapy team members, discussing mutually beneficial professional development goals, and identifying tangible action steps toward attaining those goals can be daunting for a therapy manager. Therapists new to management or those with management experience whose roles include managing and working with therapy staff may find this process challenging. The process of directing the work of others to align with organizational objectives does not require advanced management or business administration courses or degrees. The professional training of OTs and PTs allows therapy managers from either field to work through the management function of directing others from a place of familiarity. The remainder of this section will describe parallels between the therapy process and management steps: evaluating clinical competence (evaluation and assessment), setting performance expectations (mutually agreed upon goals), initiating a professional development plan (intervention planning), implementing the plan, and measuring outcomes (AOTA, 2020; APTA 2022).

Communication

Clear, effective, and relevant communication is a critical component of healthcare management and administration (Braveman, 2016a; Kent & Winston, 2016; Ledlow & Stephens, 2018; Page, 2015). Please refer to Chapter 9 of this text for communication strategies and approaches related to clients and providers. This section will focus on the communication responsibilities that therapy managers and administrators have related to internal communication such as sharing information and ideas within the therapy staff.

In the modern healthcare arena, managers and administrators must be mindful of the type or form of communication used, how the message is being received, and the message being communicated (Braveman, 2016a; Page, 2015). There are two general forms of workplace communication, oral and written. Oral communication includes interviews, one-on-one meetings, informal conversations, telephone conversations, presentations, formal group/team meetings, and virtual meetings in the postpandemic healthcare world (Page, 2015). Written forms of communication include emails, memos, letters, web pages, and reports (Braveman, 2016a; Page, 2015).

Multiple barriers exist to having any form of workplace communication received and acted upon. It is incumbent on the manager to package an idea or message efficiently into an appropriate form of communication that allows members of their team to receive, and to make sense of, the idea and then for those team members to act appropriately on the original message (Page, 2015). Managers must carefully select the words, tone, and length of the message to avoid miscommunications and errors. For example, an ongoing therapy team project update may be more effective in

FALL INCIDENT REPORT
DO NOT INCLUDE THIS FORM IN THE PATIENT'S MEDICAL RECORD

SECTION A: To be completed by clinical staff
Location at time of fall (ward, clinic, service, etc.): _____ ☐ Inpatient   ☐ Outpatient
Date of fall: Time of fall(military):
Name of Physician/ARNP/PA notified:
For inpatients, Date admitted/transferred to this ward:
Description of the event, including any obvious fall-related injuries (e.g., head trauma, change in ROM, pain, bruises, lacerations) and describe what was patient doing or trying to do that may have contributed to the fall: ☐ Found on floor   ☐ Staff lowered patient to floor   ☐ Patient lowered self to floor Was next of kin notified? ☐ Yes   ☐ No (If no why not?)

Contributory Factors (check all that apply):

Mobility:
		Cognitive & Functional factors:
☐ Up ad lib	☐ Bed rest	☐ Incontinent (circle appropriate choice(s): Bowel or bladder)
☐ Wheelchair	☐ Ambulate with wheelchair	☐ Confused/memory impaired
☐ Ambulate with assistance	☐ Ambulate with walker	☐ Altered gait/balance
☐ Restraints	☐ Other_____	☐ Altered ADL

Environmental/Equipment (check all that apply):

☐ Floor wet   ☐ Lighting poor   ☐ Needed item out of reach ☐ Cluttered area ☐ Foot wear

☐ Bed side rails (circle appropriate choice(s): all up or down 1 up (left right) top half up (left right) bottom half up (left right)

☐ Equipment faulty:

    ☐ Shower chair/commode chair   ☐ Cane   ☐ Walker   ☐ Wheelchair   ☐ Unavailable grab bars

    ☐ Stretcher   ☐ Bed   ☐ Other, please specify _____

Assistive Devices:

☐ Assistive Devices involved in fall?   ☐ No   ☐ Yes

If Yes, please complete the following:

    ☐ Assistive device(s) not appropriate?   ☐ No documentation of patient education in proper use?

    ☐ Needed transfer/mobility equipment NOT within reach?   ☐ Equipment not correctly or safely used by patient?

    ☐ Other, please specify: _____

Preventive Measures prior to incident (check all that apply):

☐ Interdisciplinary Fall Prevention Care Plan implemented & communicated to entire team

☐ Increase level of observation   ☐ Fall Alert Identifier (e.g., green armband, signage, computer alert)

☐ Patient close to nurses' station   ☐ Motion alarm

☐ Call light/bell in reach   ☐ Gait/Safety training

☐ Patient/family involved in care plan

Witnessed/Reported by: Name: Position/Title:
Report prepared by: Title:

• **Fig. 11.9** Sample Incident Report

person during individual or team meetings. Although verbal communication is often more personal, the manager's approach has the potential to cloud the message being delivered. Healthcare managers need to consider and modulate: their speaking volume, tone, and inflection; the amount of eye contact utilized; the use of body position, facial expressions, and gestures to match the size of the audience and the communication type (Braveman, 2016a).

Inherently, the manager must effectively and efficiently deliver their message to the therapy team members. Regardless of the type of communication being used, the intended message or idea needs to be clearly articulated to avoid miscommunication. For example, while some messages may be tailored to the therapy team who share a common language, other messages must have common wording (Page, 2015). The message length should match the method used to disseminate it. When sharing an important process update or information on a new piece of equipment in a team meeting, start the meeting with this information when the team is probably most focused. If a manager needs to send a message regarding coverage needs for an illness, send it as a separate email flagged important rather than tacking the coverage request onto a recurring informational email. Managers can use additional steps to ensure their message is received, starting with allowing space for questions at various points during a team meeting, asking for important points to be repeated back during individual meetings, or ending email messages stating to reply or to stop by the office with any questions. This process can shift workplace communication from a one-way information pipeline to a two-way street where the manager/administrator provides information, receives a follow-up inquiry, and then shares more to clarify the situation.

Project Management

Projects have a definitive beginning and end with a specific focus. There are numerous strategies for project management. The following section will highlight a four-phase approach (Fig. 11.10) (Berger, 2015). During phase one, the project is defined, a project manager is selected, the project scope and goals are established, and the project is presented for approval. The key deliverable for this phase is a concise project overview with expected outcomes, costs, and benefits to the organization. During phase two, a step-by-step plan is established, including a schedule detailing all activities, a budget, a list of stakeholders, and a description of how success will be measured. Once the plan is approved, a kickoff meeting with the project team should be held to review all components. The key deliverable is the project plan. During phase three, the plan is executed. It is important during this phase to measure and monitor progress. The key deliverable during this phase includes a list of setbacks, failed steps, additional costs, or unanticipated changes. Lastly, during phase four, the project comes to a close. There are several deliverables during this phase; documentation, project products, team member reviews, and lessons learned.

Controlling

Braveman, 2016c describe controlling as the managerial function aimed at ensuring the performance of the physical plant and equipment that meets an expected standard. The following section of this chapter relates to human resource management or aligning each member of the therapy team's performance with an expected, known standard.

Performance Evaluation

The effective direction of a therapy manager requires clear expectations and agreed-upon development goals. The scope of performance evaluation will vary among a new graduate, a new hire with experience in other settings, and a therapist who has been with the organization for years. Performance evaluation as a process should remain consistent throughout the therapy team- a regularly occurring, private conversation that progresses through four recurring stages: (1) assessing the knowledge, skills, and abilities of the therapy team member and how that assessment supports or hinders organizational aims; (2) identifying agreed upon performance expectations; (3) discussing tangible action steps targeting each performance expectation as well as resources and supports the organization can provide; and (4) reviewing the expectations and the team member's performance at regular intervals to allow goals to shift or resources to be allocated to facilitate goal attainment (Koverman & Braveman, 2016).

Organizations, or individual managers, may utilize several different tools to help facilitate and document this evaluation process. Therapy managers are encouraged to explore options available through professional organizations or tools within your organization. No matter the format used for performance evaluation, the aim is for the manager and the therapy team member to understand the expectations, so there are no surprises by either party during review meetings.

Formal performance evaluation meetings should take place on a planned schedule. Following an initial hire, the first formal performance meeting occurs near the 90-day mark. Depending on the organizational norms, or the manager's preference, the team member's next formal review may be scheduled for six months into the position, or it may be shifted to the 12-month point and serve as the person's annual performance review. Some factors that can play into the timing of the second review can include previous clinical

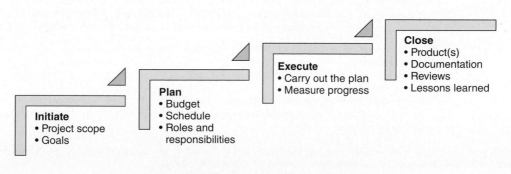

• **Fig. 11.10** Project Management Overview

experience and the status of goals during the initial review period. It stands to reason that a new graduate may require additional reviews and goal refinement compared with a clinician who has multiple years of clinical experience. All therapy managers must maintain open and consistent lines of communication with therapy team members. Performance evaluations should not be the only points of direct contact and conversation related to personal, professional, and organizational goals.

Progressive Disciplinary Action

While routine performance evaluations address growth and development over time, therapy managers are also responsible for providing timely feedback to correct actions and behaviors that do not meet the organization's standards (Braveman, 2016c). Regardless of how effective an organization's onboarding, orientation, and continuing education processes are, therapy managers will probably need to implement a formal disciplinary process. As Braveman points out, "the word *discipline* likely conjures up negative

thoughts" (2016c, p. 173); while discussions related to correcting performance can be awkward or have a negative tone, avoiding these issues can have a detrimental effect on the morale of the team and the organization as a whole.

As managers observe or receive reports of behavior that falls outside the organization's expectations, the following heuristic strategies can help to navigate the situation and correct employee performance. To provide a real-world scenario, we will utilize an example of a therapist whose client exit surveys indicate that they routinely check their smartphone during therapy sessions.

The first strategy would be for the manager to observe the behavior directly; this should be thought of as information gathering, similar to the assessment phase of the therapeutic process (AOTA, 2020). The second is timeliness; if the client exit survey is reviewed on a Tuesday, the initial conversation should occur on Tuesday or the following workday. The third strategy is for managers to align the smartphone conversation with the sequential steps of the company's progressive disciplinary action process. Table 11.6 applies a five-step

TABLE 11.6   Progressive Disciplinary Action

Step 1 **Informal conversation**	• Following the initial observation of a therapist using his smartphone for personal use during a therapy session, the manager initiates a private conversation to remind the therapist about patient care being the priority during scheduled sessions/billable time. • The manager adds a brief note to the therapist's personnel file, including the conversation's date, time, and purpose.
Step 2 **Verbal warning**	• After the second observation of smartphone use within a short time of the initial instance, the manager again initiates a private conversation. • This time the focus is on the organization's policy on personal device use and that this is the second known occurrence. • The manager again reminds the therapist about the expectations for patient care time and adds a brief written account of the conversation to the employee's file after both parties sign or initial the document.
Step 3 **Written warning**	• If a third instance of smartphone use occurs within a short time of the second, the private conversation and dual-signed notes in the personnel file are repeated. • The manager and therapist should move beyond a discussion of the organization's policy and work to identify if there are external factors causing smartphone use. • During this conversation, the therapist begins to recognize the severity of their behavior and that it is affecting their career and working relationships. • They disclose that they recently lost a sizable amount of money while online gambling and has been trying to recoup his losses. • The manager would have the ability to refer the therapist to a human resource-supported Employee Assistance Program (EAP) to help him work through a potential gambling addiction.
Step 4 **Suspension**	• Although smartphone use is not likely to progress this far into the disciplinary steps, the next instance of personal device use during billable therapy time would warrant an unpaid suspension of a duration determined by the manager and human resources (if the organization has an HR department). • The manager would articulate that ongoing smartphone use will lead to termination, and all observations of phone use and related conversations are recorded, signed, and filed with the previous documents.
Step 5 **Termination**	• The therapist would be terminated on the next instance of smartphone use within a short time of returning from the suspension. • Similar to previous steps, the behavior and conversation are recorded, signed, and filed with all previous employee documents. • The manager and an HR representative (if possible) meet privately with the therapist, review the disciplinary steps, timeline, and ongoing pattern of behavior, and then remain with or near the therapist as he gathers his items and leaves the premises.

Braveman, B. (2016). Roles and functions of managers: Planning, directing, organizing and staffing, directing, and controlling. In B. Braveman's (Ed.), *Leading and managing occupational therapy services: An evidence-based approach* (pp. 159–184). F.A. Davis.

disciplinary process to a therapist's ongoing use of his smartphone during scheduled therapy sessions. The fourth strategy is to remember that performance and conversations must be documented throughout each step to be legally defensible. Similar to therapy documentation, if the conversation is not written or filed, the conversation never takes place. Fifth, the same employee could have multiple disciplinary actions in process at any one time. Each form of behavior or conduct would begin a distinct disciplinary process. For example, the therapist checking his smartphone may have received a warning after three conversations with the manager regarding this policy. If that same therapist was 15 minutes late for their first scheduled session, the manager could not progress the smartphone disciplinary action to suspension; they would need to initiate a conversation regarding the company's attendance policy, then file a brief note of the day, time, and purpose of the conversation in the employee's personnel file. Finally, the severity of a transgression also needs to be factored in. For example, a manager may need to skip to a more consequential step if an employee fails to report a patient fall or steals from the company.

Conclusion

Physical and occupational therapists may take on managerial roles in various settings. No specific experience is required to become a manager, and the skills and attributes necessary to be effective vary. Therapists considering a career shift to management/administration can demonstrate readiness by intentionally analyzing the internal and external environmental factors that affect healthcare delivery; becoming aware of their managerial skillset and preferred styles of management and leadership; and developing an understanding of how the managerial functions of planning, organizing, directing, and controlling are implemented within their healthcare organization. Occupational and physical therapist managers should also consider the fit among the organization and its goals, the therapy department tasks that need to be completed, and the therapy team members. Managers in any therapy setting will be well-served to balance and align the needs of the individuals on the therapy team with those of the healthcare organization.

References

Accreditation Council for Occupational Therapy Education (ACOTE). (2022). *2018 ACOTE Standards and Interpretive Guide.* https://acoteonline.org/accreditation-explained/standards/.

American Occupational Therapy Association (AOTA). (2018). *Volume to value: Challenges & opportunities.* Slide deck presented at the 2018 Fall Academic Leadership Council.

American Occupational Therapy Association (AOTA). (2020). Occupational therapy practice framework: Domain and process (4th ed.). *American Journal of Occupational Therapy, 74*(Suppl. 2), 7412410010. https://doi.org/10.5014/ajot.2020.74S2001.

American Physical Therapy Association (APTA). *Standards of physical therapy practice.* https://www.apta.org/siteassets/pdfs/policies/standards-of-practice-pt.pdf. Accessed February 6, 2022.

American Physical Therapy Association (APTA). (2020). *The Role of the PT and PTA in disaster management.* https://www.apta.org/patient-care/public-health-population-care/emergency-preparedness/role-of-pt-disaster-management.

American Physical Therapy Association (APTA). (2022). *Guide to evidence-based physical therapist practice* (3rd ed.). https://guide.apta.org/.

APTA. (2022, January 1). *APTA strategic plan.* APTA. https://www.apta.org/apta-and-you/leadership-and-governance/vision-mission-and-strategic-plan/strategic-plan.

Berger, K. (2015). *A primer on project management for health care.* https://www.hsph.harvard.edu/ecpe/a-primer-on-project-management-for-health-care/.

Blanchard, K., & Bowles, S. (2001). *High Five! The magic of working together.* London: Harper Collins.

Brain Injury Association of Michigan. (2021). *Phase I: Provider survey results from a study tracking impact of fee changes in no-fault automobile insurance reform.* https://files.ctctusercontent.com/684f9e58001/385b5c27-0944-41ea-bbdd-0f9bd3ea1f6b.pdf?rdr=true.

Braveman, B. (2016a). Communicating effectively in complex environments. In B. Braveman (Ed.), *Leading and managing occupational therapy services: An evidence-based approach* (pp. 127–158). F.A. Davis.

Braveman, B. (2016b). Marketing occupational therapy services. In B. Braveman's (Ed.), *Leading and managing occupational therapy services: An evidence-based approach* (pp. 35–374). F.A. Davis.

Braveman, B. (2016c). Roles and functions of managers: Planning, directing, organizing and staffing, directing, and controlling. In B. Braveman's (Ed.), *Leading and managing occupational therapy services: An evidence-based approach* (pp. 159–184). F.A. Davis.

Braveman, B., & Phipps. (2016). Strategic planning. In B. Braveman's (Ed.), *Leading and managing occupational therapy services: An evidence-based approach* (pp. 235–253). F.A. Davis.

Card, A. J. (2020). What is ethically informed risk management? *AMA Journal of Ethics, 22*(11), 965–975. https://doi.org/10.1001/amajethics.2020.965.

Carver, N., Gupta, V., & Hipskind, J. E. (2022). Medical error. In *StatPearls.* StatPearls Publishing. http://www.ncbi.nlm.nih.gov/books/NBK430763/.

Catalyst, N. (2018). *What is risk management in healthcare?* NEJM Catalyst. https://catalyst.nejm.org/doi/full/10.1056/CAT.18.0197.

Centers for Medicare & Medicaid Services. (2021). *Fact sheet: CMS releases updated emergency preparedness guidance.* https://www.cms.gov/files/document/fact-sheet-cms-releases-updated-emergency-preparedness-guidance.pdf.

Centers for Medicare and Medicaid Services. (2021). *SNF PPS: Patient driven payment model.* https://www.cms.gov/Medicare/Medicare-Fee-for-Service-Payment/SNFPPS/Downloads/MLN_CalL_PDPM_Presentation_508.pdf.

Centers for Medicare and Medicaid Services. (2022). *Home health agency (HHA) center.* https://www.cms.gov/Center/Provider-Type/Home-Health-Agency-HHA-Center.

CMS. (2022). *CMS-Approved accrediting organizations.* https://www.cms.gov/Medicare/Provider-Enrollment-and-Certification/SurveyCertificationGenInfo/Downloads/Accrediting-Organization-Contacts-for-Prospective-Clients-.pdf.

Commission for the Accreditation of Rehabilitation Facilities. (2022). *ASPIRE to excellence quality framework.* Retrieved from 4/9/2022. http://carf.org/accreditation/qualitystandards/ASPIREtoexcellence/.

Corporate Screening. (2022). *Baby boomers' impact on human resources and the healthcare workforce.* https://www.corporatescreening.com/blog/baby-boomers-impact-on-human-resources-and-the-healthcare-workforce.

Fisher, T. F. (2011). Personnel management. In K. Jacobs & G. McCormack's (Eds.), *The occupational therapy manager* (5th ed., pp. 209–216). AOTA Press.

Gerber, M. (2004). *The E-myth; Why most small businesses don't work and what to do about it.* Harper-Collins.

Kent, B., & Winston, K. (2016). The Kawa model: An exploration of communication and leadership. In S. Dunbar & K. Winston's (Eds.), *An occupational perspective of leadership: Theoretical and practical dimensions* (2nd ed., pp. 99–110). SLACK, Inc.

Koverman, B., & Braveman, B. (2016). Roles and functions of supervisors. In B. Braveman's (Ed) *Leading and managing occupational therapy services: An evidence-based approach* (pp. 185–214). F.A. Davis.

Law, M., Cooper, B. A., Strong, S., Stewart, D., Rigby, P., & Letts, L. (1996). The person-environment-occupation model: A transactive approach to occupational performance. *Canadian Journal of Occupational Therapy, 63*(1), 9–23.

Ledlow, G. R., & Stephens, J. H. (2018). *Leadership for health professionals: Theory, skills, and applications* (3rd ed.). Jones & Bartlett Learning.

Martin, M. (2021, December 16). *Illegal job interview questions to avoid.* Business News Daily https://www.businessnewsdaily.com/4037-illegal-interview-questions.html.

Munoz, L., Bowyer, P., & Braveman, B. (2017). Turning theory into practice: Managerial strategies. In B. Braveman's (Ed.), *Leading and managing occupational therapy services: An evidence-based approach* (pp. 439–465). F.A. Davis.

Never Events. (2019). *Agency for healthcare research and quality.* https://psnet.ahrq.gov/primer/never-events.

Northouse, P. G. (2022). *Leadership: Theory and practice* (9th ed.). SAGE.

Occupational Safety and Health Administration. (2022a). *Hazard communication—overview occupational safety and health administration.* https://www.osha.gov/hazcom#HazcomHome_url.

Occupational Safety and Health Administration. (2022b). *Home | occupational safety and health administration.* https://www.osha.gov/.

Padilla, A., Hogan, R., & Kaiser, R. B. (2007). The toxic triangle: Destructive leaders, susceptible followers, and conducive environments. *The Leadership Quarterly, 18*(3), 176–194.

Page, C. G. (2015). *Management in physical therapy practices* (2nd ed.). F.A. Davis Company.

Patra, K. P., & De Jesus, O. (2021). Sentinel event. In *StatPearls.* StatPearls Publishing. http://www.ncbi.nlm.nih.gov/books/NBK564388/.

Pedersen, B., Delmar, C., Falkmer, U., & Grønkjaer, M. (2016). Bridging the gap between interviewer and interviewee: Developing an interview guide for individual interviews by means of a focus group. *Scandinavian Journal of Caring Sciences, 30*(3), 631–638.

Physical therapy professional liability exposure claim report (4th ed.). (2021). CNA/HPSO. https://www.cna.com/web/wcm/connect/15bdffdf-3753-45d6-abaf-a432a5cb5c14/CNA-Physical-Therapy-Professional-Liability-Exposure-Claim-Report-4th-Edition.pdf?MOD=AJPERES.

Shah, P., Thornton, I., Turrin, D., & Hipskind, J. E. (2022). Informed Consent. In *StatPearls.* StatPearls Publishing. http://www.ncbi.nlm.nih.gov/books/NBK430827/.

Singh, G., Patel, R. H., & Boster, J. (2022). Root cause analysis and medical error prevention. In *StatPearls.* StatPearls Publishing. http://www.ncbi.nlm.nih.gov/books/NBK570638/.

U.S. Department of Labor. (2022). *Employer costs for employee compensation.* https://www.bls.gov/news.release/pdf/ecec.pdf.

U.S. Equal Employment Opportunity Commission. (2022). *Prohibited employment policies/practices.* https://www.eeoc.gov/prohibited-employment-policiespractices.

12

Quality Assurance Performance Improvement

STEVEN D. EBERTH, OTD, OTR/L, CDP, CFPS;
and AMANDA SCOTT, OTD, OTR, BCG, CADDCT-CDP, CLT

LEARNING OBJECTIVES

By the end of this chapter, the reader will be able to:

1. Define relevant terminology regarding quality assurance and performance improvement.
2. Describe the relation between Continuous Quality Improvement (CQI) and Six Sigma.
3. Discuss components of developing a quality assurance plan.
4. Discuss the impact legislation and policy have on service delivery.
5. Describe the stages of project management.
6. Describe the effects of QAPI on outcomes.

CHAPTER OUTLINE

Introduction

Quality Assurance Performance Improvement (QAPI) consists of quality assurance, gathering data to understand the problem, and performance improvement, the action plan used to achieve the established goals. QAPI has its foundations in the Donabedian model, which examines the relationships between structure, process, and outcomes (Donabedian, 2005). According to Donabedian (2005), structures include the "conditions under which care is provided" (p. 46). The process focuses on the actions or "activities that constitute healthcare" (p. 46) carried out by contributors to care, such as healthcare providers, clients

receiving the care, and client support systems, including family and friends. The results of these interactions between structure and process are considered the outcomes within this model and can include desirable and undesirable outcomes attributed to the healthcare system.

The Donabedian model can be seen in the foundational principles of Continuous Quality Improvement (CQI) and Six Sigma, two philosophical approaches used in this chapter that are the most frequently and readily applied to practice. The founder of Continuous Quality Improvement (CQI), W. Edwards Deming, said, "Quality is everyone's responsibility" (1982). Considering Deming's words, managers and leaders must understand the concepts of QAPI, create a culture focused on QAPI, and foster sustainability through the commitment of others. Thus, It is essential to explore the ideas and principles related to developing the engagement of others at the level of shared values, which is also a fundamental component of interprofessional practice and cultures of change.

While CQI factors in the more intangible, qualitative data related to QAPI, Six Sigma takes on a more quantitative focus. Six Sigma originated in the 1980s for manufacturing processes to reduce variation and improve efficiency. This approach was integrated into healthcare settings, with hospital systems being the earliest adopters of this approach in the 1990s. Six Sigma emphasizes statistical analysis to inform decisions related to QAPI. Whether using CQI or Six Sigma, any QAPI initiative must have buy-in from all key stakeholders.

Stephen Covey (1989), a prolific author, American educator, businessperson, and keynote speaker, said that leadership is "inside-out (p. 42)." The philosophy of "inside-out" leadership has profound implications for the leaders of QAPI initiatives. Leadership "inside-out" is a principle-centered paradigm based on values, character, and ethics influencing each person's actions. Consider for a moment the implications of a principle-centered paradigm for leaders initiating a QAPI project. Likewise, consider how a principle-centered paradigm may affect the participation of others. If quality is the responsibility of everyone, then how do managers and leaders get the team to embrace this philosophy? If everyone is to be engaged in the process of improving and sustaining quality, then a level of accountability is required by all to support the QAPI initiative.

Responsibility and Accountability

Responsibility and accountability are two key components of examining employee participation in QAPI initiatives and work performance. Responsibility implies an obligation to perform certain required tasks and is typically outlined in a position description as minimum work requirements. Rarely is it the expressed responsibility of employees to engage in quality initiatives, as this is typically absent from position descriptions. As a result, quality initiatives are highly dependent on chosen accountability by the employee or mandated accountability on the employer's part. The willingness of the employee to act and be responsible is *chosen accountability* because willingness emanates from the employee's commitment and values related to the task. When an employee chooses not to be accountable, the employer invokes *mandated accountability*. Mandated accountability is the start of a behavior change process on the part of the employer with the employee that begins with the engagement of values and education about the benefits of change and shared goals, then taking steps to hold the employee accountable for the quality improvement process.

Employees who choose to be accountable more easily fulfill their responsibilities as participants in quality improvement initiatives to achieve the Institute for Healthcare Improvement Triple Aim (IHI, 2021). The IHI Triple Aim is the national strategy to improve healthcare quality initiated by the federal government. The three components of the Triple Aim include improving population health, improving the experience and quality of care, and optimizing the cost of care. The focus of the Triple Aim is to provide a framework to improve healthcare services through a QAPI approach that uses either CQI or Six Sigma to drive change. Quality must be the responsibility of everyone, so everyone must be involved in using CQI or Six Sigma and follow the phases of project management.

Quality Assurance Performance Improvement

QAPI has origins in manufacturing and engineering. Over the last 50 years, QAPI in healthcare has become a major focus in service delivery, including restructuring existing systems. Any QAPI initiative or paradigm aims to develop a proactive approach that sets requirements and standards for defining quality and efficiency in the products or services. Therapy-related QAPI focuses on key performance indicators (KPI), including but not limited to continuity of services, efficacy, and efficiency of therapy services provided. In order to measure KPI, the QAPI process must create auditing procedures so that quality can be assured, performance adjustments can be made, or validate that the current process is appropriate. The quality assurance process monitors outcomes and ensures accountability for key stakeholders. Peer review and performance incentives became the backbone of quality assurance mechanisms when QAPI was first introduced. As QAPI continued to evolve, performance improvement monitoring and evaluation of KPI became the pivotal sources of data. (Marjoua & Bozic, 2012).

QAPI has many theoretical constructs for approaching data collection and analysis. Key principles and terms apply universally regardless of the specific QAPI philosophical approach. One key factor in data collection is grouping data based on common denominators to improve the benchmarking process, comparing "apples to apples." An example is The International Classification of Disease (ICD-11) classification system from the World Health Organization (WHO, 2022). ICD-11 allows healthcare providers to organize data based on disease classification and assigns a numerical representation to a specific condition or disease. Uniform terminology allows organizations throughout the world to share data systematically. The WHO can compile the data to develop standards of care that can be used as practice or reimbursement guidelines (WHO, 2022). The ICD-11 is just one example of data collection used to inform healthcare.

Benchmarking is used in all QAPI processes to develop best practices based on comparing planned and actual processes. Quality audits identify gaps in knowledge and services to create effective action plans. The two rules primarily used during the audit process that can offer some measure of predictability in decision-making during change processes, regardless of using CQI or Six Sigma, include the 85/15 rule and the 80/20 rule.

85/15 Rule

The 85/15 rule states that 85% of quality is driven by leadership, management roles, and systems, while 15% of quality is directly related to the worker's actions (Sonderland, 2004). This means that the 85/15 rule focuses on leadership, systems, and resources as the main contributors to quality, not just the individual providers. There needs to be effective leadership and management providing the resources needed for the individual providers to be successful. Individuals create the organizational culture, "this is how we do things here" mentality that represents how the individual interprets expectations and practices. Individual employees are accountable for creating a sustainable culture and must buy into changes. The 85/15 rule is a top-down approach to quality because once the systems and resources have been identified and marshaled, we move to create a large impact with the least amount of resources needed.

80/20 Rule

The 80/20 rule (not the Pareto rule) states that 80% of problems stem from 20% of issues. (Sonderland, 2004). This rule means that a few issues or people can cause the largest negative impact. The rule highlights the need to efficiently identify and address those issues or people to create the greatest positive impact (Sonderland, 2004). The rule compels the notion of searching for and reducing the impact of the 20% that causes systemic disruption. This rule is often associated with the adages of "work smarter, not harder" and "focus on the low hanging fruit" to resolve the problems or data points that are easy to identify and fix.

Implementing QAPI

Data drives QAPI and many organizations focus on QAPI, yet quality attainment tends to be elusive. Healthcare systems are composed of people, policies, and practices that are very dynamic and complex. This complexity can foster ambiguity related to the potential misuse of resources. Often, a lack of accountability and inadequate resources result in higher care costs and delays in care delivery (Marjoua & Bozic, 2012). The key question related to QAPI is not solely data collection but proper interpretation of the data that can lead to purposeful change that creates a positive impact (Marjoua & Bozic, 2012).

Many early adopter organizations of QAPI identified the need to implement changes but lacked a way of effectively demonstrating and formalizing the efforts. One way of more easily demonstrating an organization's dedication to quality is through obtaining specialized organizational accreditations. In 1951, a nonprofit organization known as the Joint Commission on Accreditation of Hospitals was

established to provide hospitals with a voluntary accreditation process to demonstrate higher quality standards. The Joint Commission on Accreditation of Hospitals evaluates healthcare organizations using a preestablished rubric focused on quality and cost-benefit (Marjoua & Bozic, 2012).

The focus on formalized QAPI processes expanded into the managed care agencies and Medicare. With the inception of Medicare in 1965, greater access to healthcare services for persons over the age of 65 years facilitated the need for oversight. Utilization review committees were established in 1972 by the United States Congress to create a formal review process to ensure services provided were following best practices. (Marjoua & Bozic, 2012). In the 1980s, peer review organizations were created to monitor quality control for physicians and hospitals. The peer review organizations was charged with implementing Centers for Medicare and Medicaid Services (CMS) payment systems and reducing unnecessary client services. (Marjoua & Bozic, 2012).

In 2001, CMS initiated the Quality Initiatives program to create accountability metrics for healthcare providers to improve the quality of care and reduce costs (CMS, 2021). This quality program collaborates with CMS and the Department of Health and Human Services. The Patient Protection and Affordable Care Act (PPACA) created a payment framework based on key quality measures such as outcomes, readmission rates, client safety, and reducing care disparities. The CMS regional offices and State Survey Agencies monitor quality compliance at the organization and facility levels. These monitoring organizations assess the facilities based on established guidelines centered on the State Operations Manual to determine compliance requirements and action steps related to deficiencies (CMS, 2021). These quality initiatives aim to drive key decisions based on data-informed care.

Data-Informed Care

First, the difference between data-informed care and data-driven care must be made clear. Data-driven care focuses on using data to make decisions. The perception is that data-driven care removes the humanity of caring for individuals by reducing the person to mere data points. Data-informed care uses data metrics to make decisions while factoring in the less quantifiable human factors such as beliefs, perceptions, and feelings.

"Vs" data-driven healthcare assists in organizing components of healthcare data to avoid data overload.
- Volume: Sufficient amounts of data are important to determine prior to the onset of data collection and throughout the data collection process to ensure validity and avoid one-off situations that could result in poor decision-making (Bresnick, 2017).
- Velocity: The speed at which data is obtained and analyzed is another key component of data-driven care. The information must be transmitted and assessed quickly enough to inform decisions and effect change to maximize impact (Bresnick, 2017).

- Variety: Multiple sources for data collection are needed to capture a comprehensive picture. Data can be quantitative or qualitative. Data can be collected in an unstructured, semi-structured, or structured way depending on the data collection systems in place (Bresnick, 2017).
- Veracity: Reliability and data quality are imperative to decision-making. Decision makers must be able to trust that the data is free of bias and is complete (Bresnick, 2017).
- Validity: Trustworthiness of the data is founded on the accuracy of the data. Data validity is achieved by ensuring consistency in data collection methods (Bresnick, 2017).
- Viability: Relevant data must be accurately paired with the proper issue in order to develop an effective action plan (Bresnick, 2017).
- Volatility: This ties closely with velocity. Not only is the speed of data collection imperative, but assessing how rapidly the data changes is also important. If the data is quickly changing and in a state of flux, the challenge lies in creating stable decisions based on unstable data (Bresnick, 2017).
- Vulnerability: Data protection is essential as we collect copious amounts of data. Laws have been passed over the last two decades that focus on security and privacy due to the volume of data being collected and the risk of misuse (Bresnick, 2017).
- Visualization: Proper displaying of data through the use of charts and graphs assists decision-makers in interpreting the significance and meaning of the data (Bresnick, 2017).
- Value: Data collection must be done in a meaningful way. Identifying what needs to be measured and how to collect and measure data properly leads to better-informed decision-making (Bresnick, 2017).

Project Management

Project management is a component of any QAPI process. Project management involves planning, organizing, and managing resources to complete specific project goals and objectives to meet or exceed stakeholder needs and expectations. Pareto's 80/20 rule states that 20% of the work (the first 10% [initiation phase] and the last 10% [closing phase]) consumes 80% of the time and resources. The project management process comprises five phases (Fig. 12.1):

initiation, planning, executing, monitoring/controlling, and closing (Phillips, 2013).

The Initiation Phase

The initiation phase identifies the issue and rationale for the need to change (Berger, 2015). This phase examines retrospective data to create a narrative outlining the depth and breadth of the issue. The primary directive at this phase is to create a big-picture concept for the potential project. A key tool to assist in this process is a SWOT analysis. A SWOT analysis examines the Strengths, Weaknesses, Opportunities, and Threats. The format for a SWOT is often a 2×2 matrix with key indicators listed in bullet format (Table 12.1). Strengths and weaknesses are key internal indicators of the proposed project or organization, while opportunities and threats are key external indicators of the proposed project or organization (Phillips, 2013).

The Planning Phase

The second phase of project development is planning (Berger, 2015). During this phase, specific details are identified to accomplish the big picture. Frequently, a root-cause analysis is completed in this phase to create a deeper understanding of the elements contributing to the issue and to develop clear expectations and goals (Fig. 12.2). Goals should be created in a SMART format (Table 12.2). Another component of this phase is creating key action steps needed to accomplish each goal. The project plan should be detailed enough for the team members to understand the vision and steps needed for execution. Establishing a clear action plan creates the project's scope (Phillips, 2013).

Scope creep occurs when a project grows beyond the plan or capacity of the project leader. The scope is the project's defined parameters ensuring accuracy and controlling the project's focus. Creep occurs when aspects of the project go beyond the identified parameters and do not add value to the project. Scope creep often occurs when inadequate planning underestimates the project's complexity and the resources needed to succeed. Creep typically occurs in one of three forms: hope creep, effort creep, and gold plating. Hope creep refers to team members avoiding reporting when action item completion is falling behind schedule in the hopes that they will be able to "catch up" without the project leader becoming aware of the shortcomings. Effort

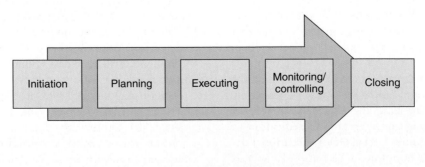

• **Fig. 12.1** The Project Management Process

TABLE 12.1	SWOT Analysis		
Strengths		**Weaknesses**	
• What do you do well? • What unique resources do you have to assist in project development? • What do others view as your strengths?		• What aspects do you need to improve? • What resources are lacking that could impede success?	
Opportunities		**Threats**	
• What opportunities does the market present? • What trends can you capitalize on?		• What does the potential competition do better? • Risks to your project success?	

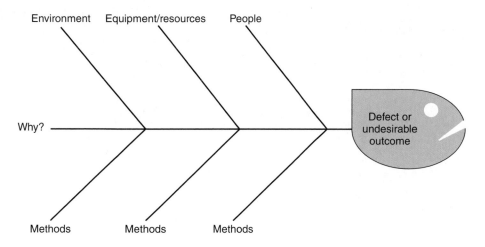

• **Fig. 12.2** Root-Cause Analysis

TABLE 12.2	SMART Goals
S	Specific
M	Measurable
A	Action-oriented
R	Reasonable
T	Time-sensitive

creep occurs when the task is more complicated than initially anticipated, thus impeding the effectiveness of the team members. Gold plating refers to the process of adding additional tasks or action items that do not significantly add value to the project. Gold plating can lead to team member frustration due to minimal impact on the value added to the project (Phillips, 2013).

All forms of creep can be avoided with proper planning and monitoring. In the project's planning phase, a clear definition of the project's scope is imperative to avoid creep from the project's onset. Also, during the planning phase, risk factors that can impede the project's success should be identified and plans made to minimize the impact of risk factors and barriers. A contingency plan should also be established to manage risk. Time management is often the

primary reason for creep setting into a project (Phillips, 2013) (Fig. 12.3).

The Execution Phase

The execution phase is the third phase of project management (Berger, 2015). This phase focuses on putting the plan into action. Project leaders will refine action items in finer detail to accomplish goals. The project leaders will then delegate the goals and action items to create an accountability chart using a Responsible, Accountable, Consulting, and Informed (RACI) matrix (Table 12.3). The execution phase also ensures that team members have the support and resources to succeed in the assigned tasks (Phillips, 2013).

The Monitoring/Controlling Phase

The fourth phase of project management is monitoring and controlling (Berger, 2015). This phase consists of project leaders assessing the efficacy and efficiency of project execution. Often, this phase consists of regularly scheduled meetings for progress review based on the RACI matrix. The monitoring and controlling phase are highly data-driven and routinely measure the current status compared with the established SMART goals. Reporting in this phase typically uses a Red, Amber, Green status report (Table 12.4). These status reports allow the project leader to adjust resources

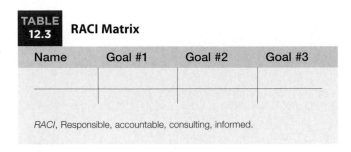

• **Fig. 12.3** Time Management Process

TABLE 12.3	RACI Matrix		
Name	Goal #1	Goal #2	Goal #3

RACI, Responsible, accountable, consulting, informed.

TABLE 12.4	RAG Status
R	Red: Progress toward goals is impeded by barriers and unlikely to achieve the goal
A	Amber: Progress toward goals is impeded by barriers and delayed goad achievement
G	Green: Progress toward goals is progressing according to schedule with no major barriers

and expectations based on team members' needs and barriers (Phillips, 2013).

The Closing Phase

The final phase of project management is the closing phase. The closing phase is closely tied to the initiation phase. This phase consists of project leaders assessing whether the big picture identified in the initiation phase was achieved. Project leaders reassess the process and analyze data to ensure all aspects of the project are addressed effectively. Following the final assessment, a finalized report is completed summarizing the overall project and key accomplishments (Phillips, 2013). Occupational and physical therapy practitioners essentially follow the common process of client care (Table 12.5).

Continuous Quality Improvement

W. Edward Deming was a statistician who advocated applying the scientific method to quality improvement processes and overall outcomes. In the 1950s, he gave a speech to Japanese business leaders in Tokyo to promote this approach embraced by industry and helped to facilitate the postwar economy the country enjoys today. The Toyota Motor Corporation was the most notable early adopter of CQI and, as a result, revolutionized quality in the auto industry that continues today, with language that can still be seen in their company vision and philosophy.

CQI is a philosophical and managerial approach to understanding and managing process variation to improve quality *and* outcomes. According to Deming (1982), the founder of CQI stated, the central problem in leadership and management is the "failure to understand the nature and interpretation of variation" (p. 465) and the ability to effectively manage the complex dynamics to reduce process deviations and quality as the customer defines this concept. The philosophy of CQI is founded on the notion that everyone in the organization needs to be afforded the same opportunity to learn and grow to develop knowledge and engage in meaningful organizational change to reduce deviations and meet the customer's needs. It is a philosophy that conveys the value of everyone's perspective and participation in QAPI initiatives.

TABLE 12.5	Project Management Rehabilitation Process	
Project Management Terminology	**Therapy Terminology**	
Initiation	Initial evaluation for a plan of care development of a client; and creating the overall picture of the client's future level of function based on the prior level and current level of function	
Planning	Goal and intervention development	
Executing	Implementing the established plan of care. Delegating action items to the client, interdisciplinary team members, and assistants creates a successful outcome.	
Monitoring and Controlling	Periodic notes and updated plans of care. The therapist assesses a client's progress toward established goals and adjusts the goals and interventions according to the client's progress.	
Closing	Discharge summary. The clinician completes a final assessment compared to prior and current levels of function. The established goals are evaluated to determine if the client achieved the goals and discuss successes and barriers to function.	

CQI is an efficient and cost-effective means of improving processes and outcomes. The selection of CQI as a means to drive change out of the recognition that while quality starts with leadership, it is the responsibility of everyone in the organization to participate (Deming, 1982). Quality initiatives require the involvement of all and the support of management to marshal the resources for change. Within a QAPI framework, it is essential to have a data-driven approach to change, and CQI is a simple means to start the process. Deming (1981), in his original work, published 14 points for the transformation of management to promote change and apply it to healthcare today.

1. Create a sense of purpose every day to improve the quality of services.
2. Learn up-to-date philosophies of management and take the lead to make a change.
3. Require statistical evidence to drive decision-making and improve quality outcomes.
4. Require statistical evidence of process control to manage the price of services.
5. Require statistical methods to identify system challenges to the quality of outcomes.
6. Institute up-to-date, on-the-job training relevant to the job and the needs of the workforce.
7. Improve supervision and institute leadership that inspires people to work together with pride to promote quality outcomes.
8. Drive out fear so that everyone can contribute to the quality of outcomes.
9. Break down barriers between departments that impede communication, handoffs, and safety and promote collaboration and streamlining.
10. Eliminate numerical goals, slogans, pictures, and posters, urging people to increase productivity as these create adversarial relationships among employees; instead, leadership needs to change the system that impedes quality improvement and outcomes.
11. Look carefully at work standards that impede quality workmanship and focus on the wrong outcome like quantity.
12. Institute a massive training program that uses simple but powerful statistical methods that empower managers to focus on quality improvement and outcomes.
13. Institute a vigorous program for retraining people in new skills that promotes growth.
14. Create a structure in top management and a plan that will orient everyone every day on the above thirteen points so that it is clear how outcomes are the responsibility of everyone.

Plan, Do, Study, Act

As a management approach, CQI is a process of continuous improvement that promotes a cyclical appraisal process called the Deming Cycle for Continuous Quality Improvement that follows Plan, Do, Study, Act (PDSA). PDSA is a systematic means of organizing the change process based on

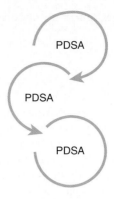

• **Fig. 12.4** Deming Cycle. *PDSA,* Plan, do, study, act.

the scientific method to manage and predict outcomes. (Fig. 12.4). The PDSA cycle can be a component of the QAPI process that deliberately transforms the process of change and outcomes. PDSA is iterative as the cycle of plan, do, study, act, when completed, can begin again for the next stage in continuous quality improvement based on the data regarding the prior outcomes. By contrast, Deming considered the Plan, Do, Check, Act cycle as a theoretical exercise by nature as it is a process of hypothesis or plausibility testing to "check" to see if the hypothesized change was true or not, see if the proposed change will work, and as a result, develop new knowledge about the proposed process change. The PDSA cycle is focused on studying the outcomes to see if they met predictions and determine why disparities may continue to exist. Plan, Do, Check, Act is theoretical, whereas PDSA is the practical application of CQI.

Plan

The *plan* stage of the Deming Cycle includes the ability to explain how quality is defined because this becomes the target outcome. Defining quality then provides a measure of knowing if the changes improve the processes and, as a result, the outcome. Defining quality and knowing if the changes improve the processes and outcome gives predictability, which provides opportunities to appraise system performance. The appraisal process provides opportunities to identify the strategies and barriers to change—to plan.

Do

The analysis continues with the *do* stage, where change is initiated in small stages to test the potential variables that may affect outcomes. It is essential to recognize that changes within a system can have a ripple effect that may be unforeseen and create negative consequences. Staging change allows for better controls and predictability. Small scale can also help the organization's human resource people adjust incrementally and contribute to the change process as it will improve their ability to report problems, which should be documented. Meaningful documentation from people who are invested in the change process promotes reflection, which may help with objectivity in reporting. Of course, documentation provides a written record of the changes or variables and enables follow-up opportunities and further analysis.

Study and Act

The *study* stage is all about data analysis to determine if predictions were accurate or not and why. This stage provides a brief look at the outcomes of the initial process changes and is a precursor to the adjusting processes. The *act* stage is the opportunity to implement the process adjustments and monitor to ensure consistent outcomes over time. Continued documentation of the efforts to embed the change process into the organizational culture is essential to further data-driven decision-making. Data provide an objective measure to appraise system performance and the opportunity to plan for necessary changes to meet market demands. This stage provides the necessary information to continue the Deming Cycle to make changes to the process that may not have been addressed in the previous evolution.

Six Sigma

Like the project management process of CQI and the Deming Cycle, Six Sigma offers a structured approach to QAPI with a systematic process. Six Sigma is an approach that began in manufacturing to increase performance and to reduce process deviations to improve quality (Fig. 12.5). Six Sigma is a standard deviation on a control chart used to determine process and tolerance limits for deviations. The approach was developed by Bill Smith, an engineer at Motorola, in 1986. The approach was later adopted by Honeywell and General Electric, finding cost savings and improved quality. It is a philosophy that emphasizes efficiency, identifies barriers to efficiency, and improves overall quality and performance through data collection and analysis by reducing variation and enhancing process control (George, et al., 2004). Six Sigma is a process that focuses on standardization and workflow by reducing non-value-adding processes known as *wastes*. The Six Sigma process is based on four pillars: quality, speed, variation and defects, and process flow (American Society for Quality, 2022).

Six Sigma applies to all aspects of healthcare as it emphasizes increased performance and reduced process deviations to increase quality because it engages employees and clients in the process improvement cycle. Also, it improves overall outcomes through data analysis to improve provider efficiency, care experience of care and satisfaction with service delivery (Henrique & Godinho Filho, 2018). Six Sigma examines data before implementation to establish a clear baseline. The next phase is to collect information on successes and barriers to client outcomes, using chart reviews, client perceptions, and healthcare provider feedback. Once the data collected is sufficient to depict the overall picture, the next step is determining barriers that fall into the "7 wastes" (Table 12.6). This phase includes root cause analysis (Chapter 11) and identifying the barriers creating the greatest impact on outcomes. Ranking barriers according to impact and the causes of the barriers moves the process into the next phase, developing action plans. These action plans, also known as performance improvement projects (PIP), include an assessment plan and tasks to remediate or minimize the barriers. Monitoring and measuring the PIPs must occur throughout the process to determine the effectiveness of the action plans and to correct the course as needed (American Society for Quality, 2022).

Data Collection

Data collection within the confines of any QAPI process requires clear, consistent collection processes. Often, a QAPI initiative will consist of multiple team members across multiple departments. Data collection guidelines allow each member to collect data to minimize the impact of confounding variables and provide consistency. Inconsistencies in data collection can lead to improper analysis and result in poor decisions due to the misinterpretation of findings. The data collection guidelines should clearly outline selecting the proper tools and statistical tests for the data and carrying those tools throughout the process.

The data collection points feed into the quantifying of outcome measures. Outcome measures create an overall mode of determining the success of the QAPI initiative. These outcome measures are established in the initial planning process and define the project's success; thus, the selection of outcome measures must reflect what is being measured. The outcome measures can also determine a person's success toward the QAPI goal.

Outcome Measures

Outcome measures come in several forms. Outcome measures can quantify success from employees, customers/clients, leadership, and systems. Becoming overwhelmed with data is a common issue in analyzing outcome measures. The key to managing this is prioritizing the outcome measures based on the highest impact with the path of least resistance. Part of the prioritization process should be based on the categories of the Lean 7 Wastes that have the most significant negative impact.

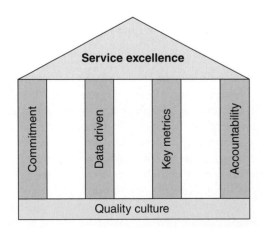

• **Fig. 12.5** Pillars of Six Sigma. (Data from American Society for Quality. [2022]. What is Six Sigma? Retrieved from: https://asq.org/quality-resources/six-sigma.)

TABLE 12.6 The 7 Wastes

Waste	Definition
Correction	• Do it right, do it once! Making corrections takes extra time away from client care, mentoring others, and learning new techniques.
Overproduction	• This can be as simple as giving too much information when answering someone's question.
Movement of material/information	• A great example is writing a note on paper and then transposing it into the computer system. It is an unnecessary extra step and leaves more room for error.
Motion of employees	• A disorganized environment creates extra steps that interrupt the process. Example: The washer and dryer are located in the basement, your dirty clothes are on the second floor, and you store your detergent in the kitchen pantry on the first floor. Is this good energy conservation or good task simplification?
Waiting	• One of the most identifiable wastes.
Inventory	• Not maximizing your utilization of resources, whether tangible items or intangible items.
Processes	• Why use 10 steps to complete a task when you can do it in 2 steps? Implementing efficient systems is crucial

Data from American Society for Quality. (2022). What is Six Sigma? Retrieved from: https://asq.org/quality-resources/six-sigma.

The most infamous measure in therapy professions is productivity or efficiency. This metric creates a percentage of billable time versus non-billable time spent with clients. Productivity can be measured daily, weekly, monthly, quarterly, or even annually. This metric is versatile because it can apply to individual employees, departments, and multiple sites within a geographic location. Productivity is used to quantify the effective use of time and allows for improved accuracy in establishing budgets.

Budget goal attainment is an outcome measure used to determine the success of management. Budgets are typically established annually and are adjusted based on past performance. This metric is easily quantifiable but has the primary drawback of being retrospective. The historical perspective on performance challenges creates a proactive approach to anticipating changes in the healthcare landscape due to changes in client acuity levels (Agency for Healthcare Research and Quality, 2017.)

Another common outcome measure is satisfaction. The satisfaction measure typically consists of employee satisfaction and customer/client satisfaction. Frequently this data is collected through surveys, focus groups, or interviews. The surveys will usually have qualitative and quantitative data using Likert scales to rate satisfaction. This outcome measure assists in determining the perceptions of the people served and fosters the identification of areas that could be improved. Employee satisfaction is often used to inform staff retention efforts. Staff turnover creates inconsistent service delivery and increases overall cost to an organization due to greater unproductive time for training. Many organizations will establish a benchmark of 10% or less for staff turnover since some turnover is expected.

Sustainability

After data collection is used to inform the outcome measures, leaders must determine the sustainability of the outcome measures and associated PIPs. The primary purpose of sustainability is to maintain gains made for the long term to become best practices. Sustainability applies to the quantifiable outcome measures and the culture change within the organization because of the successful PIP. Sustainability should be a focus in the early planning phases of a project, which enables the team to develop realistic expectations and strategies for moving the project forward. Integrating sustainability into the early planning phase also aids leaders in developing a clearer vision for the projected long-term outcome. The sustainability measurement plan is more readily defined with a clearer long-term vision. Traditionally, there are eight steps to creating sustainability (Agency for Healthcare Research and Quality, 2013). Reporting sustainability results occurs well after the initial QAPI project facilitates the maintenance of the action step in the daily routine. Communicating the results through storytelling and recognition of successes conveys the importance of the culture change and continues to empower those impacted by the sustained changes. Table 12.7 highlights steps for sustainability.

Conclusion

Whether using CQI or Six Sigma, any QAPI process requires individual and organizational support for successful launch and sustainability. Organizations must be proactive in facilitating the training of QAPI leaders and leveraging the necessary resources for PIP development and implementation. QAPI is an ongoing, team-centered process that must be agile enough to affect change in a timeframe that significantly affects the quality and efficiency of the services delivered. Many professional organizations with a QAPI focus exist to provide valuable resources, training, and networking opportunities. A QAPI list can be seen in Table 12.8, this list of organizations is not intended to be an all-inclusive list.

TABLE 12.7	Sustainability Steps
Step 1	Instill importance and haste to foster immediate action
Step 2	Assemble a project team that can take ownership of leading others in change
Step 3	Plan the work. Establish a clear vision with goals and action steps
Step 4	Attain buy-in from project team members and foster buy-in from those impacted by the PIP
Step 5	Create a culture of empowerment by enabling team members to contribute to PIP development and implementation
Step 6	Celebrate achievements. Focus on the positive results of short-term goals set in the planning process. This will maintain morale and empowerment
Step 7	Stay the course. Part of empowerment is problem-solving and minimizing barriers. Identify obstacles in the monitoring process and develop action plans for each barrier
Step 8	Develop a culture change. Create a QAPI process that is easily adapted into established routines. This enables the changes made to become more automatic, ultimately leading to generalizability

TABLE 12.8	QAPI Resources	
QAPI Organization	Website	Specialty Certification
World Healthcare Organization	www.who.int/health-topics/quality-of-care#tab=tab_1	None available
International Society for Quality in Healthcare	www.isqua.org	Multiple specialty certifications and fellowships are available
American Healthcare Quality Association	www.ahqa.org	None available
National Association for Healthcare Quality	www.nahq.org	Multiple specialty certifications are available
Agency for Healthcare Research and Quality	www.ahrq.gov	None available
American Occupational Therapy Association	www.aota.org	None available
American Physical Therapy Association	www.apta.org	None available

References

Agency for Healthcare Research and Quality. (2013). *Module 4. Approaches to quality improvement.* US Department of Health and Human Services. https://www.ahrq.gov/ncepcr/tools/pf-handbook/mod4.html.

Agency for Healthcare Research and Quality. (2017). *Module 6: Sustainability: Facilitator notes.* US Department of Health and Human Services. https://www.ahrq.gov/hai/quality/tools/cauti-ltc/modules/implementation/long-term-modules/module6/mod6-facguide.html.

American Society for Quality. (2022). *What is Six Sigma?* https://asq.org/quality-resources/six-sigma.

Berger, K. (2015). *A primer on project management for health care.* https://www.hsph.harvard.edu/ecpe/a-primer-on-project-management-for-health-care/.

Bresnick, J. (2017). *Understanding the many V's of healthcare big data analytics.* Health IT Analytics. https://healthitanalytics.com/news/understanding-the-many-Vs-of-healthcare-big-data-analytics.

Centers for Medicare and Medicaid Services (CMS). (2021). *Quality, safety & oversight - enforcement.* https://www.cms.gov/Medicare/Provider-Enrollment-and-Certification/SurveyCertification-Enforcement.

Deming, W. E. (1981). Improvement of quality and productivity through action by management. *National Productivity Review (pre-1986), 1*(1), 12.

Deming, W. E. (1982). *Out of the crisis.* MIT Press.

Donabedian, A. (2005). Evaluating the quality of medical care. *The Milbank Quarterly, 83*(4), 691–729.

George, M., Rowlands, D., & Kastle, B. (2004). *What is lean Six Sigma?* McGraw-Hill.

Henrique, D., & Filho, M. (2018). A systematic literature review of empirical research in Lean and Six Sigma in healthcare. *Total Quality Management & Business Excellence, 31*, 1–21. doi:10.1080/14783363.2018.1429259.

Institute for Healthcare Improvement. [IHI]. (2021, November 4). *Triple aim.* http://www.ihi.org/.

Marjoua, Y., & Bozic, K. J. (2012). Brief history of quality movement in US healthcare. *Current Reviews in Musculoskeletal Medicine, 5*(4), 265–273. https://doi.org/10.1007/s12178-012-9137-8.

Phillips, J. (2013). *PMP project management professional study guide* (4th ed.). New York: McGraw-Hill Education.

Sonderland, J. (2004). Building theories of project management: Past research, questions for the future. *International Journal of Project Management, 22*, 183–191.

World Health Organization. (2022). *Classification of diseases (ICD).* https://www.who.int/standards/classifications/classification-of-diseases.

13

Fundamentals of Insurance and Billing

AMANDA SCOTT, OTD, OTR, BCG, CADDCT-CDP, CLT; and JAMIE S. WAY, PhD, DPT

LEARNING OBJECTIVES

By the end of this chapter, the reader will be able to:

1. Define relevant terminology regarding payment models.
2. Describe the relationship between reimbursement and documentation.
3. Discuss the impact legislation and policy have on reimbursement of service delivery.
4. Describe the stages of appeals and denials.
5. Describe the effects of fraud and abuse on outcomes.

CHAPTER OUTLINE

Insurance-Based Business

Client's Perspective

The Employer's Perspective

The Provider's Perspective

Payor's Perspective

Fraud, Abuse, and Waste

CPT Codes – How Therapists Get Paid

Factors Affecting Payment

Medicare

Medicaid

Private Insurance and Managed Care

Claim Submission, Denials, and Appeals

Medicare Administrative Contractors

Transition to Outcome-Based Healthcare

Bundled Payments

Payment Alternatives and Considerations

Cash Practice

Pro Bono

Documenting Skill

Initial Evaluation

Daily Notes

Progress Report

Re-evaluation

Discharge Note/Summary

Medical Necessity and Medical Maintenance

Electronic Medical Records

Conclusion

Introduction

This chapter explores the types of reimbursement, also known as payors, and the requirements associated with each type. The history of federal payors and the key legislation that influences practice are outlined to offer context to the rationale for occupational therapy (OT) and physical therapy (PT) service delivery in various practice settings. As a manager and leader, the processes must be understood for reimbursing rehabilitation services. The payor type should not impact who receives rehabilitation services; however, each type dictates specific documentation requirements and processes needed to be completed by providers. In other words, from the client's perspective, they do not see a difference in how we provide services. The payor-influenced differences occur in the behind-the-scenes processes and documentation. The processes and requirements are perpetually changing as new legislation and interpretations of that legislation are implemented. Therefore it is the professional responsibility of the individual clinician to possess a strong working knowledge of the requirements. Maintaining up-to-date knowledge assists in protecting the clinician and the client ethically, legally, and clinically.

Insurance-Based Business

Insurance is the financial mechanism that shares and disperses the risk of financial loss due to an adverse event. It protects individuals and organizations against unforeseen and severe financial loss. There are a set of two contracts: the insurance company with the contract holder (policy holder) and the insurance company with the provider. This dynamic arrangement leads to considerable confusion and complexity for both clients and providers. With the rising cost of healthcare and and increasing number of clients becoming aware of their costs, health-related decisions may be altered. In light of this, as Page (2015) notes, it is important to consider the perspectives of each stakeholder: clients, employers, providers, and payors.

Client's Perspective

From the client's perspective, health insurance offers a benefit, typically obtained through their employer, that decreases their risk during changes in health. However, unlike a typical consumer environment where the customer directly pays for services, clients are one step removed from healthcare payments. In healthcare, there are three players: the client, the provider, and the insurance company. Thus the term third party payor. Even though clients have health insurance, they are not immune from incurring costs. There are insurances, premiums, deductibles, copays, and coinsurances. Each of which varies depending on the client's employer and plan. Lastly, coverage and payment differ based on provider, setting, and the payor. See Table 13.1

TABLE 13.1 **United States Healthcare Terminology**

Policyholder	• A person who has an insurance policy and pays premiums in exchange for coverage
Premium	• Payments to keep a healthcare plan active • Employer-based plans are deducted from the insured paychecks
Insured	• Any person receiving coverage under an insurance policy (e.g., the policyholder and their children)
Insurer	• Health insurance company or carrier that provides coverage to policyholders in exchange for premium payments
Uninsured	• No health insurance coverage
Underinsured	• Out-of-pocket costs, excluding premiums, over the prior 12 months equaled 10% or more of their household income
Policy limit	• Maximum amount an insurer will pay for a particular type of coverage
Plan Year	• A 12-month period (typically a calendar year) of benefits coverage
Verification	• Process of confirming coverage and benefits prior to an encounter
Preauthorization	• Providers obtain advance approval from an insurer before a service is delivered to the client • AKA precertification or prior approval
Exclusions	• Specific medical conditions or situations where an insurance policy does not provide benefits
Visit limits	• Determining how many visits the client has per year (e.g., a client has 20 OT and PT visits per year) • During the insurance verification process, it is important to determine if any visits have been used that year
Unit limits	• Determining how many units can be billed per session (e.g., insurer restricts each OT or PT session to no more than three units per session) • Determining if certain units are not covered
Deductible	• Set amount you pay for medical services before health insurance policy pays any benefits
Copay	• Set rate the insured pays for prescriptions, provider visits, and other types of care (e.g., $20)
Coinsurance	• Percentage of costs the insured pays after meeting their deductible (e.g., 20%)
Out-of-pocket maximum	• Limit the amount of money the insured pays for healthcare services in a plan year • Once met, all covered healthcare costs for the rest of the plan year are paid at 100%
In-network	• When a provider accepts the insured's health insurance • Established contract between provider and payor
Out-of-network	• When a provider does not accept the insured's health insurance • No contract between provider and payor

High deductible health plan (HDHP)	• Minimum deductible (2023)
	  • $1500 for an individual
	  • $3000 for a family

TABLE 13.1	United States Healthcare Terminology—cont'd
Health savings account (HSA)	• Requires an HDHP • Owned by individual and carries over with employment changes • Unused funds roll over every year • Employees and employers can contribute
Flexible spending account (FSA)	• Owned by the employer and lost with a job change • Funds expire at the end of the year • Employees and employers can contribute
Health reimbursement account (HRA)	• Employer-funded plan that reimburses employees for medical expenses • Only the employer can contribute
Fee schedule	• Negotiated list of payment rates by procedure (low risk for the provider) • AKA per procedure
Case rate	• Inclusive payments such as per diem, per visit, or per episode
Capitation	• Flat fee for a set period for each member of a health insurance plan (higher risk for the provider)
Cash-Based Practice	• Collection at the time of service • Limited or no insurance contracts • Provide noncovered services such as health promotion; prevention programs; educational seminars; weight loss programs; and sports performance enhancement programs
Pro Bono	• Providing therapy services at no cost to the individual • Donating professional expertise and service to charitable groups or organizations

OT, Occupational therapy; *PT,* physical therapy.

for common terminology associated with the United States healthcare system.

The Employer's Perspective

From an employer's perspective, health insurance is a benefit that helps with cost control. Instead of raising wages, employers offer health insurance, a form of compensation that is nontaxable. Unfortunately, exploding healthcare costs have strained employers, forcing them to reduce their costs by reducing the number of eligible employees, offering a variety of healthcare plans, and increasing employees' healthcare plan contributions and deductibles. The Affordable Care Act (ACA), also known as Obamacare, requires employers with 50 or more employees to offer full-time employees and their dependents health insurance. If an employer does not offer health benefits to qualified employees, the employer faces penalties and fines. The ACA also mandates that employee contributions cannot exceed 9.83% of the employee's household income. The ACA also mandates that health insurance coverage pays a minimum of 60% of the cost of covered services (Internal Revenue Service, 2022).

The Provider's Perspective

From a provider's perspective, understanding the ins and outs of health insurance is critical because, for most providers, insurance is their highest source of income. Unfortunately, payment or reimbursement is ever-changing. First, providers must establish contracts with health insurance

companies to be considered in-network. Clients typically do not seek care from providers out of network because it will cost them more. Also, healthcare plans change yearly (typically renewing on January 1 of each year). Renewing policies affects how individuals seek healthcare services. For one, deductibles reset; thus individuals may be reluctant to seek care earlier in the year. Also, the plan may be through a different insurance company. Is the provider in-network with this carrier? The new plan may carry a higher copay or coinsurance. If so, clients may be less likely to attend therapy sessions. Lastly, providers may be forced to change their care based on insurance restrictions.

Payor's Perspective

From the insurer's/payor's perspective, health insurance companies are for-profit companies with shareholders and thus need to be profitable. Therefore like any business, they work to increase revenues and control costs. Insurers increase revenue by selling as many policies as possible and they control costs by becoming more efficient administratively and decreasing reimbursement to providers. Insurance companies have significant leverage because they negotiate with employers for contracts to cover their employees and, simultaneously, negotiate with providers to provide the services to their policyholders. Furthermore, insurers/payors control costs by addressing fraud, abuse, and waste.

Fraud, Abuse, and Waste

Fraud consists of intentionally and knowingly submitting inaccurate claims for reimbursement (Centers for Medicare and Medicaid Services [CMS], 2021a). Providers who commit fraud use deceptive practices such as charging twice for a service or billing for services never provided. Abuse describes practices that result in unnecessary costs, including billing for services that were not indicated or medically necessary. Waste is unnecessary costs due to deficient management practices, overutilization of services, or misuse of resources.

Monitoring for Fraud, Abuse, and Waste

Three main federal government entities guide monitoring fraud and billing therapy-related services abuse: The Department of Health and Human Services, the Office of the Inspector General, and the Department of Justice. Legislation has been passed to combat fraud and abuse in healthcare-related billing. The Federal Civil False Claims Act (FCA) was created in 1863 during the Civil War. Many revisions have been made to this legislation, with the most recent in 2020 that updated the penalties for submitting false claims (CMS, 2021a). The purpose of the FCA has remained steady, with the focus on protecting the federal government from being overcharged. The law applied to all goods and services charged to the federal government, including healthcare-related services. Penalties for violating the FCA include fines, imprisonment, or both (CMS, 2021a). The Anti-Kickback Statute was created in 1972 as part of the Social Security Amendments. This statute broadened the FCA to make it illegal to receive or offer rewards for client referrals or other business-generating strategies. "Safe harbor" regulations within the Anti-Kickback Statute define business practices considered exempt from it (CMS, 2021a). There are numerous instances where rehabilitation providers have been investigated by the Office of the Inspector General for fraud, abuse, and waste when providing services. Box 13.1 provides an example.

Steps to Avoid Fraud, Abuse, and Waste

In light of the recent increase in legal actions against rehabilitation providers, which best practices can reduce providers' risk of fraud, abuse, or waste? The first best practice is to record the duration of a session accurately. Many of the

---

• BOX 13.1   Fraud in Therapy Settings

In May 2019, the United States Attorney's Office for the District of South Carolina found that Carolina Physical Therapy and Sports Medicine Inc. knowingly submitted fraudulent claims to Medicare and TRICARE based on a whistleblower complaint by an employee under the False Claims Act. The organization was found to have submitted claims for services provided to multiple clients simultaneously but billed for services as if the services were provided in a one-on-one format. The settlement resulted in the organization paying $790,000 to resolve the claim.

United States Department of Justice. (2019). Carolina physical therapy and sports medicine, inc. to pay $790,000 to resolve false billing allegations. https://www.justice.gov/usao-sc/pr/carolina-physical-therapy-and-sports-medicine-inc-pay-790000-resolve-false-billing

---

billing codes are time-based. By accurately recording the time spent with a client, the provider can avoid a common mistake of inflating the amount of time, also known as "rounding up." Rehabilitation providers should also accurately record if the client received a group or concurrent session versus an individual session (Table 13.2). The second-best practice pertains to the use of therapy aides. Therapy aides are not licensed providers; therefore services provided by an aide cannot be billed to Medicare and many managed care payors. Medicare states, "[services] provided by aides, even if under the supervision of a therapist, are ... not covered." (CMS, 2021b). Services provided by a physical therapy assistant (PTA) or occupational therapy assistant (OTA) can be reimbursed if properly supervised (CMS, 2021). Rehabilitation providers must know supervision requirements based on state practice acts and payor-specific requirements. Another best practice is to bill Current Procedural Terminology (CPT) codes that accurately reflect each session's services. Rehabilitation providers must possess a working knowledge of the interventions covered by each CPT code. Although many settlements pertain to organizations that have misbilled for services, the rehabilitation providers may also be held liable since they signed off on the billing. The false billing practice could jeopardize the provider's license if the rehabilitation provider's mistaken billing were done knowingly or unknowingly (American Physical Therapy Association, 2017).

Ethical Practice and Billing

Ethical practice relates not only to providing medically necessary services but also to how those services are billed. Professional organizations at the state and national levels provide documents that outline ethical practice and the consequences of unethical practice. The American Occupational Therapy Association (AOTA) provides an OT Code of Ethics document that outlines six key principles of ethical practice and provides an opportunity for any stakeholders to file an ethics complaint. AOTA has an Ethics Commission Committee that reviews complaints and enforces the procedures related to OT ethical practice (AOTA, 2020). The American Physical Therapy Association (APTA) provides a PT Code of Ethics document outlining eight key principles of PT ethical practice. If a stakeholder believes there has been a violation of the Code of Ethics for the PT or PTA, a complaint can be filed with the APTA's Ethics and Judicial Committee. In addition to the national organizations, state-specific boards related to OT and PT have an enforced ethics code of conduct with specific procedures for violations. Clinicians should review their national organization's code of ethics (Chapter 5) and all states where the clinician is licensed to comply fully with the state and national expectations for ethical practice.

CPT Codes – How Therapists Get Paid

Regardless of the payor type, reimbursement is based on the CPT billing codes developed by the American Medical

TABLE 13.2   Payor-Specific Billing

Number of Simultaneous Clients	Medicare A Med A Replacement Plans	Med B	Medicaid (varies by state)	HMO	Private Pay
1 Client	Individual	Individual	Individual	Individual	Individual
2 Clients (similar activity)	Group (MDS allows up to 25% group/concurrent per discipline)	Group	Group	Group	NA
2 Clients (different activity)	Concurrent (MDS allows up to 25% group/concurrent per discipline)	Group	Group	Group	NA
3 Clients (similar activity)	Group (MDS allows up to 25% group/concurrent per discipline)	Group	Group	Group	NA
3 Clients (different activity)	NA.	Group	Group	Group	NA
4 Clients (similar activity)	Group (MDS allows up to 25 % group/concurrent per discipline)	Group	Group	Group	NA
4 Clients (different activity)	NA	Group	Group	Group	NA

HMO, Health maintenance organization; *MDS*, minimum data set; *Med*, Medicare.

TABLE 13.3   Medicare 8-Minute Rule Chart[a]

Time Spent (min)	Number of Billable Units
8 to 22	1
23 to 37	2
38 to 52	3
53 to 67	4
68 to 82	5
83 to 97	6

[a]This chart only applies to time-based codes.

Association (AMA). Codes typically used by OTs and PTs fall under the physical medicine and rehabilitation services and procedures (97001 to 97799 codes). Thus they are not specific to OT or PT, meaning that other providers, notably physicians and chiropractors, can bill these codes depending on the payor. All CPT codes typically fall into two categories, time- or service-based. Time-based codes follow the 8-minute rule (Table 13.3). This rule states that to bill one unit of a CPT code, you must provide at least 8 minutes of that treatment to bill for that code. Medicare reimbursement of time-based codes takes (Table 13.4) the total one-on-one minutes provided and divides that number by 15. After the division, if 8 or more minutes remain, you can bill for an additional unit. Less than 8 minutes is not billable (Table 13.4).

Service-based codes are untimed. These codes can only be billed as one unit regardless of the clinicians' amount of time with the client related to the CPT code. The most well-known service-based codes are the evaluation codes (Table 13.4). Other service-based codes include unattended biophysical agent modalities and reevaluations. See

Table 13.5 for examples of calculating billable minutes using Medicare's 8-minute rule.

Clinicians may provide services to clients one-on-one or multiple clients simultaneously. The number of clients receiving services simultaneously determines if the payors are billed for individual, concurrent, or group services. Each payor determines the definitions related to these delivery modes. Generally, individual treatment is defined as services provided by one clinician to one client. Concurrent is generally defined as the treatment of two clients simultaneously, each performing different activities regardless of payor source. It is defined as concurrent therapy for the Part A resident regardless of the payor source for the second resident. Group is defined as the treatment of no more than four clients performing the same or similar activities, regardless of payor source, and being supervised by a therapist or an assistant who does not supervise any other individuals.

Factors Affecting Payment

Numerous factors will affect payment for occupational and physical therapists; however, a major factor affecting payment is related to the Centers for Medicare and Medicaid Services (CMS) processes and legislation. CMS strongly influences other payors, especially managed care, due to CMS's relationships with the managed care entities in the roles of Medicare Administrative Contractors (MACs). Other payors include private insurance, military and veteran healthcare, workers' compensation, and motor vehicle insurance (Table 13.6).

Medicare

CMS is the federally run agency that oversees Medicare and Medicaid coverage of healthcare services. Medicare was created in 1965 to provide healthcare coverage for citizens

TABLE 13.4   Common CPT Codes (AOTA, 2016)(APTA, 2016)

CPT Code	LCD Manual Description	Sample Documentation
PT-97161 OT-97165 Low complexity evaluation	A client profile and medical and therapy history, which includes a brief history including review of medical and/or therapy records relating to the presenting problem. Analysis of data from problem-focused assessment.	Assessment that identifies 1–3 performance deficits (i.e., relating to physical cognitive or psychosocial skills) that result in activity limitations and/or participating restrictions. Client presentation is stable without foreseeable complications.
PT-97162 OT-97166 Moderate complexity evaluation	A client profile and medical and therapy history, which includes an expanded review of medical and/or therapy records and additional review of physical, cognitive, or psychosocial history related to current functional performance. Analysis of data from detailed assessment.	Assessment that identifies 3–5 performance deficits (i.e., relating to physical cognitive or psychosocial skills) that result in activity limitations and/or participating restrictions. Client presentation is evolving or changing.
PT-97163 OT-97167 High complexity evaluation	A client profile and medical and therapy history, which includes review of medical and/or therapy records and extensive additional review of physical, cognitive, or psychosocial history related to current functional performance. Analysis of data from comprehensive assessment.	Assessment that identifies 5 or more performance deficits (i.e., relating to physical cognitive or psychosocial skills) that result in activity limitations and/or participating restrictions. Client presentation is unstable.
97110 Therapeutic exercise	1. Therapeutic exercise is performed with a client either actively, active-assisted, or passively participating (e.g., isokinetic exercise, stretching, strengthening and gross and fine motor movement). 2. An occupational therapist may use this code when addressing impairments of exercise tolerance due to cardiopulmonary impairments. Therapeutic exercise with an individualized physical conditioning and exercise program using proper breathing techniques can be considered for a client with activity limitations secondary to cardiopulmonary impairments. 3. Therapeutic exercise is considered reasonable and necessary if at least one of the following conditions is present and documented: a. The client has weakness, contracture, stiffness secondary to spasm, spasticity, decreased joint range of motion, functional mobility deficits, balance and/or coordination deficits, abnormal posture, muscle imbalance. b. The client needs to improve mobility, flexibility, strengthening, coordination, control of extremities, dexterity, range of motion, or endurance as part of activities of daily living training, or reeducation. 4. Documentation supporting therapeutic exercise must document objective loss of joint motion, strength, coordination and /or mobility (e.g., degrees of motion, strength grades, and levels of assistance).	Starter phrase example: (Strength) patient received therapeutic exercise, which included: level of resistance, reps/sets, to muscle(s) of extremity. Exercise upgraded by amount of (reps, sets, resistance). Clinicians provided (verbal, tactile, visual) cues to maintain proper joint alignment during therapeutic exercise. Increasing strength to -/5 resulted in improved functional performance.
97112 Neuromuscular reeducation	1. This therapeutic procedure is provided to improve balance, coordination, kinesthetic sense, posture, motor planning, body awareness, and proprioception (e.g., proprioceptive neuromuscular facilitation, Feldenkrais, and Bobath). 2. Neuromuscular reeducation may be considered reasonable and necessary for impairments, which affect the body's neuromuscular system (e.g., poor static or dynamic sitting/standing balance, loss of gross and fine motor coordination, desensitization, proprioception, hypo/hypersensitivity, hypo/hypertonicity, and neglect).	Starter phrase example: patient received neuro re-ed for the facilitation of improved (static or dynamic sitting/standing balance, loss of gross and fine motor coordination, desensitization, proprioception, hypo/hypersensitivity, hypo/hypertonicity, and neglect) during the functional performance. Techniques used were PNF, NDT, Feldenkrais, and Bobath.

Code	Description
97140 Manual therapy techniques	1. Joint mobilization (peripheral or spinal) This procedure may be considered reasonable and necessary if restricted joint motion is present and documented. It may be reasonable and necessary as an adjunct to therapeutic exercises when loss of articular motion and flexibility impedes the therapeutic procedure. 2. Soft tissue mobilization. This procedure involves the application of skilled manual therapy techniques (active or passive) to soft tissues in order to effect changes in the soft tissues, articular structures, neural or vascular systems. Examples are facilitation of fluid exchange, restoration of movement in acutely edematous muscles, or stretching of shortened muscular or connective tissue. Myofascial release/soft tissue mobilization can be considered reasonable and necessary if at least one of the following conditions is present and documented: a. The client having restricted joint or soft tissue motion in an extremity, neck or trunk b. Treatment being a necessary adjunct to other occupational therapy interventions such as 97110, 97112 or 97530 3. Manual lymphatic drainage/complex decongestive physiotherapy. The goal of this type of therapy is to reduce lymphedema by routing the fluid to functional pathways, preventing backflow as the new routes become established, and to use the most appropriate methods to maintain the reduction after therapy is complete. This therapy involves intensive treatment to reduce the size of the extremity by a combination of manual decongestive therapy and serial compression bandaging, followed by an exercise program. a. It is expected that during these sessions, education is being provided to the client and/or caregiver on the correct application of the compression bandage. b. It is also expected that after the completion of the therapy, the client and/or caregiver can perform these activities without supervision.	Starter phrase example: patient received manual therapy using (myofascial release, short stretch, neuro stretch, joint mobilization, retrograde massage, soft tissue mobilization) to (location) to facilitate (clinical indication) which resulted in (underlying impairment you were using the manual therapy for).
97760 Orthotics fitting	1. This procedure may be considered reasonable and necessary, if there is an indication for education for the application of orthotics, and the functional use of the orthotic is present and documented. 2. Generally, orthotic training can be completed in three visits; however for modification of the orthotic due to healing of tissue, change in edema, or impairment in skin integrity additional visits may be required. 3. The medical record should document the distinct treatments rendered when orthotic training for upper and lower extremity is done. 4. The client is capable of being trained to use the particular device prescribed in an appropriate manner. In some cases, the client may not be able to perform this function, but a responsible individual can be trained to apply the device.	
97761 Prosthetic training	1. This procedure and training may be considered reasonable and necessary, if there is an indication for education in the application of the prosthesis, and the functional use of the prosthesis is present and documented. 2. The medical record should document the distinct goals and service rendered when prosthetic training for upper and lower extremity is done. 3. Periodic revisits beyond the third month would require documentation to support medical necessity.	
97762 Orthotic/prosthetic checkout	1. These assessments are reasonable and necessary when there is a modification or reissue of a recently issued device or a reassessment of a newly issued device. 2. These assessments may be reasonable and necessary when clients experience a loss of function directly related to the device (e.g., pain, skin breakdown, and falls). 3. These assessments may be reasonable and necessary for determining "the client's response to wearing the device, determining whether the client is donning/doffing the device correctly, determining the client's need for padding, underwrap, or socks and determining the client's tolerance to any dynamic forces being applied."	

Continued

TABLE 13.4 Common CPT Codes (AOTA, 2016)(APTA, 2016)—cont'd

CPT Code	LCD Manual Description	Sample Documentation
97530 Therapeutic activities	1. Therapeutic activities are considered reasonable and necessary for clients needing a broad range of rehabilitative techniques. Activities can be for a specific body part or could involve the entire body. This procedure involves the use of functional activities to improve performance in a progressive manner. The activities are usually directed at a loss or impairment of mobility, strength, balance, coordination or cognition. They require the skills of occupational therapists and are designed to address a specific functional need of the client. These dynamic activities must be part of an active written plan of treatment and be directed at a specific outcome. 2. In order for therapeutic activities to be covered, the following requirements must be met: a. The client having a condition for which therapeutic activities can reasonably be expected to restore or improve functioning. B. The client's condition being such that they are unable to perform therapeutic activities except under the supervision of an occupational therapist. c. There being a clear correlation between the type of exercise performed and the client's underlying medical condition for which the therapeutic activities were prescribed.	Starter phrase example: patient received therapeutic act using activity graded at (give parameters and description of activity including time, level of complexity, level of assist) to address (underlying impairment) to facilitate improvement in (functional deficit).
97535 Self-Care/home management training	The coverage criteria and definition of self-care/home management training is found in the CMS Manual System, Pub 100-03[a], "Self-care/home management training (97535) describes a group of interventions that focuses on activities of daily living skills and compensatory activities needed to achieve independence or adapt to an evolving deterioration in health and function. These include activities such as dressing, bathing, food preparation, and cooking. The client may require adaptive equipment and/or assistive technology in the home environment. This code includes training the client and/or caregiver in the use of the equipment." This code should not be used globally for all home instructions. When instructing the client in a self-management program, use the code that best describes the focus of the self-management activity.	Starter phrase example: patient received self-care training using (adaptive equipment or adaptive strategy) graded at (give parameters and description of activity including time, level of complexity, level of assist) to address (underlying impairment that impacts the specific ADL you are addressing) to facilitate improvement in (functional deficit).
97542 Wheelchair management training	Wheelchair management "includes assessing if the client needs a wheelchair, determining what kind of wheelchair is appropriate, including its size and components, measuring the client to ensure proper fit, and fitting the client into the chair once it is received. This code is also used for reporting the time associated with training the client and/or caregiver in transfers in and out of the chair as well as propulsion on all surfaces. It is important for the therapist to provide instructions for safety so as not to risk skin breakdown or a fall." 1. This service trains the client in functional activities that promote optimal safety, mobility and transfers. Clients who are wheelchair bound may occasionally need skilled input on positioning to avoid pressure points, contractures, and other medical complications. 2. This procedure is reasonable and necessary only when it requires the skills of an occupational therapist, is designed to address specific needs of the client, and must be part of an active written plan of treatment directed at a specific goal. 3. The client and/or caregiver must have the capacity to learn from instructions. 4. Typically, three to four sessions should be sufficient to teach the client and/or caregiver these skills. 5. When billing CPT code 97542 for wheelchair propulsion training, documentation must relate the training to expected functional goals that are attainable by the client.	Starter phrase example: patient received wheelchair management training using propulsion method of (UE or LE) ft. with (verbal/tactile/visual cues, level of assist) to address functional mobility to facilitate improvement in (functional deficit). Wheelchair adaptations completed by clinician include (list wheelchair modifications done and why that modification was necessary).

[a]Medicare national coverage determinations, Chapter 1, Part 3, §170.1 https://www.cms.gov/regulations-and-guidance/guidance/manuals/downloads/ncd103c1_part3.pdf
AOTA, American Occupational Therapy Association; APTA, American Physical Therapy Association; CMS, Centers for Medicare and Medicaid Services; CPT, current procedural terminology; LCD, local coverage determination; LE, lower extremity, OT, occupational therapy; PT, physical therapy; UE, upper extremity.

TABLE 13.5 Calculating Billable Minutes Using Medicare's 8-Minute Rule

Example 1	Timed Minutes	Untimed Minutes	Medicare 8-Minute Rule	Billable Units
Therapeutic exercise 97110	25	NA	15+10	2
Therapeutic activities 97530	15	NA	15	1
Therapeutic ultrasound 97035	8	NA	8	0
Electrical stimulation unattended 97104	NA	15	NA	1
Total treatment time?	63 minutes (25 + 15 + 8 + 15)			
Total time-based codes?	48 minutes (25 + 15 + 8)			
Total billable units?	4 (3 time-based codes + 1 service-based code)			
Example 2	**Timed Minutes**	**Untimed Minutes**	**Medicare 8-Minute Rule**	**Billable Units**
Initial evaluation 97166	NA	35	NA	1
Therapeutic activities 97530	25	NA	15 + 10	2
Therapeutic ultrasound 97035	10	NA	10	0
Total treatment time?	70 minutes (35 + 25 + 10)			
Total time-based codes?	35 minutes (25 + 10)			
Total billable units?	3 (2 time-based codes + 1 service-based code)			

TABLE 13.6 Payors

Medicare A	• Automatically enrolled at no cost at age 65 or otherwise eligible • Provides health insurance for inpatient hospital services, short-term nursing home care, and home healthcare
Medicare B	• Voluntary • May have deductions made from monthly social security benefits to pay for Part B • Covers outpatient health services including OT and PT, diagnostic tests, visits to the physicians, and durable medical equipment
Medicare C	• Medicare + Choice, now known as Medicare Advantage • If already enrolled in Medicare A and B may choose alternative coordinated care plans • Requires higher premiums (social security deductions), but includes expanded benefits such as no deductibles, smaller copayments, no cost annual physical examinations • Preventative diagnostic screens, prescription drug coverage, health promotion programs
Medicare D	• The Medicare Prescription Drug, Improvement, and Modernization Act of 2003 • Includes prescription drug benefits for Medicare Part A and B enrollees
Medicaid	• Administered and managed by the state: variable state to state • The state must follow certain federal mandates to receive federal funding • Health insurance for individuals with low-income, children, or those with a disability • Income-based, means-test entitlement, enrollment limited to people below certain limited income and asset levels
Military and veteran healthcare	• Tricare • Regionally managed healthcare program for active duty and retired members of the uniformed services, their family members, and survivors
	• Veterans Affairs (VA) coverage • Pays for services available to veterans in good standing at VA approved facilities level of coverage is based upon placement into a priority group
	• Civilian Health and Medical Program of the Department of Veteran Affairs (CHAMPVA) • A comprehensive healthcare program in which the VA shares the cost of covered healthcare services and supplies with eligible beneficiaries • Secondary insurance to Medicare

Continued

TABLE 13.6	Payors—cont'd

Workers' compensation	• Varies state to state (i.e., there are state statutes governing workers' compensation)
	• Purpose ("the grand bargain")
	  • Protects employers
	    • No direct, out of pocket payment
	    • Business owners are protected from civil lawsuits related to unintentional injuries
	  • Protects workers
	    • Medical expenses
	    • Lost wages
	    • Ongoing care (e.g., vocational rehabilitation)
	    • Funeral expenses

Motor vehicle crash	• Motor vehicle crash
	• Fault vs. no-fault case
	  • Personal injury protection (PIP)
	    • Some states PIP is required, but in many it is optional
	    • Ranges from $2500 to $50,000 per person
	  • Without/beyond PIP options to pay include:
	    • MedPay supplemental coverage
	    • Client's health insurance
	    • Cash pay

Private insurance	• Any health insurance coverage offered by a private entity instead of a state or federal government • Also known as commercial insurance • Common plans include PPO and HMO • Typically provided as group-sponsored insurance, offered by an employer

OT, Occupational therapy; *PT,* physical therapy.

aged 65 years and older. In the 1970s, coverage was expanded to include end-stage renal disease and long-term disability (≥24 months) for individuals under 65 years. Medicare did not cover home health and hospice services until the 1980s (HOI, 2021). The 1990s brought the first major reimbursement changes due to the Balanced Budget Act of 1996. In the 2010s, quality assurance process improvement became part of the mandates on healthcare organizations receiving Medicare reimbursement. The most recent major changes to reimbursement occurred in 2019 with the implementation of the Patient Driven Payment Model (PDPM) and Patient Driven Grouping Model (PDGM) (CMS, 2021b).

Medicare is not free. It is funded via taxes based on the Federal Insurance Contributions Act (FICA). While working, employees and employers are taxed 1.45% of the employee's gross wages, totaling 2.9%. Medicare has two main categories, Part A and Part B. Medicare Part A is the acute and post-acute care benefit (Chapter 16), covering short- and long-term acute care (i.e., hospital care and LTACH), skilled nursing facilities, inpatient rehabilitation facilities, home health, and hospice. Medicare Part B is the outpatient benefit. Both Part A and B cover rehabilitation services provided by a licensed rehabilitation professional. Rehabilitation services are reimbursed based on CPT codes that reflect the services delivered each session. Medicare Part C or Medicare Advantage Plan collaborates between Medicare and managed care organizations. Part C offers members

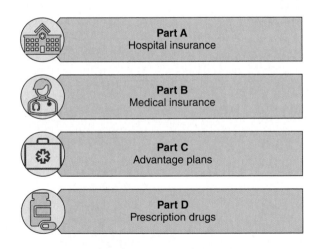

🏥	**Part A** Hospital insurance
👩‍⚕️	**Part B** Medical insurance
✚	**Part C** Advantage plans
💊	**Part D** Prescription drugs

• **Fig. 13.1** Parts of Medicare

Medicare-like services typically at a lower premium. Part C criteria for rehabilitation services varies based on the policies of each managed care organization. Part D helps cover the cost of prescription drugs (Fig. 13.1).

Medicaid

Medicaid was established in 1965 through Title XIX of the Social Security Act. Medicaid is state-run but funded by state and federal tax dollars. Each state creates and manages its own Medicaid program with state-generated taxes but must adhere to certain eligibility guidelines to qualify for matching federal money. Thus there are 51 variations of Medicaid (50 states and Washington, DC). It is traditionally a benefit for individuals who qualify for low-income status based on the federal poverty level or disability requirements.

Managed care organizations partner with each state to back the Medicaid offerings. In addition to policies and procedures, Medicaid coverage varies state by state. Some states use a process known as case-mix, which reimburses based on multiple factors such as services provided, and the level of care required. Other states use a prior authorization process. Prior authorization requires that the therapist send in a completed plan of care evaluation and then wait for the state to approve services before proceeding. Each state and process type can have specific documentation requirements.

Private Insurance and Managed Care

Private insurance (i.e., commercial insurance) is any health insurance coverage offered by a private entity instead of a state or federal government. Private insurance can be obtained via employer-based health insurance or individual plans. The latter is obtained by an individual directly from an insurance company. Employer-based or sponsored health insurance, the most common form of health insurance coverage, is purchased by an employer and offered to eligible employees and dependents. Employers typically share the cost of premiums with employees.

Most health insurance plans in the United States are managed care plans. The premise of managed care is to focus on prevention and care management to reduce costs and improve outcomes for individuals who do not qualify for Medicare or Medicaid. Managed care is an umbrella term that encompasses two main types of insurance coverage that impact rehabilitation services: health maintenance organization (HMO) and preferred provider organization (PPO). Managed care creates categories of providers known as "in-network" and "out of network." These network designations delineate contracted reimbursement rates between providers and managed care organizations. The idea is for individuals to use "in-network" providers as much as possible to control overall care costs (*Glossary*, 2022).

HMO is a health insurance plan that enforces care criteria for various healthcare providers. The focus of an HMO is integrated care that focuses on health and wellness. Often the HMOs will require providers to obtain a preauthorization or referral for healthcare services. Preauthorizations and referral requirements allow the HMO to control costs before providing services. PPO is also a health insurance plan that encourages individuals to use "in-network" providers. Unlike HMOs, PPOs typically do not require preauthorization for rehabilitation services because healthcare providers have established contracts. Each type of managed care requires different documentation requirements and requirements for CPT codes. Clinicians must know the specific requirements for the insurance plans held by their clients to minimize the risk of reimbursement denials (*Glossary*, 2022).

Claim Submission, Denials, and Appeals

When a payor refuses to pay a claim, it is known as a denial. Denials can be appealed if the provider has strong evidence to overturn the denial. The Medicare appeals process consists of five levels (Fig. 13.2). If appealing claims up to levels 3 and 5, the claim amount must exceed a specified dollar amount. Organizations have an appointed representative as the primary point of contact during the appeals process. Typically, the representative is someone in a management role who works with the organization's attorney.

First-level appeals request the MAC to make a redetermination after receiving the denial. The organization has 120 days from the denial date to request a redetermination. Each payor has a specific request form that must be completed to request a MAC redetermination. The MAC has 60 days from the date the MAC received the redetermination request to decide. The MAC must have a different staff review the redetermination than was involved with the initial denial. The MAC can dismiss a redetermination request if the organization withdraws the appeal or fails to provide the proper information and documentation.

Second-level appeals are known as the Qualified Independent Contractor (QIC) reconsideration. They occur if the organization disagrees with the MAC redetermination decision to have the denial stand. The organization must request the reconsideration within 180 days of the original denial. The organization must submit the reconsideration request within 60 days after receiving the MAC redetermination dismissal.

Third-level appeals are the Office of Medicare Hearing and Appeals (OMHA) disposition. If the organization disagrees with the reconsideration, an administrative law judge (hearing can be requested at this point if the dollar amount of the claim meets the established threshold. This hearing occurs by phone or teleconference. The hearing allows an organization to state the case for why the claim should be paid. The administrative law judge request must be filed within 60 days of receiving the reconsideration decision letter.

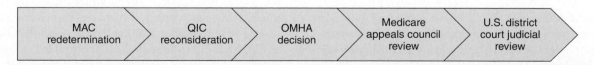

• **Fig. 13.2** Levels of Medicare Appeals Process (Centers for Medicare and Medicaid Services [2021]. *Medicare parts A & B appeals process.* https://www.cms.gov/outreach-and-education/medicare-learning-network-mln/mlnproducts/downloads/medicareappealsprocess.pdf)

Most appeals will end with the third level and rarely advance to levels 4 and 5 because of the number of resources an organization must allocate to appeal claims at each level effectively. The process discussed has been specific to CMS; however, most managed care payors follow a similar process.

The manager is typically responsible for assembling information for the appeal packets. The packets typically include medical documentation, therapy documentation, billing records, and any additional information pertinent to the denied claim. Another responsibility of managers is to mitigate risk by ensuring therapy documentation is thorough and complete (CMS 2021a).

Typically, the rehabilitation manager's responsibility is to ensure the specific requirements are met to minimize the risk of denials. To comply with rules and regulations, rehabilitation providers must remain current on Medicare and Medicaid coverage criteria. By remaining updated on payor-specific requirements, rehabilitation providers can reduce the likelihood of payment denial.

Medicare Administrative Contractors

CMS outsources the management of Medicare administration to Medicare Administrative Contractors (MAC). MACs are managed care organizations selected by CMS to process claims and denials. MACs have jurisdiction based on a geographic region. These contracts between CMS and MACs frequently change, so rehabilitation managers must be apprised of any changes to MACs since the MACs dictate policy and procedure for processing claims (CMS, 2022a).

CMS created the National Coverage Determination (NCD) and Local Coverage Determination (LCD) manuals to clarify the circumstances in which CMS will cover specific services. The LCD is in place when there is no NCD policy and is at the discretion of the MACs. The LCD is driven by specific MACs and is typically the most relevant to rehabilitation services. These manuals provide listings of diagnosis codes that allow OT, PT, and speech therapy services to be covered. Billing codes, known as CPT codes, are described in detail to assist clinicians in charging for the most accurate codes to reflect the services provided in each session. The LCD manuals are a significant resource in minimizing denials of payment by outlining key terms that should be included in rehabilitation providers' documentation for service justification. CMS regularly publishes the NCDs and LCDs updates, informed by evidence-based practice to guide payment. Based on the most recent NCD and LCD information, clinicians must stay current in billing practices (CMS, 2022b; 2022c).

Transition to Outcome-Based Healthcare

The Affordable Care Act (ACA), known as Obamacare, sought to improve overall client outcomes and increase efficiency. A report to Congress found that the service-based reimbursement system produced lower margins for clients with the following characteristics: deficits in parenteral nutrition; the presence of traumatic wounds or ulcers; requiring substantial assistance in bathing; admitted admission to home health services following an acute or post-acute stay; possess a high Hierarchical Condition Category score; certain poorly controlled clinical conditions; dually eligible. Overall, ACA emphasizes that reimbursement should be based on client characteristics instead of the number of therapy visits (CMS, 2022).

Thus CMS launched the new client-driven payment models for skilled nursing and home health, respectively known as the PDPM and PDGM, in 2019. The overarching reimbursement measures for PDPM and PDGM are outcomes for key performance areas based on the client's characteristics. Rehabilitation providers working in the post-acute care sector will significantly impact how they approach treatment delivery and outcomes measurement. Rehabilitation providers must shift the mindset to deeper clinical reasoning for treatment plan development and execution. The clinical reasoning process will be imperative in illustrating the value of rehabilitation services. The PDPM is a budget-neutral reimbursement model that impacts skilled nursing facilities caring for clients under Medicare Part A. PDPM replaced the Resource Utilization Groups (RUGs) model that had been in place since the late 1990s. PDPM is a major shift from minute-based service delivery to outcomes-based service delivery (CMS, 2018).

A common trend in skilled nursing post-acute care therapy practice has been delivering interventions individually, also known as 1:1 therapy. This 1:1 mode of service delivery was primarily due to the reimbursement constraints under the RUGs model. Employers now strongly encourage clinicians to deliver 25% of interventions using a group or concurrent model. Group delivery consists of four clients with one practitioner (4:1) and all clients performing a similar task. Concurrent delivery consists of two clients performing different tasks simultaneously with one practitioner (2:1) (CMS, 2018). This 25% rule has minimal changes between RUGs and PDPM payment models. The most relevant change under PDPM is that group and concurrent are combined within the 25% allocation. The previous RUGs model did not factor concurrent delivery into the 25% allocation. A common misconception is that the 25% group and concurrent delivery are a requirement under PDPM. The appropriateness of service delivery using individual, group, and concurrent interventions should be at the clinical discretion of the clinician based on individual client factors and the clinician's clinical reasoning.

The PDGM is a budget-neutral reimbursement model that impacts home health providers. Home Health Resource Groups (HHRGs) are the current model that began phasing out on January 1, 2020. The rationale behind the payment model change is to focus more on the client's characteristics instead of the number of visits. Success with PDGM, same as PDPM, is dependent on illustrating value through therapy services, clinical reasoning, and outcomes (CMS, 2018).

In a report to Congress, the need for value-based reimbursement was illustrated by the following report findings: the Medicare Home Health (HH) benefit is ill-defined; HH payment should not be based on the number of therapy visits; payments based on therapy thresholds create financial incentives that distract agencies from focusing on client characteristics when setting plans of care; a trend of notable shifts away from nontherapy visits; HH payment should be determined by client characteristics (CMS, 2018).

Bundled Payments

Bundled Payments for Care Improvement (BPCI) Initiative is a payment system that combines payments for multiple services for a client under a single episode of care. BPCI replaces the traditional model of healthcare reimbursement from fee-for-service to value-based care (Figs. 13.3a and 13.3b). The

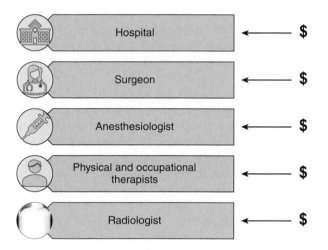

• **Fig. 13.3a** Fee for service results in payment for each service, regardless of quantity or quality.

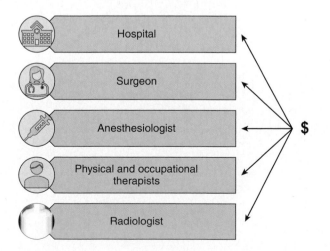

• **Fig. 13.3b** Bundled payment is a single, comprehensive payment that covers all of the services to promote comprehensive and coordinated care.

idea behind this initiative was to create financial and outcomes accountability across the continuum of care. BPCI has four models of care that can be used (Fig. 13.4). All models of care under BPCI aim to improve care quality and coordination while controlling costs. These bundled payments are shared between hospitals, post-acute care facilities, physicians, and other healthcare services reimbursable under Medicare (CMS, 2022a).

The BPCI Awardee is the entity that assumes financial responsibility for the client's episode of care, and frequently, this is the acute care organization since most clients begin episodes of care in this setting. Providers who do not assume financial responsibility can initiate the episodes of care. These are known as BPCI Episode Initiators (CMS, 2022). For example, consider a client who sustained a fall resulting in a hip fracture but has no comorbidities or complicating diagnoses. Medicare pays the BPCI Awardee $50,000 for an episode of care for this case. The acute care stay with surgical intervention for the hip fracture costs $25,000. That leaves $25,000 to be divided between the rest of the providers for that episode of care. If the remaining post-acute care costs are less than the remaining $25,000, the funds leftover are distributed by the BPCI Awardee as positive income. Now, consider that the same client has numerous comorbidities that profoundly impact the rehabilitation process. The acute care cost remains $25,000. However, the post-acute care costs totaled $35,000—the total care would result in a $10,000 loss. Because the BPCI Awardee assumed the financial risk, they are responsible for the additional $10,000 (CMS, 2022).

Payment Alternatives and Considerations

In the United States, most of the individuals receiving rehabilitation services are insured. In 2020, employment-based insurance was the most common (~54%), followed by Medicare (~18%), Medicaid (~17%), TRICARE (~3%), and Veterans Affairs-related coverage (~1%) (Note: total exceeds 100% as some individuals have more than one health insurance) (Keisler-Starkey & Bunch, 2021). For approximately 9%–13% of the population without those policies, private payor grants are options for reimbursing rehabilitation services (Keisler-Starkey & Bunch, 2021; *United States Health Insurance Coverage in 2020*, 2020). Private pay is a payment structure where the client pays for services out-of-pocket. Typically, private pay situations occur when individuals have exhausted insurance benefits or do not have any insurance or Medicare. Documentation requirements for private pay are not mandatory; however, most organizations will follow the documentation requirements established by managed care or Medicare. Grants are another option for reimbursing rehabilitation services. Frequently, grant-funded therapy programs are in a community-based model. The specific grant guidelines often determine the required documentation for grant-based reimbursement.

Model 1	Model 2	Model 3	Model 4
• Retrospective payment for all **acute care services** • This model concluded in 2016	• Retrospective payment for all **acute and post-acute care services** • Expenditures vs. target price	• Retrospective payment for all **post-acute care services** • Expenditures vs. target price	• Prospective payment for all **acute care services** • Single lump-sum payment

• **Fig. 13.4** Bundled Payments Models

Cash Practice

Cash practice includes collection at the time of service, limited insurance contracts, no insurance contracts, and noncovered services. First, providers must collect all fees (e.g., copays, deductibles) at the time of service. Second, providers can select to participate with private insurance companies who provide appropriate payment for services while avoiding private insurance contracts with those who pay poorly, which prevents the provider from covering the cost of care. This hybrid model allows providers to be in-network with some providers and out-of-network with others. Third, providers may opt out of all private insurances, thus becoming out-of-network providers for all private insurances. As an out-of-network provider, you can set your fee schedule, appointment times, visits, and services without the limitations of in-network contractual agreements. Lastly, providers may offer noncovered services such as health and wellness, sports performance, and educational services not normally covered by insurance companies (APTA, 2020a)

Federal law prevents occupational and physical therapists from opting out of the Medicare program (APTA, 2020b). Thus occupational and physical therapists have three types of relationships with Medicare. First, they can be participating providers, which means they have a contractual relationship with the Centers for Medicare and Medicaid Services (CMS) to accept all clients and provide them with any Medicare-covered services (i.e., accept assignment). Accepting assignment indicates that the provider will accept Medicare's approved amount for healthcare services as full payment. Second, OTs and PTs can be nonparticipating providers, which means they have a contractual relationship with CMS and cannot turn away Medicare clients altogether. However, they do not have to accept assignments for all Medicare-covered services. Under certain circumstances, they can charge more than the Medicare-approved amount for any covered services but not more than what is referred to as the "limiting charge" (*Lower Costs with Assignment | Medicare*, 2021).

Lastly, occupational and physical therapists do not have to enroll in Medicare, which means they are not labeled as participating or nonparticipating providers (i.e., no relationship). It is essential to note that occupational and physical therapists who are nonparticipating providers or have no relationship with Medicare do not equate to opting out. By not enrolling, occupational and physical therapists cannot treat or collect payment from Medicare beneficiaries for any Medicare-covered services. However, they could accept out-of-pocket payments from Medicare clients if it is deemed a noncovered service.

Noncovered services fall into four categories (Fig. 13.5) (CMS, 2020). First, services and supplies are not deemed medically reasonable and necessary. Not medically reasonable or necessary services include long-term nursing home/custodial care, dental care, eye exams for glasses, hearing aids, cosmetic surgery, acupuncture, and routine foot care (*What's Not Covered by Part A & Part B?*, 2021). Second, noncovered items and services are items and services provided to the client that do not meet the definition of any Medicare benefit. Covered tests, items, or services can be found on Medicare.gov/coverage. Third, services and supplies are denied as bundled or included in the basic allowance of another service, such as case management. For

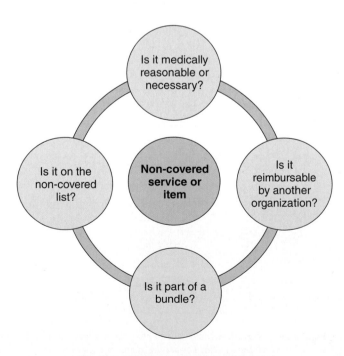

• **Fig. 13.5** Medicare's Noncovered Services

example, Medicare will not pay separately for some services and supplies because they are part of routine client care (e.g., case management services and supplies included in the basic allowance). Lastly, items and services are reimbursable by other organizations or furnished without charges, such as automobile insurance, liability insurance, and workers' compensation (CMS, 2020).

If the provider deems that Medicare is not likely to cover the service, the client must be given a waiver of liability form known as an advanced beneficiary notice (ABN) (Fig. 13.6) (CMS, 2021c). Based on Medicare coverage rules, the ABN indicates that the provider believes that Medicare will not pay for the service and that liability for charges is being transferred to the beneficiary. It must be

A. Notifier:

B. Patient name: **C. Identification number:**

Advance Beneficiary Notice of Non-coverage
(ABN)

NOTE: If Medicare doesn't pay for **D.** _____ below, you may have to pay.
Medicare does not pay for everything, even some care that you or your health care provider have good reason to think you need. We expect Medicare may not pay for the **D.** _____ below.

D.	E. Reason medicare may not pay:	F. Estimated cost:

WHAT YOU NEED TO DO NOW:

- Read this notice, so you can make an informed decision about your care.
- Ask us any questions that you may have after you finish reading.
- Choose an option below about whether to receive the **D.** _____ listed above.
  Note: If you choose Option 1 or 2, we may help you to use any other insurance that you might have, but Medicare cannot require us to do this.

G. OPTIONS: Check only one box. We cannot choose a box for you.
☐ **OPTION 1.** I want the **D.** _____ listed above. You may ask to be paid now, but I also want Medicare billed for an official decision on payment, which is sent to me on a Medicare Summary Notice (MSN). I understand that if Medicare doesn't pay, I am responsible for payment, but I can appeal to Medicare by following the directions on the MSN. If Medicare does pay, you will refund any payments I made to you, less co-pays or deductibles.
☐ **OPTION 2.** I want the **D.** _____ listed above, but do not bill Medicare. You may ask to be paid now as I am responsible for payment. I cannot appeal if Medicare is not billed.
☐ **OPTION 3.** I don't want the **D.** _____ listed above. I understand with this choice I am **not** responsible for payment, and I cannot appeal to see if Medicare would pay.

H. Additional information:

This notice gives our opinion, not an official Medicare decision. If you have other questions on this notice or Medicare billing, call **1-800-MEDICARE** (1-800-633-4227/**TTY**: 1-877-486-2048). Signing below means that you have received and understand this notice. You also receive a copy.

I. Signature:	J. Date:

CMS does not discriminate in its programs and activities. To request this publication in an alternative format, please call: 1-800-MEDICARE or email: AltFormatRequest@cms.hhs.gov.

According to the Paperwork Reduction Act of 1995, no persons are required to respond to a collection of information unless it displays a valid OMB control number. The valid OMB control number for this information collection is 0938-0566. The time required to complete this information collection is estimated to average 7 minutes per response, including the time to review instructions, search existing data resources, gather the data needed, and complete and review the information collection. If you have comments concerning the accuracy of the time estimate or suggestions for improving this form, please write to: CMS, 7500 Security Boulevard, Attn: PRA Reports Clearance Officer, Baltimore, Maryland 21244-1850.

Form CMS-R-131 (Exp. 06/30/2023)   Form Approved OMB No. 0938-0566

• **Fig. 13.6** Advanced Beneficiary Notice

given to the client and signed before providing the service. Using an ABN, you transfer liability and charges to the beneficiary if Medicare does not cover the service or services (APTA, 2020b).

Cash practice's strengths and opportunities include avoiding delays in collection, lowering administrative costs of billing, and improving cost transparency. In addition, it promotes autonomy because providers have more flexibility in their fee schedule and allow the provider and client more freedom about the care process, including length of appointments, the number of visits, and the services provided (APTA, 2020a). Potential barriers to cash practice include providers not being listed in health insurance directories, clients who only see in-network providers, loss of referrals, and Medicare requirements. The latter poses a large threat to a cash practice because occupational and physical therapists are not included in the list of practitioners who can opt out of Medicare as outlined in the Balanced Budget Act of 1997 and the Medicare Prescription Drug Improvement and Modernization Act 2003. If a Medicare beneficiary receives a service that Medicare covers, physical and occupational therapists must submit a claim to Medicare for that service. The separate Medicaid, Tricare, and Workers' Compensation regulations limit cash practice (APTA, 2021a). Lastly, cash practice does not change the necessity for proper medical malpractice liability insurance and documentation.

Pro Bono

Pro bono services include providing services at no or reduced costs, donating therapy services to charitable organizations, or volunteering (APTA, 2021b). Considering that in 2020 9%–13% of United States citizens who were uninsured and 43% were underinsured, OTs and PTs have a moral and ethical obligation to provide services to those without access to care (Keisler-Starkey & Bunch, 2021; *U.S. Health Insurance Coverage in 2020*, 2020). The AOTA and APTA list altruism as a core value, which is the unselfish concern and devotion to the best interest of others ("AOTA 2020 Occupational Therapy Code of Ethics," 2020; Core Values for the Physical Therapist and Physical Therapist Assistant, 2021). The APTA Code of Ethics explicitly refers to the ethical duty of PTs providing pro bono services in Principle 8A (American Physical Therapy Association, 2020).

Although providing pro bono services is ethical, there are many barriers. The risks of providing pro bono service do not change the necessity for proper documentation. Also, the need for medical malpractice liability insurance does not change simply because the service is provided pro bono. Therapists could be held liable for pro bono services in your employer's clinic if provided without their knowledge. Also, Good Samaritan laws differ by state and often only apply to unlicensed professionals. Lastly, occupational and physical therapists must be aware of separate regulations for Medicare, Medicaid, Tricare, and Workers' Compensation (APTA, 2020b; 2021). For instance, Medicare

---

> ### • BOX 13.2 Medicare's Definition of Reasonable and Necessary
>
> - Safe and effective;
> - Not experimental or investigational; and
> - Appropriate for Medicare clients, including the duration and frequency that is considered appropriate for the item or service, whether it is:
>   - Furnished per accepted standards of medical practice for the diagnosis or treatment of the client's condition or to improve the function of a malformed body member;
>   - Furnished in a setting appropriate to the client's medical needs and condition;
>   - Ordered and furnished by qualified personnel;
>   - Meets, but does not exceed, the client's medical need; AND
>   - Is least as beneficial as an existing and available medically appropriate alternative; OR
>   - Covered by commercial insurers unless evidence supports that differences between Medicare beneficiaries and commercially insured individuals are clinically relevant.
>
> Centers for Medicare and Medicaid Services (2021). *Medicare Program; Medicare coverage of innovative technology (MCIT) and definition of "reasonable and necessary."* Federal Register. https://www.federalregister.gov/documents/2021/11/15/2021-24916/medicare-program-medicare-coverage-of-innovative-technology-mcit-and-definition-of-reasonable-and

beneficiaries cannot receive pro bono services for *reasonable and necessary care* (Box 13.2).

Also, therapists must recognize that pro bono services *do not* include waiving copays, coinsurances, or deductibles. In addition, pro bono services do not include underbilling (i.e., not billing for services) or undercoding (e.g., billing a less expensive code than what was performed). Some states specifically discuss waivers of deductibles and copays in their statutes. For example, in Ohio, the consequences can result in disciplinary actions, including a limited, suspended, or revoked license (*Section 4755.47 - Ohio Revised Code*, 2021).

> *"the physical therapy section of the Ohio occupational therapy, physical therapy, and athletic trainers board may, except as provided indivision (B) of this section, refuse to grant a license to an applicant for an initial or renewed license as a physical therapist or physical therapist assistant or, by an affirmative vote of not less than five members, may limit, suspend, or revoke the license of a physical therapist or physical therapist assistant or reprimand, fine, place a license holder on probation, or require the license holder to take corrective action courses, on any of the following grounds: (A)(27)(a) Waiving the payment of all or any part of a deductible or copayment that a client, pursuant to a health insurance or health care policy, contract, or plan that covers physical therapy, would otherwise be required to pay if the waiver is used as an enticement to a client or group of clients to receive health care services from that provider; (A)(27)(b) Advertising that the individual will waive the payment of all or any part of a deductible or copayment that a client, pursuant to a health insurance or health care policy,*

contract, or plan that covers physical therapy, would otherwise be required to pay."

Documenting Skill

Documentation is important for all medical providers working with clients to demonstrate high-quality care, to justify the medical necessity and continuation of services, and to protect clinicians from potential fraud and abuse cases. It is expected that clinicians understand proper documentation and billing practices when they start working as licensed practitioners. Effective documentation offers clear and concise communication between healthcare providers and justification of services billed. Documentation is also used for formal reporting to CMS and other payors. The main formal assessments are the Minimum Data Set (MDS) used in skilled nursing facilities, Outcome and Assessment Information Set (OASIS) in home healthcare, and Diagnosis Related Group (DRG) in acute care.

Documentation must reflect skilled intervention as opposed to therapeutic intervention. In other words, the interventions provided must benefit the client and involve a level of complexity that only licensed clinicians can perform. If the intervention is therapeutic, although it is beneficial to the client, the intervention could be taught to any caregiver to perform. Clinicians' documentation reports include the initial evaluation, reevaluation, daily treatment notes, progress reports, and discharge notes.

Initial Evaluation

Documentation must support medical necessity, and justification of services (Fig. 13.7). Medically necessary services are "health care services or supplies needed to diagnose or treat an illness, injury, condition, disease, or its symptoms and that meet accepted standards of medicine" (Centers for Medicare & Medicaid Services, n.d.). The Centers for Medicare and Medicaid Services (CMS, 2022) provides further detail regarding medically necessary services applying to Medicare coverage. According to CMS, medically necessary services or supplies: are proper and needed for the diagnosis or treatment of the condition, are provided for the diagnosis, direct care, and treatment of the condition, meet the standards of good clinical practice in the local area, and are not mainly for the conveniences of the client or clinician.

During the initial evaluation, the history requires a systematic way of obtaining information from past and present events that led the individual to seek rehabilitation services (American Physical Therapy Association, 2018c). Demographics, social history, employment and work history, living environment, functional status, medications, clinical tests, and current complaints are some components included in the history. The client's medical diagnosis and information gained in the history benefit the therapist when hypothesizing potential causes of impairment that need further investigation using tests and measures. Another major component of the history is a review of systems to determine if symptoms warrant a referral for further medical evaluation. A review of systems will obtain information related to the major body systems including but not limited to ears, nose, throat, cardiovascular and pulmonary systems, lymphatic, integumentary, gastrointestinal, genitourinary, endocrine, neurologic, and musculoskeletal systems. The therapist synthesizes all information to make hypotheses regarding a diagnosis that will guide the hands-on examination using tests and measures. Range of motion, strength, and balance are tests used to measure impairments, while other tests may quantify function. The therapist will determine appropriate tests and measures from information gained through the

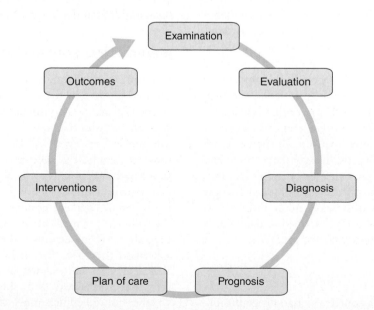

• **Fig. 13.7** Documentation Components (Reprinted from www.apta.org, with permission of the American Physical Therapy Association. © 2023 American Physical Therapy Association. All rights reserved.)

history and review of symptoms. The tests and measures will help rule out potential therapy diagnoses. The therapist considers all information gained through the history, review of symptoms, tests, and measures to develop a plan of care for the client (American Physical Therapy Association, 2018c). Only physical and occupational therapists can perform and record initial evaluations.

Daily Notes

After the plan of care is established and treatment starts for the client, the therapist or therapist assistant will document daily treatments. Documentation begins with the client and caregiver's report of the client's progress and if there have been any changes in functional abilities. The plan of care documentation also includes communication and collaboration with other providers, clients, family, caregivers, and significant other as applicable or indicated. The daily treatment note documents what was done with the client, including interventions provided with frequency, intensity, time, duration, and level of physical and cognitive assistance. The clinician should also include how the client responded to the treatment. It is not recommended to use the statement "tolerated treatment well." The clinician should describe the response, such as the client's increased knee pain with eccentric quadriceps-loading activities. The documentation should also include the plan for the next visit, including interventions with progression parameters and precautions (American Physical Therapy Association, 2018b). In the documentation for a daily treatment note, it is important to convey the skill required by the therapist or therapist assistant to administer certain interventions.

Progress Report

The progress report is like a daily note but includes more detailed information on the client's or client's status than a previous date(s) (e.g., date of initial evaluation, last reexamination, or last progress report). Progress reports should be performed regularly on all clients to support the ongoing need for rehabilitation services. The report should update the client's overall status related to the therapist's goals and plan of care. Only the therapist can write a note that requires an assessment of the client and their progression or lack of progression. Therapy assistants cannot perform a progress report per Medicare regulations, other third-party payor rules, and state law. The therapist may use data from therapy assistants to include in the progress report (American Physical Therapy Association, 2018e). Note that the daily notes and progress reports work together. If progress is described in daily notes, a progress report or summary may not be necessary.

Re-evaluation

Reevaluation codes remain a source of ongoing confusion. First, it is important to distinguish a reexamination from a reevaluation. A reexamination is performing selected tests and measures (e.g., assessing range of motion after a total knee arthroplasty) after the initial examination to determine progress toward established goals and prognosis. Reexaminations typically occur at designated points during a care episode, for example, two weeks into a four-week plan of care. This time cannot be billed as a reevaluation (American Physical Therapy Association, 2018d).

Billing a reevaluation code is indicated if there is an established and ongoing plan of care, a significant change in the patient's condition or functional status, and a change to the plan is necessary. A significant change includes new clinical findings or failure to respond to the treatment as anticipated. Reevaluation codes for physical and occupational therapists are 97164 and 97168, respectively. This code is service-based or un-timed (American Physical Therapy Association, 2018d). Only physical and occupational therapists can perform and record reexaminations and reevaluations.

Discharge Note/Summary

The discharge note concludes the OT or PT episode of care. The discharge note summarizes the client's progress toward the therapist's goals, describes the client's status, and plans for future management. The discharge note describes the outcome of the client receiving physical rehabilitation services. Many state regulations and policies require the therapist to complete the discharge note. The therapist analyzes the client's achievement toward the goals and outcomes and recommends concluding rehabilitation services. It is also important for the therapist to include client compliance or adherence issues, including the number of visits completed and if the client stopped services against the therapist's recommendation. If services are stopped before goal attainment, the therapist should explain why services were concluded (American Physical Therapy Association, 2018a). Only physical and occupational therapists can perform and record discharge notes.

Medical Necessity and Medical Maintenance

Clinicians need to understand the difference between medical necessity and medical maintenance. According to CMS, all medical services completed by a clinician must support medical necessity (Centers for Medicare & Medicaid, 2022). The medical reviewer will determine whether the services provided require the skills and knowledge of a PT, OT, or supervised PTA or OTA. CMS defines skilled care as "a level of expertise acquired through specialized training not attained by the general population." The clinician will consider the client's medical condition, but this should not be the only factor in deciding if the client requires services from a licensed therapist. The main objective in determining if skilled services are needed is whether the client needs a therapist's specialized skills, knowledge, and judgment or whether nonskilled personnel can complete the services after adequate training (APTA, 2019). The documentation must describe the services provided, including amount, frequency, duration, and services that must be considered essential for treating the client's condition. When documenting the progress report or discharge note, the therapist must demonstrate a client benefited from rehabilitation services compared with the client's condition at the onset of treatment, or the claim could be denied.

CMS describes medical maintenance as reimbursable when the individualized maintenance program is designed to improve the functional status or prevent a decline in function with rehabilitation services, improve client safety within their home, or train the caregiver in maintenance activities (Centers for Medicare & Medicaid Services, n.d.). In medical necessity and maintenance cases, clinicians still need to prove that an individual requires skilled care through documentation. Medical Maintenance has been disputed between clinical providers and insurance companies in the medical community. According to CMS (2013), Medicare contractors denied services under Medicare's skilled nursing facilities, home health, and outpatient therapy benefits based on an "improvement standard- the potential for improvement as a condition of coverage for skilled rehabilitation services." An individual with a chronic progressive disease may never improve due to their medical condition, but their ability to function at home and in the community may improve with skilled rehabilitation services. In 2013, the "improvement standard" was disputed in Jimmo versus Sebelius. The plaintiff alleged Medicare contractors inappropriately denied claims based on the beneficiary's lack of potential for improvement even though skilled care was necessary to prevent further deterioration of functional skills. CMS denied establishing the rule for the improvement standard and denying claims based on this standard. The Jimmo versus Sebelius settlement agreement did not expand Medicare coverage but clarified the existing policy. CMS revised Medicare program

manuals that contractors use to determine coverage of therapy. CMS clarified that therapy coverage is based on the need for skilled care, not the beneficiary's potential for improvement (Centers for Medicare & Medicaid Services, 2013).

Electronic Medical Records

Electronic Medical Records (EMR) are computerized systems used to streamline documentation. EMRs are specific to each setting type due to the differing requirements for documentation and billing. This setting-specific customization assists in decreasing errors; however, it creates challenges with sharing episodes of care information with providers across the continuum. The benefits of an EMR certainly outweigh the inconveniences. The primary benefits include easy access to medical records, complete documentation, sending records between providers, and ease of billing (Table 13.7).

The Health Insurance Portability and Accountability Act (HIPAA) of 1996 is a federal law that created national standards for client-protected health information (PHI). This law applies to individual providers and organizations. HIPAA essentially says that only personnel directly involved with a specific client's care can have access to relevant PHI. HIPAA also outlines circumstances when a client's permission is required to share PHI. The law also requires security safeguards to be in place to protect PHI. A common HIPAA violation by rehabilitation providers is not securing client charts, whether those charts are in hard copy or electronic format (Centers for Disease Control and Prevention, 2018). Best practice dictates that rehabilitation providers secure hard copies in locked locations when not in use. Best practice for electronic charts dictates providers to log out of electronic medical record (EMR) programs when not in use.

TABLE 13.7	Benefits of Electronic Medical Record
Benefit	Description
Ease of access	The database should be easily searchable, so clinicians can instantly pull up all the information on the client, from exercise and appointment schedules to the medications they are taking. That means no paper records to flip through, the ability to search the documents for information instantly, and no unintelligible hand-written notes.
Complete documentation	With electronic medical records (EMRs), therapists can easily document everything a client does in real-time. From arrival to billing to the appointment itself, all information can be listed in the database to give therapists a complete record of everything about the client.
Sending of records	Sending EMRs using management software typically streamlines inter-office communications. Most EMR solutions integrate seamlessly with online cloud storage and cloud storage solutions. The records can be accessed by other healthcare providers working with the client. It doesn't even matter if the other facility has fully integrated *EMRs* for physical rehabilitation services. Therapists can still access the files as long as they have a computer connected to the internet.
Ease of billing	As with all forms of accounting, syncing information with the client is difficult. Electronic medical records and therapy documentation can make the process far more comfortable. With therapy scheduling software, therapists can time alerts for when their clients are coming, keep track of how much they owe, how long it took for them to pay last time, and where to send the bill. Therapy software makes billing clients an easier procedure and reduces the chance of mistakes.

Conclusion

Clinicians must understand the similarities and differences between payors. Each payor can have specific guidelines for CPT code billing, documentation requirements for reimbursement, and reporting requirements. The NCD and LCD manuals are valuable tools to determine what is permitted under each payor. These manuals and policies and procedures are revised on a regular schedule based on current best practices and practice trends. It is the professional responsibility of the clinician to appropriately bill for services rendered based on CPT code descriptions and the delivery modes related to individual, concurrent, and group therapy. The world of healthcare is ever-changing, especially related to the payor and legislative landscape. Each clinician's professional duty is to ensure their knowledge of current payor expectations and billing practices is up to date. Up-to-date practices will help ensure that legal and ethical practices are demonstrated at the highest standards.

Activity Questions

- Are services provided by physical and occupational therapy assistants reimbursed at a reduced rate?
- Can therapists treat two Medicare beneficiaries at once?
- Can students participate in the care of clients who are Medicare beneficiaries?
- Discuss the major components required for documentation of an initial evaluation, daily treatment note, progress report, reevaluation, and discharge note.
- Discuss the similarities and differences between fraud, abuse, and waste.
- Discuss ways to avoid fraud, abuse, and waste.
- Discuss the difference between therapeutic exercise and manual therapy CPT codes.
- Compare and contrast different payor sources.
- Compare and contrast health insurance coverage provided through the Federal government versus managed care organizations.
- Discuss alternative payor sources.
- Describe the process of claim denial.
- Describe the consequence of unethical practice.
- What services might a client seek from occupational and physical therapists, yet Medicare would deem it medically unreasonable or unnecessary?

References

American Occupational Therapy Association (AOTA). (2016). *New occupational therapy evaluation coding overview.* https://www.aota.org/~/media/Corporate/Files/Advocacy/Federal/Evaluation-Codes-Overview-2016.pdf.

American Physical Therapy Association (APTA). (2017). *Preventing fraud, abuse, and waste: A primer for physical therapists.* https://www.apta.org/contentassets/1dcb4570f2294b758a94bdafb897bfad/preventing-fraud-abuse-waste-a-primer.pdf.

American Physical Therapy Association (APTA). (2018a). *Documentation: Conclusion of the episode of care summary.* https://www.apta.org/your-practice/documentation/defensible-documentation/elements-within-the-patientclient-management-model/conclusion-of-the-episode-of-care-summary.

American Physical Therapy Association (APTA). (2018b). *Documentation: Documentation of a visit.* https://www.apta.org/your-practice/documentation/defensible-documentation/elements-within-the-patientclient-management-model/documentation-of-a-visit.

American Physical Therapy Association (APTA). (2018c). *Documentation: Initial examination and evaluation.* https://www.apta.org/your-practice/documentation/defensible-documentation/elements-within-the-patientclient-management-model/initial-examination.

American Physical Therapy Association (APTA). (2018d). *Documentation: Reexamination and reevaluation.* https://www.apta.org/your-practice/documentation/defensible-documentation/elements-within-the-patientclient-management-model/reexamination-and-reevaluation.

American Physical Therapy Association (APTA). (2018e). *Medicare part b documentation requirements.* https://www.apta.org/your-practice/documentation/medicare-part-b.

American Physical Therapy Association (APTA). (2019, June 19). *Nonfederal payors that address the improvement standard.* https://www.apta.org/your-practice/payment/medicare-payment/coverage-issues/skilled-maintenance-therapy-under-medicare/nonfederal-payors-improvement-standard-skilled-maintenance.

American Physical Therapist Association. (2020, August 8). *Code of ethics for the physical therapist.* https://www.apta.org/apta-and-you/leadership-and-governance/policies/code-of-ethics-for-the-physical-therapist.

American Physical Therapy Association (APTA). (2020a). *Defining cash practice.* https://www.apta.org/your-practice/payment/cash-practice/cash-practice-defining.

American Physical Therapy Association (APTA). (2020b). *Compliance issues in cash practice.* https://www.apta.org/your-practice/payment/cash-practice/cash-practice-compliance-issues.

American Physical Therapist Association. (2021, December 21). *Core values for the physical therapist and physical therapist assistant.* https://www.apta.org/apta-and-you/leadership-and-governance/policies/core-values-for-the-physical-therapist-and-physical-therapist-assistant.

American Physical Therapy Association (APTA). (2021a). *Cash-based practice: It's complicated.* https://www.apta.org/apta-magazine/2021/08/01/apta-magazine-august-2021/cash-based-practice-its-complicated.

American Physical Therapy Association. (2021b). *Pro bono physical therapy services.* https://www.apta.org/your-practice/practice-models-and-settings/pro-bono.

AOTA 2020 Occupational Therapy Code of Ethics. (2020). *The American Journal of Occupational Therapy, 74*(Supplement_3), 7413410005p1–7413410005p13.

Centers for Disease Control and Prevention. (2018). *Health insurance portability and accountability act of 1996 (HIPAA).* https://www.cdc.gov/phlp/publications/topic/hipaa.html.

Centers for Medicare & Medicaid Services (CMS). (2013). *Jimmo v. settlement agreement fact sheet.* https://www.cms.gov/Medicare/Medicare-Fee-for-Service-Payment/SNFPPS/Downloads/Jimmo-FactSheet.pdf.

Centers for Medicare & Medicaid Services (2020). *Items & services not covered under Medicare.* https://www.cms.gov/outreach-and-education/medicare-learning-network-mln/mlnproducts/downloads/items-and-services-not-covered-under-medicare-booklet-icn906765.pdf.

Centers for Medicare and Medicaid Services (CMS). (2021a). *Medicare Parts A & Parts B appeals process.* https://www.cms.gov/outreach-and-education/medicare-learning-network-mln/mlnproducts/downloads/medicareappealsprocess.pdf.

Centers for Medicare and Medicaid Services (2021b). Chapter 15—covered medical and other health services. In *Medicare benefit policy manual*. https://www.cms.gov/Regulations-and-Guidance/Guidance/Manuals/Downloads/bp102c15.pdf.

Centers for Medicare and Medicaid Services (2021c.). *Beneficiary notices initiative (BNI)*. CMS.Gov. https://www.cms.gov/medicare/medicare-general-information/bni.

Centers for Medicare and Medicaid Services (CMS). (2022). *Bundled payments for care improvement initiative*. CMS Innovation Center. https://innovation.cms.gov/innovation-models/bundled-payments.

Centers for Medicare and Medicaid Services (CMS). (2022.) *Billing and coding: medical necessity of therapy services*. https://www.cms.gov/medicare-coverage-database/view/article.aspx?articleid=52775.

Centers for Medicare and Medicaid Services (CMS). (2022a). *What's a MAC*. CMS.Gov. https://www.cms.gov/Medicare/Medicare-Contracting/Medicare-Administrative-Contractors/What-is-a-MAC.

Centers for Medicare and Medicaid Services (CMS). (2022b). *Local coverage determinations*. CMS.Gov. https://www.cms.gov/Medicare/Coverage/DeterminationProcess/LCDs.

Centers for Medicare and Medicaid Services (CMS). (2022c). *Medicare coverage determination process*. CMS.Gov. https://www.cms.gov/Medicare/Coverage/DeterminationProcess.

HealthCare.Gov. (2022). *Glossary*. https://www.healthcare.gov/glossary/.

Healthinsurance.org, LLC (HIO). (2021, October 7). *A brief history of Medicare in America*. http://www.medicareresources.org/basic-medicare-information/brief-history-of-medicare/.

Healthcare Providers Service Organization, CNA Financial & American Physical Therapy Association. (2016). *Physical therapy professional liability exposure: 2016 claim report update*. https://www.cna.com/web/wcm/connect/2d3eaa76-aca2-4f6f-bfd8-e7706368cdac/RC_Healt_PT_Claim_Report_Update.pdf?MOD=AJPERES&CACHEID=2d3eaa76-aca2-4f6f-bfd8-e7706368cdac.

Internal Revenue Service. (2022). *Affordable care act tax provisions for employers*. https://www.irs.gov/affordable-care-act/employers.

Keisler-Starkey, K., & Bunch, L. (2021). *Health insurance coverage in the United States: 2020*. Census.Gov. https://www.census.gov/library/publications/2021/demo/p60-274.html.

Lower costs with assignment | Medicare. (2021). Medicare Costs. https://www.medicare.gov/basics/costs/medicare-costs/provider-accept-Medicare.

Page, C. G. (2015). *Management in physical therapy practices* (2nd ed.). F.A. Davis Company.

Section 4755.47—Disciplinary actions. (2021, October 9). Ohio Laws & Administrative Rules. https://codes.ohio.gov/ohio-revised-code/section-4755.47.

U.S. Health insurance coverage in 2020: A looming crisis in affordability. (2020). The Commonwealth Fund. https://doi.org/10.26099/6aj3-n655.

What's not covered by Part A & Part B? (2021). Medicare.Gov. https://www.medicare.gov/what-medicare-covers/whats-not-covered-by-part-a-part-b.

14

Starting a Business and Entrepreneurship

JENNIFER CASTELLI, OTD, OTR/L, CHT; CARL DEROSA, PT, DPT, PhD, FAPTA; and BRETT WINDSOR, PT, MPA, PhD

LEARNING OBJECTIVES

By the end of this chapter, the reader will be able to:

1. Complete a personality assessment and determine if your personality aligns with that of an entrepreneur or business owner.
2. Discover strengths, opportunities, weaknesses, and threats by completing a SWOT analysis that reflects personal desires, values, and skills.
3. Select the desired business opportunity and create a mission, vision statement, and core values to support the venture.
4. Review the steps required to complete a business plan.
5. Understand key terminology and business acumen from startup to exit strategy necessary to speak the language of small business.

CHAPTER OUTLINE

There are three things extremely hard: Steel, diamonds, and to know oneself.

BENJAMIN FRANKLIN'S 1750 ALMANAC

Are You Ready?

Suppose you are considering stepping out into the world to create employment, hoping to realize your life's purpose, or at least bring home a bigger paycheck. In that case, you will need to understand yourself and others exceptionally well, at least as well as your service or product, the current economy, and what a business owner/entrepreneur is and is not. A solid foundation of self-knowledge before jumping headfirst into owning your own business is the compass, sail, and rudder on the ship. Critical to navigation during rough weather.

Small Businesses: the Backbone of the Private Sector

Small businesses are the backbone of the United States private sector. In 2018, the Chamber of Commerce (n.d.) reported having accounted for 62% of net new jobs and 47.3% of the workforce. Small businesses create 1.5 million jobs annually. The Small Business Administration Office of Advocacy (n.d.) defines a small business as one with less than 500 employees. In 2018, 22 million of the 30.2 million small businesses were individually operated, having no other employees than the owner (Chamber of Commerce, n.d.). Given the ambition toward business ownership in the United States and globally, a new business owner/entrepreneur will be in good company whether they are the sole employee or employ 500 people.

Business Owner Versus Entrepreneur

Some would describe business owners and entrepreneurs interchangeably. However, there are subtleties in approach and mindset attributed to personality, illuminating which side a person rests naturally. Understanding the difference helps to set your compass and prepare your expectations for the journey ahead.

Legally speaking, a business owner is anyone who owns a business; usually, if someone owns a business, it means they also run it. A business owner presents in many ways. They can be the sole employee, wear all the hats, or work alongside others in their million-dollar company. Regardless of size, the business owner has ultimate control over the company's day-to-day operations and has titles such as owner, president, chief executive officer, and founder. Entrepreneurs are also business owners, but not every business owner is an entrepreneur (Law, 2021).

Business Owner

According to Law (2021), a business owner might start a business because it is a natural progression of a career or skill; they are on top of their profession and know the needs of their clientele intimately. They are good planners and prefer to grow incrementally with a to-do list to improve the business, manage employees and increase sales. Business owners are primarily present-oriented, ensuring they fully complete the day-in and day-out tasks. They are cautiously optimistic and engage in careful planning before taking calculated risks. They would not generally risk their life savings for a new, unproven idea. Business owners are often emotionally attached to their business and feel it is an extension of themselves. Because of this attachment, they generally do not have a clear exit strategy.

Entrepreneur

Law (2021) contrasts business owners with entrepreneurs. Entrepreneurs start businesses to challenge the status quo

or create a positive impact. They are dreamers and big thinkers. They are not afraid of ideas yet to be tested and love the challenge of finding a target market and teaching how the service or product will work. Think of Airbnb or Starbucks. They want to grow fast, explode into the market, and reinvent the rules to carve out a space to dominate their line of business. Like a chess player, an entrepreneur is future-oriented, thinking ten steps ahead. At first chance, an entrepreneur will hire a manager for the day-to-day operations to keep the foundation strong, allowing them to keep moving toward the future visions that pull them forward. Entrepreneurs will likely bet everything on a brand-new idea they believe will work. It is the idea an entrepreneur focuses on and the impact they want to make with the vision. The success of one vision leads to restlessness in bringing to life the next idea. That is why entrepreneurs often have an exit strategy in sight from the beginning; to realize a profit for the next investment venture. See Table 14.1 for a breakdown of the following characteristics between business owners and entrepreneurs: motivation, innovation, growth, mindset, risk, and attachment (Law, 2021).

There is no consensus on what makes an entrepreneur or business owner successful. Barrow et al. (2018) pointed out that people view entrepreneurs as highly enthusiastic, curious, and hyperactive as they burst with new ideas. Some authors have written about luck and circumstance, viewing entrepreneurship as a risk-reward system like gambling (Coad & Storey, 2021). Barrow et al. (2018) quoted Peter Drucker, the international business guru

TABLE 14.1 Characteristics of Business Owners Versus Entrepreneurs

Characteristic	Business Owner	Entrepreneur
Motivation	Natural progression of skills	Challenge status quo and create impact
Innovation	Aimed at serving customers	Big ideas that change the status quo
Growth	Local growth within the community and state	Explosive growth state, nationwide and international
Mindset	Present-focused	Future-focused
Risk	Calculated and incremental	Not afraid to risk everything for the idea they believe in
Attachment	Emotionally attached to the business, control of destiny	Rush of adrenaline bringing their vision or big idea to life

who captured the problem perfectly in his description of entrepreneurs:

> *"Some are eccentrics, others painfully correct conformists; some are fat, and some are lean; some are worriers, some relaxed; some drink quite heavily, others are total abstainers; some are men of great charm and warmth, some have no more personality than a frozen mackerel."*

Business owners can be anyone; however, they must commit to following through under potentially extreme circumstances. Generally, a successful venture is fueled by unparalleled passion and the time invested is almost always much more than a regular work week. Often, people go into business thinking they will work fewer hours when the opposite must be true: a person must be willing to put in whatever time it takes to bring the vision to life. Time is the primary building block for a business startup and mandatory to be a successful entrepreneur.

Entrepreneurs' Personality

The main attributes of an entrepreneur's personality, according to Drucker (1985), are innovation, creativity, and the willingness to create a new organization. Korunka et al. (2003) and Zhu et al. (2020) found innovativeness, risk-taking, and the need for achievement to be the top attributes. Barrow et al. (2018) add self-confidence and resilience. The common denominator across all studies is the concept of innovativeness, which is one of an entrepreneur's most central characteristics (Barrow et al., 2018; Drucker, 1985; Korunka et al., 2003; Schumpeter, 1994; Zhu, 2020). High tolerance for risk-taking also becomes a critical factor for making significant and uncertain resource commitments (Lumpkin & Dess, 1996). For entrepreneurs, the need for achievement focuses on setting goals and fueling self-esteem through constant effort, preferring to face difficulties rather than give up opportunities (Baum & Locke, 2004; Zhu et al., 2020). Table 14.2 outlines the key personality attributes of entrepreneurs.

Business Owner and Entrepreneur

Business owner or entrepreneur; the question is not which *one* you are. The real question is, what *kind* of business owner or entrepreneur are you? Individuals have within their power the opportunity to create a structure and culture that feels comfortable and fits their daily life (Ferreira et al., 2017). Every aspect of a person's life is impacted by how well their career suits them. People who are engaged in challenging and satisfying careers and use their strengths and match talents, personalities, and goals more often achieve greater success than those who are not satisfied or passionate about what they do (Lore, 1998). If people want to be healthier, live longer, and be more confident with other parts of life, finding meaning and joy, then exploring personality for job fit and business ownership is a smart idea.

When the career, or progression to ownership, does not fit talents and natural disposition, it is like wearing a shoe one size too small. The shoe can be made to fit but creates pain and discomfort. Even when the career fits, trying to be a business

TABLE 14.2	Entrepreneur Key Characteristics
Author	**Characteristic**
• Drucker (1985)[a]	• Innovation • Creativity • Willingness to create a new organization
• Parker (2018)[b]	• Self-confidence • Venturesome nature • Foresight • Unrealistic optimism
• Korunka et al. (2003); Zhu et al. (2020)[c]	• Innovation • Risk-taking • Need for achievement
• Lumpkin & Dess (1996)[d]	• High tolerance for risk-taking
• Barrow et al. (2018)[e]	• Self-confident all-rounders • Resilient • Innovative • Results-oriented • Professional risk-taker • Total commitment

[a]Drucker, P. F. (1985). *Innovation and entrepreneurship: Practice and principles* (2nd ed.). Butterworth-Heinemann.
[b]Parker, S.C. (2018) *The economics of entrepreneurship*. Cambridge: Cambridge University Press.
[c]Korunka, C., Frank, H., Lueger, M., & Mugler, J. (2003). The entrepreneurial personality in the context of resources, environment, and the startup process: A configurational approach. *Entrepreneurship Theory and Practice, 28*(1), 23–42; Zhu, F., Sun, S., & Sun, M. (2020). Influence of entrepreneurs' personality and personal characteristics on new venture performance: A fuzzy-set qualitative comparative analysis. *Social Behavior and Personality: An International Journal, 48*(12), e9199.
[d]Lumpkin, G. T., & Dess, G. G. (1996). Clarifying the entrepreneurial orientation construct and linking it to performance. *The Academy of Management Review, 21*(1), 135–172.
[e]Barrow, C., Barrow, P., & Brown. R. (2018). *The Business Plan Workbook: A step by step guide to creating and developing a successful business* (9th ed.). New York, NY, USA: Krogan Page Limited.

owner or entrepreneur without self-awareness is like wearing a shoe one size too big. The shoe can be worn but does not provide enough support for traction and agility to make big decisions. Either of these scenarios increases stress and depression and develops poor self-esteem. To quote Aristotle, "we are what we repeatedly do." If people love what they do, they love who they are. It is much easier to lead employees and develop talent in your business hen employees see the owner inspired and at peace with themself.

Step 1: Know Yourself

There are many assessments and self-help tools to know one's identity better. By understanding the building blocks of personality, one can harness opportunities quicker and minimize problems faster. The first step is to understand the dichotomy of how people take in information, make decisions on that information, reenergize, and conduct themselves in the outer world. These preferences create a type of person or business owner or entrepreneur in this case.

Katharine Briggs and Isabelle Briggs-Myers developed the Myers-Briggs type indicator (Myers et al., 2003) based on the

TABLE 14.3	Self-Assessments: Perception, Judgment, Energy, and Organization	
Assessment	**Website**	
• Myers Briggs type indicator	• https://www.mbtionline.com/	
• 16 Personalities[a]	• https://www.16personalities.com/	
• Keirsey temperament sorter[a]	• https://www.keirsey.com/	
• OKA consulting	• https://www.oka-online.com/	
• Clifton strengthsfinder	• https://www.gallup.com/cliftonstrengths/	

[a]These assessments are free.

works of Carl Jung (1921) and brought it to public use in 2003. The Myers-Briggs type indicator and theory give budding business owners an edge in understanding themselves and others in their relationship with each other and the nature of the tasks to be performed. See Table 14.3 for a list of standardized tools that help identify self-awareness metrics. These tools help a person figure out which preferences represent them best. Professional coaching is available from these sites to ensure that a person self-reports the correct type.

When creating a service or product, business owners will benefit from understanding how they best use their minds and what intrinsically motivates them compared to others. After all, these are the seeds that grow organizational culture and knowing how to prune and prime the branches will keep the culture strong and healthy. This self-discovery starts by identifying which side of each dichotomy a person prefers. A dichotomy is a division or contrast between two opposite aspects, such as a decision via thinking or feeling. In the case of personality type, the theory supports that each person uses both sides of the dichotomy but usually not with equal comfort. For example, we have two hands and use both, but not usually with equal ease and comfort. One hand is quicker, feels natural, and a person can multitask while engaged in an activity such as writing. Likewise, suppose a person makes decisions from their heart, using a feeling function. In that case, it may be effortless to empathize with someone late for work due to a family emergency but then struggle to discipline someone for missing excessive work. This scenario would have the opposite challenge for someone who uses the *thinking* function first for decision-making. People must use both sides of this decision-making process, but generally, like our dominant hand, one side feels more natural. Table 14.4 Worksheet 1 describes the steps to begin exploring personality and Table 14.5 summarizes four dichotomies essential to know about yourself and considering the perspective of others.

A combination of the four letters chosen as a preference gives business owners a framework for harnessing strengths and assessing weaknesses or blind spots in themselves and their employees. Table 14.6 summarizes all the possible preference combinations in an oversimplified format. Comprehensive teaching of personality is outside the scope of this chapter. However, much information is available on the websites listed in Table 14.3. Circle your type in Table 14.6 and temperament in Table 14.7. Explore your strengths and, on the flip side, potential blind spots.

So again, after reviewing all the information about personality, the question is, what *kind* of owner are you? Do you have a more traditional *business owner temperament*; present-focused, calculating, and planning carefully and incrementally to build skills and grow customers systematically? These owners live and breathe troubleshooting and

TABLE 14.4	Worksheet 1: Explore Your Personality Preferences	
To-Do List	**Take the Assessment**	
1.	• Go online and take the MBTI or the free 16 personalities to explore your personality. This survey should take about 12 minutes. Circle your four-letter preference. o ESTJ-ISTJ-ESTP-ISTP-ESFJ-ISFJ-ESFP-ISFP o ENTJ-INTJ-ENTP-INTP-ENFJ-INFJ-ENFP-INFP • To find your temperament, go to Keirsey Temperament Sorter, complete the indicator, and circle one of the options below. o *Guardian Artisan Idealist Rational*	
2.	• Read the type preferences given in the websites and below in Table 14.5, circle the best fit letter o E or I, S or N, T or F, J or P o Does the combination of letter preferences circled also match the indicator you took online? Yes or No o If "No," consider professional coaching from the website	
3.	• What percentage do you identify with the description? o >50% 60%–70% 70%–80% 80%–90% 90%–100% o You should be able to read the description and feel that it describes core attributes 85%–100% accurately or there is a good chance there is at least one letter misreported. o If this happens, seek coaching from the site. Use the sites to understand yourself and what motivates potential employees.	

<table>
<tr><td>TABLE
14.5</td><td colspan="3">**Simplified Breakdown of Personality to Understand Individual Preferences**</td></tr>
</table>

Type	Preferences[a]	Preferences[a]
Energy Flow	**Introversion (I)**	**Extroversion (E)**

• MBTI-type theory describes two worlds.
• Jung believed people spend time in each but prefer one to energize.
• Which do you prefer?
	• An inner world of thoughts, ideas, and concepts.
	• Characterized by:
	  o Internal directed
	  o Reflection
	  o Think to speak
	  o Contained
		• An outer world of people, actions, places, and things.
		• Characterized by:
		  o External directed
		  o Action
		  o Speak to think
		  o Expressive

Information	**iNtuition (N)**	**Sensing/Observant (S or O)**

• Jung's theory suggests people are hard-wired to notice information/data through either their five senses or a sixth sense.
• Which do you prefer?
	• Brings multiple ideas forward/imaginative.
	• Characterized by:
	  o Future focus
	  o Possibilities
	  o Theoretical
	  o Sixth sense
		• Focus on what happened and happening now.
		• Characterized by:
		  o Present focus
		  o Here-and-now
		  o Actual
		  o Five senses

Decisions	**Feeling (F)**	**Thinking (T)**

• Once information is received, a person decides on the data and prefers one of two ways.
• Which do you prefer?
	• Desires conflict resolution and personally connects to people and issues.
	• Characterized by:
	  o Harmony
	  o Circumstantial
	  o Mercy
		• Desires conflict management and analyzing issues for solutions.
		• Characterized by:
		  o Clarity
		  o Analytical
		  o Justice

Outer-World Orientation	**Perceiving (P)**	**Judging (J)**

• The persona people show to the public.
• Which do you prefer?
	• A perceiver's public persona is adaptability, open-endedness, and perception.
	• Characterized by:
	  o Options
	  o Adaptable
	  o Flexible
		• A judger's public persona is structured, orderly, and decisive.
		• Characterized by:
		  o Closure
		  o Control
		  o Scheduled

[a]Symbol in parentheses.
MBTI, Myers-Briggs type indicator.
Adapted from Jung, C. G. (1921) *Psychological types*. Princeton University Press; Myers, I. B., McCaulley, M. H., Quenk, N. L., & Hammer, A. L. (2003) *MBTI manual: A guide to the development and use of the Myers-Briggs type indicator instrument*. Consulting Psychologists Press.

<table>
<tr><td>TABLE
14.6</td><td colspan="4">**Preference Combinations Highlighting Both Temperament and 16 Type Combinations**</td></tr>
</table>

ISTJ[a] Most responsible Inspector	ISFJ[a] Most loyal Provider	INFJ[c] Most contemplative Counselor	INTJ[d] Most independent Mastermind
ISTP[b] Most pragmatic Virtuoso	ISFP[b] Most artistic Composer	INFP[c] Most idealistic Healer	INTP[d] Most conceptual Architect
ESTP[b] Most spontaneous Entrepreneur	ESFP[b] Most generous Performer	ENFP[c] Most optimistic Champion	ENTP[d] Most inventive Debater
ESTJ[a] Most hard charging Supervisor	ESFJ[a] Most harmonizing Protector	ENFJ[c] Most persuasive Teacher	ENJT[d] Most commanding Fieldmarshal

Keirsey Temperament: [a]Guardian; [b]Artisan; [c]Idealist; [d]Rational
E, Extroverion; *F*, feeling; *I*, introversion; *J*, judging; *N*, intiuition; *O*, observant; *P*, perceiving; *S*, sensing; *T*, thinking.
Adapted from the following sources Jung, C. G. (1921) *Psychological types*. Princeton University Press; Myers, I. B., McCaulley, M. H., Quenk, N. L., & Hammer, A. L. (2003) *MBTI manual: A guide to the development and use of the Myers-Briggs type indicator instrument*. Consulting Psychologists Press.

TABLE 14.7 The Business Owner: Guardian, Artisan, Idealist, or Rational

Guardian 38% Population	Idealist 12% Population
• ESTJ, ESFJ, ISFJ, ISTJ • Action is oriented toward: *procedures* • Can be seen as a: *stabilizer*	• ENFJ, ENFP, INFJ, INFP • Action is oriented toward: *personalization* • Can be seen as a: *catalyst*
Artisan 38% Population	**Rational 12% Population**
• ESTP, ESFP, ISTP, ISFP • Action is oriented toward: *The here and now* • Can be seen as a: *troubleshooter*	• ENTJ, ENTP, INTJ, INTP • Action is oriented toward: *complexity* • Can be seen as a: *visionary*

E, Extroverion; F, feeling; I, introversion; J, judging; N, intuition; P, perceiving; S, sensing; T, thinking.
Adapted from Keirsey, D. & Bates, M. (1978). *Please understand me.* Prometheus Nemesis

focus on procedures and logistics, working to stabilize the here and now. Or, do you have the temperament of a business entrepreneur; future-focused, innovative, and not afraid to risk everything to challenge the status quo with big ideas that create impact? These entrepreneurs are catalysts for change, living and breathing personalization and complexity. It is good to strive for balance.

Step 2: Getting Started—Navigate Toward Passion

The next step requires self-reflection using resources and websites in Table 14.3 and personal experience to fill in *s*trengths and *w*eaknesses, *o*pportunities, and *t*hreats (SWOT). This SWOT is an intimate breakdown of human capital that a business owner brings to the organization they hope to build. Analyzing personal strengths and weaknesses is the framework that allows one to trust instincts and build on capabilities while mitigating weaknesses. With practice, one can minimize weaknesses by gaining additional knowledge or skills in crucial areas, finding a particular kind of mentor, or hiring an employee or consultant to bridge gaps. A general overview of topics to include in the SWOT is the level of understanding regarding many aspects of the business planning, such as

mission and vision statements, potential referral sources, documentation, billing/coding, contract negotiation, credentialing if working with insurance, management skills for human resources and payroll, local and state business laws, tax laws, marketing strategies, and healthcare regulation. Refer to Table 14.8 for Worksheet 2.

Once a person understands their strengths and weakness and decides they are the best fit for being either a business owner or entrepreneur (Table 14.9 Worksheet 3), the initial planning can begin. As with all initial business planning, it is important to keep ideas realistic and scalable. Each goal should be an actionable learning goal that is specific, measurable, attainable, relevant, and time-based, known as SMART goals (Bovend'eerdt et al., 2009). Setting each goal as a SMART goal will help ensure a business plan's viability and timely completion. Along with having the right set of personal factors to start a business (self-confident, resilient, innovative, results-oriented, risk-taker, total commitment), one should complete a knowledge assessment of key issues in private practice. There are many topics a business owner must understand to comply with local, state, and federal regulations and laws. Thinking through each topic in the business plan outline (Table 14.12 Worksheet 6) will increase preparedness on paper before moving to real-life investments of time and finances.

TABLE 14.8 Worksheet 2: Strengths, Weaknesses, Opportunities, Threats (SWOT)

SWOT	Description	Example
• Strengths	• List all positive qualities of temperament and personality; learned skills, talents, competencies, assets, and capabilities	• People-person, efficient, innovative, bilingual, specialty certifications, managerial experience
• Weaknesses	• List any areas of vulnerability that need improvement, including those qualities related to your personality type/temperament that are still developing and skill deficits	• Too flexible, taking on too much work, marketing might be a challenge
• Opportunity	• List all ideas you desire to make come to life and the connections you have with people	• Interest in primary care therapy, mental health, love of horses, new reimbursement codes, spouse is an accountant
• Threats	• List things that might limit your opportunities	• Lacking finances, experience

TABLE 14.9	Worksheet 3: Self-Select Business Owner or Entrepreneur SMART goals		
Do your strengths align with those of a business owner?	Yes		No
If yes, which strengths align?			
If no, which do not align?			
Do your strengths align with those of an entrepreneur?	Yes		No
If yes, which strengths align?			
If no, which do not align?			
Practice writing a SMART goal for one area of weakness e.g. marketing	I will contact SCORE.org and sign up to receive a mentor for marketing within one month		I will spend 30 minutes on SBA.gov each day to learn about various topics starting with market research tools
SMART goal category			
SMART goal category			
Map out a timeline to achieve goals in the following phases. The more SMART goals there are, the easier and faster the steps to the big goal of starting your business.		1 year · 6 mo · 2 mo	

SMART, Specific, measurable, attainable, relevant, time-based.

Resources are abundant to improve entrepreneurial skills (Richmond & Powers, 2009). Potential business owners can attend seminars, read books, join state professional organizations, and meet with the local Service Corps of Retired Executives (SCORE) for insight into small business ownership. A person can be a volunteer to learn more about an area of practice and network with other businesses or at state and national conventions. A variety of potential business ideas and practice areas are listed in Table 14.10. This list is not all-inclusive, but these suggestions will help readers recognize opportunities.

Step 3: Defining Your Purpose—the Mission and Vision

Mission and vision statements describe a business's current or future goals and are explained later in the chapter. However, before a mission, there must be a guiding business idea. Opportunities for business ideas utilize a combination of personal desires, work experience and skills, and needed services within a community. Choose a business idea for which you are passionate. When people exercise talents and abilities they are passionate about, they experience timelessness (Kelly, 2017). Timelessness, or flow, is experienced in meaningful work and is what most people strive to achieve; work that does not feel like work. Besides a sense of timelessness, the satisfaction of doing something worthy with your

life can be more valuable than money (Kelly, 2017). Because that sense of worthiness flows from and through your temperament and character development, aligning a business idea with intrinsic values and natural strengths is prudent.

Analyze the SWOT worksheet in Table 14.8 to discover ideas that ignite your passion for a business. Cross-reference those ideas with third-party payers' reimbursement opportunities or decide to forego insurance and develop a self-pay concierge strategy to ensure the business's income and viability. Insurance companies and managed care organizations recognize new ways to address pain management or mental health programs to improve activities of daily living. There is an opportunity to create wellness programs to address obesity or cognition, particularly attached to primary care. Programs that enhance the overall quality of life by increasing functional independence are greatly valued.

There are two kinds of entrepreneurs; those who address social needs, called *social entrepreneurs*, and those who address specific medical conditions. Most therapy practices still fall in the latter category; however, social entrepreneurship has gained ground over the last 20 years (Ferreira et al., 2017). All entrepreneurship strengthens the rehabilitative profession by discovering care gaps and filling the need with a service or product. One example of social entrepreneurship is in occupational therapy. Occupational justice, occupational alienation, and occupational deprivation speak to a person's inherent right to participate in fulfilling occupations.

Exposure to prolonged isolation or lack of resources is known as *occupational alienation.* When restriction from participation is beyond a person's control, it is known as *occupational deprivation.* Both of these situations lead to a sense of meaninglessness. *Occupational justice* is the idea or theory that the right way to address this problem is to advocate and develop programs where people can understand themselves, explore and act on their environments in healthy ways, no matter what setting. Social entrepreneurship is only limited by the needs of the community. One example can be a program designed to support occupational justice in prisons and drug rehab facilities, fulfilling the American Occupational Therapy Association's Vision 2025:

"Occupational therapy maximizes health, well-being, and quality of life for all people, populations, and communities through effective solutions that facilitate participation in everyday living."
AMERICAN OCCUPATIONAL THERAPY ASSOCIATION (2017)

There are endless opportunities to invest time and talent. The prison reform bill, The First Step Act of 2018, is one example of legislature and funding that allows a profession such as OT to design programs that improve life skills, develop healthy habits for vocational training in meaningful areas, and reduce recidivism. Occupational and physical therapists have innumerable opportunities to explore and work outside the medical model. Many grant opportunities also support a business plan that raises the bar for character and skill development expectations for imprisoned individuals. The desired outcome in social entrepreneurship is increasingly valuable social capital.

Social entrepreneurship business must align well with community or global needs in addition to a business owner's intrinsic values and desires stemming from their natural temperament. The owner's temperament and character determine, at least in part, the initial organizational culture. Reflecting and communicating these values and desires in the mission, vision, and core values is worthwhile. Explore Table 14.10 for Worksheet 4 to consider various business opportunities.

The *mission statement* drives the company. It embodies the organization's goals and answers the following questions:
- *What* does the business do?
- *Whom* does the business serve?
- *How* does it serve its customers?

TABLE 14.10 Worksheet 4: Choosing a Business Idea

Type of Business Opportunity	Description of Opportunity	Number in Order of Interest
Specialty services	• Hand therapy, lymphedema, pelvic floor, low vision, or cardiopulmonary services	
Consulting	• Provide services to individuals, groups, hospitals, skilled nursing facilities, schools, or specialty physician offices • Billing for expertise rather than client care	
Independent contracting	• Negotiate a rate with multiple sources and provide services in many settings as a sole proprietor or LLC	
Health coaching	• Working with an individual or group to meet their health and fitness goals	
Direct to employer services	• Injury prevention and health promotion strategies	
Concierge practice/ subscription services	• A monthly or annual fee for unlimited access to provide services or 5–10 treatment packages around specific conditions	
Mobile services home evaluations	• Flat fee for assessing safety and accessibility in the home, safety features, and referral for remodeling bathrooms and entrances	
Integrating with other professionals	• Massage therapists, chiropractors • Occupational therapists focused on mental well-being modalities and mental health performance skills to improve occupational engagement and performance	
Partnering with a gym	• Rent space or provide consultation or personal coaching for weight loss and posture, wellness, and prevention	
Holistic or integrative care	• Offer PT or OT services within offices for functional medicine and acupuncture, serving people with chronic pain and headaches	
Chronic disease management or complex conditions	• Create programs for complex chronic disease management • Partner with primary care, internal medicine, or other medical providers	
Social entrepreneur	• Develop a nonprofit company to serve the needs of a community targeting health and wellness, youth, health disparities, seniors, or caregivers	

A solid and tangible mission motivates a team to advance toward a common goal. A strong mission statement reflects what the team aims to do every day. For example:

"At Moffitt Cancer Center, we are working tirelessly in the areas of patient care, research, and education to advance one step further in fighting this disease. We are committed to the health and safety of our patients and dedicated to providing expert cancer care"

A *vision statement* is inspirational. It focuses on what the business is not yet, but hopes to become and reflects a company's culture and core values. The vision statement highlights the future of the business. It answers the following questions:

- What are the *hopes and dreams* of the company?
- What problems are we solving for the *greater good*?
- What are we *inspired to change*?

A vision statement is powerful in creating momentum and sustaining motivation toward the next step in growing closer to achieving the greater good. For example:

"Johns Hopkins Medicine pushes the boundaries of discovery, transforms healthcare, advances medical education, and creates hope for humanity."

Core values represent the business owner or organization's highest priorities and deepest beliefs. These values are never compromised; four to five values usually guide all company actions. These examples are from Johns Hopkins:

- *Excellence in discovery: be the best. Commit to exceptional quality and service by encouraging curiosity, seeking information, and creating innovative solutions.*
- *Leadership and integrity: be a role model. Inspire others to achieve their best and have the courage to do the right thing.*
- *Diversity and inclusion: be open. Embrace and value different backgrounds, opinions, and experiences.*
- *Respect and collegiality: be kind. Listen to understand and embrace others' unique skills and knowledge.*

Refer to Table 14.11 Worksheet 5 to practice writing mission, vision, and core value statements based on a chosen business idea.

Step 4: The Business Plan: a Blueprint for Overall Business Operations

The first step requires a decision regarding the type of business to be created. The next step is to develop a mission, and a vision statement, including core values. After formulating the kind of business to build and the mission, a

TABLE 14.11	**Worksheet 5: Define Your Purpose: Mission, Vision, Core Values**

Choose a Business Idea and Create a Business Name

_____

Mission Statement: Drives the company. It embodies the organization's goals. The mission statement answers the questions: *What* does the business do? *Whom* does it serve? *How* does it help? The mission motivates a team to advance toward a common goal. Write a mission statement for your business idea.

_____

_____

_____

Vision Statement: Is inspirational. It focuses on what the business will become and reflects a company's culture and core values. The vision statement highlights the future of the business, which then provides the purpose. It answers the questions: What are the *hopes and dreams of the company*? What problems are we solving for the *greater good*? What are we inspired to *change*? Write a vision statement for your business idea.

_____

_____

_____

Core Values are four to five values representing an organization's highest priorities and deepest beliefs. Core values are never compromised and guide all company's actions.
Create core values for your business idea

_____

_____

_____

_____

_____

business plan is the next big step. A business plan defines a company's description of services, objectives, and how it plans to achieve its goals. It is essential to the foundation and framework of the business idea. It is a blueprint for others to view and begin to see the same potential as the business owner. Three aspects are generally detailed: operations, financials, and marketing. Outlining these areas highlights a strategy to secure startup financing and a roadmap to follow once up and running. A business plan outline provides this framework; see the example Worksheet 6 in Table 14.12 adapted from Richmond and Powers (2009). Visit www.sba.gov for other sources of business plan outlines.

The Business Side of Healthcare

Healthcare, while having true altruistic intentions, is a business. The business elements often seem so varied that they can appear daunting and impossible to navigate. However, business is part science and part art and thus has some foundational principles upon which it becomes possible to build. The scope of occupational or physical therapy practice has great breadth and offers numerous entrepreneurial opportunities. However, even if you are not focused on business ownership, understanding key business elements helps round out your professional identity as a physical or occupational therapist, to understand and deliver the value proposition therapy brings to the healthcare system, and provides a rich framework for communicating with others in the healthcare industry.

A chapter framed in "business" has many connotations depending on the end user. There are business owners, employees in a business, business partnerships, managers of businesses with no patient care responsibilities, managers of businesses with patient care responsibilities, independent contractors, and consultants. All serve roles within the professions of physical and occupational therapy. As a business owner, the therapist must also form business relationships with other key professionals, such as accountants, attorneys, bankers, and insurance brokers, to name just a few. In many cases, such professionals are part of your business team. It is important to develop these relationships when considering starting a new business (discussed later). Securing loans, setting up the necessary accounting structure, and developing the proper legal corporate documents are part of a startup responsibility. No matter the environment, individual members of a business organization are responsible for understanding the fundamentals of today's healthcare business environment and developing and sharing their ideas and energies to grow and strengthen the *enterprise*. An enterprise is a business or a company around which products align to create value and, in doing so, increase the overall net worth. Net worth is the result value of the assets that a corporation ultimately owns, minus the liabilities owed. Business strategies, at their simplest, are designed to increase net worth.

TABLE 14.12   Worksheet 6: Business Plan Outline

Cover Page
- Name of business
- Name of owners
- Addresses and phone numbers
- Date of the business plan prepared and by whom
- Confidentiality statement (legal document constructed to protect the business owner's information)

Executive Summary
- Brief 2- or 3-page collection of paragraph summaries of the main business plan elements

Table of Contents

Operations: Worksheets 5,7
- Business description (LLC, S-Corp, C-Corp, sole proprietorship, 501(c) non-profit)
- Mission, Vision, Core Values
- Management (day-to-day processes to balance revenue vs. costs and see a profit)
- Location (why the location supports the product or service)
- Products and services (overview of service or product and key customer benefits)
- Financial status (includes income statements, balance sheets, and cash flow)
- Long-term goals and exit plan (go public, merge, be acquired, sell, liquidate)

Marketing: Worksheet 8
- Industry Description and trends (consumer behavior)
- Target market(s) (a specific group of people that organizations want to sell services to)
- Competition (contest between organizations targeting the same consumers)
- Marketing strategies (overall game plan for creating customers)

Financials: Worksheets 9.13
- Startup costs (expenses required to plan, register, and launch a business or social venture)
- Operating costs (ongoing expenses for the normal day-to-day running of a business)
- Income statement (shows whether made or lost money during a particular period)
- Cash flow projections (run potential outcomes to estimate the impact of a decision)
- Break-even analysis (how many sales it takes to pay for the cost of doing business)
- Balance sheet (shows capital structure, i.e., a mix of debt and equity)

Appendix of Support Documents
- Resumes for the owner and key business partners
- Legal contracts and agreements (e.g., rent, vendor, insurance)
- Facility plans (e.g., the layout of the business or potential layout)
- SWOT analysis (business strengths, weaknesses, opportunities, threats)
- Marketing materials (e.g., brochure, website, business cards)
- List of business consultants, attorneys, and accountant
- Letters of reference

LLC, S-Corp, C-Corp

This section will provide an overview of several aspects of business, the value proposition, how business informatics and data mining represent the emerging highest level of "evidence" for the successful clinical practice of the future, both financially and clinically; data used to assess economic performance; key tools used in forming a business or negotiating a new business venture; developing marketing strategies; strategic planning; and practice performance indicators.

Business Terminology

There is universal applicability of language used in business, and physical and occupational therapy is no exception. Foundational definitions include:

- *Profit*: when collected revenue exceeds expenses
- *Loss:* when expenses exceed collected revenue
- *Profit and Loss Report:* an analysis of revenue compared to expenses resulting in a picture of profit or loss. Loss is often expressed in parentheses on reports.
- *Operating Profit:* revenue less all expenses
- *Cash Flow or Cash Management:* not the same as operating profit because the effect of accounts receivable and accounts payable need to be factored into cash flow reports
- *Balance Sheet:* one of the most important business tools is the balance sheet. The balance sheet considers three factors: the assets, the liabilities, and the equity. It is a financial statement that summarizes the company's assets, liabilities, and shareholders' equity at a specific time. It is an important tool for shareholders because it provides an idea of what the company owns and owes and the amount invested in the company. A balance sheet will always follow the following formula:
  - Assets = Liabilities + Shareholders' Equity
  - Each of the three balance sheet segments will have many accounts that document each value. On the asset side of the balance sheet are included items such as cash, inventory, and property. The liability side of the balance sheet is included such accounts as accounts payable and long-term debt. The accounts on a balance sheet will differ by company and industry as no single set template accurately accommodates the differences between different types of businesses. For example, there is a large difference between the balance sheet of physical therapy practice and a health club.
- *Commodity:* goods or service for which there is a demand but supplied without qualitative differentiation across the market. This concept is important in business and we will return to it in the marketing section. Although commodities can be service-based, they are more typically encountered as physical products, for example, a generator or a ladder you might purchase at a hardware store. Physical and occupational therapy are professional services on the level of those provided by lawyers (legal services), accountants (legal services), and doctors (medical services). When physical and occupational therapy allows themselves to be defined as an undifferentiated "commodity,"

they become devalued and then vulnerable to people and organizations who do not have the best interests of the therapy professions as central to their business goals.

Value Proposition

Value proposition is perhaps *the* most important term to understand in business. A value proposition is a critical element that differentiates physical and occupational therapy as professional services from an undifferentiated commodity or good. A value proposition describes the value to be delivered, providing the foundation for a belief in the customer that tangible value will be experienced and received. For the therapist looking at starting or growing a therapy business, the relationship between commodity and value proposition is of paramount importance that can provide the following guiding principle; instead of viewing physical or occupational therapy as a commodity, consider the potential to leverage *your* value to the consumer who has a value proposition. Leveraging *your* value to the consumer is the fundamental premise of marketing.

Since the value proposition is the key business element of any practice, it warrants further discussion. The value proposition can often be a differentiator in business. Remember, the value proposition is the value delivered and the customer's belief that value that will be experienced. Value includes newness and originality, performance, customization to meet a need, a unique way the work gets done, the ease with which a service can be accessed or used, accessibility and convenience, and brand and reputation. However, these examples only serve as a value proposition if the customer sees them as solving an identified problem.

An example of a value proposition in physical or occupational therapy within the musculoskeletal setting relates directly to its financial contribution to the healthcare system. When physical or occupational therapy receives access to the patient at the beginning of a musculoskeletal episode, a relatively short, active, and aggressive management plan delivered over 40-45 days can create significant functional changes sufficient to dissuade the patient from seeking additional modes of healthcare which are (a) significantly more expensive, and (b) often harmful (Frogner et al., 2018). These results in a relatively low-cost therapy episode delivering significant downstream savings to the healthcare system (Denninger et al., 2018, Horn et al., 2016) and a happy patient who tends to return when additional episodes do recur and will refer other patients to your business. This value proposition can then be leveraged towards any stakeholder needing to decrease their musculoskeletal healthcare costs, e.g., a self-insured private employer. Physical or occupational therapy can meet that need (Lentz et al., 2017; 2020).

A business model for physical or occupational therapy practice, no matter what the clinical setting, is an interdependent system consisting of four components:

1. Value Proposition: a customer's value proposition is how you create value for customers. It is how you solve a

customer's problem and meet their needs. This element of the business model is probably the most important.

2. Resources: includes people, products, money, and intellectual property. There are many different types of capital (discussed later).
3. Processes: how the value proposition gets delivered. The successful way of completing the work and the task to deliver the value proposition.
4. Profit Formula: the price point, gross and net profit margins, asset analysis, and volume of work necessary to cover the costs of the resources and deliver the value proposition.

Revenue

Since many of the above elements refer to revenue, a short discussion is warranted. Revenue in physical therapy practice includes payment per procedure aligned to the Resource Based Relative Value System (RBRVS), including timed and untimed codes, bundled payments such as payment per diagnosis, payment per visit, third-party contracts, self-pay models, and ancillary models. Physical and occupational therapists are also increasingly looking for ways to engage in "risk-based" payment systems where services are provided upfront according to a value proposition and then shared in the savings accrued by the services. Many of these payment models see the prices set by the payers, while others provide therapy with the ability to set their price, which is a critical element for therapy as it seeks to build more sustainable business models.

Price Setting

When discussing business and strategies to be successful in business, industry examples are often used, such as comparisons with Nordstroms, Toyota, or other successful businesses. The difficulty in comparing business and marketing strategies in physical or occupational therapy practice, or in most divisions of the healthcare industry, is that the provider does not set the price for the product. Except in some self-pay models, the price is largely dictated by the payor rather than the provider. This difference is why one must be careful in extrapolating tools or methods from the non-healthcare sector, which largely sets its price point. What this translates to in business language is that healthcare does not typically follow the paradigm of a "free market," ultimately determining the price point, and it also challenges the business paradigm of supply and demand. Recognizing the unique aspects of healthcare as a business helps one navigate these challenges more successfully.

Equity

Equity is an important concept in business. It is often defined as the value of an ownership interest in a business. Examples of equity include an ownership interest in a property or a business. Equity includes stock or other ownership interests, funds contributed by an owner noted on the balance sheet, and, in the context of real estate, equity is the difference between the current market value of the property and the amount the owner may still owe on the mortgage. Essentially, the amount the owner would receive after selling a property and paying off the mortgage.

The subject of equity often comes up as it relates to physical or occupational therapy practice, namely the options to become an equity owner in a therapy practice (or related business). In general, the options are to (a) buy an existing practice, (b) become a partner in an existing practice, or (c) start a new practice or new business within an existing practice. These examples will be described in detail below. Even in cases of absent interest in equity ownership, it is important that the physical or occupational therapist has an understanding of these fundamental aspects of a business. Any therapist interested in long-term financial success would do well to understand the role that equity can play in building long-term wealth.

Practice Ownership: Purchasing an Existing Practice

The purchase of an existing practice or business can be distilled simply into three types: (1) an assets purchase, (2) a business purchase, or (3) an assets and business purchase. Assets are a business's real and tangible elements, such as equipment, personnel, and property. These assets have a total value. The business also has a value, but that value is usually based on an economic formula known as the EBITDA. EBITDA refers to the company's *E*arnings *B*efore *I*nterest, *T*axes, *D*epreciation, and *A*mortization expenses. It is beyond the scope of this chapter to detail the calculation of EBITDA, but it is important to know that it is the fundamental way a business is ultimately valued. Often an industry-standard multiple is placed on the EBITDA to determine business value. The important point here is that when looking to buy an existing business, the decision is whether to buy the business and the assets or if they are just considering buying one of the two elements.

The steps that follow the decision to buy a business and the assets are generally the same. You must consider how it will be funded, such as through a business lending institution, and then create the legal communication stream for a purchase. That stream is usually in the form of two parts: a letter of intent (LOI), also known as a memorandum of understanding, and after the LOI is agreed upon, the development of an actual purchase agreement. The components of a LOI are varied but often include the following:

- A statement that a purchase agreement will be developed with sales details
- The proposed purchase price
- That what is being purchased is free of liens and claims
- Whether a noncompete is included
- That the buyer will not be responsible for any liabilities prior to closing
- That the seller cannot try and sell to others until the expiration date of the LOI confidentiality clause

The purchase agreement also has specific components, including:
- Price and the terms
- The assets the seller must provide upon closing
- Closing dates and costs
- Covenants are how the transition would occur to the buyer, non-compete clauses, confidentiality, and name changes. Essentially covenants are any additional "agreements" that need legal binding
- Representations and warranties of the buyer
- Representation and warranties of the seller
- Indemnification
- General information might need to be added because it is not covered previously. Some examples of general information include when and how the property will be transitioned to the new owner, any unfulfilled contingencies that may cancel the purchase agreement, and whether earnest money will be required of the buyer. Earnest money is simply a type of deposit made in good faith by a seller to demonstrate the sincerity of pursuing the purchase

How might this differ from simply buying into an existing business—equity ownership? The initial steps are similar to those listed in that understanding the assets, business value, and liabilities is used to determine the value. These steps are usually done with the professional expertise of an accountant and attorney. However, the key difference is the addition of an operating agreement to the discussion. When buying into an existing business, you are joining that group's operating agreement.

The operating agreement is the single most important document in a business relationship. The operating agreement typically features the following:
- The company name and type of corporation
- Definitions of terms used throughout the operating agreement
- Investment units of each member
- How profits, losses, and distributions are handled
- The manager's responsibilities and limitations
- Rights and obligations of members
- Meetings of members
- Restrictions and transferring, selling interest, or withdrawing
- How additional members may be added
- How the company is dissolved ("winding up" a company)
- Death of a member/disqualification of a member
- Other miscellaneous elements. Depending on the business, miscellaneous elements might include methods of record keeping, the rights of members to corporate records, how managers are appointed, and how capital calls (requests from the members for additional capital investment) will be handled.

For any business, an operating agreement is essential. It is a legal document that will protect an investor in a business but simultaneously spells out responsibilities. Business partnerships can sometimes sour down the line. Friends who started businesses together sometime feel a need to go separate ways. A good operating agreement helps protect everyone's investment fairly and equitably.

Sustaining A Business

Whether starting a business, buying into an existing business, or becoming an employee in an existing business, there are key drivers to assure the business remains viable and profitable. Contemporary businesses define strategy as a "pattern of resource allocation that enables a business to maintain or improve its performance." You must think broadly when considering resources because all businesses have resource capital, including financial capital, physical capital, organizational capital, and human capital. Capital is not just money; it includes people, expertise, technologies, a well-organized business structure, and more. Understanding your capital is key to being successful.

Businesses are in a continuous cycle of working to sustain their sources of strategic competitive advantage. One of the most common ways is by analyzing the environment through SWOT analysis. As previously mentioned, a SWOT refers to an analysis of the *Strengths, Weaknesses, Opportunities,* and *Threats* of a business. A good strategy neutralizes business threats, takes advantage of opportunities, capitalizes on strengths, and fixes internal weaknesses. Strategic planning is key to business success and helps determine an organization's overall goals and direction. The planning process includes the organizational design and roles needed to successfully deliver the service, the performance goals, and the resources needed to achieve those goals. Business plans and strategic plans are not the same. Business plans are management tools – they focus on finances and operations. Strategic plans are leadership tools and inventive courses of action. A successful enterprise needs sound business plans and visionary strategic plans to assure success. Refer to Table 14.13 for Worksheet 7 to begin organizing your business idea's operations. Each category identified will also need a job description to describe role responsibilities.

Marketing

It is important to note that there is a difference between marketing and advertising. Advertising is largely focused on communicating about a product or service to encourage recipients of the communication to purchase or use the product or service. Advertising uses techniques to attract and persuade customers. On the other hand, marketing focuses on activities associated with identifying the particular needs of target customers and then going about satisfying the customers better than their competitors.

Customer satisfaction is of utmost importance in healthcare and has an important influence on outcomes in patient care. At its most basic level, customer satisfaction is two-tiered. The lowest tier is simply preventing

| TABLE 14.13 | Worksheet 7: Broad Overview of Operations Responsibility Breakdown |

Create Your List Based on Company Needs

Operations Overview	Who	When	Why	Focus 1	Focus 2	Focus 3	Focus 4
Strategic planner	Owner	Monthly	Vision	Create LTGs	Develop Staff/Team	Review PI	EBITA
Compliance							
Credentialing							
Contract/management							
Staffing/timecard approval							
Technology							
Human resources – hiring, training, staffing schedules, and benefit management							
Billing							
Accounts receivable							
Inventory							
Cleaning							
Marketing							
Networking							
Advertising/events							
Branding							
Financial							
Accountant							
Accounts payable							
Payroll							
Purchasing							

EBITA, Earnings before interest, taxes, depreciation, and amortization; *PI*, performance indicators; *LTG*, long-term goals.

dissatisfaction. The higher and most important tier is securing satisfaction—developing a true partnership with the customer (the patient) so that the patient becomes an advocate for your service. Within physical and occupational therapy, there are two outcomes desired from a satisfied patient: (1) Satisfaction such that the patient will return to the business when they have a recurrence or a new problem, and (2) satisfaction great enough that they will promote or refer the business to their friends and family, who will then patronize the business as a new customer. This promotion is often referred to as word of mouth marketing.

Preventing dissatisfaction can be achieved through simple strategies such as easy-to-read billing statements, courteousness on phone calls, and not leaving patients waiting. Securing satisfaction occurs when they perceive that their goals have been achieved (i.e., they can return to doing that which caused them to seek care in the initial phase). You are truly working as a patient advocate, and the patient realizes it. However, you are also creating tangible value for that patient.

The audience for marketing efforts is wide-ranging. It includes current patients and the wider community through direct access, past patients, and referral sources. Note that each value proposition can be very different but should always be focused on a central theme. The social proof principle is of great value in marketing to your patients. Social

proof is communicating to your existing and prospective new clients about how you have helped others in similar situations. When you understand the value you have brought to others who have used your services and you use this knowledge to apply the social principle approach in your marketing messages, you will connect powerfully with prospective clients who will, in turn, choose your clinic as their clinic of choice. Focus intently on achieving patient goals.

It is important to maintain relations with past patients. There is a significantly greater cost in starting a new patient versus a returning patient. Consider implementing direct mailers, email messages, birthday cards, offering seminars, and even sponsoring appreciation events to keep past patients connected to you and your practice. Too often, physical and occupational therapists view patients very transactionally. That is, they look at patients as a single episode of care with a defined beginning and end rather than viewing the patient as someone who can turn to the therapist for advice and management throughout their entire lifespan, not only for the management of existing and future problems but also for the prevention of problems that typically develop as we age.

Many physical and occupational therapists have difficulty in marketing efforts with referral sources. Often, this reflects a deficiency in developing a meaningful connection with not only their value proposition but also because of a fundamental lack of understanding of the tangible financial and human value that therapy can deliver to the healthcare system. Because marketing is a critically important and necessary skill, physical and occupational therapists who cannot communicate a tangible value proposition to those we seek to refer to their business are unlikely to build a sustainable, profitable business model capable of building wealth.

A very common marketing strategy deployed by therapists is to visit the offices of a referring healthcare provider who has a preexisting relationship with a patient and who can choose (or not) to refer that patient to the therapy practice. The purpose of a referral source visit is simple: to develop and improve the relationship with the referral source, to identify the "needs" and the "wants" of the referral source, and most importantly, to establish the next appropriate reason for contact. It is not to "teach" a referral source about physical or occupational therapy or the new equipment you have in your clinic. After visiting a referral source, conducting a retrospective review of your visit is wise. Key questions to ask yourself include:

- What new information do I have regarding this referral source that helps me better understand and target my marketing efforts? What are the referral source's important value propositions?

- What information did I share that met the referral source's needs?
- What would have made the visit more productive?
- Was I successfully establishing an expectation that I would return with more information?

Marketing oneself differs from marketing therapy as a commodity (i.e., a good or service for which there is a demand but supplied without qualitative differentiation across the market). Marketing the expert knowledge and critical reasoning of the physical or occupational *therapist* fundamentally differs from marketing physical or occupational *therapy*. Increased awareness of the profession is an essential by-product of successful marketing activities. Consider the previously mentioned value proposition example. Describing physical or occupational *therapy* as a service that can tangibly decrease downstream healthcare costs and create patient satisfaction while simultaneously delivering true functional gains allowing an individual to resume a previously unattainable activity represents a true value. True value makes it very hard to pigeonhole physical or occupational *therapy* as a generic commodity that may or may not add value. See Table 14.14 to begin to create your marketing strategy.

TABLE 14.14	Worksheet 8: Marketing Strategies to Consider	
Analyze Needs Create a Plan	**Marketing Objectives** Think	**Communication Tool** Do
• Target market	• Who is your target market, and where are they located?	• Describe your target market.
• Product or service	• List ways to create awareness of your product or service that showcase your location. (open house, golf tournament ads, pens)	• Target market need(s) that I fulfill.
• Price point/value	• How is your product or service different than competitors in the area?	• Describe the added value of the product or service compared to what is already available.
• Where does the service happen?	• List ways to create awareness of your product or service that showcase your location (e.g., open house, golf tournament ads, pens).	1. 2. 3.
• Persuade (network, advertise, educate)	• List opportunities within the community to persuade customers to seek out your product or service (e.g., free screenings, seminars).	1. 2. 3.
• Plan—set SMART goals	• Develop at least three goals that will drive the target market to your services.	1. 2. 3.
Assess and Revise		**Implement Ideas**
• Process of evaluating product share of the market.	• How does the community or my target market see you? What is your rank? • Are you mentioned in the newspaper, given awards, or thought of as an expert? • Is your practice busy and productive as it can be?	• What are my achievements? • If they are not what was expected, we need to modify the marketing strategy. • What changes will you make?

Note: repeat the process—analyze needs, create a plan, implement, reassess and revise as needed. Repeat the process.

Evaluating Your Practice: Economic and Culture

There are several important economic indicators for evaluating a practice:

- Referrals are one indicator: Referrals include the number of new evaluations over previous months and years and the number of different referral sources per month versus the previous month and year. Rolling averages are often used to establish meaningful baselines for referral analysis.
- Patient visits are another indicator: Often referred to as visits per day. Patient visits include visits per month versus previous months and years, the number of visits per evaluation, often referred to as the length of stay, the charges and revenue per visit, and the labor cost per visit. Again, rolling averages are often used to establish sound baselines. Patient satisfaction studies, conducting thorough chart reviews for clinicians, and doing billing audits can assess the quality of care.
- Units per visit: Given the relatively high frequency of physical or occupational therapy practices using CPT codes as a basis for billing for revenue, it can often be helpful to keep track of the average number (and types) of units that are billed by visit or even by day, or by the total episode of care. A therapist who sees 12 patients daily with an average of three units per visit is often no less profitable than a therapist who sees nine patients daily but averages four units per visit. Different patient contexts can dictate different practice patterns.
- Net revenue per visit: One of the best measures of the tangible value of a visit to practice is the net revenue per visit, or the actual revenue realized by the business after a visit is completed. As previously discussed, a therapist can bill whatever amount they wish to a payer or customer, but ultimately, it is usually the payer who sets the amount that will be received for any given visit. For this reason, a combination of visits per day, units per visit, and net revenue per visit are often used as a combined metric to assess the financial health of a practice. Remember that the net revenue per visit can fluctuate widely from location to location, largely due to insurance contracts, resulting in different requirements for the number of visits required in a day to facilitate financial viability and sustainability.

Individual physical and occupational therapists can and should be assessed through an economic and a clinical lens. The good news for the clinical physical and occupational therapist is that when good clinical metrics are achieved, excellent operational metrics are usually achieved, which in turn means that a healthy, viable, and sustainable financial business model can be maintained, one which builds meaningful equity and the accumulation of wealth, that such success provides. It is a key feature to remember that consistently delivering excellence in care usually results in excellent operational and financial results.

Operational metrics such as new evaluations per month, the accuracy (and timeliness) of billing and charging, and a review of cancellations and no-shows for physical and occupational therapists are valuable economic indicators. Cancellations and no-show rates are often the "secret sauce" in evaluating a therapist's economic impact on the practice. While there are valid reasons for cancellations of appointments by patients, it is also valid to consider that a patient with a value proposition for care that places a high priority on their physical and occupational therapy care will less often cancel an appointment or be a no-show. A common way of reflecting the meaningful impact of cancellations and no-shows is found within the "drop rate." The drop rate is calculated by looking at the number of patients on a clinician's schedule at the beginning and end of the week. The drop rate reflects the difference between the two numbers. For example, if a clinician has 60 patients scheduled at the beginning of a Monday morning and sees 48 patients by the end of the day Friday, the drop rate is calculated as 12/60, or 20%. This means that 20% of the available patient slots for that clinician for that week went unfilled, resulting in a significant negative financial impact on a therapy practice. Therefore, strategies should be enacted at the practice level to ensure that all available spots are filled for any given week.

It is also important to measure the clinical effectiveness of a clinician, as a deterioration of clinical metrics is correlated and causative of a deterioration in operational and financial performance. A common method of evaluating a clinician's clinical performance is through a package of measures designed to assess (1) the functional gains a patient makes during their episode of care, e.g., the Single Alpha-Numeric Evaluator, (2) a measure of general patient satisfaction, e.g., the Net Promoter Score, and (3) a measure of the patient's perception of whether or not their goals have been achieved (e.g., percentage of patient goals achieved). If we again refer to the example value proposition discussed earlier in this chapter, we could suggest that the mix of the Single Alpha-Numeric Evaluator, the Net Promoter Score, and the patient goals achieved could be an accurate measure of whether or not the value of decreasing downstream healthcare costs has been achieved.

Strategies to evaluate a complete practice or clinic are similar to the metrics used to evaluate individual physical and occupational therapists, but additional data should be gleaned. Global practice indicators, the practice as a whole, would include payer mix percentages, no-shows/cancellations for a complete clinic, collections percentage/accounts receivable days, and cash flow. That is, any metrics used to evaluate individual clinicians should also be evaluated at a whole practice level. Doing this will help to establish benchmarks that can then be given to individual clinicians as examples of best practices most likely to benefit the practice as a whole. However, when considering an individual clinician's performance, care should be taken to ensure that the values are "risk-adjusted" to account for differences in patient populations. For example, a clinician who sees mostly high school athletes in a high socioeconomic area where most patients have excellent insurance should be expected to have very different operational and clinical outcomes than the clinician who sees mostly patients with chronic illnesses or long histories and who live in a lower socioeconomic area.

As previously mentioned, the influence of the payer (i.e., the insurance company) should also be considered when considering the ultimate value of a visit to the business. Any bill submitted to an insurance company is subject to contractual adjustments, that is, an amount agreed to between the insurance company and the therapy practice and defined in a written contract. Contractual adjustment is the difference between your charges for service as a physical or occupational therapist and the actual insurance payment. Historically, physical therapy has often been its worst financial enemy because competing physical therapy practices have offered lower amounts per visit to receive favored provider status. In markets where the amounts paid to providers per visit are relatively low, physical therapists must see more patients daily than average to break even financially. Remember that costs (e.g., salaries, rent, utilities) must be considered before a visit can be seen as profitable. If the net revenue per visit is low, more visits must be scheduled for a practice to collect enough revenue to achieve and maintain profitability. If we then return to the drop rate, we can see also how the combination of a low net revenue per visit, the resulting high visits per day required, and a >20% drop rate can cause significant financial problems for a physical or occupational therapy practice. Constant vigilance is required in a very low margin (i.e., percentage of revenue considered as profit) business, where there is very little ability to set prices when margins become too low.

Bad debt can also be considered a contractual adjustment, often due to clinician error. Examples of errors include inaccurate documentation (e.g., not adequately describing the services provided and billed for), exceeding the number of authorized patient visits, or billing codes or combinations of codes that are not allowed according to the contract. There are also administrative errors, such as not submitting billing on time or failing to secure appropriate authorizations. All contractual adjustments need to be considered in determining the financial health of a therapy practice and preventable errors need to be minimized as much as possible, remembering that a zero error rate is not a realistic expectation.

The culture of a clinical physical or occupational therapy practice is extremely important in determining its clinical and financial health. Evidence continues to accumulate to suggest that the overall context in which patients receive their care is critical in predicting their eventual outcome (McBee et al., 2017; Oostendorp et al., 2020). Many elements of a patient's eventual outcome can be due to factors not within the direct control of the physical or occupational therapist. Every contact with the patient should be considered an important contribution to the patient's eventual outcome. A practice can have the most efficient economic systems in place, but if the organization's culture is problematic, it will be difficult for a business to succeed. In the immortal words of Peter Drucker, foremost author and management consultant, "culture eats strategy for breakfast."

Leadership in an organization is largely about building the right culture for success.

Healthcare is a unique business in which the bond between a patient and a provider is very special. As a result, a good provider knows that although patient satisfaction is important, patient loyalty is the ultimate goal. This knowledge is why the first order of business in establishing a culture in a physical or occupational therapy practice is creating a patient-centered environment. There are many opportunities to create such an environment; often, some are so simple that it is easy to forget their importance. For example, training and teaching staff how to handle phone calls is critical in establishing a patient-centered culture. Administrative staff must understand that the administrative responsibilities of their job are second to welcoming patients into the practice. Small things such as greeting and acknowledging patients instead of just calling out their names in the waiting room go a long way. A physical or occupational therapist should have the staff inform the patient if they are running late and the therapist should never hesitate to apologize to patients if they are running late. Most importantly, a physical or occupational therapist should give patients undivided attention and must continually work to create an environment where the patients are always right or successful.

In order to create the optimal culture for business success, a leader in any business organization must know what is important to employees in the organization. While most think that high wages, job security, and promotion are most important to the employee, nearly every study on employee behavior and preferences reveal. While those are important, it is that the work is interesting and meaningful, and that there is a full appreciation of the work done, that is often more important (Rath & Clifton, 2004). To understand the basics of the business financials, refer to Figs. 14.1–14.5.

Sustaining Your Sources of Strategic Competitive Advantage

The previous sections focused on an overview of starting, building, and running a business, but how can a business be sustained and remain strategically competitive? A business must not have a unique and compelling value proposition but must have the resources and strategies available to make people aware of the value that can be delivered. The business must then also focus on executing the tasks required to deliver the proposition while simultaneously measuring, reflecting, and adapting to ensure the work is best aligned with the successful execution of the value proposition.

From a business standpoint, strategy includes a pattern of resource allocation that enables a business to maintain or improve performance. A good strategy focuses on neutralizing threats to business, taking advantage of opportunities promptly, capitalizing on strengths, and fixing identified internal weaknesses. As discussed earlier in the chapter, it also includes effectively recognizing and using all categories of resources, that is, your capital.

Category Start-Up Expenses	Amount ($)
Legal	1,000
Personnel (costs prior to opening)	0/Self
Office supplies/furniture	3,500
Brochure/business supplies	3,000
Clinical supplies	5,000
Consultants/accounting fee	2,000
Insurance	500
Rent/utilities	2,100
Website/telephone	5,000
Expensed equipment	15,000
Licenses/permits/advertising/bank fee	2,000
Total start up expenses	39,100
Start-up assets needed	
Cash balance on start date	50,000
Other short term assets	10,000
Total short term assets	60,000
Long term assets	0
Total assets	60,000
Total requirements	98,100

• **Fig. 14.1** Worksheet 9: Startup Costs

Category operating costs	Amount ($)	Category operating costs	Amount ($)
General fixed		**General variable**	
Rent		Marketing	
Utilities		Outsourcing fees	
Depreciation		Salaries	
Insurance		Medical/clinical supplies	
Loan repayments		Maintenance/repair	
Accounting service and fees		Education	
Consultants		Travel	
Clerical salaries and wages		Other	
Benefits		**Total**	
Office supplies		**General purchase**	
Business license		Office equipment	
Cleaning service		Clinical equipment	
Telephone		Business auto	
Other		Other	
Total		**Total**	

• **Fig. 14.2** Worksheet 10: Operating Costs: Fixed Versus Variable

Income statement for 3 years income	Year	Year	Year
Gross income from service or products			
Less bad debt			
Net income			
Cost of general fixed expenses			
Gross profit			
General fixed expenses			
Salaries and wages			
Payroll tax			
Benefits			
Equipment			
Maintenance and repairs			
Lease/rent			
Utilities			
Office supplies			
Telecommunication			
Medical supplies			
Marketing			
Professional fees/licenses and permits			
Depreciation			
Total expenses			
Net income before taxes			
Provision for taxes on income			
Net income after taxes (net profit)			

• **Fig. 14.3** Worksheet 11: Income Statement: Profit/Loss

Cash flow projection	Jan	Feb	Mar	Apr	May	June	...Dec
Opening cash balance							
Cash receipts							
Accounts receivable							
Collections							
Loans/interests							
Total cash in							
Cash payments							
Start up costs							
Rent							
Utilities							
Depreciation							
Insurance							
Loan repayments							
Lease payments							
Clinical salaries							
Office salaries							
Benefits							
Payroll wages							
Office supplies							
Medical supplies							
Postage							
Laundry/cleaning							
Telephone/fax/internet							
Licenses and permits							
Professional fees							
Marketing							
Outsourcing fees							
Maintenance/repair							
Education/ceus							
Travel							
Income							
Misc							
Total payment							
Opening cash balance							
Cash receipts							
Cash payments							
Ending cash balance							

Cash flow projection for 1 year

A cash flow projection or pro forma cash flow statement is a financial document that forecasts what cash or income is being received and what cash is being paid out.

If you are already in business for yourself (and now applying for a loan) you will have numbers to use. If you are just starting, your projected numbers will be estimated based on real probabilities.

In healthcare, unlike retail, income or cash flow can be delayed several weeks, especially if you are billing third party payors or federal or state insurers.

This is where some rehab owners miscalculate. You cannot pay for operational expenses if you don't have enough monthly cash (reimbursement) flowing in a timely manner. A general rule of thumb is to have enough funds to cover your start up costs and operating costs for 6 months.

• **Fig. 14.4** Worksheet 12: Cash Flow Projection for 1 Year

Assets		Liabilities	
Current assets		**Current liabilities**	
Cash	$	Account payable	$
Accounts receivable	$	Short term notes payable	$
Inventory	$	Federal income tax	$
Prepaid expenses	$	Self-employment tax	$
		State income tax	$
Total current assets	$	Sales tax accrual	$
Fixed assets		Property tax	$
Land	$	Payroll accrual	$
Building	$	Long term liabilities	$
Improvement	$		
Equipment	$		
Furniture	$		
Automobiles	$		
*less accrued depreciation**			
Total fixed assets	$	**Total liabilities**	$
NETWORTH (equity)			
Proprietorship	$		
Partnership			
Name _____, 51%	$		
Name _____, 49%	$		
Corporation			
Capitol stock	$		
Retained earnings	$		
Total net worth	$		

• **Fig. 14.5** Worksheet 13: Balance Sheet

Financial capital includes accounting and legal input and the analysis of economic data. *Physical capital* includes physical technology, the physical plant itself, equipment, geographic location, and access to needed materials. *Human capital* refers to training, experience, judgment, intelligence, relationships, and effective collaborations. *Organizational capital* refers to the administrative framework of the organization.

A strong administrative framework matching organizational needs is critical to ensuring business success. Using capital wisely contributes strongly to business sustainability. A business remains competitive when it implements value-creating strategies that are not being implemented as effectively and efficiently by others in the industry.

Summary

This chapter describes and discusses the essential elements required to embark on the journey of self-awareness as a business owner or entrepreneur, develop a business idea along with mission, vision, and core values to support it, as well as the concepts to understand the business of therapy practice. An overview of personality indicators, key business fundamentals, and processes is reflected in the specific tasks and reflections required to sustain and grow a business. All physical and occupational therapists have the ethical responsibility of understanding the key business elements of physical or occupational therapy practice, whether they are employees or business owners, regardless of the practice setting. While ongoing skill and professional development are important and cannot be underestimated, the physical or occupational therapy business can be summarized succinctly: it is a people-skill and knowledge-based industry. Keeping this as the "north star" helps assure success in practice.

References

Barrow, C., Barrow, P., & Brown. R. (2018). *The Business Plan Workbook: A step by step guide to creating and developing a successful business* (9th ed.). New York, NY, USA: Krogan Page Limited.

Baum, J. R., & Locke, E. A. (2004). The relationship of entrepreneurial traits, skill, and motivation to subsequent venture growth. *Journal of Applied Psychology, 89*(4), 587–598.

Bovend'eerdt, T., Botell, R., & Wade, D. (2009). Writing SMART rehabilitation goals and achieving goal attainment scaling: A practical guide. *Clinical Rehabilitation, 23,* 352–361.

Chamber of Commerce. (n.d.). Frequently Asked Questions About Small Business, 2021 (sba.gov). Retrieved from September 21, 2022. https://advocacy.sba.gov/wp-content/uploads/2021/12/Small-Business-FAQ-Revised-December-2021.pdf

Coad, A., & Storey, D. J. (2021) Taking the entrepreneur out of entrepreneurship. *The International Journal of Management Reviews, 23,* 541–548.

Denninger, T. R., Cook, C. E., Chapman, C. G., & McHenry, T. (2018). The influence of patient choice of first provider on costs and outcomes: Analysis from a physical therapy patient registry. *Journal of Orthopaedic and Sports Physical Therapy, 48*(2), 63–71.

Drucker, P. F. (1985). *Innovation and entrepreneurship: Practice and principles.* Butterworth-Heinemann.

Ferreira, J., Fernandes, C., & Kraus, S. (2017). Entrepreneurship research: mapping intellectual structures and research trends. *Review of Managerial Science, 13,* 181–205.

Frogner, B. K., Harwood, K., Andrilla, C. H. A., Schwartz, M., & Pines, J. M. (2018). Physical therapy as the first point of care to treat low back pain: An instrumental variables approach to estimate impact on opioid prescription, health care utilization, and costs. *Health Services Research, 53*(6), 4629–4646.

Horn, M. E., Brennan, G. P., George, S. Z., Harman, J. S., & Bishop, M. D. (2016). A value proposition for early physical therapist management of neck pain: a retrospective cohort analysis. *BMC Health Services Research, 16,* 253.

Jung, C. G. (1921). *Psychological types.* Princeton University Press.

Kelly, M. (2017). *Perfectly yourself: Discovering God's dream for you.* Beacon.

Korunka, C., Frank, H., Lueger, M., & Mugler, J. (2003). The entrepreneurial personality in the context of resources, environment, and the startup process: A configurational approach. *Entrepreneurship Theory and Practice, 28*(1), 23–42.

Law, T. J. (2021, February 6). *Question: Are you a business owner or an entrepreneur?* Oberlo. https://www.oberlo.com/blog/business-owner-vs-entrepreneur.

Lentz, T. A., Goode, A. P., Thigpen, C. A., & George, S. Z. (2020). Value-based care for musculoskeletal pain: Are physical therapists ready to deliver? *Physical Therapy & Rehabilitation Journal, 100*(4), 621–632.

Lentz, T. A., Harman, J. S., Marlow, N. M., & George, S. Z. Application of a value model for the prevention and management of chronic musculoskeletal pain by physical therapists. *Physical Therapy & Rehabilitation Journal, 97*(3), 354–364.

Lore, N. (1998). *The Pathfinder: How to choose or change your career for a lifetime of satisfaction and success.* Simon & Schuster.

Lumpkin, G. T., & Dess, G. G. (1996). Clarifying the entrepreneurial orientation construct and linking it to performance. *The Academy of Management Review, 21*(1), 135–172.

McBee, E., Ratcliffe, T., Picho, K., Schuwirth, L., Artino, A. R., Jr., Yepes-Rios, A. M., Masel, J., van der Vleuten, C., & Durning, S. J. (2017). Contextual factors and clinical reasoning: differences in diagnostic and therapeutic reasoning in board certified versus resident physicians. *BMC Medical Education, 17*(1), 211.

Myers, I. B., McCaulley, M. H., Quenk, N. L., & Hammer, A. L. (2003) *MBTI manual: A guide to the development and use of the Myers-Briggs Type Indicator instrument.* Consulting Psychologists Press.

Oostendorp, R. A. B., Elvers, J. W. H., van Trijffel, E., Rutten, G. M., Scholten-Peeters, G. G. M., Heijmans, M., Hendriks, E., Mikolajewska, E., De Kooning, M., Laekeman, M., Nijs, J., Roussel, N., & Samwel, H. (2020). Relationships between context, process, and outcome indicators to assess quality of physiotherapy care in patients with whiplash-associated disorders: Applying Donabedian's model of care. *Patient Preference and Adherence, 14,* 425–442.

Rath, D., & Clifton, D. (2004). *How full is your bucket?* (1st ed.). New York: Gallup Press.

Richmond, T., & Powers, D. (2009). *Business fundamentals for the rehab professional* (2nd ed.). Thorofare, NJ: SLACK.

Rutledge, H. (2008). *The Four Temperament Workbook.* OKA Otto Kroeger Association

Schumpeter, J. A. (1994). *Capitalism, socialism & democracy.* Routledge.

Small Business Administration Office of Advocacy. (2021). *Frequently Asked Questions About Small Business (sba.gov.)* https://advocacy.sba.gov/wp-content/uploads/2021/12/Small-Business-FAQ-Revised-December-2021.pdf

Zhu, F., Sun, S., & Sun, M. (2020). Influence of entrepreneurs' personality and personal characteristics on new venture performance: A fuzzy-set qualitative comparative analysis. *Social Behavior and Personality: An International Journal, 48*(12), e9199.

15

Outpatient Setting

**BLAIR CARSONE, PhD, MOT, OTR/L;
and JONATHAN ULRICH, PT, DPT, OCS**

LEARNING OBJECTIVES

After reading this chapter, you should be able to:

1. Understand what populations can be served in an outpatient clinic
2. Comprehend what services can be provided in an outpatient clinic
3. Acknowledge what legislation impacts an outpatient clinic
4. Recognize the responsibilities of management in an outpatient clinic
5. Appreciate the responsibilities of therapists in an outpatient clinic

CHAPTER OUTLINE

History and Background

Outpatient therapy has existed since the inception of the therapy profession itself. In the United States, outpatient therapy was most greatly impacted in 1965 by the Social Security Act. This landmark legislation established both Medicare (Title XVIII) and Medicaid (Title XIX), which are major insurance providers for clients receiving outpatient therapy (Klees et al., 2009). The Commission on Accreditation of Rehabilitation Facilities (CARF) soon followed in 1966, establishing quality guidelines (CARF, 2022). The

Social Security Act and CARF remain prevalent forces in providing outpatient services.

Today, outpatient clinics continue to be unique from other therapeutic settings. They cater to clients who are considered community mobile. An outpatient setting generally requires the client to visit a defined location for therapy services, physically or virtually. Traditionally, outpatient clinics are in hospitals, skilled nursing facilities, schools, neighborhoods or community centers, or private practice (i.e., standalone clinics) but may also include home visits. As of 2015, outpatient was the most common setting for physical therapists (33%), occupational therapists (22%), and speech-language pathologists (17%) (MyPTsolutions, 2015). Outpatient clinics vary greatly based on the services offered and the populations served.

Accreditation and Regulation

The regulatory bodies below are not all-inclusive. Outpatient managers should seek the counsel of qualified legal and human resources specialists to ensure they comply with all the applicable federal, state, and local laws that may impact the outpatient clinic. Laws governing clinical practice, labor, safety, and the consumer must all be considered. Several laws and regulations impact outpatient therapy services and business practices. Most notably, the Commission on Accreditation of Rehabilitation Facilities (CARF), the Centers for Medicare and Medicaid Services (CMS), and the Health Insurance Portability and Accountability Act of 1996 (HIPAA) regulate the provision of services. The Patient Protection and Affordable Care Act of 2010 (PPACA), Fair Labor Standards Act (FLSA), and Occupational Safety and Health Administration (OSHA), have laws against discriminatory practices and state licensure and practice act requirements that regulate business practices.

Commission on Accreditation of Rehabilitation Facilities

Outpatient clinics may be accredited through the CARF, an international organization founded in 1966 to provide a framework for business practice and service delivery. A qualifying clinic must provide a Quality Improvement Plan as part of its application (CARF, 2022). Unlike hospital-based outpatient therapy, outpatient clinics are not accredited by Joint Commission. Hospital-based outpatient programs can also seek CARF accreditation (CARF, 2022; Joint Commission, 2022). Overall, CARF accreditation offers distinction to an outpatient clinic.

Centers for Medicare and Medicaid Services

The CMS dictate requirements for Medicare and Medicaid. Outpatient rehabilitation is covered under Medicare Part B,

including home-health services for those who qualify (e.g., Table 15.1). Medicare establishes minimum health and safety standards mandatory for participating providers and imparts specialized regulations depending on the designation of a therapy clinic (CMS, 2022c). For instance, an outpatient clinic classified as a Comprehensive Outpatient Rehabilitation Facility (CORF) has additional standards and regulations (Legal Information Institute, 2022). For all clinics, occupational and physical therapists are considered mandatory "suppliers" per the Medicare Mandatory Claims Submission Rule (Jackson LLP Healthcare Lawyers, 2022). Therefore even if the clinician is not enrolled as a Medicare provider, they must submit claims and follow Medicare protocols when working with a potential Medicare beneficiary. Additionally, Medicare requires that timed Current Procedural Terminology (CPT) codes are only billed if the time spent with the beneficiary is one-on-one, which may require adjusted staffing ratios (CMS, 2022c).

Medicaid may also impact outpatient practice. Medicaid provides certain benefits mandated by the Federal government but varies by state. For instance, occupational therapy and physical therapy are considered optional benefits, which may make Medicaid participation unavailable in some states (CMS, 2022a). Conversely, in other states, Medicaid participation may be necessary if it is available and prevalent in the population served. For example, a pediatric therapist who works with children enrolled in Medicaid will need to enroll as a Medicaid provider. In general, Medicaid participation is dictated by its availability and clientele.

Health Insurance Portability and Accountability Act of 1996 (HIPAA)

HIPAA established several rules that impact the delivery of healthcare services in all settings. The Privacy Rule set standards for the use and disclosure of protected health information (PHI) and the rights of the client to understand and control how their health information might be used (Centers for Disease Control and Prevention, 2018). Clients must be given a Notice of Privacy Practices during the first appointment or have access to it through display in an accessible and prominent location.

TABLE 15.1 Home Health: Part A or Part B?

Billed Under	Setting	Factors	Considerations
Medicare Part A	• Traditional home health	• Homebound and under the care of a physician; in need of skilled yet intermittent nursing • Other home health services are provided by physical therapists, occupational therapists, home health aides, speech-language pathologists, and social workers	• Home health services provided under Medicare Part A are covered at 100%
Medicare Part B	• Outpatient home-based therapy	• Medicare Part A is exhausted • Covers medically necessary therapy services under the standard fee schedule, whether therapy is provided in the home or the clinic	• Home health services provided under Medicare Part B are covered at 80% • Medicare Part B will not pay for therapy services if the patient is simultaneously receiving care under Part A

The Transaction and Code Set Rule requires all covered entities to communicate using the same standards: *International Classification of Diseases, 10th edition, Clinical Modification* (ICD-10CM) for diagnosis coding, Procedure Classification System (PCS) for billing of inpatient hospital services, Current Procedural Terminology (CPT-4) for billing of physician services, and HCFA Common Procedural Coding System (HCPCS) for billing of ancillary services and procedures. CPT-4 codes commonly used in outpatient therapy billing are divided into timed and service codes. Timed codes are billed in 15-minute increments, including codes for treatments rendered (Table 15.2). Service codes are billed once, if applied, regardless of the time spent on the service, and do not require constant attendance (Table 15.3).

The Security Rule specifically addresses the protection of electronic PHI through administrative, physical, and technical safeguards (United States Department of Health & Human Services, 2020). Administrative safeguards include identifying and analyzing risks to electronic protected health information (e-PHI), implementing policies and procedures to limit exposure to e-PHI, and providing training and supervision for those who work with e-PHI. Physical safeguards include facility access and workstation/device security, such as thorough locks and passwords. Technical safeguards include tracking access to e-PHI and encryption of transmitted e-PHI to prevent unauthorized access by unintended recipients (United States Department of Health & Human Services, 2020). Managers and therapists of outpatient therapy clinics must ensure that all aspects of HIPAA are satisfied or risk monetary fines and civil or criminal penalties.

Patient Protection and Affordable Care Act of 2010 (PPACA)

The PPACA covers several aspects of health policy that affect outpatient clinic employees (CMS, 2010; Ullmann, 2015). Under the PPACA, an "employer with 50 or more full-time employees (or full-time equivalent employees) must offer minimum essential coverage to at least 95% of the employees and dependents" (Sheen, 2021, p.1). The law also expands the coverage of clinical preventative benefits (Rosenbaum, 2011). Additionally, managers may choose to

TABLE 15.2 **Commonly Used Timed Codes**

CPT Code	Name	CPT Code	Name
97032	Electrical stimulation, manual	97124	Massage
97033	Iontophoresis	97140	Manual therapy
97034	Contrast bath	97530	Therapeutic activities
97035	US/phono	97535	Self-care/home management
97039	Laser/other	97542	Wheelchair management
97110	Therapeutic exercise	97750	Physical performance testing
97112	Neuromuscular reducation	97760	Orthotic initial
97113	Aquatic therapy	97761	Prosthetic initial
97116	Gait training	97763	Orthotic/prosthetic management

TABLE 15.3 **Commonly Used Service Codes**

CPT Code	Name	CPT Code	Name
97010	Moist heat/cryotherapy	97026	Infrared
97012	Traction, mechanical	97161	Physical therapy evaluation, low complexity
97014	Electrical stimulation, unattended	97162	Physical therapy evaluation, medium complexity
97016	Vasopneumatic	97163	Physical therapy evaluation, high complexity
97018	Paraffin	97164	Physical therapy reevaluation
97022	Whirlpool	97165	Occupational therapy evaluation, low complexity
97024	Diathermy	97166	Occupational therapy evaluation, medium complexity
97028	Ultraviolet	97167	Occupational therapy evaluation, high complexity
97150	Group therapy	97168	Occupational therapy reevaluation

be involved in accountable care organizations which incentivize providers to improve quality, reduce healthcare costs, or navigate the bundled payments associated with specific diagnoses (McLawhorn & Buller, 2017). Overall, the employer of an outpatient setting may need to ensure that all aspects of PPACA are met when providing healthcare insurance benefits for employees.

Fair Labor Standards Act (FLSA)

The FLSA is a law that determines "minimum wage, overtime pay, recordkeeping, and youth employment standards" (United States Department of Labor, 2022b). For instance, outpatient therapy managers must monitor their non-salaried employees' hours to ensure proper pay. Additionally, a state may have more stringent laws than federal laws (California Department of Industrial Relations, 2021). The manager must ensure compliance with all federal and state labor laws.

Occupational Safety and Health Administration (OSHA)

OSHA establishes regulations for all businesses in the United States to ensure the health and safety of workers (United States Department of Labor, 2022a). Standards regarding bloodborne and respiratory pathogens, hazardous chemical exposures, and emergency action plans are needed for the outpatient setting. OSHA protects the worker, and managers must abide by its guidelines.

Laws Against Discriminatory Practices

Outpatient clinic managers should be aware of laws that address discriminatory practices. Title VII of the Civil Rights Act of 1964 prohibits discriminatory employment practices based on race, color, religion, sex, or national origin (United States Equal Employment Opportunity Commission, 2009). Section 501 of the Rehabilitation Act of 1973 and the Americans with Disabilities Act of 1990 (ADA) extended the prohibition of discriminatory practices to those with disabilities (ADA, 2009 2020; United States Equal Employment Opportunity Commission, 1992). The CRA and ADA also extend to clients and discrimination impacts access to care. In particular, the ADA has provisions for physical access (e.g., door widths, elevator access, seating requirements) that must be met. Outpatient clinics must adhere to these guiding laws for their employees and clients.

State Licensure and Practice Act Requirements

Finally, outpatient managers must be aware of state licensure and practice act requirements. Managers and therapists must ensure that licensed employees maintain active licensure. Although each state's practice act varies, typical requirements include reapplication, payment of fees, completion of required continuing education, and jurisprudence exams. Practice act requirements may also dictate staffing needs or specific risk management requirements. For example, some states require that assistants be supervised by "direct on-premise supervision" at all times or unless the assistant has a specific license (Pennsylvania Code, 2022; Pennsylvania State Board of Physical Therapy, 2008). Therefore outpatient managers in each state will have different requirements based on the nuances of their state practice act.

Patient Population

Outpatient therapy services can be provided to anyone who is community-mobile with cognitive, physical, neurological, and congenital disabilities. Although some outpatient clinics treat clients across the lifespan, many differentiate between pediatric and adult populations. Outpatient pediatric clinics typically provide services for newborns to 18 or 21 years of age, depending on insurance. Adult clinics usually provide services for ages 18 years and older.

The clients' age and diagnoses greatly influence pediatric outpatient therapy. Infants may receive services through state-based early intervention programs or their health insurance. Infants receiving services may have general developmental delays or a defined diagnosis (e.g., cerebral palsy, Downs syndrome, or Klumpke palsy). Children and adolescents receive services through their health insurance and will have a defined diagnosis (e.g., autism, attention-deficit/hyperactivity disorder, dyspraxia, dysarthria, or dysgraphia).

Adults receiving therapy typically have a defined diagnosis (e.g., knee replacement, cancer, dementia) to justify services. Uniquely, employed adults may receive services specifically for a job-related injury through Workers' Compensation with the primary goal of returning to work. The adult population can vary greatly in their needs, and a clinic's ability to serve clients will depend on its services.

Services

Outpatient clinics may offer comprehensive, specialized, or a combination of both services. Therapist pursuit of specialization or other certifications is much more common in outpatient settings. Certifications in manual therapy or other treatment techniques are widely available with the commitment of financial and time resources. The certifications can, in turn, be used to market a clinic or clinician to a specialized patient population. Specialized pediatric outpatient services tend to focus on a specific diagnosis or delay (e.g., feeding difficulties, sensory processing). Specialized adult outpatient services tend to focus on a body system (e.g., orthopedic, cardiac, neurological). Clinics will try to find their "niche" area by being unique and distinguished to create a consistent caseload for the therapists on staff.

Clinic owners and managers must determine if their population requires generalized or specialized services. Specialized clinics can have knowledge and resources that general clinics do not. For instance, the pediatric STAR Institute (2021) specializes in one specific type of treatment, sensory processing. However, specialized clinics have limiting factors such as: requiring clients to follow a demanding treatment schedule, lacking other specialties/approaches leading clients to either attend multiple clinics or leave to seek out more general clinics, and losing clients to early discharge if the specific approach does not benefit the client. Conversely, general clinics may have a greater diversity of services to address clients' needs, but they may need more knowledge and resources to handle complex cases. Some clinics attempt to remain generalized while providing specialty services. Although this is often seen as a beneficial combination, a general clinic may not maintain the resources and support needed for multiple specialized therapists. The clients' needs, the interests of the therapists, and the capability of the clinic and its managers must be considered when determining services in the outpatient setting.

Setting Characteristics

Outpatient clinics are distinctive from other settings. Outpatient clinics can serve clients across their entire lifespan with extensive diagnoses. The broadness of outpatient clinics can be a draw for therapists who enjoy the variation in their practice. Outpatient therapists can also specialize, attracting practitioners who want to develop specific expertise.

Outpatient clinics are distinctive in the types of interventions offered. For children and adults, outpatient clinics can provide group therapy services. Although other settings may have greater access to clients (e.g., inpatient, school), outpatient clinics generally have the space and equipment needed for efficacious individual treatment or group sessions. Lastly, outpatient adult services can provide unique services (e.g., driving rehabilitation, prosthetic training, adaptive sports) that may not be readily available elsewhere.

Outpatient clinics have more significant opportunities to develop therapeutic relationships and family-centered care (Smeulers et al., 2019). Clients in an outpatient setting commonly attend therapy a few days a week, for weeks to several months, depending upon the condition(s) for which the client is being treated. In general, clients attend outpatient therapy for longer than in other settings. The ability to build a therapeutic relationship appeals to outpatient therapists.

Providers and Care Coordination

Therapy providers are vital contributors to the success of each client. They can include occupational therapists, occupational therapy assistants, physical therapists, physical therapy assistants, speech-language pathologists, and speech-language pathology assistants. Outpatient clinics can offer one (e.g., occupational therapy), multiple therapies (e.g.,

occupational, physical, and speech therapy), or additional services in conjunction with therapy (e.g., neuropsychology, family counseling, applied behavior analysis, or nutrition counseling). Outpatient settings can also include non-medical providers, such as exercise physiologists, strength and conditioning specialists, and massage therapists. Over 38,000 outpatient clinics in the United States offer multiple therapy services (LaRosa, 2019).

Outpatient therapy providers can address a variety of performance skills. Occupational therapy can address activities of daily living and instrumental activities of daily living, focusing on the unique needs of the community-mobile client. Occupational therapists and assistants facilitate the development and refinement of fine motor coordination, visual perceptual, visual-motor integration, upper extremity strength, upper extremity coordination, and sensory processing skills. Physical therapy can address motor skills. Physical therapists and assistants facilitate the development and refinement of gross motor skills, balance, coordination, strength, range of motion, and movement patterns. Speech-language pathologists can facilitate the development and refining of language, communication, speaking, listening, voice use, and social skills. Therapy services often overlap regarding implementing techniques, strategies, and carryover but remain true to their scope of practice.

Therapy providers within the same field (e.g., occupational therapists and occupational therapy assistants) work towards the therapeutic goals established for each client. Therapists must perform the examination, evaluation, as well as reevaluation and discharge. Both therapists and assistants deliver treatment. It is beneficial for the therapist and assistant to collaborate, particularly if the assistant provides treatment and has in-depth knowledge of the client's abilities.

Responsibilities of a Manager/ Administrator

Managers (i.e., administrators) of outpatient facilities hold many responsibilities. Managers often must balance complex managerial and leadership roles. Management and leadership are commonly confused. Both are concerned with influence, employees, and goal accomplishment (Northouse, 2019). However, a manager's primary function is to provide order and consistency, whereas a leader promotes change that affects order (Kotter, 1990).

There are many different styles of management and leadership. Although these styles have been explored in social science, there has been limited research regarding implementation in the therapeutic setting. Transformational leadership or servant leadership are most applicable, based on limited findings and generalizations made from research in nursing (Alkassabi et al., 2018; Desveaux et al., 2016; Fleming-Castaldy & Patro, 2012; Gersh, 2006; Keisu et al., 2018; Kouzes & Posner, 2012). Due to the limited evidence, management and leadership styles can vary greatly between outpatient clinics and are determined by a clinic's unique individual needs.

Management in an outpatient setting depends on the size of the clinic(s) and the administration structure (Fig. 15.1). Responsibilities will evolve for any manager in an outpatient clinic setting due to the changing needs of the clients, staff, and families. Managers are responsible for the successful operation of the clinic(s); ensuring therapy providers are completing all their necessary tasks promptly, clients are receiving the best therapy, support staff understand and perform the necessary tasks expected, and families are involved and supportive of their loved ones' therapy services.

The manager is responsible for the clinic's success, largely judged by the client and family satisfaction. The clinic must maintain a customer service focus when working in an outpatient setting. Maintaining a customer service focus can sometimes conflict with the most appropriate clinical action. For example, if a patient/client has progressed to discharge but still has authorized visits through their insurance, the client may wish to schedule additional visits even if they are not medically necessary. In this case, the therapist must communicate why further visits are not in the patient's best interest while avoiding negatively impacting the patient's experience. Managers can play a supportive role in these situations by providing advice or training, such as advising therapists to address this potential issue during the evaluation. If needed, the manager may need to address the situation themselves (Fig. 15.2).

Overall, the manager is responsible for quality service delivery and client satisfaction in the outpatient setting and must contend with and resolve many obstacles through proper administrative channels. Most obstacles can be categorized as internal or external. Internal management issues arise directly from the clinic operations, whereas external management issues occur outside the clinic system but still greatly influence its function (see Chapter 11).

Referral Sources

Outpatient therapy referral sources vary but largely depend on the client's insurance. Typically, a client will be referred by a physician and have a signed order for therapy (CMS, 2019; Pendergast et al., 2012). The physician may recommend a clinic to the client, provide a list, or let the client determine a clinic for rehabilitation on their own. Most insurance companies cover direct access privileges to physical therapy, which allows the client to attend physical therapy without a referral from a physician (American Physical Therapy Association, 2021). Direct access to occupational therapy services is less common (American Occupational Therapy Association, 2021).

Workers' compensation requires preauthorization in addition to the physician's order (Bureau of Workers' Compensation, 2022). Some commercial insurance plans, such as health maintenance organizations (HMO), also require insurance preauthorization and a physician referral.

Pediatric clinics have unique exceptions for referrals. For pediatric outpatient clinics, a client receiving early intervention services (i.e., children under 3 years of age) may do so without a physician referral. Anyone can refer a child under 3 years of age to be evaluated by the early intervention team to determine eligibility.

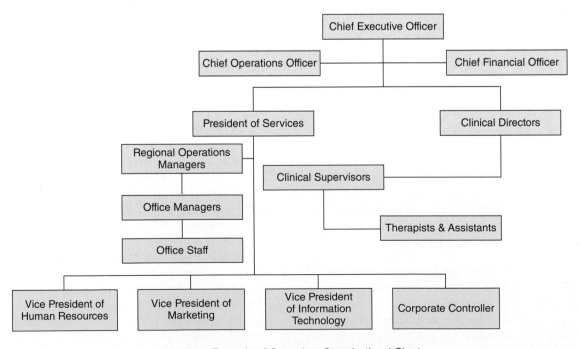

• **Fig. 15.1** Example of Outpatient Organizational Chart

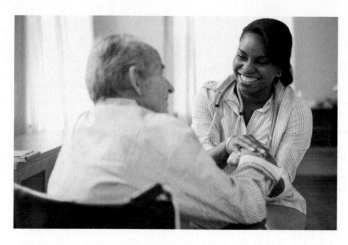

• **Fig. 15.2** Anticipating and addressing client expectations is key to optimal care. (From https://www.flickr.com/photos/52041471@N04/6052491503.)

Marketing

An outpatient manager is also responsible for marketing. Marketing for an outpatient clinic often involves a combination of online and in-person presence. Online marketing may include a website, social media, searchability, and advertisements. In-person presence might involve visits to physicians' offices, community events, and community service. Ensuring potential patients/clients know about the clinic is vital to ensuring a steady clinic volume. For more information on marketing strategies, refer to Chapter 14.

Staffing

It behooves a clinic to have proper staffing to meet the need generated through marketing and referral sources. Staffing depends on the size of the clinic, the clients served, and the services provided. The physical size of the clinic dictates the number of staff, therapy providers, and clients that can be accommodated at any given time following occupancy limits. The number of clients determines the potential increase or decrease needed for staffing. The services provided significantly impact staffing. If a clinic offers multiple therapy services or additional services, sufficient staffing to assist clients, answer questions, and schedule clients are critical to the outpatient clinic's successful flow and operation.

Client volume and demand can change throughout the week and time of day. Clinics must be open for business during a time that meets the needs of their clients. A pediatric clinic will need to have after-school availability. An adult clinic may need to have before and after work hours. Clinics may have part-time or pro re nata (PRN) staff for higher-demand slots to meet this demand.

Pediatric and adult outpatient clinics have unique staffing needs. Pediatric therapy has changed dramatically in the last few decades as the prevalence of autism and developmental disabilities have increased (Centers for Disease Control and Prevention, 2021; Durkin, 2019). This increase in demand will likely impact staffing needs. Various adult clinics may provide services to two or more non-Medicare clients at the same time. These concurrent treatment sessions can reduce therapist staffing needs but increase the need for support staff. As the landscape of therapy changes, so will staffing needs.

Productivity Expectations

Productivity standards for outpatient therapy are often dependent on staffing. For instance, a therapist who is the only one providing a very specialized service may have more flexibility in their productivity standards than a general therapist. The most notable difference, however, exists between pediatric and adult clinics.

Pediatric outpatient clinics need to have flexibility in productivity standards. Pediatric therapists often treat one-on-one due to the intensive nature of the sessions. Due to the nature of this population (e.g., reliance on others for transportation, need for multiple healthcare appointments, proclivity to illness), cancellations and "no-shows" are common. Luckily, regarding treatment efficacy, intensive episodic therapy is similar to continuous, less intensive therapy (Newman et al., 2016). Although these absences may not ultimately harm the client, they pose a challenge for outpatient productivity. Pediatric clinics usually have an attendance policy to prevent multiple cancellations or "no-shows" to therapy. The responsibility of tracking and enforcing those policies depends on who is scheduling the client. In general, attendance policies help pediatric therapists to remain productive.

Adult outpatient clinics have more rigorous productivity standards. Adult therapists often treat more than one non-Medicare client at a time, known as a concurrent, simultaneous, or overlapping schedule (Aegis Therapies, 2019). Therefore if one client does not show or cancels, the therapist can treat other clients for billable time. Clinics who use a single-booked schedule may adopt a double-booked schedule if a client arrives late or needs to reschedule. Managing multiple patients requires skill by the clinician to maintain clinical excellence and customer service. Although there are productivity advantages to a simultaneous schedule, some therapists find it too challenging or dissatisfying.

Medicare requires that treatment be provided one-on-one to its beneficiaries in adult clinics (CMS, 2019). This standard can help reduce therapists being overwhelmed and increase care quality, but it has implications for productivity. At the time of this writing, a code that was previously discarded to treat clients in groups, is being currently utilized. The use of appropriate codes should be thoroughly understood so the most appropriate approach to billing is taken for the client and the organization. For therapists who primarily treat Medicare beneficiaries, flexibility in productivity is needed, but usually not to the extent seen in pediatrics. The productivity requirements can differ because adults receiving outpatient therapy are community-mobile, meaning they usually have transportation and means to get to scheduled therapy appointments. Managers must still be aware of this possible challenge to productivity and implement attendance policies.

The manager of an outpatient clinic must responsibly address staffing and productivity standards. The manager must ensure that the staff is competent, available, and meets the clinic's standards. These requirements may fluctuate as clientele, insurance coverage/standards, and therapists' abilities change. Changes in productivity and staffing as a business shrinks or grows will ultimately impact reimbursement and the overall financial achievement of the clinic. Overall, staffing needs and productivity must be balanced regularly to ensure the clinic's success.

Reimbursement

An outpatient manager may be responsible for the financial management of the clinic. Managers must manage both revenue and expenses. In a non-profit business, ultimately, the two should balance. In a for-profit business, the manager's goal is to bring in more revenue than is spent through expenses. The manager can attempt to control labor, supplies, cost of the physical space (either lease or mortgage), and utilities. The cost of the physical space and utilities is often relatively fixed, so careful consideration when selecting a space for a clinic is important. A manager has more flexibility with variable costs such as supplies and labor.

Managers must ensure that billing is accurate and claims are processed. Underbilling results in less income for the clinic and can make supporting a clinic's expenses difficult. Overbilling puts the clinic at risk of legal action by federal, state, or local governments, and violates ethical responsibilities. Incorrect coding or documentation that does not support skilled care can result in rejected claims or payment retraction. Although the manager has many important financial responsibilities, everyone in the outpatient clinic impacts billing and payment and can be impacted *by* billing and payment. Proper billing and payment are critical to an outpatient clinic's financial success and longevity. The manager may be responsible for training staff, performing routine chart audits, and providing support as clinic staff navigate ever-changing requirements for appropriate billing.

Providing proper billing and documentation begins before therapeutic services are initiated. Prior to the initial assessment, referral source, insurance verification, and coverage of services should be completed. Insurance will often not pay for services if a referral was not received prior to an initial evaluation. If a clinic fails to verify insurance and coverage, the client may be responsible for all services out-of-pocket. Verification also informs the client of potential co-payments and an approximate number of sessions insurance will provide (if approved). This process may not be necessary for clients or families who wish to pay for their services out-of-pocket. If clients pay out-of-pocket, they often use insurance

coverage initially and then personally cover expenses once insurance funds have been fully utilized. A growing segment of clinics choose to forgo insurance as payment altogether and only accept cash payments. Although choosing cash payment may avoid the challenges associated with insurance companies, it may greatly limit who can afford to attend that clinic.

Reimbursement requirements create the opportunity for management issues to occur. For instance, if a therapy provider incorrectly bills for a session, the clinic can incur those costs if the office staff does not collect a co-payment or if the client no longer has insurance coverage. Generally, management will oversee the finances; however, payment problems can be overlooked depending on whom management expects to mitigate possible problems. A manager may need to delegate and implement policies to solve several common conundrums: (1) who is responsible for catching documentation errors, (2) who is responsible for calculating, collecting, and documenting co-payments, (3) who is responsible for verifying insurance coverages. Unclear responsibilities, lack of checks and balances, and poorly managed front offices can contribute to payment problems that impact the business's bottom line.

Therapy providers are responsible for billing units accurately and correctly. Billing units for the appropriate time and correct code(s) is required for ethical and legal practice. Billing is submitted promptly to the client's insurance to ensure reimbursement for services rendered. Therapy providers are also responsible for selecting the appropriate diagnosis (ICD-10) code(s), avoiding unspecified codes. More than one diagnosis may be appropriate to capture the comorbidities impacting treatment. All billing claims must be supported through accurate and descriptive documentation.

Code selection is important for a therapist to consider to best reflect the care's complexity and maximize potential revenue. The three codes that require the most consideration are therapeutic exercise (97110), neuromuscular reeducation (97112), and therapeutic activities (97530). Each of the previously mentioned codes can be used to code exercise activities. However, each code is selected based on the therapist's intent when prescribing the activity (Table 15.4). Therapeutic exercise should be selected when a therapist intends for an activity to improve range of motion, strength, endurance, or flexibility. Neuromuscular reeducation should be selected when the therapist intends to improve a patient's balance and posture, reeducate a muscle, or elicit cocontraction of muscles. Therapeutic activities should be selected by the therapist when the intent is to improve the patient's capacity to perform a functional task, such as sitting to stand from a chair or an overhead reaching activity to retrieve an object from a shelf (i.e., "ing" codes). Therapy must be intentional, purposeful, and justified, reflected in the chosen codes.

Reimbursement in outpatient settings has more nuances than in other settings because of the variety of payment methods and the increased likelihood that the same provider is treating multiple patients simultaneously. The clinician must know whether the CPT code used for the

TABLE 15.4	Therapeutic Exercise, Neuromuscular Reeducation, Therapeutic Activity–Which Code to Bill?	
CPT Code	**Rationale**	**Example**
97110 - Therapeutic Exercise	Therapist intent to improve a single parameter, such as range of motion, flexibility, strength, etc.	Squat exercise to improve strength of the gluteus maximus
97112 - Neuromuscular Reeducation	Therapist intent to improve posture, balance, coordination, co-contraction, etc.	Squat exercise to improve co-contraction of the quadriceps and hamstrings during weight bearing
97530 - Therapeutic Activity	Therapist intent to improve the patient's capacity in a functional activity	Squat exercise to improve patient's capacity to perform sit to stand

treatment provided is a timed or service code to determine whether the clinician can bill for multiple units or a single unit per encounter (Table 15.5). The clinician must also know whether the insurance payor follows the "total time rule" or not. If a payor follows the "total time rule," a unit of billing may be charged if greater than 8 minutes, up to 22 minutes, of direct one-on-one treatment time was spent with a patient (MedicareFAQ, 2021). If a payor does not follow the "total time rule," a unit can be billed if the clinician spends 1–15 minutes for a billing unit, often without requiring the care to be one-on-one.

Medicare

In clinics that treat an adult population, different insurance payors have unique rules and factors that can influence reimbursement. Medicare has the most rules, regulations, and factors to consider. As previously discussed, Medicare only reimburses for care provided one-to-one unless a specified group code is active and can be utilized. Therapists must manage their schedules to ensure that patients who use Medicare as their payor are scheduled alone to maximize their time and, in turn, their revenue.

Multiple Procedure Payment Reduction

The Multiple Procedure Payment Reduction (MPPR) pays a reduced rate for each subsequent unit of the same CPT code billed in the same treatment session (Clinicient, 2022). Medicare determines the reimbursement price for a unit by three factors: work value, practice expense, and malpractice expense, which is defined as a relative value unit (RVU) (Clinicient, 2022). The RVU is multiplied by a geographical adjustment and a standardized conversion factor to determine the payment amount (Table 15.6). The rationale for the reduction of payment is that the therapist/clinic does not need to spend the same amount of money on overhead to deliver the treatment and therefore does not require payment to cover non-existent overhead costs.

Therapy Cap

The Balanced Budget Act of 1997 established an annual per-beneficiary Medicare spending limit or "therapy cap" (American Physical Therapy Association, 2018). A Medicare beneficiary had a limited amount of dollars to spend on occupational therapy, physical therapy, and speech therapy. Due to the lack of a grammatical nuance, known as the Oxford comma, the Medicare cap was interpreted to apply to occupational therapy separately while applying to physical and speech therapy combined.

The therapy cap was permanently repealed in 2018 (American Physical Therapy Association, 2018). Although there is no longer a cap, Medicare will continue to monitor the utilization of therapy services. For instance, if a therapist deems treatment is medically necessary for a Medicare beneficiary after exceeding a defined amount (i.e., soft cap),

TABLE 15.5	Medicare 8-Minute Rule Chart[a]
Time Spent (min)	**Number of Billable Units**
8 to 22	1
23 to 37	2
38 to 52	3
53 to 67	4
68 to 82	5
83 to 97	6

[a]This chart only applies to time-based codes.

TABLE 15.6	Components of the Relative Value Unit
Category	**Included Factors**
Work value	Required knowledge, technical ability required for skill
Practice expense	Overhead costs related to operation of practice
Malpractice expense	Overhead costs related to malpractice coverage

the therapist must place a -KX modifier after each CPT code, notifying Medicare that the beneficiary has exceeded that amount ($2150 for 2022) (Clinicient, 2022, CMS, 2022e).

Targeted Review

If a Medicare patient receives therapy and exceeds $3000 of care in a year, the case will undergo a "targeted review" (Clinicient, 2022). During the targeted review, a Medicare auditor will review the case, in its entirety, for medical necessity. The auditor may determine that none, some, or all the care was medically necessary and withdraw payment accordingly. A therapist may not bill a patient for care deemed medically unnecessary unless an Advanced Beneficiary Notice (ABN) has been put into place (Chapter 13). Only care rendered after the ABN was provided and signed, specifically listed within the Notice of Medicare Non-Coverage (NOMNC), may be billed directly to the patient (Fig. 15.3). Of note, providing a routine, or blanket, ABN for each patient at the onset of care is considered fraudulent behavior and may be prosecuted (Medicare Interactive, 2022).

Advance Beneficiary Notice

If a therapist determines that therapy is no longer medically necessary or Medicare does not cover a particular service, then the therapist must provide the beneficiary with a NOMNC and an ABN. The NOMNC notifies the Medicare beneficiary of what is specifically not covered by Medicare and why it is not covered (CMS, 2022f). The ABN notifies the Medicare beneficiary of the three options available to them and their acknowledgment of the risks and consequences of their choice and allows the provider to transfer financial risk to the patient (CMS, 2022f).

The first option the beneficiary can choose is that they understand the treatment is not covered and they would like the therapist to submit the claims for consideration of coverage by Medicare and acknowledge they may have to pay for the uncovered care if Medicare denies the claim. The second option is that the beneficiary understands the treatment is not covered, wishes to receive it, and will pay for it without submitting claims to Medicare. The third option is that they understand the treatment is not covered, but do not want to assume the risk of paying for it, so they decline to receive the treatment at this time.

Therapy Assistant Payment Reduction

A new development in 2022 is a 15% reduction in payment for care rendered by a physical or occupational therapy assistant (American Occupational Therapy Association, 2022; American Physical Therapy Association, 2022). Any care provided to a Medicare beneficiary by a physical or occupational therapy assistant must be labeled with a -CQ or a -CO modifier, notifying Medicare that the care is subject to the 15% reduction in payment. Due

to this change, outpatient clinics may choose not to employ as many occupational or physical therapy assistants.

Medicare and Group Therapy

If a therapist must see two Medicare beneficiaries simultaneously, the therapist must decide how to bill for the care. As previously discussed, Medicare only reimburses for care provided one-to-one. The therapist must track when they spent meaningful one-on-one time with each patient. The therapist can then aggregate the time spent with each patient to determine how many units are appropriate to bill to each one. However, if two, or more patients are engaged in activities that may or may not be the same activity, and the therapist did not spend meaningful time with either patient, then the therapist may choose to bill the "group therapy" (97150) code (CMS, 2022g). "Group therapy" is a service code and may only be billed once per treatment session, regardless of the time spent completing the group therapy. Group therapy reimburses at a lower rate than the one-to-one timed codes but may be better than receiving no reimbursement.

Bundled Payment

A final consideration for the therapist is that certain groups of patients may fall into a bundled payment system (Chapter 13). Within a bundled payment system, all providers are paid a lump sum for all the care necessary for the patient. Bundled payment systems are most common in patients after total joint replacement surgeries but are also present in other patient populations (Kaiser Family Foundation, 2018). Therapists treating a patient that falls into a bundled payment group will need to ensure that they are treating the patient as efficiently as possible to minimize the risk of underpayment through overutilization.

Commercial Insurance

Commercial payors, such as Aetna or Blue Cross Blue Shield, have significantly fewer considerations when compared to Medicare. However, therapists must still be aware of factors affecting their patients and their ability to pay for services. Commercial insurance plans are often provided through a patient's employer, although they can be purchased by the patient directly. The patient and their employer pay a monthly premium for an insurance plan. Within each plan, there are three cost-sharing mechanisms that the insurance plan may use to reduce the overall cost of health care. The first is a deductible. The deductible is the amount the consumer must pay before the health insurance pays for coverage (Healthcare.gov, 2022). The second mechanism is a co-payment. A co-payment is a flat fee the consumer must pay each time they utilize a health care service (Healthcare.gov, 2022). The third mechanism is called co-insurance. Co-insurance is a percentage consumers must pay each time they utilize a health care service (Healthcare.gov, 2022). Insurance plans may utilize all three mechanisms or

{Insert provider contact information here}
Notice of Medicare Non-Coverage

Patient name: Patient number:

The effective date coverage of your current **{insert type}**
Services will end: **{insert effective date}**

- Your Medicare provider and/or health plan have determined that Medicare probably will not pay for your current {insert type} services after the effective date indicated above.
- You may have to pay for any services you receive after the above date.

Your right to appeal this decision

- You have the right to an immediate, independent medical review (appeal) of the decision to end Medicare coverage of these services. Your services will continue during the appeal.
- If you choose to appeal, the independent reviewer will ask for your opinion. The reviewer also will look at your medical records and/or other relevant information. You do not have to prepare anything in writing, but you have the right to do so if you wish.
- If you choose to appeal, you and the independent reviewer will each receive a copy of the detailed explanation about why your coverage for services should not continue. You will receive this detailed notice only after you request an appeal.
- If you choose to appeal, and the independent reviewer agrees services should no longer be covered after the effective date indicated above;
  ○ Neither Medicare nor your plan will pay for these services after that date.
- If you stop services no later than the effective date indicated above, you will avoid financial liability.

How to ask for an immediate appeal

- You must make your request to your Quality Improvement Organization (also known as a QIO). A QIO is the independent reviewer authorized by Medicare to review the decision to end these services.
- Your request for an immediate appeal should be made as soon as possible, but no later than noon of the day before the effective date indicated above.
- The QIO will notify you of its decision as soon as possible, generally no later than two days after the effective date of this notice if you are in Original Medicare. If you are in a Medicare health plan, the QIO generally will notify you of its decision by the effective date of this notice.
- Call your QIO at: {insert QIO name and toll-free number of QIO} to appeal, or if you have questions.

If you miss the deadline to request an immediate appeal, you may have other appeal rights:

- If you have Original Medicare: Call the QIO listed on page 1.
- If you belong to a Medicare health plan: Call your plan at the number given below.

Plan contact information _____

_____

Additional information (optional):

Please sign below to indicate you received and understood this notice.

I have been notified that coverage of my services will end on the effective date indicated on this notice and that I may appeal this decision by contacting my QIO.

_____   _____
Signature of Patient or Representative   Date

Form CMS 10123-NOMNC (Approved 12/31/2011)   OMB approval 0938-0953

• **Fig. 15.3** Notice of Medicare non-coverage (NOMNC)

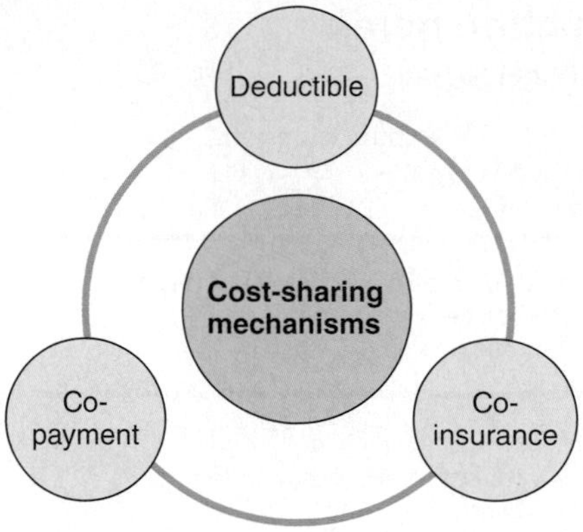

• **Fig. 15.4** Insurance Cost-Sharing Mechanisms Affecting Care. Can you define each?

none, depending upon the contract established between the beneficiary and the payor (Fig. 15.4).

Some commercial payors use a third party to authorize healthcare services, such as United Health Care, which uses United Medical Resources to authorize its therapy services (United Health Care, 2022). After completing the evaluation, a therapist must submit a form with the required information to the third party. A reviewer will provide authorization for several visits based on the information provided. A peer review can be requested if a patient or therapist disagrees with the number of visits provided. A successful peer review may increase visits allotted for the recommended care.

A final consideration for the therapist working with a commercial insurance beneficiary is the negotiated rate agreed upon between the provider and the insurance payor. Some contracts specify a fee-for-service model, in which each CPT code billed is paid at an agreed-upon rate. Other contracts utilize a case rate, in which a flat amount is paid for the care provided. The flat amount can be paid per day, visit, or episode of care, depending on the contract. Finally, contracts can utilize a capitation model, in which a lump sum is paid to care for a group of people. The lump sum is paid in full, regardless whether all the people in the group need care or if none needs care.

Workers' Compensation

Clients using workers' compensation insurance are another group commonly seen in outpatient clinics. Workers' compensation insurance covers the medical care necessary to return an injured worker to work. As a result, all the therapist's treatment and documentation must support the goal of returning the patient to work-related activities. The care of an injured worker may require more frequent communication with related medical team members, such as the referring physician, the employer, the insurance auditor, or the case manager. The documentation requirements of the employer or the payor may require more frequent progress notes, such as bimonthly or daily. Employers or workers' compensation insurers may utilize a third-party authorizing service, such as some commercial insurance

plans, to control healthcare costs. Despite the administrative burden required to treat injured workers successfully, therapists often seek to increase the percentage of injured workers on their caseload due to the higher reimbursement rate.

Automobile or Home Insurance

Clients who utilize the medical benefits allotted by automobile or home insurance may also be seen in the outpatient clinic. Automobile and home insurance provide a medical benefit, a dollar amount selected by the insured to cover medical costs in the event of an injury sustained through a covered event. Automobile and home insurances do not have contracts with providers and do not, therefore have negotiated rates. Any care provided is subject to the clinic's established fee schedule at the determined gross rate per CPT code. Therapists must know that the cost of their care is significantly higher for those choosing to use the medical benefit from their home or automobile policy. The care provided may quickly exhaust the medical benefit if the benefit was not already exhausted by the care provided by other health care providers. Due to the rapid accruement of charges, patients may make an uninformed decision to receive services and become upset when they receive the bill for the care they assumed was covered.

Pediatrics

Some reimbursement considerations are unique to pediatric clinics. For example, a pediatric clinic that provides early intervention will need to designate credentialed therapists who will bill the state. A pediatric clinic contracting with a charter or private school may still need to bill through the client's insurance. In addition to specific types of therapy (e.g., early intervention, contracted, simultaneously scheduled), therapists must also be aware of insurance coverage of certain interventions and diagnoses. For instance, some states do not reimburse for sensory integration even with ample documentation of its effectiveness. Some diagnoses, such as scar adherence, cannot be the primary diagnosis because they are considered "cosmetic" even if a client is postoperative. Therapists need to be aware of their setting's unique exceptions so that claims do not get denied and reimbursement is not delayed.

Self-Pay

Clients who self-pay may also be treated in an outpatient setting. Such patients have very few rules, regulations, and factors that must be considered by the therapists working with them. Occupational and physical therapists are compulsory providers within the Medicare program (CMS, 2019; WebPT, 2018). Therefore the therapist must bill Medicare if a Medicare beneficiary has available benefits (Fig. 15.5). As a result, therapists may not bill patients for services that qualify for payment through Medicare and are not eligible for cash-based services. An additional consideration is the No Surprises Act, passed as part of the Consolidated Appropriations Act of 2021 (CMS, 2022d). The No Surprises Act requires a provider to provide a good faith

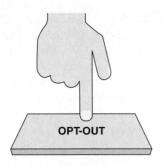

• **Fig. 15.5** Occupational and physical therapists are unable to "opt-out" from Medicare. If a therapist is not enrolled with Medicare, they must refer to Medicare providers when treatment is reasonable and necessary.

estimate of the expected charges if not using insurance. While not a bill and not final until the care has been rendered, providers need to justify excess charges if disputed by the consumer. Consumers can request a "dispute resolution entity" to review the case and resolve charges exceeding $400 compared with the good faith estimate.

Documentation

Appropriate and timely documentation is also essential to reimbursement in any outpatient clinic setting. Incorrect or inaccurate documentation is unethical, fraudulent, and detrimental to a clinic. Essential documentation begins with comprehensive evaluations that justify the need for skilled therapy services (Fig. 15.6). Descriptive reasoning in the evaluation and plan of care is more likely to be approved by the referring physician and the insurance company.

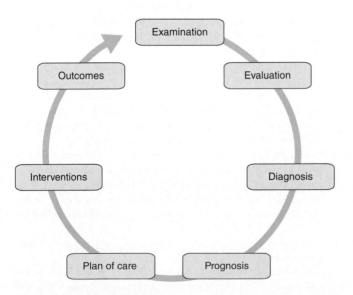

• **Fig. 15.6** Documentation Components. Elements of documentation within the patient/client management model. (Reprinted from www.apta.org, with permission of the American Physical Therapy Association. © 2023 American Physical Therapy Association. All rights reserved.)

Accurate and clear documentation of each interaction through a daily note is important for reimbursement and recording progression or regression in the client. Documentation must include all aspects required per the profession's guide to practice. A daily note still often includes the components of SOAP (subjective, objective, assessment, and plan) even if an electronic medical record system is utilized.

Patient-reported outcome measures (PRO) are important for each client's episode of care. PRO can assess the patient's subjective perspective about how their condition impacts their functional abilities. The PRO is scored and converted into a numerical value that can be used for easier comparison and combined with other data to support skilled therapy. Some insurance payors require scores to be submitted with authorization requests. The percentage of change from initial scores can be compared with other patients with similar conditions, allowing the therapist to judge whether a client is progressing as expected. All percentages of change in patients treated by a therapist can be aggregated and compared with other therapists and their scores with similar diagnoses. Managers may find it beneficial to enroll with a database, such as the Focus on Therapeutic Outcomes (FOTO) or the Physical Therapy Outcomes Registry, which has the client complete each questionnaire at set intervals and compares outcomes to other enrolled clinicians across the country (American Physical Therapy Association, 2017).

Reevaluations occur based on the insurance and most are every 2 to 6 months. Additionally, therapists are subject to reevaluation regulations per their state practice act, of which many require reevaluation every 30 days. Medicare Part B requires a progress report every 10 visits or reevaluation when the plan of care expires (CMS, 2019). Clients covered by workers' compensation may need more frequent reevaluations, either from the insurance carrier, a third party that manages claims, or the employer. Thorough documentation of the client's progress, strengths, and weaknesses in the reevaluation dictates whether insurance will approve continued services. A clinician's documentation must demonstrate a clear need for skilled therapy to restore function if therapy continues; otherwise, the client must be discharged.

Some documentation considerations are unique to pediatric or adult clinics. For instance, pediatric therapists often need to document state-provided services. Most Medicaid programs and early intervention programs are based on a family education model, and all documentation must reflect a family-centered perspective from the goals, to the intervention delivery, to the outcome measures. Adult therapists often need to document federally funded services.

Medicare Part B requires that the plan of care be certified by the patient's physician (or physician's team) within 30 days of the first encounter (CMS, 2019). Medicare defines a physician as a medical doctor (MD), doctor of osteopathy (DO), nurse practitioner (NP), or physician assistant (PA). It is important to note that doctors of dental surgery (DDS) and doctors of chiropractic (DC) are not considered physicians by Medicare and may not sign off on plans of care for Medicare beneficiaries (Fig. 15.7). Per

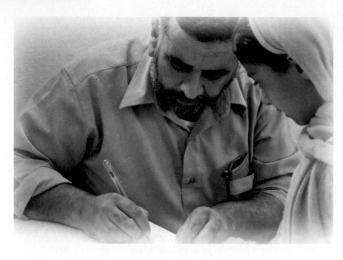

• **Fig. 15.7** Although state practice acts may allow therapists to evaluate and treat without a referral, Medicare Part B requires that the plan of care be certified by the patient's physician within 30 days of the first encounter. (From https://www.flickr.com/photos/29456680@N06/4709092642).

Medicare Part B, a care plan can last up to 90 days (CMS, 2019). The length of the care plans in the outpatient adult setting also makes reevaluations more likely to require documentation.

Maintaining accurate documentation, being professional, and communicating with all parties can prevent scheduling difficulties and unrealistic expectations from becoming greater. Issues cannot always be avoided but being aware and diligent is critical to the success of the therapy provider and client-family relationship. Accurate and thorough documentation is essential to reimbursement, but it can also be utilized to improve the outpatient clinic. Clinics and providers are responsible for providing safe and effective therapy services. Managers and therapists must continue to reassess the evolving needs of the clinic and the clientele served. Serving the growing number of clients who require advocacy, documentation, and research is critical to continuing best practices in an outpatient setting.

Quality Improvement

Consistently assessing clinic needs from both a business and consumer perspective is important to the quality of services. Ensuring employee satisfaction through regular review of pay, productivity, and benefits is important to employee retention. Ensuring customer satisfaction through frequent surveys, comment boxes, and reviews is important. Clinics also need to judge whether the clientele to whom they offer therapy services have new or growing needs. For example, outpatient pediatric clinics must provide therapy service(s) for the growing number of infants, children, adolescents, and young adults who need assistance. The incidence and prevalence of developmental disabilities are increasing and outpatient clinics need to adjust to meet the growing demand for services (Centers for Disease Control and Prevention, 2021; Zablotsky et al., 2019).

Data regarding patient improvement are necessary because of continued efforts to pay for quality health care services, not just the quantity. Medicare launched its quality payment effort called the "Merit-based Incentive Payment System" or MIPS (CMS, 2022b). Therapists who participate in MIPS submit evidence of the quality of their care. Those data are compared with the national average collected by CMS. Providers who perform above the national average receive a payment boost, while those below the national average have some payment rescinded. Overall, managers have many avenues to pursue when maintaining and improving the quality of outpatient clinics. Refer to Chapter 12 for more information on quality assurance performance improvement.

Discussion Activity

1. What are the pros and cons of working in an outpatient pediatric setting?
2. What are the pros and cons of working in an outpatient adult setting?
3. Compare and contrast the benefits of a child with a disability receiving services in an outpatient setting with a home health setting
4. Compare and contrast the benefits of an adult with a condition and/or disability receiving services in an outpatient setting with a home health setting

References

Aegis Therapies. (2019). *Group and concurrent therapy FAQs.* https://aegistherapies.com/wp-content/uploads/2019/06/AegisTherapies-GroupConcurrentFAQs.pdf.

Alkassabi, O., Al-Sobayel, H., Al-Eisa, E., Buragadda, S., Alghadir, A., & Iqbal, A. (2018). Job satisfaction among physiotherapists in Saudi Arabia: Does leadership style matter? *BMC Health Services Research, 18,* 422.

Americans With Disabilities Act. (2020). *A guide to disability rights laws.* https://www.ada.gov/cguide.htm#anchor65610.

Americans With Disabilities Act of 1990. (2009). *Americans with Disabilities Act of 1990, as amended.* https://www.ada.gov/pubs/adastatute08.htm.

American Occupational Therapy Association. (2021). Occupational therapy profession- scope of practice definitions. *American Journal of Occupational Therapy, 75*(Suppl. 3), 7513410030.

American Occupational Therapy Association. (2022). *Medicare OTA payment differential.* https://customerservice.aota.org/hc/en-us/articles/4413460452763-Medicare-OTA-Payment-Differential.

American Physical Therapy Association. (2017). *Outcomes measurement.* https://www.apta.org/your-practice/outcomes-measurement.

American Physical Therapy Association. (2018). *A permanent fix to the therapy cap: Improved access for Medicare patients comes with pending APTA-opposed cut to PTA payment.* https://www.apta.org/news/2018/02/09/a-permanent-fix-to-the-therapy-cap-improved-access-for-medicare-patients-comes-with-pending-apta-opposed-cut-to-pta-payment.

American Physical Therapy Association. (2021). *Levels of patient access to physical therapists services in the U.S.* https://www.apta.org/advocacy/issues/direct-access-advocacy/direct-access-by-state.

American Physical Therapy Association. (2022). *Medicare payment differential for services provided by PTAs.* https://www.apta.org/advocacy/issues/pta-differential.

Bureau of Workers' Compensation. (2022). *About.* https://info.bwc.ohio.gov/.

California Department of Industrial Relations. (2021). *Minimum wage.* https://www.dir.ca.gov/dlse/faq_minimumwage.htm.

Centers for Disease Control and Prevention. (2021). *Data & statistics on autism spectrum disorder.* https://www.cdc.gov/ncbddd/autism/data.html.

Centers for Disease Control and Prevention. (2018). *Health Insurance Portability and Accountability Act of 1996 (HIPAA).* https://www.cdc.gov/phlp/publications/topic/hipaa.html.

Centers for Medicare & Medicaid Services (CMS). (2010). *The Patient Protection and Affordable Care Act.* https://www.cms.gov/Regulations-and-Guidance/Legislation/LegislativeUpdate/Downloads/PPACA.pdf.

Centers for Medicare & Medicaid Services (CMS). (2019). *Outpatient rehabilitation therapy services: Complying with documentation requirements.* https://www.cms.gov/Outreach-and-Education/Medicare-Learning-Network-MLN/MLNProducts/Downloads/OutptRehabTherapy-Booklet-MLN905365.pdf.

Centers for Medicare & Medicaid Services (CMS). (2022a). *Benefits.* https://www.medicaid.gov/medicaid/benefits/index.html.

Centers for Medicare & Medicaid Services (CMS). (2022b). *Participation options overview.* https://qpp.cms.gov/mips/overview.

Centers for Medicare & Medicaid Services (CMS). (2022c). *Quality, safety & oversight – certification & compliance.* https://www.cms.gov/Medicare/Provider-Enrollment-and-Certification/CertificationandComplianc.

Centers for Medicare & Medicaid Services (CMS). (2022d). *Surprise billing & protecting consumers.* https://www.cms.gov/nosurprises/Ending-Surprise-Medical-Bills.

Centers for Medicare & Medicaid Services (CMS). (2022e). *Therapy services.* https://www.cms.gov/Medicare/Billing/TherapyServices.

Centers for Medicare & Medicaid Services (CMS). (2022f). *Beneficiary notices initiative (BNI).* https://www.cms.gov/Medicare/Medicare-General-Information/BNI.

Centers for Medicare & Medicaid Services (CMS). (2022g). *11 Part B billing scenarios for PTs and OTs.* https://www.cms.gov/medicare/billing/therapyservices/downloads/11_part_b_billing_scenarios_for_pts_and_ots.pdf.

Clinicient. (2022). *Understanding multiple procedure payment reduction (MPPR) for rehab therapists.* https://www.clinicient.com/guide/mppr/.

Commission on Accreditation of Rehabilitation Facilities (CARF). (2022). *Who we are.* http://www.carf.org/About/WhoWeAre/.

Desveaux, L., Chan, Z., & Brooks, D. (2016). Leadership in physical therapy: Characteristics of academics and managers: A brief report. *Physiotherapy Canada. Physiotherapie Canada, 68*(1), 54–58.

Durkin, M. S. (2019). Increasing prevalence of developmental disabilities among children in the US: A sign of progress? *Pediatrics, 144*(4), e20192005.

Fleming-Castaldy, R., & Patro, J. (2012). Leadership in occupational therapy: Self-perceptions of occupational therapy managers. *Occupational Therapy in Health Care, 26*(2/3), 187–202.

Gersh, M. R. (2006). Servant-leadership: A philosophical foundation for professionalism in physical therapy. *Journal of Physical Therapy Education, 20*(2), 12–16.

HealthCare.gov. (2022). *Glossary.* https://www.healthcare.gov/glossary/deductible/.

Jackson LLP Healthcare Lawyers. (2022). *Cash-pay physical therapy: Ensuring compliance with the Medicare Mandatory Claims Submission Rule.* https://jacksonllp.com/cash-pt-mandatory-claims-submission/#_ftnref1.

Joint Commission. (2022). *Joint Commission FAQs.* https://www.jointcommission.org/about-us/facts-about-the-joint-commission/joint-commission-faqs/#:~:text=The%20Joint%20Commission%20accredits%20and,and%20nursing%20care%20center%20services.

Kaiser Family Foundation. (2018). *8 FAQs: Medicare bundled payment models.* https://files.kff.org/attachment/Evidence-Link-FAQs-Bundled-Payments.

Keisu, B., Ohman, A., & Enberg, B. (2018). Employee effort – reward balance and first level manager transformational leadership within elderly care. *Scandinavian Journal of Caring Sciences, 32,* 407–416.

Kids SPOT Rehab. (2021). *Who we are.* https://www.kidsspotrehab.com/who-we-are/.

Klees, B., Wolfe, C., & Curtis, C. (2009). *Brief summaries of Medicare & Medicaid: Title XVIII and Title XIX of the Social Security Act.* https://www.cms.gov/research-statistics-data-and-systems/statistics-trends-and-reports/medicareprogramratesstats/downloads/medicaremedicaidsummaries2009.pdf.

Kotter, J. (1990). *A force for change: How leadership differs from management.* Free Press.

Kouzes, J., & Posner, B. (2012). *The leadership challenge* (5th ed.). Jossey-Bass.

LaRosa, J. (2019). *U.S. physical therapy clinics constitute a growing $34 billion industry.* https://blog.marketresearch.com/u.s.-physical-therapy-clinics-constitute-a-growing-34-billion-industry.

Legal Information Institute. (2022). *42 CFR § 485.62 - Condition of participation: Physical environment.* https://www.law.cornell.edu/cfr/text/42/485.62.

McLawhorn, A., & Buller, L. (2017). Bundled payments in total joint replacement: Keeping our care affordable and high in quality. *Current Reviews in Musculoskeletal Medicine, 10*(3), 370–377.

MedicareFAQ. (2021). *Medicare and the 8-minute rule.* https://www.medicarefaq.com/faqs/medicare-8-minute-rule/.

Medicare Interactive. (2022). *Advanced beneficiary notice (ABN).* https://www.medicareinteractive.org/get-answers/medicare-denials-and-appeals/original-medicare-appeals/advance-beneficiary-notice-abn.

MyPTsolutions. (2015). *Spotlight on outpatient therapy.* https://myptsolutions.com/outpatient-therapy-spotlight-physical-therapy-jobs/.

Newman, R., McGarvey, K., & Hoppe, L. (2016). Episodic versus continuous care in outpatient pediatric clinics. *School of Occupational Master's Capstone Projects, 6,* 1–89. http://soundideas.pugetsound.edu/ot_capstone/6.

Northouse, P. (2019). *Leadership: Theory and practice* (8th ed.). SAGE.

Pennsylvania Code. (2022). *State board of physical therapy.* http://www.pacodeandbulletin.gov/Display/pacode?file=/secure/pacode/data/049/chapter40/chap40toc.html&d=reduce.

Pennsylvania State Board of Physical Therapy. (2008). *Physical therapy practice act.* https://www.dos.pa.gov/ProfessionalLicensing/BoardsCommissions/PhysicalTherapy/Documents/Applications%20and%20Forms/Non-Application%20Documents/PTM%20-%20Physical%20Therapy%20Practice%20Act.pdf.

Pendergast, J., Kliethermes, S., Freburger J., & Duffy, P. (2012). A comparison of health care use for physician-referred and self-referred episodes of outpatient physical therapy. *Health Services Research, 47*(2), 633–654.

Rosenbaum, S. (2011). The patient protection and affordable care act: Implications for public health policy and practice. *Public Health Reports, 126*(1), 130–135.

Sheen, R. (2021). *ACA affordability for 2022 tax year to decrease.* https://acatimes.com/aca-affordability-for-2022-tax-year-to-decrease/.

Smeulers, M., Dikmans, M., & van Vugt, M. (2019). Well-prepared outpatient visits satisfy patient and physician. *BMJ Open Quality*, *8*(3), 1–3.

STAR Institute. (2021). *Vision, mission, & history*. https://sensoryhealth.org/basic/vision-mission-history.

Ullmann, S. G. (2015). Access to rehabilitative care in the Affordable Care Act era. *AMA Journal of Ethics*, *17*(6), 553–557.

United Health Care. (2022). *UMR*. https://www.uhc.com/employer/employer-resources/umr.

United States Department of Health & Human Services. (2020). *Notice of privacy practices*. https://www.hhs.gov/hipaa/for-individuals/notice-privacy-practices/index.html.

United States Department of Labor. (2022a). *Occupational safety and health administration*. https://www.osha.gov/.

United States Department of Labor. (2022b). *Wages and the Fair Labor Standards Act*. https://www.dol.gov/agencies/whd/flsa.

United States Equal Employment Opportunity Commission. (1992). *The Rehabilitation Act of 1973*. https://www.eeoc.gov/statutes/rehabilitation-act-1973.

United States Equal Employment Opportunity Commission. (2009). *Title VII of the Civil Rights Act of 1964*. https://www.eeoc.gov/statutes/title-vii-civil-rights-act-1964.

WebPT. (2018). *5 Medicare compliance issues for cash-based PTs*. https://www.webpt.com/blog/5-medicare-compliance-issues-for-cash-based-pts/.

Zablotsky, B., Black, L. I., Maenner, M. J., Schieve, L. A., Danielson, M. L., Bitsko, R. H., Blumberg, S. J., Kogan, M. D., & Boyle, C. A. (2019). Prevalence and trends of developmental disabilities among children in the United States: 2009-2017. *Pediatrics*, *144*(4), e20190811.

16

Acute Care Settings

JEFF HARTMAN, DPT, MPH, SARAH NECHVATAL, PT, DPT;
MEREDITH BURD, OTR/L, MOT, MBA, CBIS; AILEEN GORMAN, MOT, OTR/L;
and JANICE HANSHAW, MOT, OTR/L

LEARNING OBJECTIVES

By the end of this chapter, the reader will be able to:

1. Identify accreditations and regulations driving processes, policy, and operations in short-term acute care settings.
2. Recognize the unique pace of short-term acute care settings and rehabilitation evaluation and intervention.
3. Understand reimbursement structure for short-term acute care settings.
4. Understand the key role rehabilitation professionals play in discharge planning in the short-term acute care setting.
5. Identify the common settings patients discharge to after a short-term acute care stay.
6. Compare and contrast the role of a physical therapist working in the emergency department from other areas in the healthcare system

7. Differentiate the role of physical therapists in the emergency department from other medical providers
8. Understand the benefit of employing physical therapists in the emergency department
9. Recognize the types of patients seen by physical therapists in the emergency department
10. Understand a manager's role in overseeing physical therapy in the emergency department

CHAPTER OUTLINE

Short-Term Acute Care Hospital

History and Background

Short-term acute care refers to services such as surgery or treatment for acute medical conditions and injuries. Patients receiving acute care services are typically admitted to a hospital and referred to as "bedded" for a short-term illness or condition (Centers for Medicare & Medicaid Services [CMS], n.d.). Acute care plays a vital role in preventing death and disability. Within health systems, acute care also serves as an entry point to health care for individuals with emergent and urgent conditions (Hirshon et al., 2013).

Accreditation and Regulations

Several accrediting and regulatory bodies provide oversight and direction for acute care operations. The Joint Commission is one of the most notable accreditation groups serving as independent bodies. The Joint Commission has accredited hospitals for nearly 70 years and today accredits nearly 4,000 community, academic, pediatric, long-term acute, psychiatric, rehabilitation, and specialty hospitals (Joint Commission, 2022a). This accreditation validates that the facility has met a rigorous set of standards for care delivery, personnel management, and the environment.

The Centers for Medicare & Medicaid Services (CMS) also provides regulatory direction to acute care settings (CMS, 2021a). These health and safety requirements are mandated for hospitals to participate in Medicaid and Medicare programs. Specific requirements can vary slightly based on geographic location within the country because regions and markets are managed by different jurisdictions.

Patient Population, Services, and Setting Characteristics

Short-term acute care incorporates care for patients hospitalized across the lifespan. Depending on the size and structure of the hospital, typical units may include the following:
- Neonatal Intensive Care (NICU)
- Pediatric Intensive Care (PICU)
- Neuroscience Intensive Care (NSICU)
- Pediatrics
- Behavioral Health
- Medical/Surgical
- Intermediate or Stepdown Care
- Critical Care (CCU) or Intensive Care (ICU)
  - There may also be specialty critical care units, including Surgical Intensive Care, Cardiovascular Intensive Care, and Medical Intensive Care.
- Further specialties with dedicated units may include Oncology, Burns, Observation, Orthopedics, and Trauma.

The American College of Surgeons (ACS) recognizes three levels of trauma center certifications: Level I, Level II, and Level III. Each level's terminology describes the services available to patients at each facility. State or local municipality typically designates the trauma center level while the ACS verifies specific standards. The ACS verifies research support, disaster management planning, trauma patient volumes, operating room availability, trauma surgeon/neurosurgeon/orthopedic response time, and transfer protocols. Level 1 trauma center hospitals have the most stringent qualifications and must be capable of treating patients across the spectrum of injuries from the most to least severe (*American College of Surgeons,* 2022).

Facilities referred to as critical access hospitals can also provide short-term acute care. Critical access hospitals must maintain no more than 25 inpatient beds or swing beds (i.e., a hospital room that can switch from in-patient acute care status to skilled care status). These facilities must average a length of stay of 96 hours or less per patient served by acute services (CMS, 2021b). Critical access hospitals are highly reliant on their surrounding geography. Only certain states maintain a program that classifies facilities as critical access hospitals, and those state requirements include a physical location no more than 35 miles from the nearest facility (CMS, 2021b). Swing beds allow flexibility to which level of care each bed is dedicated, based on hospital census needs at any given time. Flexible designations include the ability to provide skilled nursing facility–level care in the inpatient beds.

Evaluation and Treatment

Occupational and physical therapy services are consultative in the acute care setting. A physician or advanced practice provider-generated order is required for intervention. Once the order is received, the therapist must conduct a thorough chart review to ensure that the patient is medically stable for intervention. Specific precautions based on a diagnosis or surgical procedures should be identified. They may need clarification if they are outside the order set, as the surgeon or physician may have specific preferences. Considerations should be made for patient readiness for intervention, including stability of vital signs, laboratory results, imaging, respiratory status, and if activity orders are present. Open discussions with physicians and their preferences for protocols may assist with efficiencies.

Early mobility is integral to providing quality care. In one study by Corcoran et al. (2017), it was demonstrated that an early mobility program decreased the average ICU length of stay by 20%, decreased a floor bed stay by 43%, allowed for a discharge to home in 40.5% of admissions compared with 18.2% of admissions prior to the beginning of the program, and saved this particular hospital over 2.2 million dollars (not adjusted for inflation). Limited mobility can contribute to a decline in the ability to complete self-care, the need for admission into a sub-acute facility, or even death (Brown et al., 2004). Occupational and physical therapy clinicians play integral roles in promoting mobility and participation in activities of daily living during short-term acute admissions and, thus, contribute to all the above-listed benefits. Speech-language pathologists should also be involved in ICU early mobility to address areas such as swallowing, using speaking valves, communication (with or without an assistive device), and cognitive functioning (Corcoran et al., 2017).

During evaluation and treatment, the therapist should monitor the patient's current lines (e.g., IVs, PICC lines, femoral lines, and central lines), drains (e.g., chest tubes, JP drains), and airway status. These items may increase the difficulty of assessment and limit mobility without proper planning. It is important to be aware of the precautions surrounding these items (Fig. 16.1).

The intent of consultation of physical and occupational therapists in this setting is typically to provide medical providers with an assessment of the patient's prior level of function, the current level of function, and recommendations for a safe discharge destination once the patient is deemed

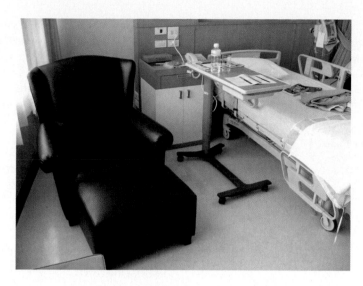

• **Fig. 16.1** Bedside care: therapists must be resourceful and creative with appropriate interventions despite sometimes facing limited space or access to rehabilitation equipment. (From https://www.flickr.com/photos/95672737@N00/936422226.)

medically stable for discharge from the hospital per the medical provider's orders.

Documentation of evaluation and treatment is typically completed in an electronic medical record (EMR). Regulatory bodies and accreditation standards are key drivers in the documentation requirements for short-term acute care providers.

The Joint Commission requires a plan to be established before treatment is initiated. The plan contains the "type, amount, frequency, and duration of physical therapy, occupational therapy or speech-language pathology services to be furnished to the individual." The plan must also include the diagnosis and anticipated goals. (Joint Commission, 2022b).

Treatment is delivered according to the originally determined plan and based on the patient's progress during admission. It is common for a therapy plan of care to require adjustment because a patient's status worsens or does not medically progress as initially projected. Occupational and physical therapists should be guided by best-practice research in formulating and delivering interventions. The American Physical Therapy Association (APTA) has published several clinical practice guidelines that should aid clinical decision-making (American Physical Therapy Association, Clinical practice guidelines). This library of clinical support includes recommendations for the interpretation of lab values and vitals in determining the appropriateness of therapeutic intervention. The American Occupational Therapy Association (AOTA) also publishes practice guidelines, statements, and position papers to underline the importance of occupational therapy practitioners in acute care and beyond.

Length of Stay, Pace, and Readmissions

Length of stay in short-term acute care settings may vary, but generally, the national average for a patient's length of stay is 5.5 days (Tipton et al., 2021). Due to the relatively short length of stay when compared with other settings, short-term acute care is considered a fast-paced environment for therapists who must provide evaluation and treatment for patients when indicated prior to their discharge from this setting.

Therapists must provide a discharge recommendation upon initial assessment/evaluation based on the patient's functional performance while considering the patient's prior level of function and support available to them in their baseline home environment. There is an emphasis on the decreased length of stay and decreasing readmission rates for patients in short-term acute care hospital settings. As a patient's length of stay increases, costs rise, patients can have more exposure to various infections, and their risk of a hospital-acquired infection also increases (Tipton et al., 2021). A reduction in hospital readmissions results in improved patient safety and outcomes and this initiative is supported by the Hospital Readmissions Reduction Program (HRRP). This Medicare program encourages hospitals to improve care coordination and discharge planning to avoid readmissions by linking reimbursement to the quality of hospital care (CMS, 2021c).

Providers and Care Coordination

Therapy services are ordered by medical providers such as physicians or advanced practice providers (physician assistants or nurse practitioners). Care coordination in the short-term acute care setting requires a multidisciplinary approach. There are several disciplines involved in the coordination of care for patients to ensure the best outcomes (Fig. 16.2).

Teamwork among all disciplines is important in assisting with proper discharge planning and ensuring the patient receives the best care. Communication with physicians and nursing staff can guide therapists when the patient is

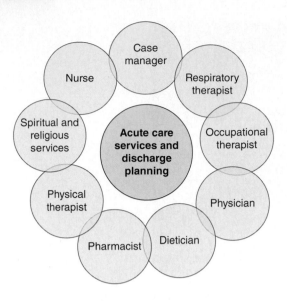

• **Fig. 16.2** Multidisciplinary Team in Acute Care

medically stable and rehabilitation therapies can be initiated. Therapists may notice trends in vitals, such as orthostatic hypotension or oxygen desaturation with mobility, that may impact the patient's medical treatment course, which should be discussed with the patient's medical team. Therapists should also provide information regarding the patient's functional and mobility status. For example, a collaborative approach with respiratory therapy is essential when attempting to ambulate a patient who requires high levels of oxygen or is intubated but demonstrates the strength and coordination required for gait activities. Therapists can use the insight they gain during therapy sessions to provide discharge or equipment recommendations for the patient. Providing timely discharge recommendations may require communication with the case manager as they work on coordinating a patient's discharge needs (Chapter 21).

Responsibilities of a Manager/Administrator

A manager or administrator in the short-term acute care setting has a wide variety of responsibilities, including direct oversight of personnel, daily staffing needs, budgeting, adherence to regulations, program development, and advocating therapy services. Short-term acute care environments are often fluid or even unpredictable. Hospital census (i.e., the number of admitted patients at any given time) drives many processes and procedures. Periods of high census might require triaging patients or prioritizing the most critical work for throughput (i.e., moving patients through the hospital system from admission to discharge). A low census might require a manager to consider calling off staff with or without pay, depending on hospital policy. Finding appropriate staffing ratios, not only in physical, occupational, or speech therapy but also with providers, nurses, and others, is a significant responsibility of hospital leadership.

Hospital managers and administrators must be mindful of patient satisfaction data specific to their department and the entire hospital. Patient satisfaction is measured by the Hospital Consumer Assessment of Healthcare Providers and Systems (HCAHPS) survey. HCAHPS surveys provide a patient's perspective on their care, allowing comparisons across hospitals, encouraging hospitals to improve the quality of services they provide, and increasing the facility's accountability. The 29-question survey is distributed to a random sampling of adult patients after discharge. It is required for hospitals to send out surveys each month throughout the year. In 2010, The Patient Protection and Affordable Care Act was enacted and utilized HCAHPS scores as one of the measures to calculate value-based incentive payments starting with discharges in October of 2012 (CMS, 2021d).

Reimbursement, Documentation, and Quality Improvement

Documentation of services must meet requirements from CMS, the accrediting body of the hospital (often Joint Commission), and any state-specific requirements. A physician can decide to admit a patient to the hospital if, due to medical necessity, they are expected to stay two or more midnights. Inpatient short-term acute care is billed under Medicare Part A. If the patient is not expected to need two or more midnights, they are treated under observation status and billed under Medicare Part B (Medicare.gov, *Inpatient or outpatient hospital status affects your costs*). Inpatient status is one of the requirements for a skilled nursing facility short-term stay to be covered under Medicare Part A at discharge (Medicare.gov, *Skilled nursing facility care*). Other payors include commercial insurance companies, employer-paid policies, or Medicaid. Organizations engage in contractual agreements with each payor defining what, when, and how the hospital is paid.

Diagnosis Related Groups (DRGs) are the basis of Medicare's hospital reimbursement system. This system considers the average case mix (i.e., patient complexity) treated by the entity concerning costs incurred by the hospital to provide the necessary level of care (CMS, n.d.). DRGs provide inpatient hospitals with predetermined singular payments rather than itemized reimbursements. DRG reimbursement is based on a set of six criteria (Fig. 16.3).

When the Deficit Reduction Act of 2005 went into effect, CMS no longer reimbursed medical facilities for costs related to HACs (CMS, 2019). Currently, 14 conditions are specified as Hospital Acquired Conditions (HACs). This list includes:

1. Foreign object retained after surgery
2. Air embolism
3. Blood incompatibility
4. Stage III and IV pressure ulcers
5. Falls and trauma
6. Catheter-associated urinary tract infection (UTI)
7. Vascular catheter-associated infection
8. Surgical site infection: Mediastinitis following Coronary Artery Bypass Surgery (CABG)
9. Manifestations of poor glycemic control

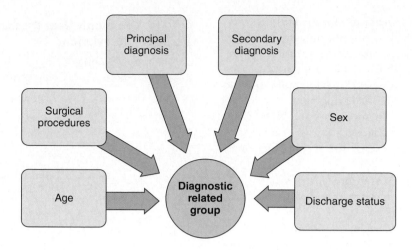

• **Fig. 16.3** DRG Reimbursement Criteria. (From Centers for Medicare & Medicaid Services. (2019). *Design and development of the diagnosis related group (DRG)*. https://www.cms.gov/icd10m/version37-fullcode-cms/fullcode_cms/design_and_development_of_the_diagnosis_related_group_(DRGs).pdf.)

10. Deep vein thrombosis (DVT)/pulmonary embolism (PE) following total knee replacement or hip replacement
11. Surgical site infection following bariatric surgery
12. Surgical site infection following certain orthopedic procedures of spine, shoulder or elbow.
13. Surgical site infection following cardiac device procedures
14. Iatrogenic pneumothorax with venous catheterization. (CMS, 2019).

In April 2021, a federal rule on "Interoperability, Information Blocking and ONC Health IT Certification" outlined the 21st Century Cures Act's requirements, ensuring patients have access to their medical records (Office of the National Coordinator for Health information Technology, n.d.). Under the Cures Act, notes completed by rehabilitation therapists are required to be shared with the patient. When documenting the point of service, therapists should converse with the patient about what they are documenting, including the therapeutic evaluation and recommendations. Access and transparency to medical records also provide patients with helpful reminders of the education provided by their providers. Some facilities may be able to pull education or home exercise programs from an external source and embed those recommendations within the documentation, which may also assist with compliance or the need to reprint patient handouts (Klein et al., 2016).

Quality improvement is site-specific and may include measurement of productivity, compliance with documentation and regulations, and timely response to therapy orders (Chapter 12). Using incident or adverse event reports data, such as falls, equipment malfunction, or patient injury, managers may identify trends in areas that need improvement. Working together as a team and dissecting the situations, new policies/procedures can be created, education provided to employees, or a closer inspection of the products in use can improve patient safety and the quality of care provided.

Discharge Planning

Discharge planning begins upon admission to a short-term acute hospital. As mentioned earlier, short-term acute care aims to treat time-sensitive or critical needs. Once those needs are met, and medical stability is achieved, the patient must move to another level of care or back to their prior disposition. Throughput is essential to short-term acute care management. If throughput is not prioritized, access to short-term acute care hospital beds may be limited and escalate into a public health crisis.

Specific to rehabilitation professionals, discharge planning begins with the initial evaluation. Therapists consider the following details to begin generating discharge recommendations:

• Prior level of function
• Current home setup
• Social support available
• Cognitive status; orientation to person, place, time, and situation
• Current precautions/restrictions such as blood pressure parameters, weight-bearing restrictions, diet
• Current health status
• Pain, if present, and impact to function
• Upper/lower extremity range of motion and strength
• Transfer status
• Ambulation status
• Ability to complete activities of daily living (ADLs)
• Ability to complete instrumental activities of daily living (IADLs)
• Sensation
• Fine and gross motor coordination
• Proprioception
• Vision

Outcome measures are important to incorporate into documentation for a multitude of reasons. First, outcome measures can provide documentation for medical necessity, a requirement from CMS. In addition, outcome measures track progress and patient response to therapeutic intervention and aid in determining the most appropriate discharge disposition. CMS calls out several rehabilitation-specific outcome measures (CMS, 2022a), including:

- National Outcomes Measurement System (NOMS) by the American Speech-language Hearing Association
- Patient Inquiry by Focus On Therapeutic Outcomes (FOTO)
- Activity Measure – Post-Acute Care (AM-PAC)
- OPTIMAL by Cedaron, through the American Physical Therapy Association

After the initial therapy evaluation, consideration of family and caregiving training implementation is important. Items to address include possible adaptive equipment recommendations (with guidance on purchase locations), how to utilize assistive devices, fall prevention strategies, completion of home exercise programs, and techniques to assist with the patient's self-care. Providing hands-on training with patients and their caregivers can ensure they feel comfortable as the discharge planning from acute care progresses, possibly reducing staff assistance.

Once deemed medically stable, there are many different discharge dispositions for patients following a short-term acute care stay (Fig. 16.4). Many factors should be considered when determining the most appropriate next level of care for these patients. For patients requiring ongoing rehabilitative services, options such as post-acute rehab are considered. Depending on regional or market-level terminology, some titles are used interchangeably to describe discharge settings. Post-acute care refers to a wide range of services, including inpatient rehabilitation facilities, skilled nursing facilities, home health, and long-term care facilities (Redberg, 2015).

Additionally, when documenting discharge recommendations, it is important to convey the medical necessity of continued therapy services if indicated for insurance authorization for post-acute care rehabilitation (Chapter 17). Healthcare terminology often includes numerous abbreviations and discharge settings are not excluded (Table 16.1). A

TABLE 16.1	Commonly Used Discharge Setting Abbreviations
Discharge Setting Abbreviations	**Full Name**
LTACH	Long-term acute care hospital
IRF, IPR, or ARU	Inpatient rehab, inpatient rehab facility, or acute rehabilitation unit
SNF, SAR, STR	Skilled nursing facility, subacute rehab, short-term rehab
HH	Home health
OP	Outpatient therapy
LTC	Long-term care

comprehensive list of common terminology to describe discharge dispositions include:

- Skilled nursing facility
- Nursing home
- Assistive living facility, independent living facility
- Inpatient rehabilitation unit (facility or hospital-based)
- Long-term acute care hospital
- Home health
- Outpatient therapy services
  - Clinic-based includes more formal programs such as day rehab
- Hospice
  - Acute care therapy practitioners have an important role to play even if the patient is planning to discharge under hospice services. Some items that may be addressed before discharge under hospice services in the home environment are caregiver body mechanics, adaptive equipment, energy conservation, positioning, and modified techniques for daily tasks (Allen, 2016).

Conclusion

Short-term acute care is a fast-paced environment serving the needs of the critically ill. Time-sensitive care is not limited to medical interventions; rehabilitation professionals are key in delivering acute care. Hospitalized patients benefit from the skilled interventions of rehabilitation professionals while admitted and long after discharge because of the significant role physical and occupational therapists play in defining the path of health management after the hospital stay.

Physical Therapists in the Emergency Department

History and Background

During the 1990s and 2000s, the annual number of emergency department (ED) visits rose 31% and wait times to

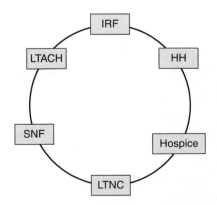

• **Fig. 16.4** Post-Acute Care Discharge Dispositions. *HH,* Home health; *IRF,* inpatient rehabilitation facility; *LTACH,* long-term acute care hospital; *LTNC,* long-term nursing care; *SNF,* skilled nursing facility.

see a physician increased significantly. Patient satisfaction decreased and there was a decreased ability to provide safe care (Magid et al., 2009; Nawar et al., 2007; United States Government Accountability Office, 2009; Tang et al., 2010). Patients with acute or severe musculoskeletal pain or dizziness presenting to the ED were treated with medications (Jones et al., 2018; United States Department of Health and Human Services, n.d.). If the symptoms were still uncontrolled, they would be admitted to the hospital for further symptom management. Once the patient could safely mobilize, they would often be discharged with a prescription for medication and a recommendation to follow up with their primary care provider (PCP). It was not uncommon for patients to return to the ED for symptom management while they waited for an appointment with their PCP (Benbassat & Taragin, 2000).

Similarly, patients would go to urgent care (UC) settings for musculoskeletal and vestibular complaints and then be referred to their PCP for follow-up care. The PCP might offer medication management, lifestyle modifications, imaging, or labs and ultimately refer to specialty care if symptoms persist. Whether initially seen through the ED or UC, patients typically gain access to a physical therapist several weeks after the onset of severe symptoms (Walk et al., 2015).

This inefficient and costly use of healthcare forced hospitals in the United States to find creative solutions to these problems. Among these solutions was the utilization of nurse practitioners and physician assistants, known as physician extenders (Hooker & McCaig, 1996; Sturmann et al., 1990). The United States was a late adopter of staffing physical therapists in the ED (Fleming-McDonnell et al., 2010; Kim et al., 2018; Lebec & Jogodka, 2009). Other countries such as Australia and the United Kingdom have had physiotherapists practicing as first-contact providers in their EDs and UCs for much longer (Anaf & Sheppard, 2007; Hattam, 2004; Kilner, 2011; Kilner & Sheppard, 2010; Nall, 2009). These countries were the first to produce scientific evidence demonstrating the benefit of providing physical therapy in the ED and inspired research in the United States. Specifically, they were the first to demonstrate that primary contact physiotherapists reduce wait times and treatment times compared to other providers when addressing musculoskeletal conditions (Bird et al., 2016).

In 1998, Carondelet Hospital in Tucson, AZ, was the first in the United States to implement physical therapists in the ED (Woods, 2000). By 2010, it was estimated that 15 facilities had full-time physical therapists working in the ED (Guy et al., 2014). Evidence demonstrating the value of physical therapy in these programs started to spread in the United States, resulting in more hospital systems adopting the practice (Fleming-McDonnell et al., 2010; Kilner, 2011; Kilner & Sheppard, 2010; Lebec et al., 2010; Lebec & Kesterloot, 2010). In 2020, it was estimated that the total number of EDs that staffed physical therapists had tripled and many believe this number continues to rise at a similar rate today. In addition to licensed clinicians in the ED, physical therapist students are rotating through EDs for clinical

education experiences (Strickland & Hartman, 2019), and formal groups within the American Physical Therapy Association are being formed to support physical therapists who are working or are interested in working in the ED.

Regulations

In 1986, President Ronald Reagan created and the United States Congress enacted the Emergency Medical Treatment and Labor Act (EMTALA), which "requires hospitals with emergency departments to provide a medical screening examination to any individual who comes to the emergency department and requests such an examination and prohibits hospitals with emergency departments from refusing to examine or treat individuals with an emergency medical condition" (Medicaid, 2022). This "antidumping" law was created to ensure that patients receive a medical screening examination regardless of their ability to pay. While ensuring public access to emergency services, EMTALA does not ensure access to a physical therapist, thus limiting a patient's direct access to the ED (CMS, 2022b). Patients are typically referred to a physical therapist by a medical provider who has medically screened the patient and deemed physical therapy necessary. However, EMTALA does not apply to UC settings that are not on a hospital campus; therefore, patients can potentially have direct access to a physical therapist in those types of UC settings.

When practicing in the ED, a physical therapist's scope of practice is guided by three components: jurisdictional, professional, and personal scopes (APTA, Scope of Practice). The state where the ED is located has a practice act that governs what physical therapists can do legally under their professional license, which sets the jurisdictional scope of practice while practicing in the ED or any area within the healthcare system. The professional scope of practice is grounded in the profession's unique body of knowledge and training, while the personal scope is what the individual provider is competent and comfortable performing (APTA, Scope of Practice). While physical therapists in the ED experience unique situations related to complexity, acuity, or psychosocial challenges (Ciccarella et al, 2016), their scope of practice is the same as other physical therapists practicing in the same state.

Providers and Care Coordination

The emergency department provides team-based care where professionals with different areas of expertise work together within their unique scope of practice to provide a multi-disciplinary approach to addressing patients' needs (Ciccarella, et al., 2016; Moss et al., 2002; Muntlin Athlin et al., 2013; Reddy & Spence, 2006). Emergency PTs may collaborate with the following:

- Emergency medicine providers (medical doctors, doctors of osteopathic medicine, nurse practitioners, physician assistants, and emergency medicine technicians)
- Registered nurses

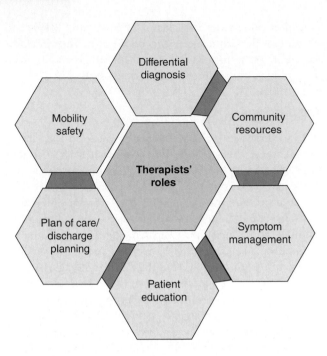

• **Fig. 16.5** Emergency Department and Urgent Care Roles

- Certified nursing assistants or emergency technicians
- Occupational therapists
- Pharmacists
- Respiratory therapists
- Social workers and nurse case managers (discharge planners)
- Other specialists (e.g., surgeons, prosthetists, orthotists)

A physical therapist in the ED and UC settings provides immediate access to a physical therapy evaluation and treatment for acute or severe symptoms. The goals of the physical therapy session include collaborating with the medical team for diagnostic clarity, plan of care development, and often direct intervention, typically involving symptom management and safe mobilization (Ciccarella et al., 2016). Additionally, physical therapists can offer patient and family education, assist in creating a safe discharge plan, and coordinate community resources as needed (Fig. 16.5). A significant contribution of the physical therapy experience, especially in the ED, consists of providing reassurance to the patient and family and assisting in a complete understanding of their medical situation, typically decreasing anxiety and stress (Ciccarella et al., 2016). It has been shown that patients spend more time with clinicians when physical therapy is integrated into their ED visit (McClellan et al., 2006) and have access to the care they need. This additional time decreases the risk that their acute issue will evolve into a chronic issue necessitating additional use of the health care system and a possible return to the ED (Walk et al., 2015). Providing physical therapy services in the ED has also decreased the overall cost of care for symptom management (Walk et al., 2015).

Additional benefits of emergent and urgent access to physical therapy:

- Reduces unnecessary admissions to the hospital (Gurley et al., 2020; Morphet et al., 2016)

- Reduces the need for imaging (Fleming-McDonnell et al., 2010; Lebec & Jogodka, 2009; Pugh et al., 2020)
- Reduces use of medications (opioids, which are highly addictive, and sedating medications, which increase the risk of falls) (Pugh et al., 2020; Thackeray et al., 2017)
- Increases patient satisfaction (Fruth et al., 2013; Lau et al., 2008)
- Decreases the burden of PCP care/follow-up (Lebec & Jogodka, 2009; Morris & Hawes, 1996)
- Decrease unnecessary referrals to specialists (Walk et al., 2015)
- Improves patient outcomes (Kilner, 2011; Sakamoto et al., 2018)
- Increases ED/UC staff satisfaction (Lebec et al., 2010)
- Decreases risk of fall-related revisits to ED within 30 days (Kilner, 2011; Lesser et al., 2018)

While patients who present to the ED are very similar to those seen elsewhere in physical therapy from a diagnostic perspective, the main differences may be the intensity and urgency of the physical problem they are experiencing or the intensity and urgency of the psychosocial challenges they face may be facing (Ciccarella et al., 2016). Physical therapists spend, on average, 30–45 minutes with each patient (McClellan et al., 2006) but time can vary considerably depending on the patient's needs and the complexity of the situation (Ciccarella et al., 2016). The chief complaints most frequently seen by physical therapists in the ED are as follows:

- Musculoskeletal pain (Ciccarella et al., 2016; Lebec & Jogodka, 2009)
  - Spine pain (most common)
  - Limb pain
  - Non-cardiac chest pain
- Vertigo/vestibular dysfunction (Lebec & Kesterloot, 2010; Lebec & Jogodka, 2009)
- Non-surgical fractures (Taha et al., 2021)
  - Extremities (mobility recommendations and Durable Medical Equipment assignment)
  - Splinting
  - Ribs (patient education)
- Falls/Gait instability (mobility recommendations and set up with community resources) (Anaf & Sheppard, 2007; Ball et al., 2007)
- Failure to thrive/Frailty (mobility recommendations and set up with community resources) (Anaf & Sheppard, 2007)
- Chronic and persistent pain (Dépelteau et al., 2020; Poulin et al., 2016)
- Migraines (Dodson et al., 2018; Vinson, 2002)
- Concussion (Bryan et al., 2016; Deichman et al., 2019; Mistry & Rainer, 2018)
- Wounds and burns (Taira et al., 2010)

Upon entry into the ED, patients will be triaged into one of five levels according to the severity or urgency of the situation and sent to one of three general areas of the ED: emergent care, urgent care, and observation (Ciccarella et al., 2016; Iserson & Moskop, 2007). This triage process enables the ED to manage clinical risk and safely handle patient flow so that the more urgent patients will be attended to first. Levels I and II are typically critical and require emergent care due to life-threatening concerns. Levels III–IV are not life-threatening yet require urgent care to prevent complications. Level V patients are non-urgent and are seen when time permits. An observation unit is a specialized unit designed to assess a patient's situation before deciding on discharge or admission (Baugh et al., 2011). Patients typically stay less than 24 hours in these units. Physical therapists typically see Level III–V patients in all three settings and may even be called for Levels I–II to assist the team with splinting or other procedures before transportation to surgery.

Responsibilities of Manager/Administrator

Managers and administrators are responsible for the systems that are in place in hospitals and EDs. They oversee the models of care delivery and ensure an optimal balance of cost, quality, and access for patients who come to their facilities (Ciccarella et al., 2016). There are different ED staffing models across the country, including full-time physical therapists who spend most of their day, 8–12 hours, in the ED, including weekends (Lebec et al., 2010; Lebec & Kesterloot, 2010; McClellan et al., 2006). There are also on-call physical therapy services in which the physical therapist is based in either the acute care setting or an outpatient clinic but can be called to see patients in the ED during their hours of availability. Some models are diagnosis-specific, in which the physical therapists are only consulted for one or two diagnoses, such as acute back pain, falls, or vestibular disorders. Other models focus more on people groups, such as the geriatric population (Dresden et al., 2020). Typically, the staffing model depends on the average volume of patients in the ED or the priorities established by department leadership (Ciccarella et al., 2016; Lebec & Jogodka, 2009).

Each healthcare system calculates productivity differently, depending on the manager or administrators to determine the productivity standards for their clinicians. While research has shown that 3.7 patients are needed to cover the cost of a full-time physical therapist (Gross et al., 2016), productivity standards are typically the same as the other physical therapists in their rehabilitation department. Managers and administrators monitor productivity and identify barriers and facilitators to meeting established standards.

Typically, physical therapists in the ED work independently and are more isolated from colleagues, including their manager/administrator, compared with other settings within a hospital system. Because of this, a physical therapist working in the ED needs to be an independent and responsible employee who can adequately represent and advocate the physical therapy department in the hospital (Ciccarella et al., 2016). The manager's role is to balance being accessible and providing the employees adequate autonomy to do their job.

Referral Sources and Marketing

In the ED, all emergency providers are potential referral sources for physical therapy. Because physical therapy in the ED is a relatively new and growing practice area, many emergency providers are unaware of how valuable a physical therapist can be. As a result, physical therapists must constantly market their knowledge and skills to other emergency providers (Ciccarella et al., 2016). Bringing awareness may involve the physical therapist finding new cases that have the potential of benefitting from their services and then directly advocating a referral. Although time-consuming, this direct contact and advocacy is an opportunity to market the physical therapist's knowledge and skills and is a reminder of how we can assist with symptom management, assessing for home safety, and facilitating the connection with community resources. Even when the medical provider initiates a referral, a strong model implemented by some programs is to make direct contact with the referring provider before and after every physical therapy evaluation and treatment. This communication allows the therapist to demonstrate their knowledge and skill and reminds the provider of the physical therapist's contribution to the patient experience. A common saying in the ED is "out of sight, out of mind," therefore the more visible physical therapists are and interact with other providers, the more likely they will be utilized in the ED.

Reimbursement and Documentation

Documentation for physical therapy in the ED is the same as providing physical therapy elsewhere in the same hospital system (Ciccarella et al., 2016). While documentation requirements are unique to each healthcare system and vary greatly between hospitals, depending on the division of physical therapy in which the physical therapist works (i.e., inpatient, outpatient), the physical therapist working in the ED is responsible for following the guidelines of their department, hospital by-laws, and state practice act (APTA, 2014).

Insurance varies greatly in the ED; the typical payor mix in the ED is federal, private, and self-pay (Ciccarella et al., 2016). Unique to the ED, patients are guaranteed to see a medical provider within hours of arrival, no matter the condition or insurance status (CMS, 2022a). With many barriers preventing people from easily accessing their PCP or specialist care, people will choose to go to the ED for convenience. In addition, with 31.6 million people uninsured in the United States (Cha & Cohen, 2022), the ED may be the only healthcare option. While patient socioeconomic demographics vary among healthcare systems and geographic areas, there is generally a higher level of uninsured patients who present to the ED. Despite this, independent audits performed by one of the largest ED physical therapy programs in the United States demonstrated equivalent reimbursement rates for physical therapy services in the ED compared to outpatient physical therapy services within the same system (Gross et al., 2016). Regardless of how the patient is billed or their insurance covers, physical therapy is often not considered a revenue-generating service in the ED or acute care setting (Lebec & Jogodka, 2009).

Occupational Therapists in the Emergency Department

Occupational therapists can provide specialized training, prepare the patient for discharge to home, or determine the patient's readiness for discharge (Hendricksen & Harrison, 2001). Based on the assessment and recommendations made by the occupational therapist, the ordering provider will have increased insight into the patient's baseline and current level of functioning. This information can help avoid admission to the hospital or decrease the overall length of stay if the patient is eventually admitted for inpatient care (Carlill et al., 2002).

Occupational therapists in the ED provide specialized education and training for ADL or IADL, adaptive equipment, assistive devices, and recommendations for durable medical equipment. Depending on the therapy department, some recommended equipment may be dispensed to the patient directly following the evaluation and treatment. Other times, the recommended equipment may be obtained outside the hospital setting.

One visit from an occupational therapist in the emergency department may be sufficient for the patient to return to their prior living environment. However, the occupational therapist may also recommend continued therapy in another setting, such as outpatient or home health. If an inpatient rehab or skilled nursing facility stay is recommended, the patient will likely require admission to the hospital and consultation with social services to assist in discharge planning and reimbursement purposes.

Functional assessments should be utilized as a part of occupational therapy assessment due to evidence that a measure of poor function is related to adverse outcomes following a stay in the emergency department. Use of the Identification of Seniors at Risk (ISAR) and the Triage Risk Screening Tool (TRST) are recommended screening tools as these assessments have had the most extensive psychometric testing compared with other similar screening tools (Bissett et al., 2013). Discharge recommendations are typically communicated to the hospital team through the EMR. However, due to the fast pace of the emergency department, therapists may need to communicate their discharge recommendations directly. Social services consult may also be warranted depending on the patient's needs and facility protocol.

Although current practice does not often utilize occupational therapists in EDs in the United States, occupational therapists should advocate their role in the ED and emphasize the benefits to the patient. Medical providers in the emergency department can find value in the unique skill set occupational therapists possess as there is evidence that patients who receive occupational therapist assessment in the hospital setting have a lower likelihood for readmission due to their emphasis on the patient's functional and social needs (Rogers et al., 2017).

Conclusion

Emergency departments today face many of the same challenges as two decades ago. Some have successfully utilized creative staffing solutions, while others have been slow to adopt evidence-based solutions, such as using physical and occupational therapists in the ED. While momentum is gaining, more needs to be done. Regardless of where a patient presents with urgent and emergent symptoms or poor access to healthcare, they should be able to have rapid and convenient access to a physical or occupational therapist to manage their symptoms better and develop a rehabilitative plan of care. Without physical and occupational therapists in the ED and UC settings, patients will have a delay in effective care which may prolong their discomfort and increase the cost of managing their condition.

References

Allen, M. (Ed.), (2016). Role of Occupational therapy in end-of-life care. *Am J Occup Ther, 70*(Suppl 2), 7012410075p1–7012410075p16. https://doi.org/10.5014/ajot.2016.706S17.

Anaf, S., & Sheppard, L. A. (2007). Describing physiotherapy interventions in an emergency department setting: An observational pilot study. *Accident and Emergency Nursing, 15*(1), 34–39.

American College of Surgeons. (2022). *Resources for optimal care of the injured patient 2022 standards.* Chicago, IL.

American Physical Therapy Association (APTA). (n.d). *Clinical practice guidelines.* https://www.apta.org/patient-care/evidence-based-practice-resources/cpgs.

American Physical Therapy Association (APTA). (n.d.). *Scope of practice.* https://www.apta.org/your-practice/scope-of-practice.

American Physical Therapy Association (APTA). (2014). *APTA guidelines: Physical therapy documentation of patient/client management.* https://www.apta.org/siteassets/pdfs/policies/guidelines-documentation-patient-client-management.pdf.

Ball, S. T., Walton, K., & Hawes, S. (2007). Do emergency department physiotherapy practitioner's, emergency nurse practitioners and doctors investigate, treat and refer patients with closed musculoskeletal injuries differently? *Emergency Medicine Journal: EMJ, 24*(3), 185–188.

Baugh, C. W., Venkatesh, A. K., & Bohan, J. S. (2011). Emergency department observation units: A clinical and financial benefit for hospitals. *Health Care Management review, 36*(1), 28–37.

Benbassat, J., & Taragin, M. (2000). Hospital readmissions as a measure of quality of health care: Advantages and limitations. *Archives of Internal Medicine, 160*(8), 1074–1081.

Bird, S., Thompson, C., & Williams, K. E. (2016). Primary contact physiotherapy services reduce waiting and treatment times for patients presenting with musculoskeletal conditions in Australian emergency departments: An observational study. *Journal of Physiotherapy, 62*(4), 209–214.

Bissett, M., Cusick, A., & Lannin, N. A. (2013). Functional assessments utilized in emergency departments: A systematic review. *Age and Ageing, 42,* 163–172.

Brown, C. J., Friedkin, R. J., Inouye, S. K. (2004). Prevalence and outcomes of low mobility in hospitalized older patients. *Journal of the American Geriatrics Society, 52,* 1263–1270.

Bryan, M. A., Rowhani-Rahbar, A., Comstock, R. D., & Rivara, F. (2016). Sports- and recreation-related concussions in US youth. *Pediatrics, 138*(1), e20154635.

Carlill, G., Gash, E., & Hawkins, G. (2002). Preventing unnecessary hospital admissions: An occupational therapy and social work service in an accident and emergency department. *British Journal of Occupational Therapy, 65*(10), 440–445.

Centers for Medicare & Medicaid Services (CMS). (n.d.). *Data navigator glossary of terms.* https://www.cms.gov/Research-Statistics-Data-and-Systems/Research/ResearchGenInfo/Downloads/DataNav_Glossary_Alpha.pdf.

Centers for Medicare & Medicaid Services (CMS). (2019). *Design and development of the diagnosis related group (DRG).* https://www.cms.gov/icd10m/version37-fullcode-cms/fullcode_cms/Design_and_development_of_the_Diagnosis_Related_Group_(DRGs).pdf

Centers for Medicare & Medicaid Services (CMS). (2021d). *HCAHPS: Patients' perspectives of care survey.* https://www.cms.gov/Medicare/Quality-Initiatives-Patient-Assessment-Instruments/HospitalQualityInits/HospitalHCAHPS.

Centers for Medicare & Medicaid Services (CMS). (2021a). *Hospitals.* https://www.cms.gov/Regulations-and-Guidance/Legislation/CFCsAndCoPs/Hospitals.

Centers for Medicare & Medicaid Services (CMS). (n.d.). *Design and development of the diagnosis related group.* https://www.cms.gov/icd10m/version37-fullcode-cms/fullcode_cms/Design_and_development_of_the_Diagnosis_Related_Group_(DRGs).pdf.

Centers for Medicare & Medicaid Services (CMS). (2021c). *Hospital readmissions reduction program (HRRP).* https://www.cms.gov/Medicare/Medicare-Fee-for-Service-Payment/AcuteInpatientPPS/Readmissions-Reduction-Program.

Centers for Medicare & Medicaid Services (CMS). (2021b). *Critical access hospitals.* https://www.cms.gov/Medicare/Provider-Enrollment-and-Certification/CertificationandComplianc/CAHs.

Centers for Medicare & Medicaid Services (CMS). (2022a). *Medicare Benefit Policy Manual - Centers for Medicare & Medicaid Services.* https://www.cms.gov/Regulations-and-guidance/guidance/manuals/downloads/bp102c15.pdf.

Centers for Medicare & Medicaid Services (CMS). (2022b). *Emergency Medical Treatment & Labor Act* (EMTALA). https://www.cms.gov/regulations-and-guidance/legislation/EMTALA.

Cha, A. E., & Cohen, R. A. (2022). *Demographic variation in health insurance coverage: United States,* 2020 (Number 169). https://www.cdc.gov/nchs/data/nhsr/nhsr169.pdf.

Ciccarella, S., Deusinger, S. S., Fincham, S., Jogodka, C., Krautner, G., Lebec, M., McDonnell, D. F., Poirier, N., TenBarge, L., & Tompkins, J. (2016). *Incorporating physical therapist practice in the emergency department: A toolkit for practitioners.* https://fptcu.com/Gep%20Files/Emergency%20PT/Reading%205%20EmergencyDepartment_Toolkit%20for%20PT.pdf.

Corcoran, J. R., Herbsman, J. M., Bushnik, T., Van Lew, S., Stolfi, A., Parkin, K., McKenzie, A., Hall, G. W., Joseph, W., Whiteson, J., & Flanagan, S. R. (2017). Early rehabilitation in the medical and surgical intensive care units for patients with and without mechanical ventilation: An interprofessional performance improvement project. *PM & R, 9*(2), 113–119.

Deichman, J. J., Graves, J. M., Klein, T. A., & Mackelprang, J. L. (2019). Characteristics of youth who leave the emergency department without being seen following sports-related concussion. *Concussion (London, England), 4*(4), CNC68.

Dépelteau, A., Racine-Hemmings, F., Lagueux, É., & Hudon, C. (2020). Chronic pain and frequent use of emergency department:

A systematic review. *The American Journal of Emergency Medicine, 38*(2), 358–363.

Dodson, H., Bhula, J., Eriksson, S., & Nguyen, K. (2018). Migraine treatment in the emergency department: Alternatives to opioids and their effectiveness in relieving migraines and reducing treatment times. *Cureus, 10*(4), e2439.

Dresden, S. M., Lo, A. X., Lindquist, L. A., Kocherginsky, M., Post, L. A., French, D. D., Gray, E., & Heinemann, A. W. (2020). The impact of geriatric emergency department innovations (GEDI) on health services use, health related quality of life, and costs: Protocol for a randomized controlled trial. *Contemporary Clinical Trials, 97*, 106125.

Fleming-McDonnell, D., Czuppon, S., Deusinger, S. S., & Deusinger, R. H. (2010). Physical therapy in the emergency department: Development of a novel practice venue. *Physical Therapy, 90*(3), 420–426. https://doi.org/10.2522/ptj.20080268.

Fruth, S., Slaven, E. J., Brickens, M. J., Hartman, J., Gentry, N., Hicks, A., Hahn, L., Schaumberg, M. (2013). *Patient perceptions of the value and efficacy of interventions provided by physical therapists in the emergency department.* San Diego, CA: American Physical Therapy Association Combined Sections Meeting. https://www.researchgate.net/publication/288488662_Patient_perceptions_of_the_value_and_efficacy_of_interventions_provided_by_physical_therapists_in_the_emergency_department.

Gurley, K. L., Blodgett, M. S., Burke, R., Shapiro, N. I., Edlow, J. A., & Grossman, S. A. (2020). The utility of emergency department physical therapy and case management consultation in reducing hospital admissions. *Journal of the American College of Emergency Physicians Open, 1*(5), 880–886.

Guy, R., Kesteloot, L., & Lebec, M. (2014, February 3-6). *Physical therapists in the emergency department: A national survey.* Poster presentation at the combined sections meeting of the American Physical Therapy Association, Las Vegas, NV.

Gross, A., Flint, K., & Brichler, K. (2016). Orthopaedic section poster presentations (Abstracts OPO1–OPO236). *Journal of Orthopaedic and Sports Physical Therapy, 46*(1), A58–A157.

Hattam, P. (2004). The effectiveness of orthopaedic triage by extended scope physiotherapists. *Clinical Governance: An International Journal, 9*(4), 244–252. https://doi.org/10.1108/14777270410566661.

Hendricksen, H., & Harrison, R. A. (2001). Occupational therapy in accident and emergency departments: A randomized controlled trial. *Journal of Advanced Nursing, 36*(6), 727–723.

Hirshon, J. M., Risko, N., Calvello, E. J., Stewart de Ramirez, S., Narayan, M., Theodosis, C., O'Neill, J., & Acute Care Research Collaborative at the University of Maryland Global Health Initiative. (2013). Health systems and services: The role of acute care. *Bulletin of the World Health Organization, 91*(5), 386–388.

Hooker, R. S., & McCaig, L. (1996). Emergency department uses of physician assistants and nurse practitioners: A national survey. *The American Journal of Emergency Medicine, 14*(3), 245–249.

Iserson, K. V., & Moskop, J. C. (2007). Triage in medicine, part I: Concept, history, and types. *Annals of Emergency Medicine, 49*(3), 275–281.

Joint Commission. (2022b). *Comprehensive accreditation manual for hospitals.* Oak Brook, IL: Joint Commission Resources.

Joint Commission. (2022a). *What is accreditation?* https://www.jointcommission.org/accreditation-and-certification/become-accredited/what-is-accreditation/?utm_content=dm-c-135#b6621ea07c4d48d68c1a8bdde62ff5e4_31ad6e2af27640458cf473ab797281a8.

Jones, M. R., Viswanath, O., Peck, J., Kaye, A. D., Gill, J. S., & Simopoulos, T. T. (2018). A brief history of the opioid epidemic and strategies for pain medicine. *Pain and Therapy, 7*(1), 13–21.

Kilner, E. (2011). What evidence is there that a physiotherapy service in the emergency department improves health outcomes? A systematic review. *Journal of Health Services Research & Policy, 16*(1), 51–58.

Kilner, E., & Sheppard, L. (2010). The 'lone ranger': A descriptive study of physiotherapy practice in Australian emergency departments. *Physiotherapy, 96*(3), 248–256.

Kim, H. S., Strickland, K. J., Mullen, K. A., & Lebec, M. T. (2018). Physical therapy in the emergency department: A new opportunity for collaborative care. *The American Journal of Emergency Medicine, 36*(8), 1492–1496.

Klein, J. W., Jackson, S. L., Bell, S. K., Anselmo, M. K., Walker, J., Delbanco, T., & Elmore, J. G. (2016). Your patient is now reading your note: Opportunities, problems, and prospects. *The American Journal of Medicine, 129*(10), 1018–1021.

Lau, P. M., Chow, D. H., & Pope, M. H. (2008). Early physiotherapy intervention in an accident and emergency department reduces pain and improves satisfaction for patients with acute low back pain: A randomised trial. *The Australian Journal of Physiotherapy, 54*(4), 243–249.

Lebec, M., & Kesterloot, L. (2010). Physical therapist consultation in the emergency department for patients with musculoskeletal disorders: A descriptive comparison of programs in the American southwest. *International Journal of Orthopaedic and Trauma Nursing, 4*(14), 224–225.

Lebec, M., Cernohous, S., Tenbarge, L., Gest, C., Severson, K., & Howard, S. (2010). Emergency department physical therapist service: A pilot study examining physician perceptions. *Internet Journal of Allied Health Sciences and Practice, 8*(1), 1–12.

Lebec, M., & Jogodka, C. E. (2009). The physical therapist as a musculoskeletal specialist in the emergency department. *The Journal of Orthopaedic and Sports Physical Therapy, 39*(3), 221–229.

Lesser, A., Israni, J., Kent, T., & Ko, K. J. (2018, Nov). Association between physical therapy in the emergency department and emergency department revisits for older adult fallers: A nationally representative analysis. *Journal of the American Geriatrics Society, 66*(11), 2205–2212.

Magid, D. J., Sullivan, A. F., Cleary, P. D., Rao, S. R., Gordon, J. A., Kaushal, R., Guadagnoli, E., Camargo, C. A., Jr., & Blumenthal, D. (2009). The safety of emergency care systems: Results of a survey of clinicians in 65 US emergency departments. *Annals of Emergency Medicine, 53*(6), 715–723.e1.

McClellan, C. M., Greenwood, R., & Benger, J. R. (2006). Effect of an extended scope physiotherapy service on patient satisfaction and the outcome of soft tissue injuries in an adult emergency department. *Emergency Medicine Journal: EMJ, 23*(5), 384–387.

Medicare.gov. (n.d.). *Skilled nursing facility (SNF) care.* https://www.medicare.gov/coverage/skilled-nursing-facility-snf-care.

Medicare.gov. (n.d.). *Inpatient or outpatient hospital status affects your costs.* https://www.medicare.gov/what-medicare-covers/what-part-a-covers/inpatient-or-outpatient-hospital-status.

Mistry, D. A., & Rainer, T. H. (2018). Concussion assessment in the emergency department: A preliminary study for a quality improvement project. *BMJ Open Sport & Exercise Medicine, 4*(1), e000445.

Morphet, J., Griffiths, D. L., Crawford, K., Williams, A., Jones, T., Berry, B., & Innes, K. (2016). Using transprofessional care in the emergency department to reduce patient admissions: A retrospective audit of medical histories. *Journal of Interprofessional Care, 30*(2), 226–231.

Morris, C. D., & Hawes, S. J. (1996). The value of accident and emergency based physiotherapy services. *Journal of Accident & Emergency Medicine, 13*(2), 111–113.

Moss, J. E., Houghton, L., Flower, C. L., Moss, D. L., Nielsen, D. A., & Taylor, D. M. (2002). A multidisciplinary care coordination team improves emergency department discharge planning practice. *Medical Journal of Australia, 177,* 435–439.

Muntlin Athlin, Å., von Thiele Schwarz, U., & Farrohknia, N. (2013). Effects of multidisciplinary teamwork on lead times and patient flow in the emergency department: A longitudinal interventional cohort study. *Scandinavian Journal of Trauma, Resuscitation and Emergency Medicine, 21*(1), 76.

Nall, C. (2009). Primary care physiotherapy in the Emergency Department. *The Australian Journal of Physiotherapy, 55*(1), 70.

Nawar, E. W., Niska, R. W., & Xu, J. (2007). National hospital ambulatory medical care survey: 2005 emergency department summary. *Advance Data,* (386), 1–32.

Poulin, P. A., Nelli, J., Tremblay, S., Small, R., Caluyong, M. B., Freeman, J., Romanow, H., Stokes, Y., Carpino, T., Carson, A., Shergill, Y., Stiell, I. G., Taljaard, M., Nathan, H., & Smyth, C. E. (2016). Chronic pain in the emergency department: A pilot mixed-methods cross-sectional study examining patient characteristics and reasons for presentations. *Pain Research & Management, 2016,* 3092391.

Pugh, A., Roper, K., Magel, J., Fritz, J., Colon, N., Robinson, S., Cooper, C., Peterson, J., Kareem, A., & Madsen, T. (2020). Dedicated emergency department physical therapy is associated with reduced imaging, opioid administration, and length of stay: A prospective observational study. *PLoS One, 15*(4), e0231476.

Redberg, R. (2015). The role of post–acute care and variation in the medicare program. *JAMA Internal Medicine, 175*(6), 1058.

Reddy, M., & Spence, P. R. (2006). Finding answers: Information needs of a multidisciplinary patient care team in an emergency department. *AMIA Symposium, 2006,* 649–653.

Rogers, A. T., Bai, G., Lavin, R. A., & Anderson, G. F. (2017). Higher hospital spending on occupational therapy is associated with lower readmission rates. *Medical Care Research and Review: MCRR, 74,* 668–686.

Sakamoto, J. T., Ward, H. B., Vissoci, J. R. N., & Eucker, S. A. (2018). Are nonpharmacologic pain interventions effective at reducing pain in adult patients visiting the emergency department? A systematic review and meta-analysis. *Academic Emergency Medicine: Official Journal of the Society for Academic Emergency Medicine, 25*(8), 940–957.

Strickland, K., & Hartman, J. (2019). *Characterizing a novel clinical education experience in the emergency department/observation unit of an urban academic hospital.* Washington, DC: American Physical Therapy Association Combined Sections Meeting.

Sturmann, K. M., Ehrenberg, K., & Salzberg, M. R. (1990). Physician assistants in emergency medicine. *Annals of Emergency Medicine, 19*(3), 304–308.

Taha, R., Leighton, P., Bainbridge, C., Montgomery, A., Davis, T., & Karantana, A. (2021). Protocol for surgical and non-surgical treatment for metacarpal shaft fractures in adults: An observational feasibility study. *BMJ Open, 11*(6), e046913.

Taira, B. R., Singer, A. J., Thode, H. C., Jr., & Lee, C. (2010). Burns in the emergency department: A national perspective. *The Journal of Emergency Medicine, 39*(1), 1–5.

Tang, N., Stein, J., Hsia, R. Y., Maselli, J. H., & Gonzales, R. (2010). Trends and characteristics of US emergency department visits, 1997-2007. *JAMA, 304*(6), 664–670.

Thackeray, A., Hess, R., Dorius, J., Brodke, D., & Fritz, J. (2017). Relationship of opioid prescriptions to physical therapy referral and participation for medicaid patients with new-onset low back pain. *The Journal of the American Board of Family Medicine: JABFM, 30*(6), 784.

The Office of the National Coordinator for Health information Technology. (n.d.). *ONC's cures act final rule.* https://www.healthit.gov/curesrule/overview/about-oncs-cures-act-final-rule.

Tipton, K., Leas, B. F., Mull, N. K., Siddique, S. M., Greysen, S. R., Lane-Fall, M. B., & Tsou, A. Y. (2021). *Interventions to decrease hospital length of stay.* Rockville (MD): Agency for Healthcare Research and Quality (US). (Technical Brief, No. 40.) https://www.ncbi.nlm.nih.gov/books/NBK574435/.

US Department of Health and Human Services. *What is the U.S. opioid epidemic?* https://www.hhs.gov/opioids/about-the-epidemic.

US Government Accountability Office. (2009). *Hospital emergency department: Crowding continues to occur, and some patients wait longer than recommended time frames.* https://www.gao.gov/assets/gao-09-347.pdf.

Vinson, D. R. (2002). Treatment patterns of isolated benign headache in US emergency departments. *Annals of Emergency Medicine, 39*(3), 215–222.

Walk, M. E., Mehta, A., Katipally, B., Frei, C., Du, L. (2015). Integrating a physical therapist into the urgent care team: An administrative case study of collaborative seamless, and cost-effective care pathway for neuromusculoskeletal problems. *Physical Therapy Journal of Policy, Administration and Leadership, 15*(2), 3–13.

Woods, E. (2000). The emergency department: A new opportunity for physical therapy. *PT-ALEXANDRIA, 8*(9), 42–47.

17

Post-Acute Care Settings

STEPHANIE L. BONK, OTD, OTR/L; RENÉE LACH-SHARON, PT, GCS, CEEAA, MSCS, CPHQ; DANIEL MILLER, MSPT, MBA; JENNIFER EDWARDS, MSPT; RACHAEL FRAKES SPANN, MOT, OTR/L, CDIS; and WILLIAM R. VANWYE, PT, DPT, PhD

LEARNING OBJECTIVES

By the end of this chapter, the reader will be able to:

1. Distinguish between the post-acute care settings.
2. Identify the different prospective payment systems by setting.
3. Discuss rehabilitation frequency for each post-acute care setting.
4. Determine the appropriate discharge destination.

CHAPTER OUTLINE

Introduction

Post-acute care offers various medical services at home or in specialized facilities to support recovery from a recent injury or illness, typically after a short-term acute care hospital (STACH) stay (Chapter 16). Each post-acute care setting offers varying levels of medical and rehabilitative care with the overall goal of preventing rehospitalizations. Since STACH stays are measured in days, discharge planning begins at admission. Physical (PT) and occupational therapists (OT) are essential players in the multidisciplinary team approach to determining discharge disposition.

Research has found that when discharge recommendations from therapists are followed, re-admission rates are lower (Smith et al., 2010). Thus PTs and OTs need to understand each of these settings to make accurate discharge recommendations (see the chapter activities at the end of the chapter). In addition, therapists must recognize the evolving healthcare landscape from a volume-based system to a value-based system. An important step in this process was passing the *Improving Medicare Post-Acute Care Transformation* or IMPACT act of 2014 (Box 17.1). This act aimed to improve Medicare's post-acute care services via standardized data submission.

• BOX 17.1 **The IMPACT Act**

In 2014, the Improving Medicare Post-Acute Care Transformation (IMPACT) Act was signed into law.

The Act requires the submission of standardized data by inpatient rehabilitation facilities (IRF), skilled nursing facilities (SNF), home health agencies (HHA), and long-term acute care hospitals (LTACH).

- LTACH: Long-Term Care Hospital CARE Data Set (LCDS)
- SNF: Minimum Data Set (MDS)
- HHA: Outcome and Assessment Information Set (OASIS)
- IRFs: Inpatient Rehabilitation Facility-Patient Assessment Instrument (IRF-PAI)

From Center for Medicare and Medicaid Services. (2021). *IMPACT Act of 2014 Data standardization & cross setting measures.* CMS.Gov. https://www.cms.gov/medicare/quality-initiatives-patient-assessment-instruments/post-acute-care-quality-initiatives/IMPACT-Act-of-2014/IMPACT-Act-of-2014-data-standardization-and-cross-setting-measures.

TABLE 17.2 Activities of Daily Living (Self-Care)

ADLs	IADLs
• Ambulating	• Transportation
• Feeding	• Shopping
• Dressing	• Meal preparation
• Personal hygiene	• Home maintenance
• Continence	• Communication
• Toileting	• Managing medications
	• Managing finances

ADLs, Activities of daily living; *IADLs,* instrumental activities of daily living. Data from https://www.ncbi.nlm.nih.gov/books/NBK470404/

TABLE 17.1 Key Factors When Selecting a Discharge Destination

Destination	Key Factors
Home	• The patient can safely perform all ADLs and IADLs (I), with supervision, or 24-hour assistance
IRF	• The patient has medical needs and can tolerate intensive rehabilitation equating to 3 hours per day or 15 hours in a week
SNF	• The patient requires 24-hour skilled nursing services with general physician supervision (e.g., weekly) • The patient is unable to tolerate intensive rehabilitation
HH	• The patient can return home but must be homebound, requiring in-home nursing or rehabilitation services
LTACH	• The patient requires complex medical care with daily physician involvement, 24-hour skilled nursing services, and rehabilitation as tolerated
Hospice	• The patient is expected to live 6 months or less • End-of-life palliative care for comfort and quality of life
Long-term nursing care	• The patient requires long-term, indefinite unskilled nursing care via private pay or Medicaid

ADLs, Activities of daily living; *HH,* home health; *I,* independently; *IADLs,* instrumental activities of daily living; *IRF,* inpatient rehabilitation facility; *LTACH,* long-term acute care hospital; *SNF,* skilled nursing facility.

An important question for any therapist as part of discharge planning is to ask: is this patient safe to go home (Table 17.1)? Typically, most patients would prefer to return to the familiarity of their own homes. Thus discharge planning requires a comprehensive approach to ensure patient safety. If a patient can perform activities of daily living (ADLs) and instrumental activities of daily living (IADLs) independently and safely, discharge to home would be indicated (Table 17.2). Some patients can be discharged home with occasional to 24-hour assistance from family, friends, or private pay in-home services, depending on the level of assistance they need for ADLs and IADLs. However, patients commonly require ongoing medical and rehabilitation services after a STACH stay due to post-hospital syndrome and hospital-associated deconditioning (Falvey et al., 2015; Krumholz, 2013).

Skilled post-acute care settings include inpatient rehabilitation facilities (IRF), skilled nursing facilities (SNF), home health (HH), and long-term acute care hospitals (LTACH) (Table 17.3). The patient's medical status, physical functioning, and contextual factors help determine the most appropriate discharge setting. Patients tolerating intensive rehabilitation would be most appropriate for an IRF, with rehabilitation specialists leading the care. SNFs are most appropriate for patients with ongoing medical care directed by nursing and require general physician supervision. HH is appropriate for individuals who are well enough to return home; however, they are considered homebound and require ongoing medical or rehabilitation care. If a patient needs ongoing complex medical care that a physician directs daily, they would be most appropriate for an LTACH. Lastly, patients receive end-of-life, palliative care during hospice care for comfort and quality of life. IRF, SNF, HH, and LTACH services are considered skilled and thus covered by Medicare Part A and most private insurances. Medicare covers hospice care under Part A if the provider is Medicare-approved. In contrast, long-term nursing care in the home or at a facility is considered unskilled and thus typically requires private pay. Individuals who cannot afford long-term nursing care can apply for Medicaid assistance to help cover the costs.

Inpatient Rehabilitation Facilities/Acute Rehabilitation Units

History and Background

Acute rehabilitation is a specialized post-acute practice area in IRFs or acute rehabilitation units (ARUs). This setting is

<table>
<tr><td>TABLE 17.3</td><td colspan="5">Overview of Post-Acute Care Settings</td></tr>
</table>

	Average LOS	Rehabilitation Frequency	Average Session Length/ Discipline	Productivity Standards[a]
IRF[b]	12 days	2 sessions/day	60–90 min	5–6
SNF[b]	28 days	1 session/day	30–45 min	8–10
HH[b]	30-day periods	1-2 sessions/week	45 min	5–6
LTACH[b]	25 days	As tolerated	As tolerated	8–10

[a]Average number of patients a physical therapist or occupational therapist is expected to treat/day
[b]Payer is Medicare Part A or Private Insurance
HH, Home health; *IRF*, inpatient rehabilitation facility; *LOS*, length of stay; *LTACH*, long-term acute care hospital; *SNF*, skilled nursing facility.

crucial in caring for, treating, and recovering patients with disabling injuries or illnesses. Inpatient rehabilitation facilities are stand-alone hospitals offering acute rehab services versus acute rehabilitation units located within a hospital. These rehab facilities and units specialize in improving function and restoring independence after illness or injury. The American Academy of Physician Medicine and Rehabilitation describes rehabilitative medicine as "not just physical medicine approaches, but also multidisciplinary interventions and medications with the goal of restoration of a person's function after injury or illness" (*History of the Specialty*, 2022).

The first acute rehabilitation unit was opened at Temple University in 1929 by Dr. Frank Krusen. After contracting tuberculosis in medical school, Dr. Krusen realized the importance of physical medicine and dedicated his career to promoting the significance of the specialty. In 1936, Dr. Krusen moved to the Mayo Clinic, developed the Department of Physical Medicine & Rehabilitation (PM&R), and started the first physiatry residency program. Although PM&R treatments were utilized prior to WWII, their prominence greatly increased with many injured soldiers returning home throughout the war. Rehabilitative medicine was unique at that time in that it included multidisciplinary interventions to improve a person's function. As WWII ended, organized medicine began recognizing the field and realizing its importance for patient care. The American Medical Association established a Section on PM&R in 1945 (*History of the Specialty*, 2022).

In the 1980s and continuing for several decades, inpatient rehabilitation programs expanded across the United States. In the 1990s, the International Classification of Diseases (ICD) coding system, used across multiple settings, expanded to include codes based on diagnoses, functioning, and disability. The Medicare Inpatient Rehabilitation Facilities Prospective Payment System (PPS) was enacted in 2001. Changes, clarifications, and addendums to the IRF-PPS continue today (Sandel, 2017).

Acute rehabilitation is a post-acute care setting with various diagnoses and patient populations. It is a heavily regulated setting with specific guidelines by Center for Medicare and Medicaid Services (CMS). Due to these specific regulations and intensive therapy requirements, functional gains may be seen in a relatively short length of stay. The specialized training of the multidisciplinary team in the acute rehabilitation setting allows patients to receive a high quality of care and medical oversight needed during their recovery. The anticipated discharge destination from acute rehabilitation is home, where patients can continue their recovery in a less structured environment.

Accreditation and Regulations

Most inpatient rehabilitation facilities are accredited by the CMS because it is recognized and accepted by third parties nationally. CMS accreditation may be a condition of reimbursement for certain insurers or payers beyond Medicare and Medicaid. It also helps demonstrate an acute rehabilitation facility's commitment to excellence in quality, accountability, and patient safety. CMS accreditation improves risk management, aids in risk reduction, and provides ongoing education and training opportunities. It can provide a framework for creating an organizational structure and standardization and consistency for processes across the organization. CMS accreditation assures that the organization is current with healthcare regulations and supports continuous quality improvement efforts (*What Is Accreditation | The Joint Commission*, 2022).

Patient Population, Services, and Setting Characteristics

Acute rehabilitation serves patients across their lifespans. There are specialty pediatric acute rehabilitation centers and acute rehabilitation centers that specialize in the care of adult patients. Like other post-acute care settings, the goal is to transition from attaining medical stability in the STACH setting to addressing the long-term functional needs of the patient. Post-acute care aims to improve the patient's quality of life and function. The main difference between post-acute settings is the intensity of therapy. CMS has specific criteria each patient must meet to fulfil the requirements for admission into acute rehabilitation (*Medicare Benefit Policy Manual* Chapter 1 - Inpatient Hospital Services Covered Under Part A, 2021).

1. Pre-admission screening (PAS): Acute rehabilitation admits patients from several different settings. Patients are frequently admitted from acute care hospitals but can also be admitted from LTACHs, SNFs, assisted living facilities, HH, or the emergency room. Clinical liaisons receive the patient referral and screen the patient in collaboration with the physician using the PAS to determine whether the patient would be an appropriate rehabilitation candidate.
2. History and physical and three face-to-face physician visits: The rehabilitation physician must evaluate and examine each patient within 24 hours of admission. Following the examination, the physician must write a history and physical (H&P) plan to manage the patient's rehabilitation needs. In addition to the H&P, the rehabilitation physician must have three face-to-face weekly visits with the patient to document their progress.
3. Individualized plan of care (IPOC) and interdisciplinary team (IDT) meeting: During the patient's evaluation period, each discipline involved in the patient's care will complete evaluations and develop an individualized plan of care. The patient's medical and functional needs and goals are synthesized into the plan of care. The plan must be agreed upon and signed within the first 4 days of the patient's rehabilitation stay. IDT meetings must be held at least once weekly throughout the patient's acute rehabilitation stay. All providers participating in the care of each patient must be in attendance. A weekly IDT meeting allows team members to assess the patient's progress, identify barriers to meeting goals, and monitor and revise the patient's plan of care as needed.
4. Admission orders: Each patient must have an order from the physician stating they are being admitted to acute rehabilitation upon admission to the IRF or ARU.
5. IRF-patient assessment instrument (PAI): The IRF-PAI must be completed for each patient during an acute rehabilitation stay. This document collates medical, functional, and quality data submitted to CMS for reimbursement.
6. Multiple therapy disciplines: Each patient admitted to acute rehabilitation must require two or more therapy disciplines. One of the therapy disciplines required must be PT or OT.
7. Intensive rehabilitation therapy program: Patients in acute rehabilitation must participate and tolerate 3 hours of therapy daily for at least 5 out of 7 days per week. Patients are scheduled for PT, OT, and speech language pathology (SLP) daily, depending on their specific needs. In certain situations where patients cannot tolerate a full 3 hours of therapy a day, they may qualify for a modified schedule of 15 hours spread over the entire week.
8. Medical necessity: Patients in acute rehabilitation must be medically complex and require close medical management and oversight. To qualify for acute rehabilitation, the patient should not be managed at a lower level of care.
9. CMS 13: To be reimbursed through IRF-PPS, 60% of all patients admitted to the IRF or ARU each year must have at least one of 13 conditions (Fig. 17.1) (*Specifications for Determining IRF "60% Rule" Compliance*, 2017).

Patients in the IRF setting must participate in 3 hours of therapy, 5 days per week, equating to 900 billed minutes weekly. A patient's week is defined, with day one being their day of admission through their seventh day in acute rehabilitation. To ensure that the patient is seen for the entirety of these minutes, patients are typically scheduled for 3 hours of therapy Monday through Friday and will have therapy on the weekend days as necessary (*Medicare Benefit Policy Manual* Chapter 1 - Inpatient Hospital Services Covered Under Part A, 2021).

Patients are scheduled for PT, OT, and SLP according to their care plan and goals. Patients who do not have SLP needs will typically be treated for 90 minutes of PT and OT each day. Patients with SLP needs will usually be treated daily for 60 minutes of each discipline. The time each discipline treats

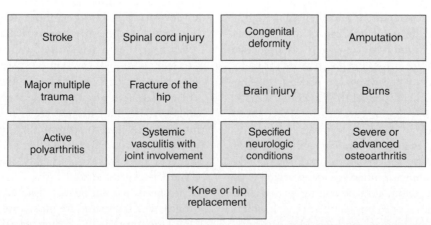

*If bilateral, BMI >50, or age 85+

• **Fig. 17.1** Centers for Medicare and Medicaid Inpatient Rehabilitation Facility Conditions

each patient can be customized based on their specific needs in their plan of care. If the patient cannot tolerate lengthy sessions, the time may be broken up throughout the day. Low activity tolerance or other extenuating circumstances impact a patient's ability to tolerate three hours of therapy daily. In these situations, an order can be written to extend the 900 minutes across 7 days rather than the typical 5 days. A common example of this would be patients who require hemodialysis two or three times a week in acute rehabilitation. Due to the time needed to complete dialysis and fatigue level, the physician typically writes an order to support the intensity change.

Providers and Care Coordination

One of the key facets of the acute rehabilitation setting is the multidisciplinary approach to treatment. Facilities may differ slightly with the interdisciplinary team members, but the key players include a PM&R physician (i.e., physiatrist), medical physicians, PTs, OTs, SLPs, case managers, and nursing staff. Other disciplines include respiratory therapists, dietitians, social workers, and pharmacists.

- The PM&R physician is responsible for overseeing the care and progress of patients throughout their stay in acute rehabilitation. This specialty focuses on the treatment of the musculoskeletal system. Physiatrists diagnose, manage, and treat pain and functional deficits from injury, illness, or medical conditions.
- Internal medicine doctors are also key to a patient's recovery. In acute rehabilitation, internal medicine providers focus on the patient's medical needs. Some examples may include medication management, multisystem support, and managing the overall medical prognosis of the patient.
- PT, OT, and SLP are integral to the rehabilitative process. These disciplines collaborate with medical team members and nursing staff to ensure patients' progress toward their goals.
- Case Managers are critical to managing a patient's rehab stay (see Chapter 21). They coordinate patient needs alongside the therapy, medical, and nursing teams. They also collaborate with each patient and their support system for discharge planning. Discharge planning begins when a patient is admitted or during the referral process. Case managers frequently speak with patients throughout their stay to ensure the discharge plan meets their needs and goals. Another aspect of this discipline is managing authorizations with the patient's insurance company or payer source.
- Nurses assist patients in acute rehabilitation by providing 24-hour care, including collaboration regarding managing medical issues, hands-on nursing care, working with the interdisciplinary team, and educating patients on nursing-specific topics. For example, nurses in rehabilitation frequently address bowel and bladder concerns, medication, pain management, skin integrity, and chronic disease education.

Depending on the medical needs of the patients in each facility, it is helpful to have respiratory therapists, dietitians, wound care specialists, and dialysis partnerships. Access to these disciplines allows more medically complex patients (e.g., post mechanical ventilation, hemodialysis, post-tracheostomy, post-COVID-19) to be admitted. These disciplines help address the specialized needs of those who are more medically complex; hence, these patients are more likely to be successful in their transition home. Additional specialties frequently consulted in acute rehabilitation include neuro-optometry, prosthetics/orthotics, neuropsychology, recreational therapy, and movement disorder physicians. Many patients come to a rehabilitation unit with new vision deficits or newly diagnosed movement disorders. A partnership with these practitioners offers patients and staff the support to ensure a proper treatment plan and the most effective rehabilitative stay.

Responsibilities of a Manager/Administrator

Therapy managers or administrators in the inpatient rehabilitation facility setting have multiple responsibilities that vary day-to-day. The role also varies depending on the leadership structure of the organization. Typically, the therapy manager is responsible for all personnel management in the therapy department. The leader also manages the department's staffing needs, budget, and daily operations. In addition to the day-to-day operations, the therapy manager develops and implements the goals, objectives, standards of performance, and overall program development to ensure the patient receives the highest quality of service and care. The therapy manager can also play a large role in the organization, helping with hospital processes, compliance, and overall operations.

Referral Sources and Marketing

IRFs take admissions from a large variety of referral sources. Most admissions come from the acute care setting after a patient has been hospitalized for an illness, injury, or surgery. Admissions may also come from an SNF when the patient would benefit from the increased intensity of therapy or an LTACH when the patient is medically stable. IRFs can also directly admit patients from the community because they are licensed as a hospital. Direct referrals and admissions for IRF can come from HH companies, emergency departments, urgent care centers, or physician offices. These referrals are typically made when a patient has had a functional decline or is not safe or successful at their current functional level in the community and at home.

Each hospital has a marketing and admissions team that manages these referrals. Facility liaisons typically have a clinical background and assist with coordinating the patient's needs for admission. They also are skilled at determining which patients are most appropriate for the setting. One large proponent of their position includes educating hospitals and providers in the community on the benefits and services offered in an IRF setting.

Staffing and Productivity Expectations

Every facility will use some form of productivity monitoring. The two most popular are productivity derived from units of service and hours per patient day. Units of service (UOS) are common in outpatient settings. UOS are used to discern how much time each employee spends per patient. It is important to know how much time the therapist will spend with each patient when scheduling patients. In 2017, tiered Common Procedural Codes (CPT) codes were established for PT and OT. Instead of one evaluation code, three codes reflect patient presentation: low, moderate, or high complexity. Although these newer PT and OT evaluation codes remain untimed, Medicare estimates average times of 20–30, 30–45, and 45–60 minutes for low, moderate, and high complexity evaluations, respectively. Facilities may use these average times as a marker for initial scheduling assessments and productivity (Andrus & Gawenda, 2016).

IRF patients are typically scheduled for 60 or 90-minute therapy sessions. A high complexity evaluation would be 45 minutes and the remaining 15 to 45 minutes could be billed as treatment using a different CPT code that reflects the intervention for that portion of the session. A typical 8-hour day would result in the billing of approximately 28 UOS. A breakdown reveals that 28 UOS in 15-minute increments equates to 7 hours of billable patient care or a caseload of five to six patients per day.

Hours per patient day (HPPD) is another method used to determine productivity; however, it is driven by the patient census. Each facility will develop a formula that will be used to decide how much staff is needed to ensure all patients are seen for 180 minutes per day to meet their plan of care. The formula does not specify how many therapists are required for each discipline but rather the total number of FTE (full-time equivalent) staff needed at each census count. HPPD allows more variability and flexibility to meet the patient's skilled needs. In an IRF using HPPD, a therapist may have four to six patients to treat each day. This number will vary depending on the involvement of the SLP and the patient's individualized plan of care. Using HPPD, therapists will have 6–7 hours of billable patient care scheduled on average.

Reimbursement, Documentation, and Quality Improvement

CMS uses case-mix groups (CMGs) to reimburse IRFs for services provided to Medicare patients (i.e., IRF-PPS). The CMG classification system ideally groups patients with similar medical and functional needs who are expected to utilize similar resources. Each CMG provides the basis for payment and the average length of stay for each patient admitted to an IRF. Three main factors contribute to the assignment of a CMG for each patient. First, the impairment group code is assigned to the patient by the rehabilitation physician. The impairment group code is the primary diagnosis and reason for the patient's admission into the IRF. Next, the patient's comorbid conditions are added.

Lastly, the patient's motor score collected by clinicians on admission is calculated and assigned based on both motor and self-care task performance. These items are combined and the patient's CMG is assigned (Barrilleaux, 2021). The facility is reimbursed the full amount of the CMG if the patient has a community discharge. If the patient cannot discharge to a community setting, the IRF is reimbursed at a per diem rate.

Several metrics and outcome measures are tracked and reported in acute rehabilitation. The medical acuity level is typically monitored to ensure appropriate patients are admitted to acute rehabilitation. The case mix index (CMI) measures the patient population's case-mix groups. As the medical complexity of the patient population increases, the CMI increases, and vice versa. Other quantitative outcomes that are frequently monitored include average length of stay and mandatory quality reporting items such as worsened pressure injuries, catheter-associated urinary tract infections, and falls.

Because the goal of acute rehabilitation is a functional improvement, analysis of outcome measures is integral to ensuring that an acute rehabilitation program is successful. Because reimbursement is closely linked to discharge disposition, patients' discharge destination is also closely monitored. Most acute rehabilitation programs have target goals for community discharge rates. Discharges to acute care and discharges to non-community settings are also typically tracked.

Another outcome measure frequently reviewed is the functional improvement of the patient population. During the first three days of admission, the clinical staff completes a functional assessment called section GG of the IRF-PAI. This is designed to collect the patient's usual performance for self-care tasks, functional mobility, and bowel and bladder continence. Each item is individually scored and added together for a combined score. This same process is completed at discharge. The difference between these combined scores demonstrates a quantifiable change in function from admission to discharge. Scoring can be further analyzed to improve self-care or mobility-specific items. These metrics may also be combined with the length of stay to see the level of improvement per patient day. Quality metrics and outcome measures may be compared to the national and regional averages using IRF-specific software. Much of this data is also reported to CMS and is available for consumers to view on medicare.gov.

Skilled Nursing Facility

History and Background

SNFs started in the 19th century. There are conditions of participation created under the Social Security Act in 1965 to which SNFs must adhere to qualify for Medicare reimbursement. There have been four payment systems for therapy reimbursement in the SNF setting. First, the PPS in 1983 increased the demand for therapy in SNFs while reducing the

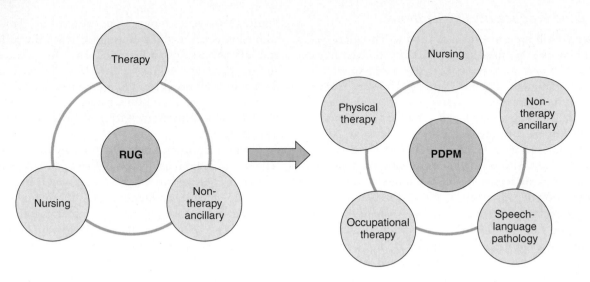

• **Fig. 17.2** Comparison of Patient Driven Payment Model (PDPM) and Resource Utilization Groups (RUGs) Payment Systems

length of hospital stay. Second, the Balanced Budget Act of 1997, refined in 1999, aimed to decrease the cost of SNFs. Third, 44 Resource Utilization Groups (RUGs) were implemented in 2010 and increased to 66 RUGs in 2011. Lastly, the current payment system is the Patient Driven Payment Model (PDPM) (Fig. 17.2), which was started in 2019 and aimed to focus less on the volume of services and more on patient characteristics (Cabigao & Cherney, 2014; Prusynski, 2021; *Skilled Nursing Facility (SNF) Prospective Payment System (PPS) Legislative History.*, 2021).

The PDPM comprises five components: PT, OT, SLP, nursing, and non-therapy ancillary (NTA). PDPM allows the patient to receive the services to meet their needs and goals, which improves payment accuracy. To assist in determining the costs of therapy, the clinical category and functional status are used. The patient's primary diagnosis and functional status determine the clinical category. The primary diagnosis is joint replacement, non-surgical orthopedic, orthopedic, acute infections, medical management, cancer, pulmonary, cardiovascular, acute neurologic, and non-orthopedic surgery. The functional status is determined by the Section GG item scores inputted by the PTs and OTs during the evaluation (CMS, 2021). SLP do not enter GG scores, but they address acute neurologic clinical classification, SLP-related comorbidities, presence of cognitive impairment, use of mechanically-altered diet, and presence of swallowing disorder (CMS, 2021).

- GG items:
  - OT
    - Self-Care, A. Eating
    - Self-Care, B. Oral Hygiene
    - Self-Care, C. Toileting Hygiene
    - Self-Care, E. Shower/Bathe self
    - Self-Care, F. Upper Body dressing
    - Self-Care, G. Lower Body dressing

- Self-Care, H. Putting on/Taking off footwear
- Mobility, F. Toilet Transfer
- Mobility, Does the resident use a wheelchair/scooter?
- Mobility, R. Wheel 50 feet with two turns
  - Mobility, Indicate the type of wheelchair/scooter used (50 ft/2 turns)
- Mobility, S. Wheel 150 feet
  - Mobility, Indicate the type of wheelchair/scooter used (150 feet)
- PT
  - Mobility, A. Roll left and right
  - Mobility, B. Sit to lying
  - Mobility, C. Lying to sitting on bed side
  - Mobility, D. Sit to stand
  - Mobility, E. Chair/bed to chair transfer
  - Mobility, G. Car transfer
  - Mobility, I. Walk 10 feet
  - Mobility, J. Walk 50 feet with two turns
  - Mobility, K. Walk 150 feet
  - Mobility, L. Walking 10 feet on uneven surfaces
  - Mobility, M. 1 step (curb)
  - Mobility, N. 4 steps
  - Mobility, O. 12 steps
  - Mobility, P. Picking up object
- GG scores are numbered 1–7, 88, 09, or 10:
  - 06 – Independent – can the client complete the task with no assistance? (with or without adaptive equipment)
  - 05 – Setup or clean-up assist – can the person be left alone to do the task after setup?
  - 04 – Supervision or touching assistance – does the helper provide only supervision (verbal cues) or light touch?
  - 03 – Partial/moderate assistance – does the helper provide less than half of the effort to complete the task?

- 02 – Substantial/maximal assistance – does the helper provide more than half, but less than 100%, of the effort to complete the task?
- 01 – Dependent – does the helper need to do 100% of the task, or are two or more helpers needed at any time?
- 07 – Resident refused
- 88 – Not attempted due to medical condition or safety concerns
- 09 – Not applicable – not attempted, and the resident did not perform this activity prior to the current illness, or injury
- 10 – Not attempted due to environmental limitations (i.e., lack of equipment, weather constraints)

Accreditation and Regulations

In 1987, the Federal Nursing Home Reform Act (OBRA) regulated almost all nursing homes. At the state level, state agencies license SNFs and federal governments certify SNFs for Medicare/Medicaid reimbursement. Licensing started in the late 1960s with the passage of Medicare/Medicaid. Many states follow the federal requirements, but some update regulations to fit their specific needs and desires. Other accrediting bodies include the Commission on Accreditation of Rehabilitation Facilities (CARF) and the Joint Commission on Accreditation of Healthcare Organizations (JCAHO). SNFs must be certified to receive reimbursement from Medicare or Medicaid. SNFs can be private (profit and nonprofit) or government-owned (Cabigao & Cherney, 2014; *Skilled Nursing Facility (SNF) Prospective Payment System (PPS) Legislative History*, 2021).

Patient Population, Services, and Setting Characteristics

The population of SNFs is primarily the geriatric population with an average age of 65 to 100 years with various diagnoses and physical and/or cognitive deficits. Residents of the SNF include long-term care who reside there permanently and patients who reside temporarily at the SNF while receiving nursing and/or rehabilitation services. In addition to nursing and rehabilitation services, other social work services, activities, dining, housekeeping, maintenance, business, and admissions are included. These services ensure a well-rounded stay for the residents and patients. The setup of the SNF varies by site and depends on the logistics of the building. Some rooms are shared, while others are single. The level of assistance the individuals at the SNF require varies, but often they receive assistance with completing ADLs, functional transfers, functional mobility, and IADLs. Another factor that varies is the facility's culture, based on geographic location, clientele, staff, and funding availability.

Often within SNFs, the long-term nursing/care population comprises residents who live at the facility due to their medical, physical, and cognitive needs. The goal for these

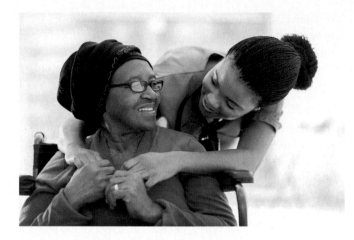

- **Fig. 17.3** Nursing care includes assistance with medical, physical, and cognitive needs for safety and to maintain independence. (https://www.flickr.com/photos/68716695@N06/29609199652/).

residents to maintain their highest level of independence and safety with assistance from the staff (Fig. 17.3). These residents pay to reside in an SNF with personal funds (i.e., savings, pensions, stocks), government programs like Medicaid, long-term care insurance, veterans' benefits, or through the Older Americans Act (*What Is Long-Term Care?* 2017).

Providers and Care Coordination

The providers at an SNF often consist of the therapy team, which is PT, OT, SLP, and respiratory therapy. They work with the nursing staff, including registered nurses, licensed practicing nurses, and certified nursing assistants (CNA). The other providers include social workers, dieticians, and medical providers such as physician assistants and physicians.

For care coordination, there is often a daily morning meeting where all the directors from the various departments meet with the administrator to discuss any overnight changes. These changes may include new admissions, incidents, changes in behavior or status of some of the patients, and any other daily occurrences. Daily meetings ensure managers can share pertinent information with their team. Also, a weekly meeting is held with the directors of therapy, admissions, business, nursing, and the physician assistants to discuss each patient receiving therapy to assist in determining a discharge plan for the patient. Lastly, if the therapy team is contracted to work at the SNF, the director of therapy often has a phone conversation with the other area directors to discuss any staffing needs or other pertinent information.

Responsibilities of a Manager/Administrator

A manager of the therapy department is responsible for the daily scheduling, daily operations, communication between all departments, completing Minimum Data Set (MDS) requirements for the billing office, participating in meetings, and treating patients. Managers of the various other departments mentioned above in the care team are responsible for their departments. The administrator oversees the facility's operations, ensuring adherence to accreditation standards, and liaising between the building and the corporate headquarters (Myers et al., 2018).

Referral Sources and Marketing

The main referral sources for the SNF include local hospitals and patients of the SNF's medical director. In most geographical areas, acute care hospitals regularly refer to and coordinate with a particular SNF; however, patients have the freedom to decide which facility to attend, including picking a location closer to their home or their family's home. Some SNFs have someone in their marketing department who regularly goes to the local hospitals to talk with patients about the SNF, provide flyers to local senior living facilities, meet with administrators and discharge planners (often social workers) at local hospitals, and host get-togethers of "graduates" of SNF to advertise services.

Staffing and Productivity Expectations

Most therapists are full-time staff. However, it is common for companies to hire therapists who are pro re nata/per diem (PRN) to support the regular staff during a high census, vacations, or sick days. If the therapy staff is part of a contract company that provides services to other SNFs in the area, the therapists may go between multiple buildings to fulfill needs or obtain full-time hours. The productivity level depends on the company and building size, but often for evaluating therapists is between 80 to 90 percent, and for assistants is 90 to 95 percent (Bennett et al., 2019).

Reimbursement, Documentation, and Quality Improvement

Reimbursement and payment of therapy at a SNF include various sources. Most patients' reimbursement is from the PDPM model for Medicare Part A, but patients may have other or additional coverage through private insurance or Medicaid. Each reimbursement type has its own rules for billing and compliance. As mentioned earlier, a qualifying inpatient admission falls under the Two-Midnight rule (CMS, 2015). However, to qualify for rehabilitation care at a SNF, Medicare requires the patient to be admitted to the hospital for a minimum of 3 days (i.e., the Three-Day Rule). The 3 days do not include time spent in the emergency department, under observation, or on the day of discharge. Individuals must be inpatients in the SNF for four days (*Medicare Benefit Policy Manual:* Chapter 8 – Coverage of Extended Care (SNF) Services under Hospital Insurance, 2019).

The Three-Day Rule was waived during the COVID-19 pandemic, so Medicare A will still reimburse if patients are medically stable to discharge to an SNF. Medicare A will also reimburse an SNF stay if a patient was at the hospital for three nights and discharged home but then requires an SNF stay within 30 days of discharge for the same reason they were hospitalized. Medicare A will cover up to 100 days per year. The average length of stay in an SNF is approximately 30 days (Chapter 7: Skilled Nursing Facility Services (March 2022 Report) – MedPAC, 2022). Length of stay depends on the patient's abilities and the payer source. For example, some private insurances (e.g., Humana, Blue Cross Blue Shield, Aetna) decide the length of stay. Lastly, there are scenarios when a patient might plateau, be discharged, and then have a change in status that could allow them to be readmitted to an SNF. If a patient is readmitted within 30 days of discharge for whatever reason, it would be reimbursed by Medicare. After a patient is discharged from an SNF, if they reenter an SNF within 30 days, they do not need another 3-day qualifying hospital stay to get additional SNF benefits. For example, a patient who is non-weight-bearing might be discharged home, but after three weeks, when their status improves to weight-bearing as tolerated, they are re-admitted to the SNF with Medicare coverage (*Medicare Benefit Policy Manual:* Chapter 8 – Coverage of Extended Care (SNF) Services under Hospital Insurance, 2019).

Billing occurs through the MDS office at the SNF. Dependent on the size of the SNF, there are usually one to three RNs who work as billing specialists and are responsible for selecting the proper codes for maximum reimbursement. Billing specialists are also responsible for compliance and must follow all guidelines to receive payment. They often communicate with third-party payers by completing insurance updates and sending and completing appeal letters when patients want to appeal the decision the insurance company (including Medicare) has made regarding the discontinuation of services within the SNF (*Minimum Data Set (MDS) 3.0 for Nursing Homes and Swing Bed Providers*, 2022; *Therapy Services*, 2021).

The documentation requirements are dependent on the payer source and the company that operates the SNF. For example, for all payer sources, the therapy evaluations are completed by the therapists. For Medicare A and some private insurances, the progress notes (PN) and discharge (DC) summaries can be completed by both the therapists as well as the assistants, but for Medicare B, PN and DC need to be completed by the therapists (*Skilled Services Requirements, 42 CFR § 409.44*, 2016). SNF electronic medical record (EMR) systems vary from site to site.

Outcomes follow the Federal Nursing Home Compare, which started in 1998, and the Five-Star rating system incorporated in 2008. Star ratings are determined by recertification survey scores, nursing staffing levels, and quality measures such as pain, urinary tract infections (UTI), pressure sores, delirium, and physical restraints. The star rating of a SNF is public knowledge and patients and their families can look at this rating to determine which SNF they will attend (Cabigao & Cherney, 2014).

The National Quality Forum (NQF) is a voluntary organization that looks at the MDS 17 measures on patients' health conditions, functioning, preferences, and wishes. Its mission is to have evidence-based and best-practice care for healthcare.

They also have a team to keep consistent with the changing healthcare environment (*What We Do*, 2022). Lastly, the standard recertification survey occurs every 9–15 months and when they come onsite, the visit is unannounced. While onsite, they thoroughly assess the quality of care and life with residents, family members, and employees. They then provide feedback to the facility on areas of concern and needs for change to comply (*Survey Protocol for Long Term Care Facilities – Part 1. State Operations Manual*, 2005).

The collected health informatics can be analyzed by running reports of the documentation system to look at productivity, margins of profit, and missing doctor signatures on documentation. Overall, this information can improve the quality of care, patient outcomes, and staff satisfaction in the SNF. Lastly, using methods to collect health information impacts the amount and quality of documented information for staff to complete all daily responsibilities (Ko et al., 2018).

Home Healthcare

History and Background

What began as providing nursing care to those who had difficulty leaving their home has blossomed into a setting that is now multidisciplinary and able to manage increasingly complex and higher acuity patients. With technology, these boundaries continue to be expanded. The following information will examine the rules, regulations, and unique challenges of this setting.

There are two main types of home care. First, care focuses on everyday activities such as dressing, bathing, grooming, and household tasks such as cleaning, cooking, and preparing meals. This care is considered unskilled and thus is private pay. The second is short-term, physician-directed care designed to help patients prevent or recover from an illness, injury, or hospitalization. HH care services are delivered by skilled healthcare providers such as nurses, PTs, OTs, SLPs, and social workers (*Medicare Benefit Policy Manual* Chapter 7 - Home Health Services, 2022). This section will explore the latter version of home care services.

Historically, healthcare began with physicians and nurses performing home services (Kub et al., 2015). With advances in medicine, there was a shift in the care setting. Advances in medical technology required space and maintenance that only hospitals could provide. Physicians started to specialize more and offer their services in centralized locations. Increased use of cars and public transportation allowed patients to travel to hospitals. By the 1930s, most care of acutely ill patients had transitioned to the hospital and visiting nurses provided long-term care in the home to chronically ill and dying patients. In the late 1950s, hospitals began to refer home care nurses to help discharge patients from the hospital to the home and provide post-acute care.

Charities and public contributions initially funded HH care agencies until the Medicare Act in 1965 (Davitt & Choi, 2008). Medicare covered care for patients sent home from the hospital under the Part A HH benefit. It was limited to 100 visits following a 3-day or longer hospital stay. Medicare also covered more chronic care. Under Part B, the general HH benefit was limited to 100 home visits per calendar year. Home care continued to expand with the Omnibus Reconciliation Act of 1980, which removed limits on the number of home care visits and prior hospitalization requirements. Also, it extended participation in the Medicare home care benefit program to include for-profit home care agencies. At this point, more than half of the patients receiving HH care did not have immediate prior hospitalizations and many received services for more than 6 months.

HH care continued to expand through the late 1980s with the hospital PPS (Davitt & Choi, 2008). PPS resulted in faster hospital discharges and increased the need for post-hospitalization home care services. Medicare HH care payments increased 33% annually between 1989 and 1996. In 1997, the Balanced Budget Act (BBA) set new limits on Medicare HH care. Limits were set on Medicare spending and a new requirement of homebound status was developed. The BBA also required agencies to report outcome data on all Medicare and Medicaid patients using the *Outcome and Assessment Information Set* (OASIS) to refocus care on post-acute and episodic care. The 1997 BBA created a HH care PPS. HH agencies would be paid a set amount for each 60-day episode, regardless of the number of visits provided, and payment was broken down into 80 separate clinical categories. Cost-based reimbursement with a PPS resulted in a 20% decline in the use of HH care, with many rural area agencies closing. The BBA reduction in HH care reimbursement led to the closure of 14% of home health agencies (HHAs) between 1997 and 1999. By 2001, approximately 33% of HHAs had closed.

PPS had a unique effect on therapy. Under PPS, the therapy provided during an episode of care was one of the three main factors used to calculate the amount an HHA would be paid for the episode. The PPS payment was based on 6, 14, and 20-visit thresholds (*CMS Announces Payment Changes for Medicare Home Health Services Improving Beneficiary Access and Quality and Efficiency of Care | CMS*, 2007). Thus this PPS threshold payment factor led to a steady increase in PT, OT, and SLP services (Medicare and Medicaid, 2018).

Although the presumption is that more care would improve outcomes, Medicare performed data analysis and found that the outcomes of patients getting more visits did not consistently match the amount of therapy provided. Overall, Medicare found that often the outcomes leveled off, but the patient visits continued. To correct this issue, Medicare made another change to the payment model. In January 2020, Medicare implemented a new payment model for HH called the Patient Driven Grouping Model (PDGM) (*Medicare and Medicaid Programs*, 2018). This model removed the amount of therapy provided as a factor in determining payment. PDGM emphasizes the patient's diagnosis while emphasizing the patient's overall function and comorbidities (Fig. 17.4). This model will be discussed further in a later section of this chapter.

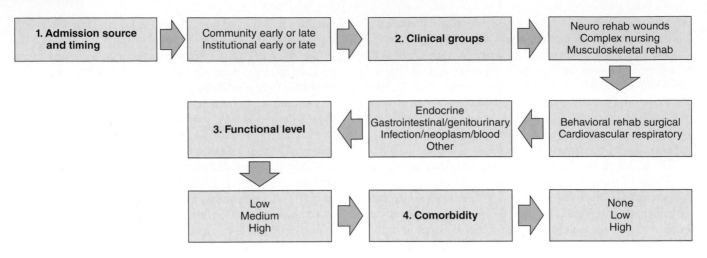

• **Fig. 17.4** The Patient-Driven Groupings Model

Accreditation and Regulations

The state must license HHAs to receive Medicare Certification. Many states require an agency to obtain a Certificate of Need before accepting an application for agency licensure. The Certificate of Need (CON) is a regulatory mechanism used by states to control healthcare costs by restricting the number of duplicate services available in the state and determining whether new facilities meet a community's needs. CON programs may also help to ensure that traditionally underserved communities receive access to health services (*Certificate of Need (CON)*, 2019).

State licensure processes vary from state to state but generally include application to the state specifying the ownership of the agency, agency's physical address, services to be provided (e.g., nursing, therapy, HH aide), name of the agency administrator, name of the governing body, and area (counties) of coverage for the agency. If a CON is required, it is generally included in the application to the state. After the application is made to the state, the agency will have an onsite initial licensure survey to ensure the agency complies with all state rules and regulations. When an HHA has obtained licensure, they can work toward Medicare Certification. The agency must have at least 10 patients who have received services from the agency before CMS will survey them. At least 7 of the 10 patients must receive services from the agency at the survey time. The CMS survey determines compliance with all the health and safety Conditions of Participation as defined in the Federal Registrar (*Home Health Agency (HHA) Center | CMS*, 2021).

CMS requires HHAs to provide nursing services and at least one other therapeutic service (e.g., PT, OT, SLP, medical social services, or HH aide) in residence used as the patient's home. At least one of the services must be provided directly by an employee of the HH agency and the other services can be provided under a contractual arrangement if needed. Further certifications can be sought by HHA, including the Joint Commission on Accreditation of Healthcare Organizations (JCAHO), the Community Health Accreditation Program (CHAP), and the Accreditation Commission for Health Care (ACHC) certifications. These are voluntary certifications that an HHA can choose to pay to participate in to show that they have achieved the quality standards of these organizations. If an HHA chooses to seek one of these certifications, it will be surveyed by the accrediting group and must pass that survey to be certified. To maintain the certification, they must pass subsequent surveys at the frequency determined by the accrediting organization.

Once an HHA is fully licensed and certified, they are expected to provide care consistent with the CMS Conditions of Participation and regulations. The Conditions of Participation outline the expectations of an HHA, from staffing regulations and required governance to licensure and training expectations of clinical staff. The Conditions of Participation also outline the rights of the patients receiving care from an HHA. The CMS regulations are built off the Conditions of Participation and contain further guidance and standards for the industry. Chapter 7 of the Medicare Benefit Policy Manual (MBPM) (2022) describes the regulations for the operation of an HHA, while Chapter 15 of the MBPM (2021) describes the expected billing practices and guidelines. It is important for any therapist working in HH to familiarize themselves with Chapter 7 of the MBPM because it describes what qualifies patients to receive HH services and what constitutes skilled level treatments from the clinicians.

The regulations set out by CMS in Chapter 7, and the National Coverage Determinations are the basis for most state regulations, and the Medicare Audit Contractors will use them to create their Local Coverage Determinations. CMS sets National Coverage Determinations to describe what types of services are covered by Medicare and are often used by private insurances as their basis for coverage. Medicare Audit Contractors are Medicare Intermediaries that manage the Medicare benefits for a specified geographical area. They are tasked with Managing the Medicare provision and ensuring compliance with Medicare Regulations. They often create Local Coverage Determinations that are used to further clarify the National Coverage Determinations and regulations from CMS concerning coverage for services and requirements that must be met for those services to be billable (*What's a MAC | CMS*, 2022).

Each state also monitors the services of HHA and is responsible for performing surveys for continued licensure and investigating any complaints filed against an HHA on behalf of a patient. The individual states may also have further regulations for HH services. For example, Illinois requires additional yearly training on Alzheimer's disease for anyone working in HH. The state regulations can also set rules regarding which services can be provided by which disciplines practicing HH. For example, certain states do not allow PTs to perform INR testing despite being within their scope of practice in many other states. Thus therapists must be aware of state regulations for their practice areas.

Therapists must understand their state practice act to determine what they can legally perform. For example, some states do not allow HH therapists to educate patients on medications. Also, therapists must determine the allowable practices of assistants and aides. Certain states require explicit documentation of therapy assistant supervision, while others have specific time requirements. Familiarity with state practice acts, rules, and regulations is vital for all therapists.

Patient Population, Services, and Setting Characteristics

Historically, HH has focused on geriatric patients. Older adults are often confronted with mobility issues immediately following an acute care stay. Mobility issues have necessitated the evolution of HH visits until the patient has sufficient strength and endurance to get to an outpatient setting. The trend toward the shortened length of hospital stays combined with the health risk of a global pandemic has escalated the demand in this area over the last several years.

Some HHAs also offer hospice services. As previously discussed, hospice care provides care to terminally ill patients. The focus is on palliative or comfort care instead of curative care. Hospice care meets the patient's medical needs and includes the patient's and family's psychosocial and spiritual needs at the end of life. Agencies must meet specific federal requirements and be separately certified as a Medicare or Medicaid-certified hospice to provide hospice care. Hospice agencies have unique regulations, guidelines, and reimbursement structures independent of those governing HHAs (*Hospice Center*, 2021).

Children with congenital pathologies require frequent care; however, not all HHAs serve pediatrics due to their unique skillset, equipment needs, and limited funding, and each state funds most pediatric cases through Medicaid (Foster et al., 2019). Since Medicaid funds come from the federal and state governments, reimbursement can vary markedly from one state to the next. Becoming a Medicaid

provider is not a HHA requirement. It is a financial decision left up to the individual agencies and can affect whether they treat pediatric patients.

Delivering care in the home presents a unique set of challenges. Travel modes vary depending on rural versus urban settings. For instance, HH therapists may utilize bush planes to access patients in Alaska, whereas a therapist in New York City may use the subway system. Rural HH therapists may cover several counties in a car and regularly travel on unmaintained roads to see patients. Reliable transportation is essential, as is driving in all weather conditions. Cell coverage may be limited in rural areas, so basic knowledge of car repairs, such as changing a flat tire, can also be useful. It is prudent to have a well-stocked car to manage any vehicle emergency.

Traditionally, HH therapists are provided with a treatment bag to carry the necessary equipment. Items tend to be limited to allow for portability. Most therapists carry personal protection equipment, vital sign equipment, basic wound care supplies, a balance pad, and resistive bands. Creativity to utilize items in the patient's home to assist with exercise and function benefits the therapist and ensures the patient has the items on hand to comply with a home program. Canned goods and plastic milk jugs can substitute as weights for resistance training.

Homes vary greatly based on socioeconomic factors. The size, structural barriers, cleanliness, family dynamics, and pets can all impact care delivery. A benefit of this setting is that clinicians can identify, rectify, or mitigate risk factors in the patient's natural environment. For example, a set of stairs to the upstairs bathroom may necessitate a bedside commode until the patient is more mobile and can safely negotiate the stairs.

Pets can be a wonderful source of emotional comfort for patients but can challenge the HH therapist. Some pets become aggressive when a stranger enters the home or lays hands on their owner. It is always best practice to ask for all pets to be secured in a separate room during your visit. If a patient is a sole caregiver for the pet, it is wise to include items such as feeding and caring for the pet as part of your plan of care to ensure the patient's mobility allows them to do it safely.

Infection control is a critical element of healthcare yet can be challenging in the home. State-mandated protocols must be followed to limit risk factors for patients. In severe cases of hoarding or unsanitary conditions, a referral to a social worker to assist with community resources or a report to Adult Protective Services may be indicated. This decision is usually made collaboratively with the rest of the interdisciplinary team.

Providers and Care Coordination

Federal and state guidelines dictate the structure and coordination of the care team in the HH setting. For patients to receive care reimbursable by Medicare, a physician must certify the need for services in the home and establish a plan of care. The primary care physician commonly certifies the need for services. The physician must certify that the patient (1) is homebound, (2) needs intermittent SNF or PT, OT, or SLP, and (3) is under the physician's ongoing care. The physician must also periodically review the home care plan, no less than every 2 months. Most physicians are not familiar with the nuances of CMS regulations and rely on an HHA for guidance on items such as homebound status. Many private insurance companies default to Medicare guidelines and therefore EMR systems tend to be set up to satisfy these requirements. Individual companies may add additional duties and responsibilities for state compliance, quality, or clinical programs (*Medicare Benefit Policy Manual* Chapter 7 - Home Health Services, 2022).

Most HH cases involve skilled nursing. Other services in order of referral volume are PT, OT, HH aide, SLP, and social worker. According to Medicare, skilled nursing, PT, and SLP are qualified stand-alone services, meaning an HH referral for any of these disciplines allows that discipline to open the case and be the sole discipline to follow for the treatment plan. In contrast, OTs were first granted the right to open a HH case in 2021 under a temporary COVID-19 Emergency Health Measure (*COVID-19 Emergency Declaration Blanket Waivers for Health Care Providers*, 2021). Congress passed the HH Flexibility Act that allowed OT to open a Medicare patient case permanently during the same time frame (Doggett, 2019). CMS updated the Conditions of Participation regulations in January 2022 to reflect the new law. However, for the case to be reimbursable, there must also be the need for another qualifying therapy service (i.e., PT or SLP) to establish a plan of care after the initial assessment (Doggett, 2019). Allowing OT to open the case can aid an agency when a PT or SLP is not immediately available, such as staffing shortages, and ensure timely initiation of care until the other qualifying discipline can start. Social workers can only treat the patient after one of the qualifying disciplines has opened the case. HH aides require the plan of care to be developed and regularly supervised by nursing, PT, or OT (*42 CFR Part 484 — Home Health Services*, 2022).

Responsibilities of a Manager/Administrator

In addition to the clinical team, CMS defines the operational roles required in each HH agency. CMS defines the roles and staff required to license an HHA in their Conditions of Participation for HH. The Conditions of Participation require that the following administrative roles are in place for all agencies:

1. Governing Body: The governing body is responsible for managing the agency and oversight of the care provided, including the financial, clinical, and quality management of the agency.
2. Administrator: The administrator is the person who oversees all day-to-day operations of an HHA and reports to the Governing Body. The administrator is not required to be a clinician, but a clinician is placed in this position in most cases.
3. Clinical Manager: The clinical manager is a clinician responsible for overseeing staffing and clinical care. The Clinical Manager is responsible for ensuring that patients receive an appropriate comprehensive plan of care. Depending on the number of patients the agency serves, there is often more than one clinical manager in an HHA (*42 CFR Part 484 — Home Health Services*, 2022).

As mentioned previously, CMS requires HHA to provide nursing services and at least one other therapeutic service (e.g., PT, OT, SLP, medical social services, or HH aide) in residence used as the patient's home. At least one of the services must be provided directly by an employee of an HHA and the other services can be provided under contractual arrangements if needed.

Most agencies hold weekly interdisciplinary team meetings to discuss patients and coordinate care. These can be held virtually or in person. Extra effort must be made in the HH setting to communicate due to the autonomous nature of the environment. Fortunately, technology continues to provide multiple avenues for this to occur. Most companies have preferences for email, text, or phone calls based on the type of information communicated, and all communication must be mindful of Health Insurance Portability and Accountability Act (HIPAA) regulations for patient privacy of information. Daily communication with fellow clinicians and patient care managers is essential for good care. If a therapist supervises an assistant, they must follow all discipline-specific state practice act requirements for supervision, including documentation of all communication.

Referral Sources and Marketing

The source of HH referrals falls into two categories: community and institutional. Community referral sources are physicians, nurse practitioners, and physician assistants. Assisted living, independent living, and group homes can also initiate referrals to HH when resident needs are identified by contacting that resident's physician. School systems can do the same for their pediatric students. Institutional referrals are from hospitals, IRFs, SNFs, and LTACHs. Hospital-based HHAs have a definite advantage with institutional referrals as many patients prefer to follow the continuum of care within the same provider network. Depending on the agency, the HH company may have a dedicated sales force focused on marketing to these referral sources or those duties may be included in the operational manager's job responsibilities.

Staffing Challenges

Patients are centrally located in most settings, such as hospitals, senior care facilities, or outpatient clinics. However, in the HH setting, patients can be spread over a wide geographical territory, creating unique staffing and productivity challenges for the agency. Considerations need to be made for the types of disciplines and services ordered or needed by the patient. Care must be taken not to overwhelm a patient with multiple services on the same day, especially if the type of visit required is of a longer duration. The agency can better monitor the patient's ongoing health status by spreading the services throughout the week.

An OASIS (Outcome and Assessment Information Set) Start of Care (SOC) visit requires 1.5 hours of in-home time with an additional 1 hour of documentation outside the home. If both nursing and PT are ordered, CMS dictates that an RN perform the OASIS SOC visit (*42 CFR 484.55 — Condition of Participation: Comprehensive Assessment of Patients.*, 2022, p. 55). Many private insurances are now requiring OASIS as well. When OASIS is not required, the required documentation is significantly less and more consistent with documentation found in the outpatient setting. Non-OASIS SOC visits are less intensive, with approximately 1 hour of in-home and documentation time. Additional discipline add-on evaluations average 1 hour. Follow-up treatment visits for nursing can vary widely depending on the care needed, such as a wound dressing change versus medication education. Nursing visits can range from 20 minutes to 1 hour, whereas therapy visits average 45 minutes.

Each HHA determines the coverage area for each clinician based on referral volume for a given geographic area, drive distances, drive times, and average visit time. The agency sets a weekly productivity expectation based on those criteria. Most agencies have a mapping tool to allow each clinician to map out the most efficient route to each patient, limiting travel overlap to aid in meeting productivity. However, coordinating with patients' preferences and other appointments (e.g., physician appointments, other HH disciplines, or haircare) can make executing the most efficient route challenging. Another staffing consideration is weekend and evening coverage. Each agency requires CMS Conditions of Participation to have a nurse on call 24 hours a day in an urgent need. The on-call nurse will often assist in triaging, including determining if an issue can be addressed over the phone or requires a next-day nursing visit. In some cases, the nurse may decide that emergent care is needed. In addition, many agencies have PTs perform a weekend call rotation to admit high-priority orthopedic patients (Medicare and Medicaid, 2017).

Reimbursement, Documentation, and Quality Improvement

HH is a covered service under the Medicare Part A benefit. It is defined as intermittent, medically necessary skilled care (e.g., nursing, PT, OT, and SLP) ordered by a physician (*Medicare Benefit Policy Manual* Chapter 7 - Home Health Services, 2022). Outpatient clinics have also been known to go into a patient's home and provide care. However, this care is limited to PT, OT, and SLP services. Nursing and social worker care are not provided; thus this service is generally inappropriate for patients with more medically-based needs. The reimbursement for this type of home care is provided under the Medicare part B benefit, which has a greater out-of-pocket cost to the patient. It also comes with different rules and regulations for the service provider.

Historically, Medicare paid for HH services under the Part A benefit fee-for-service. In other words, each visit was reimbursed individually. Then, in 1999, Congress passed legislation to improve the quality of care and limit the potential for fraud and abuse. One result of this legislation was the development of the OASIS (Medicare and Medicaid Programs, 2018). The OASIS is a data collection tool that gathers information on HH patients' clinical presentation, functional levels, psychological state, living situation, and demographic data. These data points measure healthcare quality (by tracking outcomes), guide performance improvement, and determine reimbursement. The OASIS is completed at admission, recertification, discharge, and when the patient is transferred to a different healthcare setting, like a hospital.

CMS is continually revising and improving the data tool; refer to the CMS website for the latest version (*OASIS Data Sets | CMS*, 2022). The OASIS-D1 became effective in January 2022, and due to the COVID-19 Public Health Emergency, CMS delayed the release of OASIS-E until January 2023. Agencies must plan to review and train their staff on the changes and new requirements implemented with each revised version. An OASIS is required for each 60-day certification period. As of 2020, CMS has begun to reimburse for services using the Patient-Driven Grouping Model (PDGM) every 30 days of the certification. Each period is placed into a different subgroup based on the admission source (two subgroups), timing of the admission (two subgroups), clinical grouping (12 subgroups), functional impairment level (three subgroups), and a comorbidity adjustment (three subgroups). Each period can be categorized into one of the 432 case-mix groups for payment. Periods with low visit utilization are not case-mix adjusted; they are paid on a per-visit basis using national rates. Each of the 432 PDGM payment groups has a threshold for low visits, referred to as a Low-Utilization Payment Adjustment (LUPA). Most HH providers utilize an outcome measurement tool to guide their clinicians on the best approach to patient care under the PDGM model (*Home Health Patient-Driven Groupings Model | CMS*, 2021).

Chapter 7 of the MBPM outlines documentation requirements to justify services delivered (*Medicare Benefit Policy Manual* Chapter 7 - Home Health Services, 2022). Documentation includes the traditional elements set forth by the professional therapy organizations and quality expectation minimums by CMS and its intermediaries. For instance, each visit must demonstrate the specific skills performed by the therapist and the medical necessity for the visit itself. In other words, the care provided could not be performed by a layperson.

In addition, CMS requires several additional documentation elements for its HH providers. The largest requirement is process measures. CMS wants HHAs to review these potential risk areas for the patient. If the patient is at risk, the patient's plan of care should include elements to mitigate the risk (*42 CFR Part 484 — Home Health Services*, 2022). Process measures cover areas strongly correlated with hospitalization, such as diabetic foot care. If a patient has diabetes, it is a CMS requirement that diabetic foot care and education be added to the patient plan of care. A second area is medication reconciliation. Each visit, the clinician must review all medications and compare them with the medication list to ensure accuracy, including checking for new, changed, or discontinued medications. The plan of care must also include a review of each medication to ensure the patient and caregivers understand the medication's purpose, administration, and potential side effects. Other areas covered by the process measures are pressure ulcer risk and treatment, fall risk, depression, pain, oxygen safety for those requiring supplemental oxygen, and home safety.

CMS also requires each visit to demonstrate an element of patient/caregiver education. The clinician should document the education provided, the patient/caregivers' ability to demonstrate their understanding of that education, and if ongoing instruction is indicated. Each case must also have documentation providing evidence that the patient was provided with information regarding the coverage of services. Coverage of services begins with the initial *Consent to Treat*, followed by a *Notice of Non-Coverage* when services are discontinued. Lastly, there should be evidence that the patient was provided an accurate and up-to-date medication list and discharge instructions when services were terminated (*42 CFR Part 484 – Home Health Services*, 2022).

Each Medicare-certified HHA must participate in the HH Quality Reporting Program (HHQRP). Data are gathered from the OASIS and quality measures are reported on outcomes and process measures. In addition, agencies are required to report the results of a 34-item patient survey, the Consumer Assessment of Healthcare Providers and Systems (CAHPS), and the HH Care Survey (HHCAHPS). The patient surveys address four areas of care: (1) care of patients, (2) communication between providers and patients, (3) specific care issues, (4) overall rating of care provided by an HHA (willingness to recommend an HHA to friends and family). CMS publicly reports these data on Care Compare (*Find Healthcare Providers: Compare Care Near You | Medicare*, 2022). CMS uses star ratings to summarize a provider's performance. These ratings are updated quarterly and are an easy-to-use tool for the public to choose an HH care provider.

Beginning January 1, 2016, CMS piloted a model program called HH Value-Based Purchasing (HHVBP) in nine states. The model incentivizes care efficiency while maintaining high quality by tying payment to quality performance during a given year. This initial model was determined to be effective, and a nationwide rollout was announced in the CY 2022 HH PPS proposed rule. 2023 will be the first performance year in which quality performance data will be collected and used to calculate payment adjustments (Medicare and Medicaid, 2018).

Long-Term Acute Care Hospitals

LTACHs, also known as transitional care hospitals, are similar to STACHs in that they are licensed by the state as acute care hospitals, with accreditation and certification by the Joint Commission and Medicare. They are reimbursed via the same PPS system as STACHs, diagnosis-related groups, or DRGs (*Elements of LTCHPPS | CMS*, 2021). The LTC-DRG reimbursement system calculates hospitalization costs by the patient's principal diagnosis (e.g., ICD 10 code) with adjustments based on secondary diagnoses, age, sex, and discharge status (*Long-Term Care Hospitals Payment Systems*, 2021). Qualifying for an LTACH requires a qualified hospital stay and documentation that the patient requires medically complex care after a short-term acute care hospital stay. For example, patients referred to an LTACH commonly include those with heart failure, chronic lung disease, ventilator dependence, multi-organ system failure, infection, or stroke. Most individuals have multiple comorbidities (approximately 15) and require a length of stay of approximately 25 days.

Compared with an SNF, which requires less frequent physician-patient contact (e.g., weekly), patients in LTACHs require daily physician involvement due to the complexity of their cases. Patients in LTACHs will receive rehabilitation services from PT, OT, or speech therapy based on the patient's medical status and ability to tolerate rehabilitation services. LTACH treatment session length differs from an SNF, where patients typically receive combined therapy for 60–90 minutes per day, and an IRF, where patients receive daily, intensive combined rehabilitation for 3 hours per day or a minimum of 15 hours per week. Although rehabilitation is an important component of the LTACH setting, patient complexity dictates the amount of therapy; thus therapists must adjust the frequency and duration of sessions. To augment rehabilitation, LTACHs also offer restorative care (i.e., unskilled rehabilitation), which an aide or certified nursing assistant (CAN) often provides. Restorative care can occur in isolation or with ongoing PT, OT, and speech rehabilitation (*Minimum Data Set (MDS) 3.0 for Nursing Homes and Swing Bed Providers*, 2022). As with STACHs, PTs and OTs are essential to successful discharge planning, along with physicians, nurses, dieticians, pharmacists, respiratory therapists, and case managers (see Chapter 21).

Conclusion

Each post-acute care setting has unique features, primarily balancing the need for medical care and rehabilitation. Patients who are more complex and require physician involvement daily would be most appropriate for an LTACH. Patients with medical needs that can be addressed by nursing and are medically stable enough to withstand up to 60 minutes of therapy per day would be most appropriate for an SNF. Individuals requiring intensive rehab and who can participate in three hours of therapy services per day would benefit from an IRF. Lastly, patients who can return home but continue to need ongoing medical and rehabilitation services may benefit most from HH. Therapists utilize their examination and evaluation expertise as part of a multidisciplinary team to determine the most appropriate setting for the patient, balancing the wishes of the patient and their medical and rehabilitation needs for a safe return home and to prevent rehospitalizations.

Chapter Activities and Discussion

1. Give an example of a patient that would be appropriate for LTACH, inpatient rehabilitation, skilled nursing facility, and HH services. What qualifying factors may exist that would determine eligibility in each setting?
2. What is the IMPACT act and why is it important?
3. Review each case and determine the appropriate discharge disposition.

CASE 1

The patient is a 76-year-old admitted with pneumonia. Before STACH admission, the patient lived alone in a one-story house with no steps to enter. The patient was independent with ADLs, including ambulation without a gait device in the home and short distances in the community. The patient required assistance for IADLs from their son and daughter. The patient will require ongoing medical and rehabilitation needs at discharge. Considering this and the information below, what is your discharge recommendation?
Eating/feeding: independent
Oral Hygiene: independent
Toilet Hygiene: supervision or touching assistance
Washing/bathing: partial/moderate assistance
Upper body dressing: supervision or touching assistance
Lower body dressing: partial/moderate assistance
Putting on/taking off footwear: supervision or touching assistance
Bed mobility: supervision or touching assistance
Transfers: partial/moderate assistance
Ambulation/gait: partial/moderate assistance for 50 feet with a front-wheeled walker
Steps: not applicable
Sitting balance: Independent
Standing balance: supervision or touching assistance with a front-wheeled walker
Activity tolerance/aerobic endurance: fair
IADLs: dependent

CASE 2

The patient is a 56-year-old admitted with metabolic acidosis, resulting in multi-organ failure and intubation for mechanical ventilation. Before STACH admission, the patient was independent with ADLs, IADLs, and worked full-time as an office manager. The patient lived alone in a one-story house with no steps to enter. The patient has multiple comorbidities, including diabetes, obesity, hypertension, hyperlipidemia, heart failure, sleep apnea, and asthma. The patient will need physician and nursing care daily to manage these comorbidities and hospital-acquired pressure ulcers that have become infected. Considering this and the information below, what is your discharge recommendation?
Eating/feeding: substantial/maximal assistance
Oral Hygiene: dependent
Toilet Hygiene: dependent

Washing/bathing: dependent
Upper body dressing: substantial/maximal assistance
Lower body dressing: dependent
Putting on/taking off footwear: dependent
Bed mobility: substantial/maximal assistance
Transfers: Substantial/maximal assistance
Ambulation/gait: dependent
Steps: not applicable
Sitting balance: substantial/maximal assistance
Standing balance: dependent
Activity tolerance/aerobic endurance: poor
IADLs: dependent

CASE 3

The patient is a 56-year-old admitted for right total knee arthroplasty. Before STACH admission, the patient was independent with ADLs, IADLs, and worked part-time selling antiques. The patient's spouse works full-time but will assist the patient before and after work with IADLs. They have a one-story house with one platform step to enter and no railing. The patient will need education for dressing changes and rehabilitation to return to their previous level of function. Considering this and the information below, what is your discharge recommendation?
Eating/feeding: independent
Oral Hygiene: independent
Toilet Hygiene: independent
Washing/bathing: independent with a sponge bath
Upper body dressing: independent
Lower body dressing: partial/moderate assistance
Putting on/taking off footwear: substantial/maximal assistance
Bed mobility: independent
Transfers: independent
Ambulation/gait: independent for 50 feet with a front-wheeled walker
Steps: partial/moderate assistance with a front-wheeled walker
Sitting balance: independent
Standing balance: supervision or touching assistance with a front-wheeled walker
Activity tolerance/aerobic endurance: good
IADLs: The patient can independently manage telephone communication but is dependent on transportation, shopping, finances, home maintenance, and managing medications

CASE 4

The patient is a 59-year-old admitted to the hospital after a right hemisphere stroke with left-sided hemiplegia. Before STACH admission, the patient was independent with ADLs, IADLs, and worked full-time as a bank manager. The patient lives with their spouse, who works full-time. Therefore 24-hour assistance is not possible. They have a two-story house with four steps to enter and bilateral railing. The patient will require intense rehabilitation to return to their previous level of function at discharge. Considering this and the following information, what is your discharge recommendation?
Eating/feeding: partial/moderate assistance
Oral Hygiene: partial/moderate assistance
Toilet Hygiene: partial/moderate assistance
Washing/bathing: partial/moderate assistance
Upper body dressing: partial/moderate assistance

Lower body dressing: partial/moderate assistance
Putting on/taking off footwear: dependent
Bed mobility: partial/moderate assistance
Transfers: partial/moderate assistance
Ambulation/gait: partial/moderate assistance for 150 feet with hemi-walker
Steps: dependent
Sitting balance: Independent
Standing balance: partial/moderate assistance with hemi-walker
Activity tolerance/aerobic endurance: good
IADLs: partial/moderate assistance

References

42 CFR 484.55—Condition of participation: Comprehensive assessment of patients. (2022). Code of Federal Regulations | National Archives. https://www.ecfr.gov/current/title-42/chapter-IV/subchapter-G/part-484/subpart-B/section-484.55.

42 CFR Part 484—Home Health Services. (2022). Code of Federal Regulations | National Archives. https://www.ecfr.gov/current/title-42/chapter-IV/subchapter-G/part-484.

Andrus, B., & Gawenda, R. (2016). *How to use the new PT and OT evaluation codes.* WebPT. https://www.webpt.com/blog/farewell-97001-how-to-use-the-new-pt-and-ot-evaluation-codes/.

Barrilleaux, J. (2021). *Inpatient rehabilitation facility coding. Journal of AHIMA.* https://journal.ahima.org/inpatient-rehabilitation-facility-coding/.

Bennett, L. E., Jewell, V. D., Scheirton, L., McCarthy, M., & Muir, B. C. (2019). Productivity standards and the impact on quality of care: A National Survey of Inpatient Rehabilitation Professionals. *The Open Journal of Occupational Therapy, 7*(4), 1–11. https://doi.org/10.15453/2168-6408.1598.

Cabigao, E., & Cherney, C. (2014). The skilled nursing facility. In D. Yee-Melichar, M. Flores, & E. Cabigao (Eds.), *Administration and Management: Effective practices and quality programs in eldercare* (1st ed., pp. 105–122). Springer Publishing Company.

Certificate of need (CON). (2019). Georgia Department of Community Health. https://dch.georgia.gov/divisionsoffices/office-health-planning/certificate-need-con.

Chapter 7: Skilled nursing facility services (March 2022 Report) – MedPAC. (2022, March 15). Medpac. https://www.medpac.gov/document/chapter-7-skilled-nursing-facility-services-march-2022-report/.

CMS Announces Payment changes for Medicare home health services improving beneficiary access and quality and efficiency of care | CMS. (2007). CMS.Gov. https://www.cms.gov/newsroom/press-releases/cms-announces-payment-changes-medicare-home-health-services-improving-beneficiary-access-and-quality.

CMS. (2015) *Fact Sheet: Two-midnight rule.* https://www.cms.gov/newsroom/fact-sheets/fact-sheet-two-midnight-rule-0.

CMS. (2021) *Patient driven payment model |.* CMS. https://www.cms.gov/Medicare/Medicare-Fee-for-Service-Payment/SNFPPS/PDPM.

COVID-19 emergency declaration blanket waivers for health care providers. (2021). CMS. https://www.cms.gov/files/document/summary-covid-19-emergency-declaration-waivers.pdf.

Davitt, J., & Choi, S. (2008). Tracing the history of Medicare home health care: The impact of policy on benefit use. *The Journal of Sociology & Social Welfare, 35*(1). https://scholarworks.wmich.edu/jssw/vol35/iss1/12.

Doggett, L. (2019, June 6). *H.R.3127 - 116th Congress (2019-2020): Medicare home health flexibility act* (2019/2020) [Legislation]. http://www.congress.gov/.

Elements of LTCHPPS | CMS. (2021). https://www.cms.gov/Medicare/Medicare-Fee-for-Service-Payment/LongTermCareHospitalPPS/elements_ltch.

Falvey, J. R., Mangione, K. K., & Stevens-Lapsley, J. E. (2015). Rethinking hospital-associated deconditioning: proposed paradigm shift. *Physical Therapy, 95*(9), 1307–1315.

Find Healthcare Providers: Compare Care Near You | Medicare. (2022). Medicare.Gov. https://www.medicare.gov/care-compare/.

Foster, C. C., Agrawal, R. K., & Davis, M. M. (2019). Home health care for children with medical complexity: Workforce gaps, policy, and future directions. *Health Affairs, 38*(6), 987–993.

History of the specialty. (2022). American Academy of Physical Medicine and Rehabilitation. https://www.aapmr.org/about-physiatry/history-of-the-specialty.

Home health agency (HHA) center | CMS. (2021). CMS. https://www.cms.gov/Center/Provider-Type/Home-Health-Agency-HHA-Center.

Home health patient-driven groupings model | CMS. (2021). CMS. https://www.cms.gov/Medicare/Medicare-Fee-for-Service-Payment/HomeHealthPPS/HH-PDGM.

Hospice Center. (2021). CMS.Gov. https://www.cms.gov/Center/Provider-Type/Hospice-Center.

IMPACT Act of 2014 Data standardization & cross setting measures | CMS. (2021). CMS.Gov. https://www.cms.gov/Medicare/Quality-Initiatives-Patient-Assessment-Instruments/Post-Acute-Care-Quality-Initiatives/IMPACT-Act-of-2014/IMPACT-Act-of-2014-Data-Standardization-and-Cross-Setting-Measures.

Ko, M., Wagner, L., & Spetz, J. (2018). Nursing home implementation of health information technology: Review of the literature finds inadequate investment in preparation, infrastructure, and training. *Inquiry: A Journal of Medical Care Organization, Provision and Financing, 55*, 46958018778902.

Krumholz, H. M. (2013). Post-hospital syndrome – A condition of generalized risk. *The New England Journal of Medicine, 368*(2), 100–102.

Kub, J., Kulbok, P., & Glick, D. (2015). Cornerstone documents, milestones, and policies: Shaping the direction of public health nursing 1890-1950. *The Online Journal of Issues in Nursing, 20*(2), 3.

Long-term care hospitals payment systems. (2021). MedPAC. https://www.medpac.gov/wp-content/uploads/2021/11/medpac_payment_basics_21_ltch_final_sec.pdf.

Medicare and Medicaid program: Conditions of participation for home health agencies. (2017). Federal Register. https://www.federalregister.gov/documents/2017/01/13/2017-00283/medicare-and-medicaid-program-conditions-of-participation-for-home-health-agencies.

Medicare and Medicaid programs; CY 2019 Home health prospective payment system rate update and CY 2020 case-mix adjustment methodology refinements; home health value-based purchasing model; home health quality reporting requirements; home infusion therapy requirements; and training requirements for surveyors of national accrediting organizations. (2018). Federal Register. https://www.federalregister.gov/documents/2018/11/13/2018-24145/medicare-and-medicaid-programs-cy-2019-home-health-prospective-payment-system-rate-update-and-cy.

Medicare benefit policy manual chapter 1—Inpatient hospital services covered under part A. (2021). CMS. https://www.cms.gov/Regulations-and-Guidance/Guidance/Manuals/downloads/bp102c01.pdf.

Medicare benefit policy manual chapter 7—Home health services. (2022). CMS. https://www.cms.gov/Regulations-and-Guidance/Guidance/Manuals/Downloads/bp102c07.pdf.

Medicare benefit policy manual: Chapter 8 – Coverage of extended care (SNF) services under hospital insurance. (2019). CMS. https://www.cms.gov/Regulations-and-Guidance/Guidance/Manuals/Downloads/bp102c08pdf.pdf.

Medicare benefit policy manual chapter 15—covered medical and other health services. (2021). CMS. https://www.cms.gov/Regulations-and-Guidance/Guidance/Manuals/Downloads/bp102c15.pdf.

Minimum data set (MDS) 3.0 for nursing homes and swing bed providers. (2022). CMS. https://www.cms.gov/Medicare/Quality-Initiatives-Patient-Assessment-Instruments/NursingHomeQualityInits/NHQIMDS30.

Myers, D. R., Rogers, R., LeCrone, H. H., Kelley, K., & Scott, J. H. (2018). Work life stress and career resilience of licensed nursing facility administrators. *Journal of Applied Gerontology: The Official Journal of the Southern Gerontological Society, 37*(4), 435–463. https://doi.org/10.1177/0733464816665207.

OASIS Data Sets | CMS. (2022). CMS. https://www.cms.gov/Medicare/Quality-Initiatives-Patient-Assessment-Instruments/HomeHealthQualityInits/OASIS-Data-Sets.

Prusynski, R. (2021). Medicare payment policy in skilled nursing facilities: Lessons from a history of mixed success. *Journal of the American Geriatrics Society, 69*(12), 3358–3364.

Sandel, E. (2017, March 13). *The early history of physical medicine and rehabilitation in the United States.* PM&R KnowledgeNow. https://now.aapmr.org/the-history-of-the-specialty-of-physical-medicine-and-rehabilitation/.

Skilled nursing facility (SNF) prospective payment system (PPS) legislative history. (2021). CMS. https://www.cms.gov/Medicare/Medicare-Fee-for-Service-Payment/SNFPPS/Downloads/Legislative_History_2018-10-01.pdf.

Skilled services requirements, 42 CFR § 409.44. (2016). CMS. https://www.govinfo.gov/content/pkg/CFR-2010-title42-vol2/pdf/CFR-2010-title42-vol2-sec409-44.pdf.

Smith, B. A., Fields, C. J., & Fernandez, N. (2010). Physical therapists make accurate and appropriate discharge recommendations for patients who are acutely ill. *Physical Therapy, 90*(5), 693–703.

Specifications for determining IRF "60% rule" compliance. (2017). CMS. https://www.cms.gov/files/document/specifications-determining-irf-60-rule-compliance.pdf.

Survey protocol for long term care facilities – part 1. State operations manual. (2005). CMS. https://www.cms.gov/medicare/provider-enrollment-and-certification/guidanceforlawsandregulations/downloads/som107ap_p_ltcfpdf.

Therapy services. (2021). CMS. https://www.cms.gov/Medicare/Billing/TherapyServices.

What is accreditation | The joint commission. (2022). The Joint Commission. https://www.jointcommission.org/accreditation-and-certification/become-accredited/what-is-accreditation/?utm_content=dmc-135#b6621ea07c4d48d68c1a8bdde62ff5e4_31ad6e2af27640458cf473ab797281a8.

What is long-term care? (2017). National Institute on Aging. https://www.nia.nih.gov/health/what-long-term-care.

What we do. (2022). National Quality Forum [NQF]. https://www.qualityforum.org/what_we_do.aspx.

What's a MAC | CMS. (2022). CMS.Gov. https://www.cms.gov/Medicare/Medicare-Contracting/Medicare-Administrative-Contractors/What-is-a-MAC.

18

School and Special Education

BLAIR CARSONE, PhD, MOT, OTR/L; KAREN DISHMAN, OTD, OTR, ATP;
and JESSICA BENDER, PT, EdD, PCS

LEARNING OBJECTIVES

By the end of this chapter, the reader will be able to:

1. Understand the history of occupational and physical therapy in the school setting.
2. Understand the difference between an Individualized Education Plan (IEP) and a 504 plan.
3. Describe the process of referral to special education and related services.
4. Understand the difference in goal writing between school-based therapy and medical models.
5. Understand the difference between a push-in and a pull-out therapy model in the school setting.
6. Understand the requirements of documentation of therapy services in the school setting.

CHAPTER OUTLINE

History and Background

Physical and occupational therapists have a long history of working with children with disabilities in schools, beginning in the late 1800s (Moffat, 2003). Since then, special education services for children with disabilities have evolved from focusing on physical disabilities to serving children with a wide range of intellectual, physical, and mental disabilities (Effgen & Kaminker, 2014). The advent of special education in the United States granted therapy services to students with disabilities. Special education legislation began in the 1950s when the Supreme Court case of Brown v. Topeka Board of Education ruled that separate education for students with disabilities was not equal (United States Courts, 2021). This landmark trial started a cascade of new laws and regulations that improved access to quality special education services (Fig. 18.1).

As schools began to include a broader range of children with disabilities and impairments served through special education, the role of physical and occupational therapists as related service providers also began to increase (Thomason & Wilmarth, 2015). After the 1950s, laws, and regulations were developed that required public schools to provide therapy services and free appropriate public education

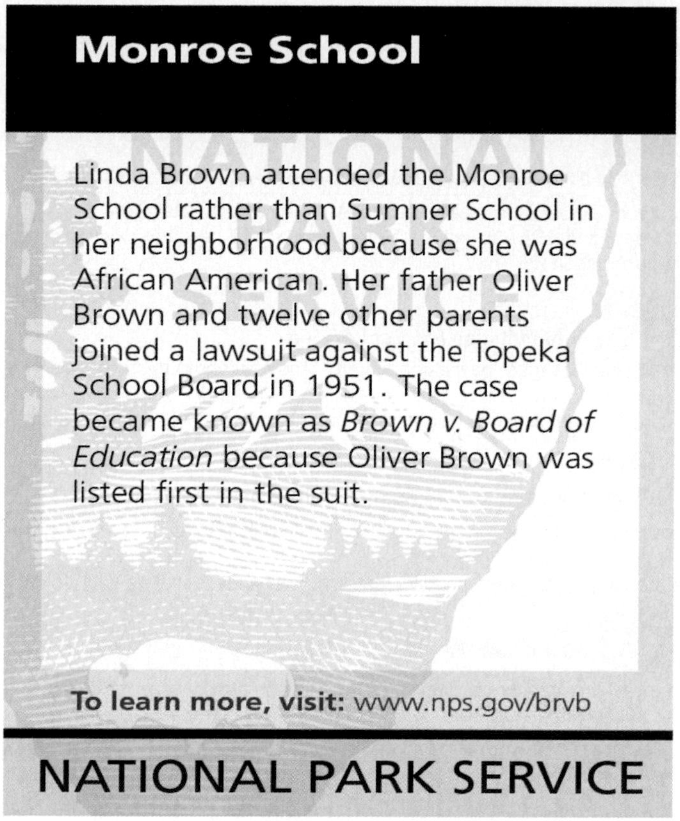

Monroe School

Linda Brown attended the Monroe School rather than Sumner School in her neighborhood because she was African American. Her father Oliver Brown and twelve other parents joined a lawsuit against the Topeka School Board in 1951. The case became known as *Brown v. Board of Education* because Oliver Brown was listed first in the suit.

To learn more, visit: www.nps.gov/brvb

NATIONAL PARK SERVICE

• **Fig. 18.1** Brown v. Board of Education

(FAPE) in the least restrictive environment (LRE) for students with disabilities (Salend & Garrick Duhaney, 2011) such as most notably, the Rehabilitation Act, Education for All Handicapped Children Act, Individuals with Disabilities Education Act (IDEA), and Individuals with Disabilities Education Improvement Act (IDEIA). The introduction of these regulations vastly improved conditions for students with disabilities (Figs. 18.2 and 18.3). Through this innovative legislation, children can now access individualized education and therapeutic services that enhance their participation in school-related activities.

Education for All Handicapped Children Act, Public Law 94-142

In 1973, legislation on nondiscrimination and equal rights for individuals with disabilities was addressed through the Rehabilitation Act (US Department of Education, 1995). Section 504 of the Rehabilitation Act is enforced under the Office of Civil Rights. It states that all individuals with disabilities in the United States must be included in all areas of programming funded by the federal government and must not be excluded or denied benefits (US Department of Education, 1995). This legislation included public schools, higher education, and other public agencies (US Department of Education, 1995).

This rapid expansion led to the passing of legislation called the Education of All Handicapped Children Act, also known as ECA (1975). This federal legislation mandated that all children aged 6–21 years were eligible to receive a FAPE and included related services, such as physical and occupational therapy and speech and language assistance (Public Law [PL] 94-142, 1975). This legislation introduced seven essential concepts that are still relevant today including, zero reject, least restrictive environment, right to due process, nondiscriminatory evaluation, individualized education program, parent participation, and related services.

Zero reject: Zero reject is the policy that no child with a disability can be excluded from any part of their education (Salend & Garrick Duhaney, 2011).

Least restrictive environment (LRE): In the LRE, children with disabilities must be educated amongst their typically developing peers as much as possible (PL 108-446).

Right to due process: Procedural due process of the law guarantees that children with disabilities and their families can participate in all identification, evaluation decisions, and educational placement efforts. The right to due process also guarantees an impartial hearing, access to educational records, and the right to have counsel (PL 99-372).

Nondiscriminatory evaluation: This ensures that testing is standardized, not biased, and is based on reliable norms (PL 94-142).

Individualized education program (IEP): Every child receiving special education must have an individualized education program that outlines the student's present

1954
Supreme Court Case of *Brown v. Topeka Board of Education*
- Separate education for students with disabilities was not equal
- New laws and regulations that improved access to special education services

1965
Elementary and Secondary Education Act (ESEA) of 1965
- Delegated resources to increase impoverished students' access to education
- In 1966, congress amended ESEA to include a provision to fund new and existing programs for students with disabilities in public schools

1973
Rehabilitation Act-Section 504
- All individuals with disabilities must be included in all areas of programming funded by the federal government
- This legislation included public schools, higher education, and other public agencies

1975
Education for all Handicapped Children Act (EHA)
- Public school districts were required to provide all children with disabilities access to free and appropriate public education (FAPE)
- Did not require states to provide appropriate educational services to children with disabilities under six

1986
Public Law 99–457
- States must guarantee services for children with disabilites between ages three and five
- Public law 99–457 became the individuals with disabilities education act (IDEA)

• **Fig. 18.2** Timeline of Special Education (1950s to 1980s)

1990
Individuals with Disabilities Education Act (IDEA)
- Special education services were expanded to include students 18–21 years; students with autism and traumatic brain injury diagnoses
- Added the provision of transition services, assistive technology, and related rehabilitation counseling and social work

1997
Individuals with Disabilities Education Act (IDEA)
- Part H becomes part C: Required states to provide services for children from birth to three years and FAPE to children with disabilities from three to five years
- Changed the age of transition planning from 16 to 14 years old and transformed the way schools received funding for special education

2001
No Child Left Behind (NCLB)
- Children should have a fair, equal, and significant opportunity to obtain a high-quality education

2004
Individuals with Disabilities Education Improvment Act (IDEIA)
- 7 principles: Child find and zero reject, nondiscriminatory assessment, IEP, LRE, due process, parental participation, and transition
- Identification of specific learning disabilities without significant discrepency between IQ and achievement

2015
Every Student Succeeds Act (ESSA)
- Replaced the no child left behind act
- Under ESSA, some students with disabilities are exempt from taking standardized tests with their peers 2018

2018
Omnibus Spending Bill
- Addtional state funding for IDEA

• **Fig. 18.3** Timeline of Special Education (1990s to 2000s)

level of performance, services, and supports necessary for educational success (PL 94-142).

Parent participation: Parents are encouraged to participate in the special education process, must consent to any evaluations, and have the right to access their child's school records (PL 94-142).

Related services: Services such as physical therapy, occupational therapy, speech-language pathology, psychological services, recreation, transportation, and medical and counseling services are to be provided if these services will facilitate the student benefitting from special education (PL 94-372).

Individuals with Disabilities Education Act

In 1990 and 1997, the ECA underwent revisions and reauthorizations to become the Individuals with Disabilities Education Act or IDEA (IDEA, 2021). In IDEA (1990), special education services were expanded to include students aged 18-21 with autism and traumatic brain injury diagnoses. IDEA (1990) also added the provision of transition services, assistive technology, and related rehabilitation counseling and social work (Selend & Garrick Dulaney, 2011).

Reauthorization of IDEA in 1997, Part C, required states to provide services for children from birth to 3 years and FAPE to children with disabilities from 3 to 5 years (Doubet & Quesenberry, 2011). IDEA (1997) also changed the transition planning age from 16 to 14 years, including students with emotional or behavioral disabilities, and transformed how schools received special education funding (Salend & Garrick Dulaney, 2011). As a result, transition planning is an integral part of special education. The multidisciplinary team comes together with the student and family to create an outline of the student's long-term goals and the support necessary to succeed after high school. The focus is on employment, community engagement, self-efficacy, and quality of life.

In 2004, the IDEA was amended and passed into federal law with an increased focus on accountability and outcomes (Effgen, 2013). It is now known as the Individuals with Disabilities Education Improvement Act (IDEIA); however, it is still referred to as IDEA. The IDEA (2004) supports the public education of all children, irrespective of disability. IDEA, Part B mandates a free and appropriate public education for children between the ages of 3 and 21 years whose disability impacts their ability to access and benefit from their educational environment. Each municipality or school district is responsible for implementing IDEA Part B. Since the passing of the Education of All Handicapped Children Act, it has been amended many times. School-based physical and occupational therapists must practice according to legislation and scope of practice by the American Physical Therapy Association (APTA), American Occupational Therapy Association (AOTA), and mandated educational legislation, such as the IDEA (AOTA, 2020; CPTA, 2018).

Individualized Education Program

The IDEA (2004) states that the IEP is a living document that outlines each student's present level of performance, plan, goals, and objectives for school-age children 5 to 21 years (Effgen, 2013). The IEP determines the eligibility for special education and the specialized services necessary for the student to meet their goals (Vialu & Doyle, 2017). Therefore each child qualifying for and receiving special education in public schools must have an IEP (Table 18.1). The IEP is a legal document developed by the student's team that includes the student's present level of performance, strengths, and concerns for the student's education, along with the plan and goals for improving participation and eliminating barriers to access their education (Salend & Garrick Duhaney, 2011).

The IEP team members can include the family, educational staff, speech and language pathologists, audiologists, occupational therapists, and physical therapists when appropriate (Fig. 18.4). Physical therapy, occupational therapy, and speech and language therapy services, including frequency and location, are determined collectively by the IEP team (Vialu & Doyle, 2017). The team should consider whether the student will positively respond to therapy intervention resulting in improved educational access when determining the need for each therapy service (Vialu & Doyle, 2017).

Special education services, including school-based therapies, are provided under Part B of IDEA (2004). Physical therapy, occupational therapy, and speech and language therapy are services offered to support the student's IEP. Related service support aims to help the child with a disability to progress towards educationally based goals and participate in school-related activities (IDEA, 2004). This law requires special education and related services, such as physical and occupational therapy, to be provided in the least restrictive environment (Thomason & Wilmarth, 2015). In addition, the IDEA mandates that special education services, including related services, are provided to the student at no cost.

Section 504 of the Rehabilitation Act

The IDEA (2004) also mandates that children who do not qualify for special education services may be eligible to receive school-based physical and occupational therapy under Section 504 of the federally mandated Rehabilitation Act (1973). Section 504 ensures that all children with disabilities are given the same access to their educational environment as their nondisabled peers. The definition of disability is much broader under Section 504 than the IDEA and includes children with impairments that limit one or more life activities. Section 504 also provides specific details of services and equipment that must be accessible, including assistive technology, auxiliary aids (interpreter services), physical accommodations, and behavioral modifications (Table 18.1) (Doubet & Quesenberry, 2011; United States Department of Education, 1995).

TABLE 18.1 Individualized Education Plan (IEP) vs. 504 Plan	
Individualized Education Plan (IEP)	**504 Plan**
• Evaluations performed by a multidisciplinary school team or outside evaluator depending on the child's needs to determine eligibility	• Diagnosis from the child's doctors and information from family members, teachers, and service providers are used to determine whether a 504 plan is needed
• Must qualify for services under one of the following disability categories: • Autism, deaf, deaf-blind, emotional disability, hearing impairment, intellectual disability, multiple disabilities, orthopedic impairment, other health impairment, specific learning disability, speech or language impairment, traumatic brain injury, and visual impairment • The disability must significantly impact the student's educational progress	• Students who do not qualify for special education services through an IEP may qualify for services through a 504 plan instead • For students who have medical needs or a disability that requires support or accommodations but not specialized instruction
• Qualifying for an IEP ensures access to special education and related services (if eligible)	• Qualifying for a 504 plan ensures access to accommodations and related services (if eligible)
• The IEP is a legal document that provides specially designed instruction based on the child's needs and outlines accommodations, goals, objectives, services, and placement in the least restrictive environment.	• 504 plans provide accommodations and equipment and can include related services
• IEPs must be revised at least one time per school year	• 504 plans may be revised each year, but it is not required
• Example 1: A student is determined eligible for special education services under the autism disability category, and their disability is significantly affecting their educational progress. The student requires specialized instruction for 60% of the day in a special education classroom.	• Example 1: A student diagnosed with ADHD does not qualify for special education services. • However, the student still requires accommodations for fine motor and sensory needs.
• Example 2: A student with a diagnosis of cerebral palsy is eligible for special education services under other health impairments. The student's disability is significantly impacting access to education. The student requires specialized instruction, assistive technology, adaptive seating, and power wheelchair training. Also, the student requires support from a special education teacher, physical therapist, occupational therapist, and speech-language pathologist.	• Example 2: A student with a diagnosis of muscular dystrophy may not qualify for special education based on testing in the areas of academics (cognition), receptive and expressive language, or adaptive skills; however, the student requires accommodations for gross and fine motor performance, including functional mobility and functional upper extremity skills to participate in classroom tasks. • These might include writing, turning pages in a book, managing materials and personal items, navigating the school's physical environment, and participating in physical education.

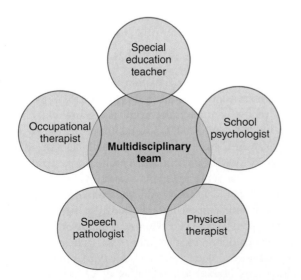

• **Fig. 18.4** Students with disabilities have various needs that may require several individuals' expertise

Special Education Process

The prevalence of developmental disabilities is increasing (Zablotsky et al., 2019). Schools must provide physical and occupational therapy as a related service for students determined eligible for these services. However, the increased need for special education services has increased the need for regulations. Public schools have the greatest regulation due to government oversight (US Department of Education, 2022).

Referral and IEP process

School-based therapy providers serve a diverse population. School-based therapy services can be provided to students with cognitive, physical, neurological, and congenital disabilities. For example, the National Center for Education Statistics (2021) reported that 33% of all public-school students who received special education services had specific learning disabilities, 19% had speech or language impairments, and between 2% and 15% had other health impairments (such as strength deficits, heart condition, or epilepsy). In addition, student populations with autism spectrum disorder, developmental delays, intellectual disabilities, and emotional disturbances make up approximately 5% to 11% of students. In comparison, 2% or less of those served under IDEA included students with multiple disabilities, hearing impairments, orthopedic impairments, visual impairments, traumatic brain injuries, and deaf-blindness (National Center for Education Statistics, 2021).

Students with disabilities who have difficulties participating in school-related activities, such as academic learning, lunchtime, physical education, and recess, can qualify for physical and occupational therapy services if they meet eligibility criteria. (Fig. 18.5).

Referrals in a public-school setting are made in several different ways and processes may vary from state to state and district to district. If a child is 3 to 5 years old and has not yet started kindergarten, the parent/caregiver or teacher may contact the local public school agency and request an evaluation (Fig. 18.6). As specified by IDEA, the public school will initiate an evaluation if the child is suspected of having a disability (IDEA, 2022). A similar process occurs for children receiving early intervention services who turn 3 years old and become too old for these services. These children are referred by the early intervention providers for special education evaluation.

Special education services typically begin through the student's general education teacher in school-age children, ages 5 to 21 years. The teacher's concerns are reported to a response intervention team consisting of the student's parents or caregivers, an administrator, the teacher, and any

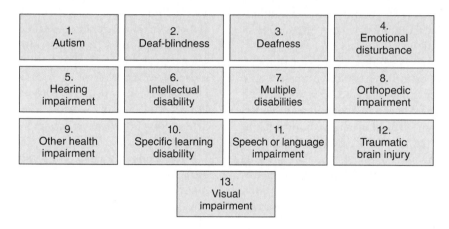

• **Fig. 18.5** IEP Eligibility Categories

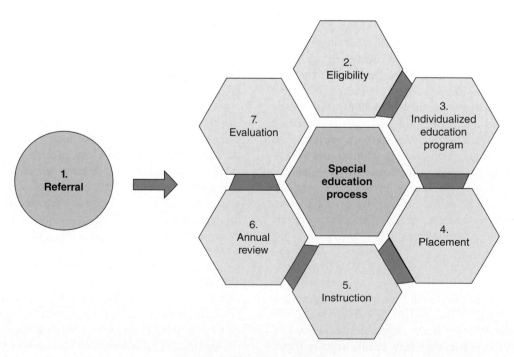

• **Fig. 18.6** Special Education Process

other faculty working with the child (Project IDEAL, 2022). Response to Intervention is a model to address problem areas based on a three-tier system: Tier 1: core curriculum and behavioral strategies; Tier 2: targeted group instruction or remediation; and Tier 3: individualized, intensive strategies (Project IDEAL, 2022). If the Response to Intervention model does not improve the student's performance, the child is referred to the special education team for an evaluation to determine eligibility for special education (Project IDEAL, 2022).

Parental consent must be received to begin the student's evaluation and the testing must be completed within 60 days of the referral date. The special education teacher initiates the evaluation and collects data from faculty and staff. They may also initiate a referral to have related services evaluate the child, including occupational therapy, physical therapy, speech-language pathology, and psychology. After all testing information is completed and analyzed, an IEP meeting is scheduled to share the results of the evaluations and determine whether the student meets the eligibility criteria for special education.

In public schools, an IEP is required documentation that specifies the special education instruction, supports, and services the student needs to progress, access, and participate in school. Physical and occupational therapy providers contribute to the IEP team, including education professionals, school personnel, and parents. Students who are 14 years and older are invited to attend their IEP meeting for an opportunity to explain their educational needs. Other services, such as speech-language pathology, psychology, audiology, counseling, interpreting, recreation therapy, and social work, may collaborate with or serve as IEP team members.

Unlike occupational and physical therapy, a student can receive speech therapy services in public schools without meeting the state eligibility criteria (Ireland & Conrad, 2016). The student may receive speech and language services as a related service under the student's IEP, provided that the student meets the eligibility criteria for at least one disability category. Speech-language pathologists are also responsible for evaluating students for eligibility for special education services but only for the category of speech or language impairment. If a student receives special education for only speech or language impairment services, the speech-language pathologist is responsible for managing the IEP. Physical and occupational therapies cannot be standalone services on an IEP. The team can consider a 504 plan to meet the student's needs if the student does not qualify for an individualized education plan.

Evaluation

The first step in special education is evaluation. A multidisciplinary team evaluates the student's eligibility for special education services and uses many different assessments and checklists to gather information from family, teachers, staff, and other related services. Based on the student's unique needs, the IEP team will recommend the corresponding discipline(s) to evaluate the need for therapeutic intervention. The IEP must relate to the educational needs of the student. The evaluation results from each discipline will be reported at the IEP meeting and the need for services will be discussed as a team. The IEP team should consider whether the student will positively respond to therapy intervention resulting in improved educational access when determining the need for each therapy service (Vialu & Doyle, 2017). For example, a physical and occupational therapy evaluation aims to determine which interventions improve a student's ability to access their educational environment.

Typically, a standardized gross and fine motor test is administered to establish a performance baseline and document progress. Common standardized tests used by physical therapists in the school setting include the Peabody Developmental Motor Scales-2, the Bruininks Oseretsky Test of Motor Proficiency-2, the Gross Motor Function Measure, and the School Function Assessment. In addition, school-based occupational therapists commonly use Peabody Developmental Motor Scales-2, Test of Handwriting Skills-revised, Sensory Processing Measure, the Beery-Buktenica Developmental Test of Visual Motor Integration, Sensory Profile-2, Bruininks Oseretsky Test of Motor Proficiency-2, School Function Assessment, and Test of Visual Perceptual Skills-4.

After being evaluated and determining eligibility, therapists create educationally relevant goals to be included in the student's IEP. The IEP team participates in yearly IEP meetings where present levels of performance, goals, and objectives are updated. A review is required every 3 years, including comprehensive evaluations to document progress and determine continued eligibility for special education. However, state practice acts require that reexamination occur every 30–90 days (Effgen, 2013)

Determining the Need for School-Based Therapy

Therapists work collectively with the planning and placement team to provide screening, evaluations, and therapy intervention for children with disabilities (CPTA, 2018). School-based therapists (physical, occupational, and speech) develop and provide therapeutic interventions and treatment plans to achieve students' IEP goals; services are also provided to children with disabilities to improve their access to their educational environment (Vialu & Doyle, 2017).

The IEP team considers several factors when determining the need for school-based therapy. First, the IEP team should discuss how the student's disabilities affect their educational performance and whether school-based therapy is an educational and not a medical need (Thomason & Wilmarth, 2015). It is essential to consider whether the student requires the therapist's expertise to attain their IEP goals and improve their educational access (Vialu & Doyle, 2017). Finally, school districts, physical therapists, and occupational therapists must look to their state guidelines to provide school-based physical therapy services because the IDEA does not provide guidance specific to physical therapy (Vialu & Doyle, 2017).

The APTA defines best practices for school-based physical therapy as providing children with disabilities services to enhance the benefit of special education (CPTA, 2018). Following best practices, school-based physical therapists provide services in the least restrictive environment, including classrooms, physical education classes, playgrounds, and the cafeteria, to fully support the student's IEP goal achievement (Thomason & Wilmarth, 2015). The emergence of motor learning research has directed physical therapists to provide intervention that is more functional and inclusive (Thomason & Wilmarth, 2015).

Therapy Services and Goals

Occupational and physical therapy are related services and, therefore must assist a child to benefit from their special education. The services and goals must be related to the student's performance in the school environment. Occupational and physical therapy caseloads vary tremendously from school to school and from state to state. The IEP goals are based on the child's needs in all areas of development and are determined by the child's present level of academic achievement and functional performance (PLAAFP). The student's IEP goals and objectives are established first to determine if the therapist's expertise is needed to address any of these goals (Vialu & Doyle, 2017). Then, the discipline(s) will construct appropriate school-related goals if intervention is warranted. School-related activities must be addressed when services are provided in a school setting. Physical and occupational therapy goals should be educationally relevant and measurable. The timeline for goal achievement is the school year.

Intervention and Setting Characteristics

Children receiving special education services often do so in the context of the typical classroom. Of the more than seven million students receiving special education services, 64.8% of children (6–21 years) spend at least 80% of the day in general education (Riser-Kositsky, 2019). The inclusion of students with disabilities in general education classrooms has increased from 33.1% since 1989 (Riser-Kositsky, 2019). Special education teams are progressing from a more contained model to providing services in the student's natural environment.

Best practice suggests that therapists provide a combination of direct, indirect, and consultation services to the students they treat (Thomason & Wilmarth, 2015). This service provision allows physical and occupational therapists one-on-one treatment of children with disabilities, staff training, and

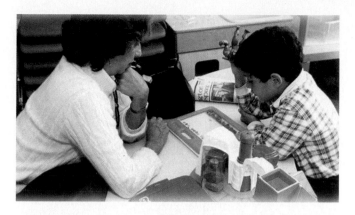

• **Fig. 18.7** An occupational therapist providing push-in service in a general classroom. (From https://upload.wikimedia.org/wikipedia/commons/1/1e/Special_ed_teacher.jpg.)

collaboration in the student's best interest. Therapies can facilitate participation and progression in typical school-related routines and activities, ensuring inclusion with same-aged peers to the greatest extent possible. Participation may be enhanced through good collaboration with outpatient therapies for continuity between the two settings.

Therapy services may be provided in the general education classroom, lunchroom, gymnasium, special education classroom, or a private room, depending on the student's goals and needs (Fig. 18.7). Contemporary practice for occupational and physical therapists is to provide services during typical school and classroom-related activities and routines. Therapies are provided in a push-in or a pull-out model. A push-in model suggests that the student participates in therapy in their regular classroom. In contrast, with a pull-out model, therapy is provided to the student outside their classroom. Pull-out therapy usually occurs in a private room, in a one-on-one setting, or a small group. The recommended therapy setting is written on the IEP and must be followed when providing services.

Providers and Care Coordination

Providers vary among educational settings. Providers may be employed directly by the school or a therapy company with whom the school contracts. School-based therapy providers must collaborate to best meet the needs of the students they serve. Based on the scope of practice and the state practice act, school therapists will provide therapy services along a continuum of prevention, promotion, and interventions. The team members work together to help students with disabilities meet their educational goals. In public schools, therapy providers are vital contributors to the education team and include occupational therapists, occupational therapy assistants, physical therapists, physical therapy assistants, and speech-language pathologists.

Physical therapists address supports and barriers that enable or hinder a student's ability to navigate the school environment during curricular and extracurricular activities. They support academic and nonacademic outcomes, including

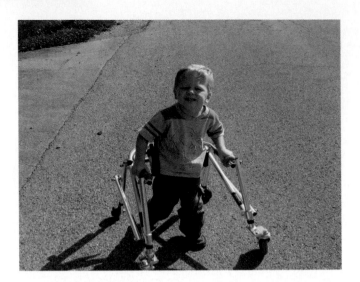

• **Fig. 18.8** Physical therapists use their movement and gait analysis expertise to design effective interventions. (From https://www.flickr.com/photos/56833981@N00/260912724.)

physical access to the school building, recess, physical education, sports participation, self-help skills, and transportation. Physical therapists use their movement and gait analysis expertise to design effective interventions (American Physical Therapy Association, 2021). They deliver a variety of interventions to assist students in routine activities. Some examples include driving a power wheelchair safely in the auditorium to attend school functions, climbing stairs to access the library, playing at recess, and helping students learn to walk through the lunch line to select their food (Fig. 18.8).

Physical therapists also assess the equipment and mobility needs of children. For children with moderate to severe physical disabilities, physical therapists provide appropriate positioning strategies and specialized equipment for postural control deficits to enable better access to curriculum materials, classroom, and school-wide activities (Barr, 2021). Mobility needs and positioning strategies may be accomplished through collaboration with the multidisciplinary team, including occupational therapists, speech-language pathologists, and teachers of the visually impaired.

School-based physical therapists have the training and skills to promote health and wellness, provide specialized exercise intervention, facilitate participation in an adapted sports program, and consult with other school staff regarding modifications and accommodations to improve the accessibility of the school setting (APTA, 2019a; Jeffries et al., 2019; Lindqvist, 2017; Rowland et al., 2015). They are the experts in environment and task modification and adaptation to increase students' access to the educational environment (Academy of Pediatric Physical Therapy [APPT], 2012a). Physical therapists in the school setting should advocate for "prevention, wellness, fitness, health promotion, and management of disease and disability" (APTA, 2019b, p. 2). Physical therapists should also support and advocate for inclusive physical education and reduce inequities

of social determinants of health among children with disabilities (APTA, 2019b).

Occupational therapists address supports and barriers that enable or hinder a student's participation during curricular and extracurricular activities in a school setting. Occupational therapists and occupational therapy assistants support academic and nonacademic outcomes, including social skills, math, reading, writing, behavior management, recess, participation in sports, self-help skills, prevocational/vocational participation, and transportation (American Occupational Therapy Association, 2016). Occupational therapists utilize their activity and environmental analysis expertise to design effective interventions and modify the environment. Occupational therapists and assistants deliver a variety of interventions such as assistive technology to complete classwork assignments, playing games to promote social skills, improving the mechanics of handwriting, and sensory activities to increase tolerance of the classroom environment. They also serve to educate teachers, staff, and families to encourage an inclusive, safe school setting for all students.

Speech-language pathologists address supports and barriers that enable or hinder a student's speech, language, or communication in a school setting. They also support academic and nonacademic outcomes, including social skills, math, reading, writing, comprehension, self-help skills, and prevocational/vocational participation. Speech-language pathologists utilize their speech, language, and communication expertise to design effective interventions. Some examples include small groups to increase communication skills, practicing target sounds, and utilizing oral motor exercises to improve feeding and swallowing skills (American Speech Language Hearing Association, 2021). All therapy services strive to facilitate successful engagement in all school-related activities.

Service Overlap

There is often overlap in skills and services offered by various disciplines, including the physical therapist, occupational therapist, physical education teacher, or adapted physical education teacher (Vialu & Doyle, 2017). Collaboration between disciplines is key to meeting the needs of the student. Both physical and occupational therapists promote health and wellness in the school setting. The school-based physical therapist is the practitioner of choice when functional mobility and gross motor skills are the main factors limiting the student's participation in their educational experience (APPT, 2012b). In the school setting, physical therapists provide expertise in movement and function for children with disabilities. Physical therapists are also experts in environment and task modification and adaptation to increase students' access to the educational environment (APPT, 2012a). Occupational therapists are the practitioner of choice for analysis of the activity, the environment to facilitate student access, support sensory needs, and successful participation in the school setting (AOTA, 2014).

The IDEA (2004) does not allow the substitution of physical education with school-based physical or occupational therapy to increase physical activity. Physical and occupational therapists should collaborate with adaptive physical education teachers to provide students with disabilities inclusive opportunities to participate in physical activity, health, and wellness programs. Students with disabilities can engage in physical activity that meets the recommended guidelines with appropriate accommodations, modifications, and support (NCHPAD, 2017).

Discharge

Discontinuing physical or occupational therapy in the school setting is a team decision. Considerations for discharge include whether the student's deficits continue to impact their ability to access their education and if functional goals have been attained (Effgen, 2013).

Adapted Sports

Transitioning from school-based therapy to adapted sports programs offered in most school districts could facilitate a lifelong healthy fitness routine for those with disabilities. Adapted sports, also known as unified sports, are an inclusive opportunity for students with disabilities (Fig. 18.9).

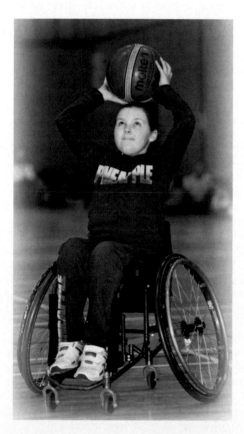

• **Fig. 18.9** Students with disabilities can transition from school-based therapies to adapted sports. (From https://www.flickr.com/photos/58447039@N07/8680809040.)

This program can promote increased participation in physical activity and help overcome societal barriers for this population (Queralt et al., 2016). Physical therapists have the skills and knowledge to facilitate this transition. Adams et al. (2018) studied pediatric physical therapists' role in promoting sports participation in children with developmental coordination disorder. The researchers found that 46% of pediatric physical therapists were involved in transitioning from physical therapy to sports for children with this condition. Barriers to sports participation included motor impairments and a lack of knowledge regarding inclusion. The facilitators of participation were determined to be parental and school support (Adams et al., 2018).

Documentation and Quality Improvement

Documentation is as essential in school settings as it is in others. Therapists document each student session, consultation visits with teachers or staff, equipment or strategy preparation, communication with family, and IEP meetings. Session documentation includes the date, time, session length, subjective, objective, assessment, and plan information. School-based therapists should always follow their state practice act on proper documentation, which is often more specific and rigorous than individual school districts.

Documentation in the school setting is also used to communicate with other members of the student's educational team and is necessary for the student's success. In addition, documentation can be utilized for quality improvement. Thorough documentation can shine a light on solutions or issues that need to be addressed by quality efforts. In public schools, documentation is essential for deciding if services will help students benefit from special education and provides evidence of progress toward their IEP goals. Documentation is also important for special education teachers, who need regular therapist feedback to determine each student's progress toward goals.

Support from Administration and Management of IEP

As a related service provider, physical and occupational therapists need the endorsement of administration and teachers to advocate the benefits of their services and repertoire of skills. Support from parents and caregivers can ensure the carryover of learned skills in the home. Related service providers should educate administration and staff on their role and scope of practice (Bender et al., 2021). Support for related service providers can be accomplished in several ways: disseminating literature on the importance of therapy; participating in professional development to educate administration, staff, and parents on the breadth and depth of physical and occupational therapy practice; and providing strategies for teachers and parents to collaborate with therapists to encourage fitness activities for students with disabilities (Bender et al., 2021).

Depending on the hierarchy at individual schools, related service providers may report to the director of Special Education, the school principal, or the lead special education teacher. Services should be scheduled so that therapy does not conflict with or distract from classroom instruction. Collaborative meetings with teachers should be scheduled to discuss the student's progress in therapy and address any new concerns. Meetings and regular communication with parent(s)/caregiver(s) should also address student progress and concerns.

Management of a student's IEP includes ensuring that all services and equipment are supplied and available; monitoring and collecting data on progress toward goals; educating faculty and staff on services and equipment, and planning and leading annual IEP meetings to revise the student's plan. The student's special education teacher oversees the management of the IEP and ensures the delivery of services.

Caseload refers to only the number of students a therapist is treating, but workload "refers to all activities in which a school-based practitioner engages in that support students directly and indirectly" (Seruya & Garfinkel, 2020, p. 1). The change in semantics allows therapy practitioners to spend time with the student in their natural environment providing direct service, setting up equipment/strategies, educating teachers and staff, and communicating with families.

Reimbursement

School districts may not charge parent(s)/legal guardian(s) for the costs of related services included in the student's IEP. The school receives federal, state, and local funding to cover the costs of these services so that the child may receive an FAPE as required by law. However, school districts that enroll as Medicaid providers can receive reimbursement for school-based services. Criteria to apply for Medicaid reimbursement include determining the following:
1. If the child is Medicaid-eligible.
2. If each service is specifically identified in the IEP.
3. If services are medically necessary for the child to benefit from their educational program.
   Medicaid varies from state to state and the local laws should be checked.

Private and Charter Schools

During the 2020–21 school year, 95% of students ages 6 to 21 years were enrolled in traditional schools, while 3% were in public or private schools for students with disabilities (National Center for Education Statistics, 2021). Most charter schools are publicly funded, thus are bound by the same laws as public schools. Private schools do not receive public funding; therefore they are not required to follow the same regulations as public schools.

Although private schools are exempt from providing therapy services, they may decide to become voluntarily accredited and provide therapy services. Agencies, such as the National Commission for the Accreditation of Special Education Services (2022), provide quality standards like those in public schools. Private schools that do not receive federal funding are not required to implement an IEP. However, they must refer the student to a local public school district if a parent requests an evaluation. The public school district will determine the frequency and duration of special education and related services provided to the student. Some private schools may offer school-based therapy by contracting with a therapy agency.

Summary

Today, over 7 million students between the ages of 3 and 21 years receive special education services (National Center for Education Statistics, 2021). School-based therapy supports the student's successful engagement in school-related activities. Occupational, physical, and speech-language therapy, among other supports and services, are available to help eligible students fully benefit from their education (IDEA, 2017).

Discussion Activities

1. What services can be provided under an IEP?
2. What services can be provided under a 504 plan?
3. What are the eligibility differences between an IEP and a 504?
4. How are goals and objectives different in a school model compared with a medical model of physical and occupational therapy?

References

Academy of Pediatric Physical Therapy. (2012a). *Fact sheet. The role of school-based physical therapy: Successful participation for all students.* https://pediatricapta.org/includes/fact-sheets/pdfs/12%20Role%20of%20SchoolBasedPT.pdf.

Academy of Pediatric Physical Therapy. (2012b). *Resource/fact sheet: The pediatric physical therapist as the practitioner of choice.* https://pediatricapta.org/includes/fact-sheets/pdfs/12%20Ped%20PT%20as%20Practioner%20of%20Choice.pdf.

Adams, I. L. J., Broekkamp, W., Wilson, P. H., Imms, C., Overvelde, A., & Steenbergen, B. (2018). Role of pediatric physical therapists in promoting sports participation in developmental coordination disorder. *Pediatric Physical Therapy: The Official Publication of the Section on Pediatrics of the American Physical Therapy Association, 30*(2)106–111.

American Occupational Therapy Association, American Physical Therapy Association, & American Speech-Language-Hearing Association. (2014). *Workload approach: A paradigm shift for positive impact on student outcomes.* http://www.aota.org/-/media/Corporate/Files/Practice/Children/APTA-ASHA-AOTA-Joint-Doc-Workload-Approach-Schools-2014.pdf.

American Occupational Therapy Association. (2016). *Occupational therapy's role with school settings* [Fact sheet]. https://www.aota.

org/-/media/Corporate/Files/AboutOT/Professionals/WhatIsOT/CY/Fact-Sheets/School%20Settings%20fact%20sheet.pdf.

American Occupational Therapy Association. (2020). Guidelines for supervision, roles, and responsibilities during the delivery of occupational therapy services. *American Journal of Occupational Therapy, 74*(Suppl. 3), 7413410020.

American Physical Therapy Association. (2019a). *Association's role in advocacy for prevention, wellness, fitness, health promotion, disease and disability management: HOD P06-19-26-11.* https://www.apta.org/siteassets/pdfs/policies/association-role-advocacy.pdf.

American Physical Therapy Association. (2019b). *Physical therapists' role in prevention, wellness, fitness, health promotion, and management of disease and disability: HOD P06-19-27-12.* https://www.apta.org/apta-and-you/leadership-and-governance/policies/pt-role-advocacy.

American Physical Therapy Association. (2021). *School based physical therapy.* https://www.apta.org/your-practice/practice-models-and-settings/school-based-physical-therapy.

American Speech Language Hearing Association. (2021). *School-based service delivery in speech-language pathology.* https://www.asha.org/SLP/schools/School-Based-Service-Delivery-in-Speech-Language-Pathology/.

Barr, A. (2021). *School-based physical therapy: Taking on our role during a pandemic.* https://www.apta.org/article/2021/04/21/school-based-physical-therapy-taking-on-our-role-during-a-pandemic.

Bender, J., Cale, C., Groff, S., & Panesar-Aguilar, S. (2021). A critical examination of school-based physiotherapists' perceived aptitude and willingness to facilitate health and wellness promotion. *World Journal of Social Science Research, 8*(4), 1–17.

Connecticut Physical Therapy Association. (2018). *Physical therapy in Connecticut schools: Best practices and resources.* https://www.ctpt.org/Customer-Content/WWW/CMS/files/CT_School_Based_Guidelines_2018.pdf.

Doubet, S., & Quesenberry, A. C. (2011). History of early childhood special education. In A. F. Rotatori, F. E. Obiakor, & J. P. Bakken (Eds.), *Advances in special education Volume 21: History of special education* (pp. 47-60). Emerald Group Publishing Unlimited. https://eds.b.ebscohost.com/eds/ebookviewer/ebook/bmxlYmtfXzM1NTczOF9fQU41?sid=a3e3a88e-0ff2-49c5-bbdc-ac678392a07c@sessionmgr103&vid=4&format=EB&rid=2.

Effgen, S. K. (2013). *Meeting the physical therapy needs of children* (2nd ed.). F. A. Davis.

Effgen, S. K., & Kaminker, M. K. (2014). Nationwide survey of school-based physical therapy practice. *Pediatric Physical Therapy, 26*(4), 394–403.

Individuals with Disabilities Education Act. (1990). *Sec. 901. terminology and technical amendments.* https://www.govinfo.gov/content/pkg/STATUTE-104/pdf/STATUTE-104-Pg1103.pdf.

Individuals with Disabilities Education Act. (1997). *Sec. 101. Amendments to the individuals with disabilities education act.* https://www.govinfo.gov/content/pkg/PLAW-105publ17/html/PLAW-105publ17.htm.

Individuals with Disabilities Education Act. (2017). *Sec. 300.34 related services.* https://sites.ed.gov/idea/regs/b/a/300.34.

Individuals with Disabilities Education Act. (2019). *Section 1414.* https://sites.ed.gov/idea/statute-chapter-33/subchapter-ii/1414

Individuals with Disabilities Education Act, 20 U.S.C. § 1400 (2004). https://www2.ed.gov/policy/speced/leg/idea/idea.pdf.

Individuals with Disabilities Education Act. (2021). *About IDEA.* https://sites.ed.gov/idea/about-idea/#:,:text=On%20November%2029%2C%201975%2C%20President,Disabilities%20Education%20Act%20(IDEA).

Individuals with Disabilities Education Act. (2022). *A history of the individuals with disabilities education act.* https://sites.ed.gov/idea/IDEA-History/.

Ireland, M., & Conrad, B. J. (2016). Evaluation and eligibility for speech-language services in schools. *Perspectives of the ASHA Special Interest Groups, 16*(1) 78–90.

Jeffries, L. M., McCoy, S. W., Effgen, S. K., Chiarello, L. A., & Villasante-Tezanos, A. G. (2019). Description of the services, activities, and interventions within school-based physical therapist practices across the United States. *Physical Therapy, 99*(1), 98–108.

Lindqvist, A. K. (2017). Physiotherapist enabling school children's physical activity using social cognitive theory, empowerment, and technology. *European Journal of Physiotherapy, 19*(3), 147–153.

Moffat, M. (2003). The history of physical therapy practice in the United States. *Journal of Physical Therapy Education, 17*(3), 15–25.

National Center for Education Statistics. (2021). *Students with disabilities.* https://nces.ed.gov/programs/coe/indicator/cgg.

National Center for Health, Physical Activity and Disability. (2017). *Discover inclusive school wellness.* https://www.nchpad.org/fppics/NCHPAD_Discover%20Inclusive%20School%20Wellness(1).pdf.

National Commission for the Accreditation of Special Education Services. (2022). *Accreditation information.* http://ncases.org/.

Public Law 94-142: Education of all handicapped children act, 89 Stat.773-796, 1975. http://www.gpo.gov/fdsys/pkg/STATUTE-89/pdf/STATUTE-89-pg773.pdf[6].

Public Law 99-372: Handicapped children's protection act, 20 USC §, 1986.1415 (e)(4)(f). http://www.gpo.gov/fdsys/pkg/STATUTE-100/pdf/STATUTE-100-Pg796.pdf.

Public Law 108-446: Individuals with disabilities education improvement act of 2004. http://www.copyright.gov/legislation/pl108-446.pdf.

Project IDEAL. (2022). *The special education referral process.* http://www.projectidealonline.org/v/special-education-referral-process/.

Rehabilitation Act of 1973, § 504, 29 U.S.C. § 701 (1973). https://www.dol.gov/agencies/oasam/centers-offices/civil-rights-center/statutes/section-504-rehabilitation-act-of-1973.

Riser-Kositsky, M. (2019). *Education week: Special education: Definition, statistics, and trends.* https://www.edweek.org/teaching-learning/special-education-definition-statistics-and-trends/2019/12.

Rowland, J. L., Fragala-Pinkham, M., Miles, C., & O'Neil, M. E. (2015). The scope of pediatric physical therapy practice in health promotion and fitness for youth with disabilities. *Pediatric Physical Therapy, 27*(1), 2–15.

Salend, S. J., & Garrick Duhaney, L. M. (2011). Historical and philosophical changes in the education of students with exceptionalities. In A. F. Rotatori, F. E. Obiakor, & J. P. Bakken (Eds.), *Advances in special education Volume 21* (pp. 1–20). Emerald Group Publishing Unlimited.

Seruya, F. M., & Garfinkel, M. (2020). Caseload and workload: Current trends in school-based practice across the United States. *American Journal of Occupational Therapy, 74*(5), 1–9. https://research.aota.org/ajot/article/74/5/7405205090p1/8417/Caseload-and-Workload-Current-Trends-in-School?searchresult=1.

Thomason, H. K., & Wilmarth, M. A. (2015). Provision of school-based physical therapy services: A survey of current practice patterns. *Pediatric Physical Therapy, 27*(2), 161–169.

United States Courts. (2021). *History- Brown v. Board of Education.* https://www.uscourts.gov/educational-resources/educational-activities/history-brown-v-board-education-re-enactment.

United States Department of Education. (1995). *The civil rights of students with hidden disabilities under Section 504 of the Rehabilitation Act of 1973* [Online Pamphlet]. U.S. Government Printing Office. https://www2.ed.gov/about/offices/list/ocr/docs/hq5269.html.

United States Department of Education. (2022). *Frequently asked questions*. https://www.ed.gov/answers/#.

Vialu, C., & Doyle, M. (2017). Determining need for school-based physical therapy under IDEA: Commonalities across practice guidelines. *Pediatric Physical Therapy, 29*(4), 350–355.

Zablotsky, B., Black, L. I., Maenner, M. J., Schieve, L. A., Danielson, M. L., Bitsko, R. H., Blumberg, S. J., Kogan, M. D., & Boyle, C. A. (2019). Prevalence and trends of developmental disabilities among children in the United States: 2009-2017. *Pediatrics, 144*(4), e20190811.

19
Mental Health Settings

PATRICIA LAVERDURE, OTD, OTR/L, BCP, FAOTA; BRIDGETTE LeCOMPTE, MS, OTR/L;
AMY ESTES MILLER, PT, DPT; and MICA MITCHELL, PT, DPT

LEARNING OBJECTIVES

By the end of this chapter, the reader will be able to:

1. Examine the collaborative and comprehensive continuum of mental health care.
2. Identify the federal, state, and local laws governing mental health services and protecting individuals with mental health conditions.
3. Define the roles and responsibilities of occupational and physical therapy practitioners and the interprofessional

healthcare team in treating clients with mental health disorders.
4. Identify how mental health disorders may manifest in clients with physical and mental health needs.
5. Examine evidence-based evaluation and intervention approaches for people with mental health conditions.

CHAPTER OUTLINE

History and Background

Accreditation and Regulations

Patient Population, Services, and Setting Characteristics
    Mental Health Continuum
    Diversity Differences
    Mental Disorders
    Response to Illness and Injury
        Coping
    Mental Health and Chronic Pain
        Contemporary Pain Management
    Trauma
        Adverse Childhood Experiences
        Trauma and Treatment Implications

Childhood Mental Disorders
Substance Use
Mental Health Disorders in Incarcerated Populations

Providers and Care Coordination
    Collaboration and Care Coordination
    Therapeutic Use of Self
    Evaluation and Intervention Planning

Responsibilities of a Manager/Administrator
    Reimbursement, Documentation, and Quality Improvement

Discussion

Activities

History and Background

Addressing clients' mental health status has long been challenging for healthcare providers. Mental health influences an individual's ability to participate meaningfully in life roles, routines, and activities and may also lead to significant social challenges and physical health issues. The National Alliance on Mental Illness estimates that one in five Americans experiences mental illness each year (2020), and mental illness accounts for one-third of the world's disabling conditions (Anderson et al., 2011; Nguyen & Davis, 2017). Severe mental health problems (e.g., schizophrenia,

bipolar disorder, and major depressive disorder) and substance use disorders impact individuals of all age groups. Suicide is the second leading cause of death in 15- to 29-year-olds (Nguyen & Davis, 2017). Socioeconomic challenges such as poverty, food and housing insecurity, educational deprivation, and financial stress are closely linked to mental health issues and illness (Lund et al., 2010). However, access to mental health care is significantly limited due to scarce resources, financial burdens, or social stigma (Lake & Turner, 2017).

The challenges associated with mental health have been observed throughout history, evident through the elusive understanding of the etiology, impact, and treatment of those challenges until late into the 20th century. Early societies viewed mental health issues as demonic possessions or physical illnesses requiring invasive treatments such as bloodletting or trephination, a procedure involving removing a small part of the skull (Faria, 2013). In almost all cases, individuals with mental illness were isolated from society and cared for by family members or assigned members of the community. Often, individuals with mental illness were incarcerated in jails as convicted criminals or confined to almshouses (Fig. 19.1). By the late 17th to early 18th century, public and charitable institutions known as insane or lunatic asylums began to proliferate in Europe and the colonial Americas. Though purported to be treatment facilities, many were overcrowded with poor sanitation conditions. Restraint and ice water baths were not uncommon. As the asylums grew larger and housed more individuals, clients were conscripted into roles of arduous work to support institutional living in response to the societal value of activity and productivity or as punishment for wrongdoing (Ernst, 2018).

In the mid to late 1800s, Dorothea Dix (Fig. 19.2), a teacher and rigorous advocate for individuals with mental illness in the United States, challenged the societal view of the time that individuals with mental illness could not be cured and were destined to a lifetime of suffering with their condition (Parry, 2006). She is credited with developing or expanding more than 30 hospitals designed to treat individuals with mental illness. Based on her exposure to the moral treatment and mental hygiene movements taking hold in Europe and the United States at the time, Dix drew attention to the poor conditions and maltreatment of individuals with mental illness in asylums, almshouses, and prisons and facilitated the development of treatment facilities that could better meet the mental healthcare needs of these individuals (Gollaher, 1995; Levin & Gildea, 2013). While still entwined with institutional profit, engaging clients in productive activity became increasingly aligned with client self-improvement (Ernst, 2019).

Early to mid-20th century treatment approaches were based upon the expanding understanding of the body and the brain and the connections between them. Mental healthcare providers of the time considered mental illness an issue of body function, resulting in expanding biomedical treatment approaches. The development and proliferation of insulin coma therapy (ICT) as a form of psychiatric treatment illustrates the deeply rooted belief that the etiology of mental illness could be found in the body and, more specifically, the brain (Doroshow, 2007). Shortly after the discovery of the medicinal properties of insulin for individuals with diabetes, mental healthcare providers began using it with individuals with severe mental health disorders such as

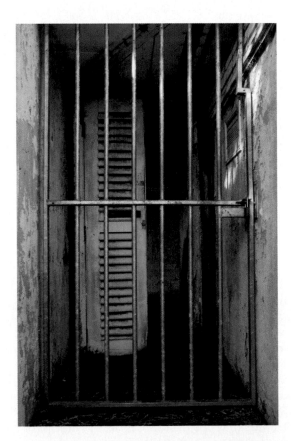

• **Fig. 19.1** The stigma of mental illness left many locked away until deinstitutionalization in the late 20th century. (From https://www.flickr.com/photos/21228143@N03/7459751850.)

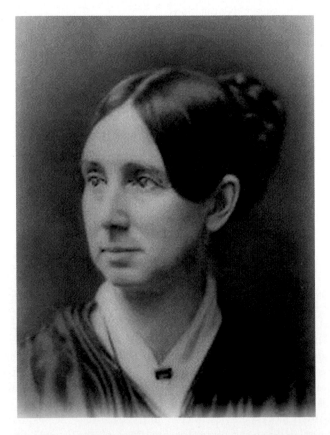

• **Fig. 19.2** Dorothea Dix is credited with developing or expanding more than 30 hospitals designed to treat individuals with mental illness. (From https://www.flickr.com/photos/28826830@N00/24668446186.)

schizophrenia. Clients were administered large doses of insulin to induce hypoglycemic coma. Dosages were manipulated to maintain clients in a coma for minutes to hours before being administered a sugar solution. Consciousness would return along with anticipated periods of lucidity that were not supported in published evidence, only described anecdotally. Clients often underwent this treatment protocol five to six times per week for several weeks or months until they were considered either recovered or incurable (Doroshow, 2007).

Other biomedical approaches, such as the use of stimulant medications to induce seizures (Cooper & Fink, 2014), electroconvulsive therapy (Guimarães et al., 2018), and lobotomy (Faria, 2013), were increasingly popular for treating serious mental illnesses. As the research on the etiological factors of mental illness, the aggregation of outcomes of biomedical approaches, the development and implementation of psychopharmaceuticals, and humanitarian and rehabilitation approaches to mental illness expanded through the 1950s, the outcomes for individuals with severe mental illness began to improve (Davidson et al., 2010). Simultaneously, societal demands for humanitarian approaches and deinstitutionalization (i.e., a shift of treatment of individuals with mental illness from the asylum to the community) (Salime et al., 2022) were heeded and community-based treatment models emerged. While advances in neuroscience and psychopharmacology continue to contribute valuably to the biomedical treatment of individuals with mental illness, rehabilitation, public health, empowerment, and recovery models offer complementary and alternative approaches to meet mental health needs across the continuum of severity and functional impact.

Post-World War I and polio rehabilitation models, adopted early in their professional histories, enabled occupational and physical therapy practitioners to address the mental health needs of society. Recognizing the impact of mental health needs on recovery, occupational and physical therapy practitioners used the Rehabilitation Frame of Reference (Gillen, 2014) to modify environments, promote engagement in meaningful daily activity, promote personal improvement and social participation, and support the return to productive life (Cioppa-Mosca, 2019; Cockburn, 2016). As deinstitutionalization accelerated and clients transitioned from the asylums to community-based treatment, adaptive, compensatory, and modifying interventions were used by occupational therapy practitioners to promote improved community living, self-determination, and autonomy (Cockburn, 2016; Gillen, 2014). Physical therapy practitioners addressed mobility, accessibility, and physical activity.

Professionals working with this population began to recognize that paradigms such as phases of illness (e.g., acute, maintenance and continuation), disease profiles (e.g., relapse, recurrence, remission, and recovery) (Jacob, 2015), and the specialist healthcare framework (Evans & Bufka, 2020) could not fully support the development of effective treatment approaches for this group of individuals now living in the community, often for the first time. Conceptual

structures emerged to examine the factors associated with and the consequences of disease that provided a foundation from which healthcare professionals and researchers could examine mental health and healthcare from a broader lens of groups and populations. The Nagi Disability Model, a seminal structure describing the relationships of illness, function, and participation published in 1964, carefully linked health and disability and provided epidemiological definitions and processes to examine these constructs on the population level (Altman, 2016; Jette, 2006).

Population and public health approaches recognizing the array of factors that influence or even determine the health status of individuals and populations became valuable to providers implementing services for this population. These factors include genetics, physical health, stable living conditions (e.g., shelter, food, relationships), education, socioeconomic status, and social justice. Programs addressing safety, food and housing security, work transition, healthcare management, and leisure pursuits emerged and are still available to individuals with mental health care needs today (Grajo et al., 2020; Gutman, 2021; Marshall et al., 2021).

In the late 1970s, the World Health Organization (WHO) published the International Classification of Impairments, Disabilities and Handicaps (ICIDH), a conceptual and complementary framework designed to formally link the consequences of illness on function (WHO, 1980) and to examine the relationship of the myriad of influences on health and wellness. The ICIDH is credited with founding a common nomenclature to examine the factors associated with illness, disability, and participation that fueled research across the spectrum of healthcare (Disability Data Briefing, 2002; Fisher, 1994). These models and the population-based intervention approaches derived from them empowered individuals with mental health needs to become more actively involved in their healthcare and their community (Fisher, 1994). Nelson and colleagues (2001) suggest that empowerment models in mental health include:

- Promoting choice and control: Creating opportunities for individuals and populations to take the initiative and assert control increases confidence, self-esteem, self-efficacy, and independence.
- Facilitating community integration: Creating and implementing responsive organizations and integrated mental health supports strengthens supportive relationships and enhances participation in the community.
- Creating valued resources and pathways to access them: Advocacy efforts to create and provide access to resources such as education, employment, and housing enhances mental health and wellbeing.

In 2002, the WHO released a revision to the ICDIH called the International Classification of Functioning, Disability and Health (ICF) (WHO, 2022a). The ICF is a classification of health and health-related domains. The ICF places human function at its center and describes its levels of function as the individual's body or body parts, the individuals and their lived experience, and the ecological system in which they function. "Within the ICF, contextual factors include aspects of the [individual,] built, social, and attitudinal environment that create the lived experience of functioning and disability as well as personal factors such as sex, age, coping styles, social background, education, and overall behavior patterns that may influence how disablement is experienced by the individual" (Jette, 2006, p.730).

Over time, holistic and client-centered approaches embodied in the ICF led to adoption of a recovery framework that empowers individuals experiencing mental health challenges to exert choice in their healthcare. The recovery framework conceptualizes recovery as a process that involves building resilience and control over one's life challenges and emphasizes that individuals experiencing mental health issues can achieve a meaningful life despite persistent symptoms (Jacob, 2015; Liberman & Kopelowicz, 2005). Like many who live productively with chronic illness, symptom remission alone is an insufficient indicator of recovery for people with mental illness. Psychosocial functioning may continue to be impaired even when mental health symptomatology has been reduced or eliminated (Koran et al., 1996; Tohen et al., 2000). While symptom remission is valuable, the premise of the recovery framework is therefore not curative, but rather framed to (American Occupational Therapy Association [AOTA], 2020; Liberman & Kopelowicz, 2005):

- Enhance social relationships.
- Promote function across occupational domains of self-care, independent living (e.g., home and money management), and health management (e.g., sleep, rest, and medication management).
- Enhance productive participation in school or work.
- Promote active and restorative participation in recreational activities.

Liberman and Kopelowicz (2005) argue that mental health recovery is dependent upon a continuous, "comprehensive, coordinated, competent, and consumer-oriented" (p. 739) service delivery system that flexibly addresses healthcare needs across a hierarchical continuum of levels. Recovery models are applied across client populations (individuals, groups, and communities), settings (e.g., hospitals, rehabilitation, and long-term healthcare facilities, community-based setting, schools, and criminal justice systems), and types of services (e.g., residential, inpatient acute care, partial hospitalization, intensive or routine outpatient [telehealth], peer-support systems [e.g., anonymous programs such as 12-step programs, support groups]). Today, recovery models enable practitioners to focus efforts on creating pathways to fulfilling relationships and participation in meaningful occupations with their clients.

Assessment and intervention focus on identifying risk and protective factors, identifying at-risk populations (e.g., combat veterans, individuals who have experienced trauma; prodromal or first-episode psychosis), and developing individual, group, and community-based mental illness prevention programs. Matching individual needs to resources and supports results in optimal function and positive mental health. Physical, behavioral, and mental health are interconnected, and it is within the scope of physical therapy practitioners to screen for and address associated conditions (APTA, 2020). Positive mental health is achieved when individuals participate meaningfully in occupations of values, routines, and roles and achieve a sense of well-being (AOTA, 2020; Huppert, 2005). Occupational and physical therapy practitioners promote positive mental health across the spectrum of service delivery by helping clients take care of their physical and mental health needs, engage in physical activity, and interact and build connections with people in their lives.

Accreditation and Regulations

Due to the expansive and varied contexts in which mental health services are provided, it is imperative that practitioners investigate, understand, and operate within the essential accreditations, laws, regulations, and professional standards of practice tailored to their specific practice setting. At the national and state level, various organizations accredit behavioral health and human service organizations, setting high-quality care and safety standards. These standards are important for practitioners to uphold as direct contributors to quality improvement, risk management, reimbursement of services, and client outcomes. Occupational and physical therapy practitioners must also ensure the alignment of organizational policies, procedures, and practices with laws and regulations on mental health.

Federal, state, and local laws/regulations govern mental health services and the protection of individuals with mental health and substance conditions, including the rights of those receiving services, privacy/confidentiality, and community inclusion (Mental Health America [MHA], n.d.). The federal government is responsible for establishing and enforcing minimum standards for regulating mental health systems and providers, protecting the rights of individuals, funding services, and supporting research and innovation (MHA, n.d.). The federal government collaborates with states to support mental health services; however, states have flexibility with expanding and enforcing their standards if they meet the required minimums set forth by the federal government. As a result of this flexibility, enforcement and practices not only vary state by state but may also vary between local governments. Furthermore, practitioners should also be aware of funding structures and how they impact access to services, the social determinants of health, required documentation practices, reimbursement for agencies and individuals, and ethical decision-making for service provision.

Occupational and physical therapy practitioners must use their foundational knowledge, professional guidance, and laws/regulations governing occupational and physical therapy practice to guide their current and future scope of practice in alignment with the broader context. This means simultaneously navigating various national, state, and local influences, which may complement or compete with professional reasoning, the scope of practice, and ethical decision-making. Table 19.1 situates common mental health laws/regulations, accreditations, funding structures,

TABLE 19.1 Common Laws, Regulations, Accreditation, and Funding of Mental Health Services in the United States

Level	Laws and Regulations, Accreditation and Funding
Professional Foundational Documents & Guidance	**American Occupational Therapy Association (AOTA)** • Vision 2025: Occupational therapy *maximizes health, well-being, and quality of life for all people, populations, and communities through effective solutions that facilitate participation in everyday living.* • Standards of Practice for Occupational Therapy (2021) • Occupational Therapy Practice Framework - 4th Edition (OTPF-4) (2020) • AOTA Code of Ethics (2020) • Mental Health Promotion, Prevention, and Intervention in OT Practice (2017) **American Physical Therapy Association (APTA)** • Position Statement 2020: *The APTA supports interprofessional collaboration at the organizational and individual levels to promote research, education, policy, and practice in behavioral and mental health to enhance the overall health and well-being of society, consistent with APTA's vision.* • Core Values for the Physical Therapist and Physical Therapy Assistant • Code of Ethics for the Physical Therapist

National Level Regulation and Policy	**Federal Laws and Regulations**
	• Americans with Disabilities Act (ADA)
	• The Rehabilitation Act of 1973
	• Protection and Advocacy for Individuals with Mental Illness Act (PAIMI Act)
	• Health Insurance
	  • Affordable Care Act (ACA)
	  • The Mental Health Parity and Addiction Equity Act (MPHAEA)
	• Education
	  • Individuals with Disabilities Education Act (IDEA)
	  • Every Student Succeeds Act (ESSA)
	• Privacy
	  • Family Educational Rights and Privacy Act (FERPA)
	  • Health Insurance Portability and Privacy Act of 1996 (HIPAA)
	
	Accreditation
	• Joint Commission
	• Commission on Accreditation of Rehabilitation Facilities (CARF)
	• Council on Accreditation (COA)
	
	Funding
	• Centers for Medicare and Medicaid Services (CMS)
	• Department of Veterans Affairs (VA)
	• Children's Health Insurance Program (CHIP)
	• Mental Health Block Grants

State Level Regulation and Policy	**State Laws and Regulations** • OT and PT State Licensure/Practice Act • Statutes (e.g., restraint and seclusion, Qualified Mental Health Professional (QMHP)) • Education (e.g., students with disabilities, school mental health) • Incarceration and Jail Diversion Programs • Involuntary Commitment **Accreditation** • Facility licensure or accreditation (e.g., Certified Community Behavioral Health Clinic) **Funding** • Medicaid & CHIP • Mental Health Block Grants
Local Level	• Local laws and regulations (e.g., emergency/crisis response) • Facility policies and procedures

American Occupational Therapy Association. (2017). Mental health promotion, prevention, and intervention in occupational therapy practice. *American Journal of Occupational Therapy, 71*(Suppl. 2), 7112410035. https://doi. org/10.5014/ajot.2017.716S03

American Occupational Therapy Association. (2020). AOTA 2020 occupational therapy code of ethics. *American Journal of Occupational Therapy, 74*(Suppl.3), 7413410005. https://doi.org/10.5014/ajot.2020.74S3006

American Occupational Therapy Association. (2021). Standards of practice for occupational therapy. *American Journal of Occupational Therapy, 75*(Suppl.3), 7513410030. https://doi.org/10.5014/ajot.2021.75S3004

American Occupational Therapy Association. (2023). Vision 2025. https://www.aota.org/about/mission-vision

American Occupational Therapy Association. (2020). Occupational therapy practice framework: Domain and process (4thed.). *American Journal of Occupational Therapy, 74*(Suppl.2), 7412410010. https://doi. org/10.5014/ajot.2020.74S2001

American Physical Therapy Association. (2023). Vision, Mission, and Strategic Plan. https://www.apta.org/apta-and-you/leadership-and-governance/vision-mission-and-strategic-plan

American Physical Therapy Association. (202o). Code of Ethics for the Physical Therapist. chrome-extension://efaidnbmnnnibpcajpcglclefindmkaj/https://www.apta.org/siteassets/pdfs/policies/codeofethicshods06-20-28-25.pdf

and professional influences at the national, state, and local level (MHA, n.d.; SAMHSA, 2022a). This list is not exhaustive and further investigation will be necessary for a more comprehensive understanding of how these are applied in various settings.

Patient Population, Services, and Setting Characteristics

Mental Health Continuum

Mental health is a dynamic state of functioning that occurs along a continuum and varies throughout an individual's life due to biological, environmental, or situational factors. It is a "state of mental well-being that enables people to cope with the stresses of life, realize their abilities, learn well and work well, and contribute to their community" (WHO, 2022b, para 1.). Positive mental health can be strengthened with or without mental illness (Keyes, 2006, 2007, as cited in Miles et al., 2010). The absence of mental health challenges does not necessarily indicate positive mental health, nor does the absence of positive mental health indicate mental health challenges (Keyes, 2005, as cited in Miles et al., 2010). Viewing mental health as a continuum and an important aspect of health for all helps reduce the stigma around mental health and mental illness (Peter et al., 2021).

The Centers for Disease Control's (CDC) Whole School, Whole Community, Whole Child Model (WSCC) is one example of how positive mental health can be addressed in schools using a health promotion and prevention framework (CDC, 2022). The WSCC model aims to promote active learning and establishment of healthy behaviors for all students by focusing on aspects of the environment (e.g., social and emotional climate, physical environment), access to mental and physical health education and services (e.g., physical education, nutrition, counseling), employee wellness, community partnerships, and family engagement. This model is well aligned with occupational and physical therapy scope of practice using a public health approach to mental health in education; however, practitioners can instill the mental health continuum mindset to promote positive mental health for all regardless of their practice setting. Practitioners can use their knowledge and expertise to recognize shifts in client and colleague mental health, facilitate mental health care access/programming, and respond to individuals' diverse mental health needs regardless of the absence or presence of mental illness.

Diversity Differences

Practitioners' awareness of their biases, prejudices, stereotypes, and discrimination toward historically excluded and marginalized groups will help address the gap in access and utilization of mental health care services (Mongelli et al., 2020). The diversity of individuals and communities exists in socioeconomic status, race, color, religion, sex, gender,

gender expression, age, national origin (ancestry), neurodiversity, disability, marital status, sexual orientation, and military status (Loden& Rosener, 1991). Individuals from historically excluded and marginalized groups are less likely to use mental health services (Mongelli et al., 2020). Individuals from racial/ethnic historically marginalized groups are 20%–50% less likely to seek mental health services for themselves and 40%–80% more likely to stop treatment before recommended (Mongelli et al., 2020). The disparities in receiving and continuing mental health services can be attributed to cultural stigma and lack of resources (Mongelli et al., 2020). These differences in the beliefs and perceptions of mental health diagnoses and treatment may impact an individual's involvement in their care and the staff's perceptions of their client's illness.

Gender-responsive and culturally relevant strategies should be considered across all mental health settings to minimize the effects of stigma (Parcesepe & Cabassa, 2013; Wirth & Bodenhausen, 2009). Sources of disparities in lesbian, gay, bisexual, transgender, queer, questioning, or intersex (LGBTQI) youth are likely caused by high levels of social isolation, lack of parental support, bullying, and increased stigma, discrimination, and violence (National Alliance on Mental Illness [NAMI], 2020; Tordoff et al., 2022). Important risk factors for LGBTQI people are the impact of coming out, rejection, trauma, substance use, homelessness, suicide, and inadequate mental health care (King, 2015; NAMI, 2020). Gender-affirming care mitigates depression, anxiety, and suicidal ideation in transgender and non-binary youth, improving mental health outcomes (Tordoff et al., 2022). A practitioner that is knowledgeable of the struggles and the experiences of marginalized groups can be proactive when providing mental health support to meet the individual's needs.

The cooccurrence of physical and mental health problems via invisible disabilities may be unknown to health care providers. For example, Mazi and colleagues (2019) found a significant correlation between pelvic floor dysfunction and depression. Similar relationships have been found between pelvic pain syndromes and anxiety, depression, and mood disorders (Alonso & Coe, 2001; Dorn et al., 2009; Iacovides et al., 2015). The normalization and systematization of discrimination based on these factors may negatively influence an individual's awareness of their needs and a provider's provision of services (VanPuymbrouck et al., 2021). Individuals from marginalized groups are less likely to find adequate mental health services and may experience discrimination or stigma, further increasing the disparity of mental health service utilization. Other groups of individuals that have been marginalized in society are homeless and incarcerated individuals. Of the 2.5 to 3.5 million Americans who experience homelessness, approximately 33% have a mental illness (Mongelli et al., 2020). The intersection or presence of multiple marginalized identities increases the negative impacts of bias and discrimination in an individual's life. Awareness of and advocacy for differences in mental health perceptions and viewpoints that exist for individuals can

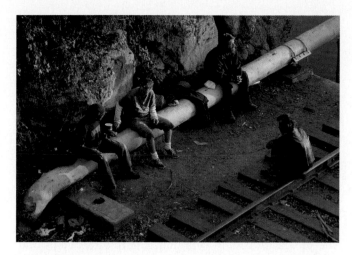

• **Fig. 19.3** Approximately one-third of the homeless population in the United States has a mental illness. (From https://www.flickr.com/photos/78425154@N00/1487002016.)

assist the interdisciplinary team in providing services, resources, and treatments that meet their unique needs. When designing staff training programs, individual, responsive, and relevant information should be incorporated across all mental health settings (Fig. 19.3).

Numerous models for building cultural competence to reduce health disparities provide a basis for education within the mental health system (Butler et al., 2016). Many frameworks present a continuum from cultural denial or destructiveness to cultural competence or proficiency. Other frameworks consider cultural competence a constantly evolving self-awareness process, not an endpoint (Foronda et al., 2015). An example of educational awareness of gender-responsive strategies would be the acknowledgment of the differences between the reception of mental health treatment between males and females. Men are less likely to seek help for mental health problems (Oliver et al., 2005). In a National Health Interview Survey by the National Center for Health Statistics conducted in 2020, significant differences were found between women and men receiving mental health treatment. It was reported that 25.6% of women received mental health treatment in the past 12 months versus 14.6% of men; 21.2 % of women had taken medication for their mental health versus 11.5% of men; and women (12.1 %) were more likely to have received counseling or therapy from a mental health professional versus men (7.9 %) in the past 12 months (Smith et al., 2018). Not seeking treatment for men includes stigma and socialization of asking for help being a weakness.

Mental Disorders

Mental disorders are organized and classified in a standardized manual used widely throughout the healthcare community entitled The Diagnostic and Statistical Manual of Mental Disorders, Fifth Edition (DSM-5) (American Psychiatric Association [APA], 2013). The manual provides concise and explicit criteria to promote effective and consistent review of symptomatology, identification of diagnostic classifications, and precise coding for data collection and billing purposes for conditions affecting children and adults. For each mental health disorder, the DSM-5 offers a review of symptoms, possible differential diagnoses, and descriptive text that includes topics such as diagnostic and associated features, risk factors and prevalence, disease development (age of onset) and course, gender and diversity factors, common co-occurring conditions, and functional impacts.

The DSM-5 defines a mental disorder as a syndrome characterized by a clinically significant disturbance in an individual's cognition, emotion regulation, or behavior that reflects a dysfunction in the psychological, biological, or developmental processes underlying mental functioning (APA, 2013). The DSM-5 is an iterative document constantly updated through the collaboration of researchers and clinicians working with clients with mental health disorders. In fact, in 2009, the National Institute of Mental Health (NIMH) launched the Research Domain Criteria Initiative (RDoC), which provides a research framework to support the advancement of knowledge addressing mental health diagnosis, prevention, treatment, and cure (NIMH, 2022). The DSM-5 categorizes mental health disorders into the following classifications:

- Neurodevelopmental disorders
- Schizophrenia spectrum and other psychotic disorders
- Bipolar and related disorders
- Depressive disorders
- Anxiety disorders
- Obsessive-compulsive and related disorders
- Trauma- and stressor-related disorders
- Dissociative disorders
- Somatic symptoms and related disorders
- Feeding and eating disorders
- Elimination disorders
- Sleep-wake disorders
- Sexual dysfunctions
- Gender dysphoria
- Disruptive, impulse-control, and conduct disorders
- Substance-related and addictive disorders
- Neurocognitive disorders
- Personality disorders
- Paraphilic disorders
- Other mental disorders
- Medication-induced movement disorders and other adverse effects of medication
- Other conditions that may be a focus of clinical attention

The DSM-5 and the RDoC offer occupational and physical therapy practitioners valuable resources to identify and develop effective interventions for individuals with mental health disorders. Additional resources include the AOTA Mental Health Special Interest Section, the AOTA Psychosis Community of Practice, the Psychiatric Occupational Therapy Action Coalition, and the International Organization of Physical Therapists in Mental Health (IOPTMH). Box 19.1 Clinical Spotlight illustrates the role and responsibilities of

• BOX **19.1** Clinical Spotlight

A 42-year-old male is referred for physical therapy at a state psychiatric hospital for abnormal head and neck positioning. He is on multiple medications for depression and anxiety and is independent with ADLs and ambulation. Upon observation, the client ambulates in the hallway with his head in significant right cervical rotation and maintains this position even when eating. He has had multiple medical tests, including a radiograph of his spine, and reports are negative for a medical cause of his neck position. Nursing staff who check on the client throughout the night report that his head and neck seem to have full movement when he is asleep. Upon entering the clinic, the client paced around the room, was very hesitant to speak about his neck, and would not allow the therapist to palpate or passively move his head. After building rapport within the session, the client was able to lie supine but allowed no further intervention for short periods (1–2 minutes). He continued to have his head in right cervical rotation. Through multiple treatment sessions, he began to perform active left cervical rotation while supine on a plinth. He was given encouragement and positive feedback and the therapist always acknowledged his pain. By the third session, the client cried as he revealed that his neck had been in this position since he was assaulted in a previous treatment facility. After eight sessions, the client could complete full active cervical range of motion in all planes and allowed the therapist to perform soft tissue mobilization.

Consider the following questions:
- What differential diagnoses do you think were considered by the referring physician?
- What billing codes could be used for the initial sessions?
- What interpersonal skills can be used during a treatment session with clients with Functional Neurological Symptom Disorder and how might you build rapport with this client?
- What environmental modifications could be used in the clinic?
- What might be helpful and purposeful instructions for support staff?

occupational and physical therapy practitioners in addressing their clients' mental health in a psychiatric health facility. Read the scenarios and reflect on the questions provided.

Response to Illness and Injury

Serious and chronic illness, traumatic injury, or prolonged hospitalization can lead to mental health challenges and diminish the long-term quality of life outcomes in clients (Herrera-Escobar et al., 2021; Kellezi et al., 2017). Depression, anxiety, and post-traumatic stress disorder are common post-injury, illness, and the onset of disability conditions. Mental health challenges are common among those experiencing chronic illness and disability but rarely are they referred to a mental healthcare provider as a part of their treatment plan (CDC, 2021). A person's experience of disability is derived from an array of experiences, which may include their (1) cultural, social, and religious background and their views of health and disability, (2) personality, temperament, and tolerance for discomfort and change, and (3) the onset and the progressive nature of the condition and subsequent disabling impacts. When individuals are able to exert control and choice (i.e., self-determination) and have confidence that they can master

the realistic and meaningful goals they set (i.e., self-efficacy), their performance, participation, and sense of well-being are enhanced (Baum et al., 2015). The WHO purports, "To reach a state of complete physical, mental, and social wellbeing, an individual or group must be able to identify and realize aspirations, to satisfy needs, and to change or cope with the environment" (1986, p.1). Well-being is altered when an individual is impacted by disability, and either cannot effectively exert control or choice, set or achieve goals, or meaningfully engage in the social, physical, or cultural environment due to health and participation challenges (Pizzi & Richards, 2017).

Coping

The process of coping with and adjusting to serious and chronic illness or disability has been studied for decades and numerous psychosocial models of adaptation have been explored (Jensen et al., 2011; Livneh, 2001; Livneh & Martz, 2016; Savage, 2005). *Stage phase models* align psychological reactions in an overlapping process of separation (shock and denial), liminality (anxiety and anger), and reorganization (acceptance and adjustment). *Linear models* similarly organize responses in stages; however, there is an additional emphasis on positive and negative mediating factors, such as the type, severity, and duration of the condition, the personality characteristics of the client, and the physical, social, and cultural environmental characteristics. These factors influence emotional regulation and coping adaptation through the recovery process. *Pendular models* posit that coping with serious and chronic illness and disability requires a reorganization and reconstruction of one's self-image, which results in many of the psychological responses described in stage phase and linear models. However, pendular models account for the constant swing back and forth of a pre- to post-disability image of self and back again.

Coping with serious and chronic illness and disability is often more complex and less predictable than the preceding models suggest. The psychological trauma associated with these conditions often renders the individual's normal coping patterns inaccessible or inadequate to manage overwhelming anxiety (Parker et al., 2003). Perceptions, emotions, and behaviors become disorganized and ineffective, and anxiety, depression, personality disorders, or dissociative reactions can occur (Savage, 2005). The recovery process through rehabilitation provides a gradual but continual interaction between one's limitations and residual and emergent abilities and mastery within carefully constructed physical, social, and cultural environments. Occupational and physical therapy practitioners who engage their clients in spontaneous, creative, problem-solving, and risk-taking tasks promote self-regulation and reorganization of self-image and adaptive patterns of coping.

Coping challenges may be additionally exacerbated by individuals who have experienced illness and injury requiring critical care and mechanical ventilation in their medical course. Post-intensive care syndrome (PICS) is a collection of physical, cognitive, and emotional characteristics that persist in many clients into subacute and post-hospitalization (Fernandes et al., 2019). Physical characteristics such as fatigue, difficulty sleeping, decreased appetite, and impaired respiratory function have been reported. Cognitive and emotional characteristics include memory impairments, difficulty concentrating and making decisions, and anxiety and depression. Symptoms of posttraumatic disorder have been documented. Reducing the risk factors associated with PICS requires careful attention to pain, agitation, sedation, and glycemic management. In addition, delirium in postoperative and acute care settings is a significant risk factor for poor mental health and rehabilitation outcomes (Lee et al., 2020). Occupational and physical therapy practitioners offer valuable contributions to the healthcare team in identifying and preventing agitation and delirium, promoting adequate pain control, educating staff, clients, and their families, and advancing supportive discharge plans.

Mental Health and Chronic Pain

The history and current management of chronic pain are replete with examples of team development and collaboration. Dissatisfied with the results of using regional anesthesia to manage chronic pain in soldiers returning from military service following World War II, Dr. John Bonica led an interprofessional team to examine the medical literature addressing pain (Ballantyne et al., 2018). In the early 1950s, he and his team of professionals from the fields of neurology, psychiatry, and orthopedics developed the first multidisciplinary pain clinic, co-locating healthcare team members in one place and increasing the efficiency of their consultative and collaborative practice. The success of Bonica's and colleagues' collaborative success in treating chronic pain and their founding of a national organization and professional journal dedicated to pain research led to heightened attention to pain and pain management and the proliferation of interprofessional pain clinics around the globe by the 1970s (Ballantyne et al., 2018).

In 20 years, the team approach to chronic pain management advanced treatments from a focus on correcting an injury that caused pain and the anesthetization of the nociceptors surrounding the region to an interprofessional client-focused approach to pain management. The work of behavioral psychologist Wilbert Fordyce in the late 1970s reinforces the value of the biopsychosocial model still used in pain clinics today (Fordyce, 1982). The components of the model, to which a team of physicians, psychologists, social workers, and occupational and physical therapy practitioners contributed, include (Andrasik et al., 2005; Dickinson et al., 2007; Gatchel, 2007; Miaskowski et al., 2020):

- Administering medicine on a predetermined schedule versus responding to changes in perceived pain.
- Rewarding client behaviors associated with pain reduction or increased engagement in functional activity and movement (e.g., improved exercise tolerance, increases in work and social activities).

- Reduction in or extinction of pain-related behaviors (e.g., facial grimaces, verbal complaints, reliance on pharmaceuticals, sedentary behavior).
- Resting after exercise regimens or functional activities are completed instead of when pain increases.

This revolutionary and valuable approach to chronic pain management of the 1960s and 1970s eroded by the end of the 1990s; however, when payment models shifted to fee-for-service, the growth of managed care shifted from team to point-of-service care, and the development of medical subspecialty situated pain management on nerve blocks, ablations, and insertions of spinal cord stimulators. Interprofessional pain clinics closed, leaving chronic pain management to primary care providers and their arsenal of pharmaceutical options, primarily opioids, and modality-specific chronic pain treatment centers. The availability and marketing of exogenous opioids (e.g., oxycodone, hydrocodone, morphine, and methadone), their widespread effect on the central and peripheral nervous system, and a lack of evidence regarding their addictive qualities made them a treatment of choice for many healthcare providers (Berrettini, 2016).

Concerned with undiagnosed pain, misguided treatments, and inappropriate client goals, in 1996, the American Pain Society began its campaign to educate healthcare providers to assess and address their clients' pain (Campbell, 2016). Shortly after, the Joint Commission on Accreditation of Healthcare Organizations established guidelines mandating pain assessment and treatment in all accredited settings (Curtiss, 2001). Simultaneously, Purdue Pharma introduced OxyContin, a sustained-release opioid-based formulation. Since that time, scientists have discovered the addictive quality of opioids, but also the brain may reduce the natural pain-killing neurotransmitters to compensate for the saturation of opioids, requiring increased frequency and dosage of opioid medication. The United States Department of Health and Human Services (2022) reports that in 2019, an estimated 10.1 million individuals aged 12 years or older misused opioids in the past year.

Contemporary Pain Management

Contemporary efforts by the International Association for the Study of Pain include bringing scientists, healthcare providers, and policymakers together to study pain and translate knowledge into improved pain relief for clients worldwide. Advances in neuroscience have improved the understanding of the neurophysiology of pain, nociceptors and nociceptive signal transmission, pain modulation mechanisms, and the perception of pain (Berrettini, 2016). Occupational and physical therapy practitioners play a central role in the advances in non-pharmacological approaches to pain management, particularly in the case of chronic pain. The criteria for chronic pain include (Balagué et al., 2012; Butler & Moseley, 2020; Nijs et al., 2014):

- Pain persistence longer than 4 months.
- Pain intensity that is unrelated to the physical severity of the original injury.

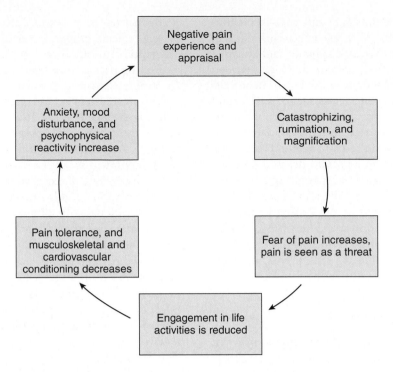

• **Fig. 19.4** The Cyclical Process From Pain to Psychophysiological Reactivity

- The lack of presence of ongoing damaging processes.
- The presence of psychological variables (e.g., somatic focus, depression, impaired sleep, anxiety, hopelessness, withdrawal).

The Fear Avoidance Model describes how individuals experiencing pain become trapped in this cycle resulting in chronic pain and disablement (Crombez et al., 2012; Vlaeyen & Linton, 2012). Fear-avoidance may lead to increased pain or reinjury, resulting in decreased engagement in life activities, disuse deconditioning, and, paradoxically, increased pain. When clients have a negative experience and appraise their pain, they reduce their daily activity in anticipation of pain. A cyclical process leading from pain to psychophysiological reactivity ensues (Leeuw et al., 2007; Vlaeyen & Linton, 2000) and is illustrated in Fig. 19.4.

Fear-avoidance reactivity is not uncommon in those who experience musculoskeletal conditions or falls. When a client experiences a fall, the fall experience may result in fear of falling. As a result, clients may avoid physical activity to prevent future falls. In 2015, the Joint Commission issued Sentinel Event Alert 55 to prevent and reduce fall-related injuries in healthcare facilities, and since its publication, addressing falls and fall-related injuries has also been at the forefront within mental health facilities (Joint Commission, 2015). Fall risk and prevention in mental health facilities, particularly in acute settings, is critically important due to numerous risk factors, including polypharmacy or medication use with side effects of dizziness or orthostatic hypotension, poorly fitting footwear, decreased or ineffective use of assistive devices, aggressive events or behavioral concerns, cognitive impairments, or confusion, and decreased impulse control and balance problems (Abraham, 2016).

A team approach must be taken to prevent and reduce falls and the responsibility does not lie solely with the nursing staff. Occupational and physical therapy practitioners have an important role to play in fall prevention and reduction, including staff and client education, team communication, client assessment and treatment, and system-level data collection and analysis. Occupational and physical therapy practitioners should be considered for involvement in mental health facility design to address factors influencing fall risk and preventing falls.

Occupational and physical therapy interventions focus on disrupting the chronic pain cycle that leads an individual experiencing pain from avoidance of activity to increased negative emotions, from withdrawal and further avoidance to deconditioning, distress, and disability, and finally catastrophizing and leading to further chronic pain responses (Murphy et al., 2014). The adoption of the biopsychosocial model is once again the theoretical framework of choice because it promotes the team's interaction with the biological and psychosocial aspects of pain. It acknowledges the interaction between the physical body and the mind and social context and it emphasizes teaching clients how to address these issues effectively in their pain management. Evaluation and intervention focus on the client's functioning and aim to change how the client reacts to pain by providing pain education, illuminating hurt versus harm, and highlighting pain's impact on thoughts, feelings, and behaviors. By leveraging this model, occupational and physical therapy practitioners can introduce safe and consistent activities and build active coping skills throughout their interventions. Chronic pain interventions may include:

- Sleep hygiene
- Lifestyle redesign

- Gradual exposure to safe physical activities
  - Finding and engaging in meaningful activity
  - Diversifying activity options
  - Whole body reconditioning
  - Establishing activity pacing structure
- Learn, implement, and practice relaxation techniques
  - Diaphragmatic breathing
  - Visualization
  - Relaxation and breathing apps
  - Mindfulness meditation

Pain neuroscience education is a promising biopsychosocial approach that uses simple narratives and images, metaphors, and drawings to educate clients about the nervous system's neurobiology and neurophysiology of pain and pain processing (Louw et al., 2011; Zimney et al., 2014). Pain neuroscience education has been shown to change the perception of pain and the pain experience, reduce fear and catastrophizing, increase physical activity, increase pain thresholds during activity, and improve adherence and outcomes of therapeutic exercise in clients with chronic pain.

Occupational and physical therapy practitioners are critical partners in developing evidence-based non-pharmaceutical pain management interventions for the future. Interprofessional client-centered care is again at the forefront, and involving clients in the care decision-making process is a hallmark of the provision of services. The 2021 ACPA-Stanford Resource Guide to Chronic Pain Management (American Chronic Pain Association [ACPA], 2021) includes numerous interventions that are included in the scopes of occupational and physical therapy practice, such as functional activity training, active exercise (e.g., range of motion, stretching, strength training, cardiovascular conditioning), Pilates, Tai Chi, Qigong, yoga, Feldenkrais Method, art activities, and mindfulness and imagery activities.

Box 19.2 Clinical Spotlight illustrates the role and responsibilities of occupational and physical therapy practitioners in addressing their clients' mental health in an outpatient orthopedic health facility. Read the scenarios and reflect on the questions provided.

Trauma

Trauma is the physical and emotional response individuals experience following an event that threatens physical or emotional harm. Single or repeated exposure to deeply distressing events often overwhelms an individual's ability to cope and may result in acute or long-term effects on mental, physical, emotional, social, and spiritual well-being (SAMHSA, 2022b). While more about the subjective experience of trauma rather than what happened, trauma affects individuals of all ages, gender, socioeconomic, race, ethnicity, and affinity. Common physical symptoms include nausea, dizziness, disturbed sleep patterns, insomnia, changes in appetite, headaches, and gastrointestinal problems and may mask trauma exposure and emotional responses (Rueness et al., 2020; Schnurr et al., 1998). Additionally,

---

• BOX 19.2 Clinical Spotlight

An 18-year-old female presents in an outpatient clinic with an 8-month history of severe right leg pain, weakness, and decreased active range of motion. There were concerns about contractures, but under anesthesia, she has full range of motion in all joints of her right leg. She now uses a wheelchair for mobility and does not bear weight on her right leg. She sits with her right leg flexed at the hip and knee with her right foot resting on the wheelchair. She has received many medical diagnostic tests, none revealing a medical cause for her symptoms. Her quality of life and independence have decreased significantly since the onset of her symptoms. Her prior level of function included competitive volleyball; however, no known leg injury occurred preceding the onset of symptoms.

A review of her medical records reveals that she has a history of sexual abuse at 17 years old. During the first physical therapy appointment, she would not allow the physical therapist to touch her leg and screamed if she believed someone might touch her leg.

Consider the following questions:

- How would you discuss the client's symptoms with the rest of the team? Would you suggest that the client is "faking" her symptoms?
- Given her prior level of function and the known symptomology, what are some examples of short-term or long-term goals?
- What would be your first treatment approach?
- If you had access to a pool for aquatic therapy, would you consider it for this client?
- What phrases could be said to the client to promote trust and self-confidence?

---

individuals who have experienced trauma may be at higher risk of several physical health conditions and poor health outcomes (Pietrzak et al., 2012). Emotional signs of trauma exposure include sadness, anger, denial, fear, and shame, which can result in psychological disorders such as post-traumatic stress disorder, depression, anxiety, dissociative disorders, and substance abuse problems (SAMHSA, 2022b).

Acute exposure to trauma activates the survival response of fight-flight-freeze, which can include increased heart rate, sweating, shallow breathing, and decreased digestion (Murison, 2016; Vyas et al., 2016). Over time, trauma leads to hypervigilance and hyper or hypo arousal, decreased attention, memory, and problem solving, emotional numbing and social withdrawal and relationship issues, and, for some, near constant fight-flight-freeze responses. Structural changes in the brain have been reported that result in emotional dysregulation and dissociation (Murison, 2016; Perry & Szalavitz, 2017; Rodenbush, 2015; Vyas et al., 2016). Challenges in attention and activity regulation, executive functioning, motor planning, and social participation are often experienced. In children, the root of these functional challenges can be masked by diagnoses with similar presentations, such as attention deficit hyperactivity disorder and learning disability (The National Child Traumatic Stress Network, 2016; Rodenbush, 2015).

Adverse Childhood Experiences

Early adversity and trauma exposure can have lasting effects on physical health and quality of life outcomes and contribute to significant public health issues (Ranjbar & Erb, 2019). To understand these impacts, Felitti and his colleagues (1998) undertook an expansive retrospective study at Kaiser Permanente from 1995 through 1997 of the impact of adverse childhood and disruptive household experiences on individual and community health through the lifespan. In what became known as the Adverse Childhood Experiences (ACE) study, the researchers examined the relationship between abuse and household dysfunction occurring during the first 18 years of life and disease risk factors, incidence, and mortality, healthcare utilization, and quality of life through the lifespan. Medical records were reviewed and health outcomes were compared with subjects' responses on a questionnaire examining childhood exposure to psychological abuse, physical abuse, contact sexual abuse, exposure to substance abuse, mental illness, violent treatment of mother or stepmother, and criminal behavior (Felitti et al., 1998). Felitti and his team (1998) discovered that an ACE score has both a strong and cumulative effect on the health of adults, and a score of four or above increased the occurrence of the health risk factors such as smoking, severe obesity, physical inactivity, depressed mood, suicide attempts, alcoholism, use of illicit drugs, injection of illicit drugs, and incidence of sexually transmitted disease. The higher the ACE score, the higher the risk of poor health (Anda et al., 2006; Deighton et al., 2018).

The ACE study demonstrated a correlation between childhood trauma exposure and later engagement in health-risk behaviors typically associated with coping strategies (Deighton et al., 2018; Felitti et al., 1998). Smoking, alcohol use, overeating, overtly sexualized behaviors, and many sexual partners are commonly used to cope with abuse, violence exposure, and family dysfunction (Felitti et al., 1998). The early and prolonged engagement in health-risk behaviors as a response to trauma exposure may manifest itself as chronic diseases and poor health outcomes (Felitti et al., 1998).

Trauma and Treatment Implications

Attention to the prevalence of trauma exposure and treating all clients with sensitivity is critical for all rehabilitation professionals (Ranjbar & Erb, 2019). Primary prevention of childhood trauma exposure will minimize the long-term health effects and require sociopolitical change (Felitti et al., 1998). When exposure is present, implementing behavioral coping strategies is a way to prevent childhood and adolescent health-risk behaviors (Felitti et al., 1998). An adult dealing with the effects of ACE will need assistance to change the health-risk behaviors they have adopted and engaged in throughout their life (Felitti et al., 1998). Client-centered care may be insufficient; following principles of trauma-informed care may be critical to meeting the healthcare needs of this population. The CDC Center for Preparedness and Response, in collaboration with SAMHSA's National Center for Trauma-Informed Care, offers the following guiding principles to guide treatment for individuals who have experienced trauma (CDC, 2020):

- Safety: Ensure physical and emotional safety for individuals throughout the system of care. Create an environment that is predictable, easy to navigate, and calm. Avoid known and expected triggers and retraumatization/revictimization.
- Trustworthiness and transparency: Focus on the relationship and show empathy. Communicate clearly and slowly and without judgment. Consider the power imbalance and be respectful of client boundaries. Take every opportunity to educate clients and ask permission for interventions and procedures.
- Empowerment and choice: Provide an opportunity for choice and decision-making with autonomy. Educative interventions are valuable to the client, though information may need to be broken down depending on the client's level of arousal and dysregulation.
- Collaboration and mutuality: Facilitate opportunities to collaborate and share power. Work with clients on collaboratively identifying and responding to signs of stress and co-develop strategies to address feelings of vulnerability. Recognize when the client's needs are beyond the scope of occupational or physical therapy practice and refer to other qualified professionals.
- Cultural, historical, and gender issues: Be attentive to how policy, procedure, process, and procedures impact and influence the quality of care of individuals and groups of varying gender, cultural, and historical associations.

Childhood Mental Disorders

Analysis of the 2016 National Survey of Children's Health conducted by the Data Resource Center for Child and Adolescent Health. Child and Adolescent Health Measurement Initiative revealed that at least one in six children and youth in the United States (7.7 million) have both an identifiable and treatable mental health disorder (Whitney & Peterson, 2019). Mental health disorders in childhood often result in significant impacts on emotional, behavioral, and learning development and can impair transition to and quality of life during adulthood (Global Burden of Disease Pediatrics Collaboration et al., 2016), yet 49% of children and youth with a mental health condition do not receive needed care (Whitney & Peterson, 2019). Children and youth with mental health disorders can have difficulty managing emotions (e.g., persistent sadness) and forming and maintaining relationships (e.g., withdrawal) at home, school, and in the community, engaging effectively in routines and activities, difficulty sleeping and concentrating, and wide mood and behavioral swings (e.g., outbursts).

Common mental health disorders seen in childhood include autism spectrum disorders (16.1%), depression (6.2%), attention deficit and hyperactivity disorder (5.5%), conduct disorder (5.0%), eating disorders (4.4%), and anxiety (3.2%) (Erskine et al., 2017). Other, more severe mental health conditions such as pediatric bipolar disorder, avoidant-restrictive food intake disorder, oppositional defiant disorder, disruptive mood dysregulation disorder, and childhood schizophrenia are less prevalent but require an intensive array of services across the

As a school-based occupational or physical therapist, you are informed of a student with an Individualized Education Program (IEP) who may need a therapy evaluation and are invited to attend the IEP meeting. The student is a 12-year-old female who is finishing 6th grade. She has chronic low back pain and left ankle pain. The team has concerns regarding the student's decreased ability to ambulate between locations in the building and participate in gross motor activities, such as physical education and field trips. The student struggles with fatigue during the day, computer skills, and executive functioning. She is falling behind on schoolwork, and it is affecting her grades and social aspects of her school day. She was adopted from an orphanage in Russia at two and is identified under the educational category of Speech-Language Impairment and Other Health Impairment. Depending on symptoms, the student alternates between independent ambulation, using forearm crutches, and self-propelling a manual wheelchair. There are no known injuries and the symptoms began gradually 10 months ago. The student has lost voluntary left ankle control and complains of numbness. A few weeks ago, she started to have tremors and weakness in her left hand.

Medical records indicate the student has received multiple diagnostic tests, including radiographs, MRIs of the brain, spine, arm, and leg, EMGs, and blood tests. The working diagnosis is Functional Neurological Symptom Disorder. She receives outpatient physical, occupational, and speech therapies.

Consider the following questions:

- What would you recommend to the IEP team regarding an evaluation for school physical or occupational therapy? Should any other data be collected?
- What are possible accommodations?
- How would you educate the school staff regarding the student's physical limitations and diagnosis?
- If the team decided to proceed with evaluations, what possible outcome measures or tests could you perform?
- In what settings of the school environment would you want to observe the student?

continuum of care. Services include play therapy, cognitive-behavioral therapy, parent education, family therapy, intensive behavioral intervention, and medication (Waddell et al., 2015). Engaging children and youth with mental health disorders in prosocial activities and occupations of meaning, such as self-care, play, leisure, and social participation, can significantly improve occupational performance, behavior, and social participation (Brooks & Bannigan, 2021). Box 19.3 Clinical Spotlight illustrates the role and responsibilities of occupational and physical therapy practitioners in addressing their clients' mental health in an educational setting. Read the scenarios and reflect on the questions provided.

Substance Use

NIMH defines substance use disorder (SUD) as "a mental disorder that affects a person's brain and behavior, leading to a person's inability to control their use of substances such as legal or illegal drugs, alcohol, or medications" (NIMH, n.d.). NIMH suggests that SUDs can range from mild to moderate to severe, with substance dependency and addiction characterizing the most severe form. Nearly half of all individuals who develop SUDs experience co-occurring mental illness (Kelly & Daley, 2013; Ross & Peselow, 2012). This co-occurrence may be attributed to overlapping risk factors for both mental disorders and SUDS, such as genetics and environmental factors (e.g., stress, trauma), use of substances to self-medicate for individuals with mental disorders, or changes in brain structure and function due to substance use in individuals with SUDs which may contribute to the development of a mental disorder (NIMH, n.d.) Additionally, high rates of substance use are seen in clients with anxiety disorders and mental disorders such as depression, bipolar, attention-deficit hyperactivity, psychotic illness, borderline personality, and antisocial personality (National Institute on Drug Abuse [NIDA], 2020).

Treatment for SUDs should be comprehensive, well-coordinated, inclusive of mental disorder treatment, and individualized to meet the individual's unique needs. Treatment may be provided along a continuum, ranging from substance use/relapse prevention and early intervention/identification to outpatient and inpatient/residential treatment. NIDA (2020) proposes that comprehensive substance use care includes comprehensive case management and substance use monitoring, recovery support programs offered over the full continuum of care, and evidence-based interventions that provide mental and physical health, educational, vocational, and legal services, and family systems support. According to NIDA (2019), common evidence-based treatments for SUDs include:

- Detoxification
- Medication to treat opioid, tobacco, or alcohol use
- Behavioral therapy (e.g., cognitive behavioral therapy, multidimensional family therapy, motivational interviewing/incentives)
- Evaluation/treatment for co-occurring mental disorders
- Relapse prevention

Occupational and physical therapy practitioners can support individuals with SUDs as part of an interdisciplinary team with unique expertise in medication management, physical and mental well-being, the establishment of healthy habits and routines (e.g., physical exercise), daily living and work skill development, building and maintaining healthy relationships, and discovering/engaging in meaningful occupations (Wilburn et al., 2021). Research indicates occupational therapy services for individuals with addiction typically focus on skills training, occupation-based intervention, and supporting individuals with establishing and maintaining sobriety through community-based programming/routines, with the most effective being prioritization of occupational engagement and client-centered practice in addition to skills training (Ryan & Boland, 2021). Physical therapy practitioners often focus on addressing SUDs through stress and pain management (emphasis on nonopioid pain treatment) and motivational interviewing (APTA, 2018).

Mental Health Disorders in Incarcerated Populations

Serious mental health disorders are overrepresented in prison populations, with an estimated one in seven individuals experiencing clinical depression or psychosis (Fazel et al., 2016). Studies of prevalence rates indicate that serious mental illness affects an average of 14.5% of men and 31.0% of women imprisoned in the United States justice system (Steadman et al., 2009). The percentage of women who are incarcerated and have a history of sexual or physical abuse is reported to be as high as 60%–80% (Browne et al., 1999; Jordan et al., 1996; Owen & Bloom, 1997). Mental illness among prisoners increases their risk of self-harm and suicide attempt, victimization, and violence (Fazel, 2016), issues that might prompt a referral to occupational and physical therapy services. Practitioners working with imprisoned individuals should collaborate with the care team to identify mental health problems and incorporate trauma-focused and gender-specific interventions to meet their unique needs.

The complex dynamic between jail or prison systems and psychiatric hospitals is evidenced in some states when an individual is found not mentally fit to stand trial (Stringer, 2019). At that time, the person awaits evaluation or transfer to an inpatient facility to receive treatment. The interconnections between the justice system and mental health resources are complicated and persistent issues that require effective processes and proper resources (Stringer, 2019). Failures in mental health resources being available to individuals who are incarcerated can have serious consequences for the person and the community (Stringer, 2019). Clients may be referred to occupational or physical therapy practitioners at any point in their justice-system involvement for various reasons, including assistive device evaluations, daily living skills, and chronic pain.

Providers and Care Coordination

Providing care for clients with mental health needs requires the coordination of the client, their caregivers/family, and an array of healthcare professionals who serve their unique and diverse needs. Care provision is generally provided across a continuum of increasing complexity from self-care to peer support, to community-based (e.g., health and wellness centers and employee wellness resources), to primary care, to hospital-based (e.g., emergency room, inpatient acute psychiatric care, inpatient long-term psychiatric care) service delivery. Care is recovery-focused and person-centered (Davidson et al., 2010; Jacob, 2015). However, in the US health system, there are generally two distinct systems of care: one for diagnosing and treating mental illness and one for physical.

As outlined throughout this chapter, separating these often-co-occurring conditions is difficult and inadequate. Separating them influences the effectiveness of intervention and impacts health outcomes. In a recent New England Journal of Medicine (NEJM) Catalyst Insights Council

survey of 565 healthcare executives, clinical leaders, and healthcare practitioners from health systems, hospitals, and provider organizations, 14% of respondents indicated that their healthcare organizations do not offer mental health services and, of those that did, 61% indicated that their healthcare system services are not adequate to meet the need (Compton-Phillips & Mohta, 2018). A range of barriers, including absent or inadequate insurance coverage and costs, access to appropriate care, and care fragmentations, prevents the effective delivery of mental health care across many healthcare systems (Compton-Phillips & Mohta, 2018). To improve patient outcomes, the NEJM Catalyst Insights Council suggests that mental health must be integrated and coordinated across healthcare, including primary, ambulatory, specialty, and acute care settings. All providers must actively identify and collaborate to address each client's mental health needs (Compton-Phillips & Mohta, 2018).

Collaboration and Care Coordination

Effective care providers work in partnership with other members of the team. Understanding the roles and goals of team members, developing, and employing effective communication skills, and participating in shared decision-making are essential skills of members of the care team (Institute of Medicine [IOM], 2006). Providers strive to coordinate and integrate care "across people, functions, activities, and sites over time to maximize the value of services delivered to patients" (Shortell et al., 2000, p. 129). Integration must occur across the levels of the client, the program, and the systems to ensure effective care (IOM, 2006). The APA describes the Collaborative Care Model as an integrated client treatment that results from care providers intentionally coordinating services to address the client's individual and often co-occurring needs (see Chapter 20). Integrated programs are characterized by closely linked infrastructure that promotes access to and communication with care providers across the care context. Finally, integrated systems ensure an organizational structure that supports programming and treatment across the care continuum through infrastructure tools such as diverse funding mechanisms, data collection, and reporting, needs assessment and planning, program development, and collaborative operational functions.

Occupational and physical therapy practitioners are essential providers in the service delivery continuum of integrated care and can effectively address the intersecting co-occurring mental and general health challenges in mental health care. The Collaborative Care Model highlights five key priorities: client-centered team care, measurement-based treatment, evidence-based care, population-based care, and accountable care (APA, 2022). Client-centered care focuses the entire care team on the client's unique goals and integrates services to avoid duplication and discomfort. Using a measurement-based treatment framework, care providers and clients collaborate on developing client-centered goals, and progress and outcomes are regularly monitored. Treatments are based upon the best available evidence to ensure efficacy and positive, cost-effective outcomes. Population-based care tracks groups of clients across the care continuum to ensure that clients' progress and services are efficiently adjusted and implemented as needed. Finally, in the Collaborative Care Model, providers are accountable for the quality of their care and the outcomes for their clients. Reimbursement is based on clinical outcomes versus volume of care.

Therapeutic Use of Self

Therapeutic use of self (TUS) is an integral part of the therapeutic process for individuals needing mental health care (Currid & Pennington, 2010). Healthcare providers use TUS as a tool across the continuum to focus support on client strengths and collaborative goal setting (Arnd-Caddigan & Pozzuto, 2008). Taylor and colleagues (2009) describe TUS as a practitioner's planned use of their personality, perceptions, and insights as integral components of the therapeutic process. TUS is commonly used therapeutically in the following ways (Dewane, 2006):

- Use of personality: Using knowledge of the characteristics and traits of oneself to interact successfully with others.
- Use of belief system: Strengthening understanding of one's belief system and identifying how our worldview and biases may influence the therapeutic process.
- Use of relational dynamics: Using knowledge of how individuals interact in the context of relationships to facilitate effective interaction. The Intentional Relationship Model helps practitioners learn to navigate interpersonal events that occur in relationships to strengthen their therapeutic value (Taylor et al., 2009). In addition, forming clear boundaries and professional codes of conduct support the effective use of relational dynamics therapeutically (Zur, 2004).
- Use of anxiety: Attending to anxiety-provoking experiences can lead to valuable insights regarding the effectiveness of mental healthcare.
- Use of self-disclosure: Though somewhat controversial, Dewane (2006) suggests that using appropriate self-disclosure in which the focus remains on the client can support the formation of a trusting and authentic relationship.

Providers can enhance their skills in the use of TUS by examining their belief systems and assumptions (Cooper, 2007) and attending to skills that promote emotional intelligence (listening, empathy, self-control) (Bar-On, 2010; Cooper, 2007; Leahy, 2008; Roberts et al., 2010), and establishing mentorship and supervisory relationships (Milne & James, 2002; Wheeler & Richards 2007). In addition, taking care of oneself is critical. High stress and poor psychological well-being of healthcare providers can negatively impact the effectiveness of TUS (Robertson & Flint Taylor, 2010).

Evaluation and Intervention Planning

Clients experiencing mental health disorders are often referred to occupational and physical therapy practitioners for co-occurring conditions and those referred due to their mental illness symptoms often find it challenging to identify how their symptoms impact their everyday function. These challenges can lead to inaccurate diagnosis and implementation of effective intervention. Occupational and physical therapy practitioners can be instrumental to the healthcare team in identifying the functional challenges experienced by their clients. The AOTA OTPF-4 (AOTA, 2020) and the APTA Guide to Physical Therapy Practice 3.0 (PT Guide) (APTA, 2014) guide the collection of evaluative data occupational and physical therapy practitioners can use to evaluate clients. The process of evaluation during which the practitioner gathers data on what the client can do (capacity), what they do daily (habits and routines), and how they perform it is illustrated by Rogers & Holm (2016).

As illustrated in Fig. 19.5, the evaluation process is ongoing. Throughout the therapy process, the practitioner constantly gathers and assesses data regarding the client's strengths, limitations, interests, and participation. The range of participatory challenges changes as the client progresses through the therapy process, and careful data collection and analysis are required to measure progress and to modify intervention approaches.

Evidence-based occupational and physical therapy interventions have been developed and implemented across various mental health challenges (AOTA, 2010; D'Amico, 2018). Common interventions include the following:

- Environmental adaptation and modification: Adapting and modifying the environment reduces physiological and psychological triggers, promotes organization and control, and reduces physical and social participation barriers.
- Sleep hygiene: Promote effective sleep hygiene routines and effective sleep/rest patterns. Clients may find that engaging in activity supports sleep-rest patterns.
- Exercise: Engage in various physical activities that promote physical engagement and regulate activity, emotional responses, and connection to others (Danielsen et al., 2021).
- Pilates, Tai Chi, Qigong, yoga, Feldenkrais Method: Movement-based rehabilitation therapies that engage the mind and body concurrently have been shown to be effective in reducing pain and improving range of motion, strength, balance, coordination, cardiovascular health, physical fitness, mood, and cognition (Phuphanich et al., 2020).
- Mindfulness/guided imagery: Meditation that promotes nonjudgmental awareness, attention, and acceptance of the sensory details of the body and environments to reduce the emotional and physiological responses to stress, anxiety, and depressive symptoms to promote healing (Gu et al., 2015; Janssen et al., 2018; Kabat-Zinn, 2015).
- Self-care and leisure activity participation: Engaging in purposeful, meaningful, and culturally relevant occupations can promote function and well-being (Ikiugu et al., 2019).
- Social participation: Positive mental health effects have been noted when individuals experiencing mental health challenges participate socially with others, and it is found to be a protective factor against mental illness in individuals experiencing neurodiversity (Brooks et al., 2021).

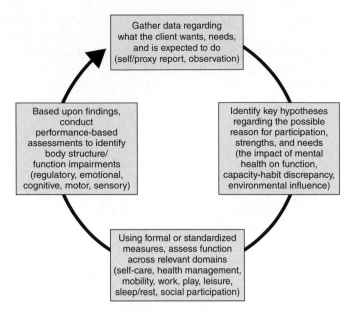

• **Fig. 19.5** The Evaluation Process

- Education and educational programs: Educative interventions are valuable tools to prevent mental illness and improve mental health outcomes. Occupational and physical therapy practitioners can educate clients on the use of evidence-based non-pharmaceutical alternatives known to support individuals with recognizing and mitigating pain and other symptoms (ACPA, 2021). In addition, instructing clients in addressing barriers and establishing routines can support medication adherence and prevent substance misuse (AOTA, 2017).
- Skills training programs: Providing training in specific skills required for participation in meaningful activity, particularly in self-care, work, and leisure, and establishing effective routines can promote positive mental health (Ryan & Boland 2021).
- Cognitive-based interventions: Using cognitive-based interventions, clients learn to recognize the signs of anxiety, disordered thoughts, and emotional dysregulation and employ strategies to regulate emotions, behavior, and participation (Nakao et al., 2021).

As noted in this chapter, mental health disorders frequently co-occur with other conditions addressed by occupational and physical therapy, such as musculoskeletal, neuromotor, movement disorders (including those caused by medication), cognitive and perceptual, and sensory impairments. Identifying and examining the best available evidence to evaluate and treat these co-occurring conditions is important.

Responsibilities of a Manager/ Administrator

The responsibilities of a mental health manager/administrator vary based on the practice setting and are often dynamic, multi-faceted, and ever-changing. The manager's primary role is to work with others to achieve the intended goals or outcomes of the organization. In mental health settings, these outcomes are typically related to client safety/well-being, client quality of life/outcomes, or quality of services. To achieve desired outcomes, managers are charged with:

- Recruiting and retaining qualified personnel through sustainable workforce planning (e.g., workloads that are equitable and feasible, competitive bonuses and salaries)
- Building capacity through training and education (e.g., crisis prevention/response, evidence-based practices)
- Appraising performance of personnel and supporting professional growth
- Ensuring quality customer service and client safety/care (e.g., access to high-quality care across the continuum of care, collaborating with the interprofessional team)
- Facilitating conflict resolution and problem-solving
- Promoting a positive work culture/climate (e.g., inclusive, safe, efficient, enjoyable)
- Engaging in continuous program evaluation and quality improvement (e.g., assessing, addressing, and influencing the social determinants of health)

It is crucial for the mental health manager/administrator to be proactive, aware, and responsive to the mental health needs of the employees working within the organization. Stress and poor mental health in the workplace are known to contribute to absenteeism, loss in productivity, burnout, poor job performance, negative mental and physical health, reduced engagement in work roles, strains on communication and relationships, impairment in daily functioning, and substance use as a coping mechanism (Adams & Nguyen, 2022; CDC, 2018). Healthcare workers are particularly vulnerable to compassion fatigue, a combination of burnout and secondary trauma (Cocker & Joss, 2016).

In their research, Wu and colleagues (2021) identified eight categories of best practices to support mental health in the workplace. Occupational therapy and physical therapy practitioners are uniquely equipped to lead effectively, model, and support these best practices:

- Culture: Eliminating stigma and prioritizing well-being in the workplace
- Robust mental health benefits: Advocating and supporting mental health care access, coverage, and quality of care through benefit plans
- Mental health resources: Addressing organizational factors which contribute to stress, providing training, incorporating stress management and mindfulness as part of the workday
- Workplace policies and practices: Advocating for and valuing diversity, equity, and inclusion; safety and ergonomic practices; policies related to harassment, violence, crisis response/prevention
- Healthy work environment: Fostering connections and social engagement; incorporating healthy habits and routines into the workday, including rest
- Leadership support: Addressing work climate; modeling healthy behaviors; facilitating conflict resolution; providing constructive performance feedback and support
- Outcomes measurement: Setting goals and monitoring for improved work climate, mental well-being, access to resources, sense of belonging
- Innovation: Incorporating creative solutions, such as using technology and other strategies to increase access and remove barriers to supporting mental health

Reimbursement, Documentation, and Quality Improvement

Measuring and improving the quality of mental health care is paramount for administrators and providers alike. Kilbourne and colleagues (2018) suggest that despite considerable commitment to do so, little progress has been made, and the quality of mental healthcare remains poor. They identified several barriers to quality improvement efforts, including "lack of standardized information technology-based data sources, limited scientific evidence for mental health quality measures, lack of provider training and support, and cultural barriers to integrating mental health care within general health environments" (p. 30) and suggest the following actions necessary to ensure continuous improvement:

- Develop and utilize validated measures of patient-centered outcomes across the spectrum of client factors (age, diagnosis, symptomatology, economic stability, education access and quality, health care access and quality, neighborhood and built environment, social and community context) to evaluate, monitor progress, and regularly measure client outcomes. Occupational and physical therapy practitioners utilize several valuable patient-centered measures that can be used to support the assessment of the quality of services, such as the Kohlman Evaluation of Living Skills (KELS) (Thompson, 1992), the Milwaukee evaluation of daily living skills (MEDLS) (Leonardelli, 1988), the Canadian occupational performance measure (COPM) (Carswell et al., 2004), the routine task inventory (RTI-E) (Allen & Katz, 2006), and the performance of self-care skills (PASS) (Rogers & Holm, 1989).

- Identify, aggregate, and analyze common data elements addressing client factors, evidence-based interventions, and clinical measures. Occupational and physical therapy practitioners carefully collect and document client evaluation, progress, and outcome data following ethical and practice guidelines and are well positioned to collaborate with their teams to evaluate relevant data to ensure quality improvement. For example, to analyze fall incident data and determine solutions for organizations, the Joint Commission Center recommends utilizing the Targeted Solutions Tool for process improvement (Joint Commission, 2015).

- Establish effective and collaborative working relationships among providers across the continuum of care. Both the OTPF-4 and the PT Guide and the professions' ethical guidelines provide clear guidance for collaboration and referral among the care team for occupational and physical therapy practitioners. Practitioners can be instrumental in designing and coordinating care across the mental health care continuum.

- Establish a wide range of evidence-based and cost-effective practices to support mental health and co-occurring conditions for clients needing services. Occupational and physical therapy practitioners are leading the way in designing and implementing evidence-based interventions that support value-based reimbursement models that demonstrate high quality and valued improvements rather than volume of service. Further work in strengthening our evidence base is needed.

Discussion

As more is learned about the classifications, etiologies, course of mental health disorders, and the impact of co-occurring health conditions, occupational and physical therapy practitioners will be increasingly called upon to address the mental health needs of the clients they treat across the continuum of healthcare, community, and educational settings. Occupational therapy has a long history of working with clients served by mental health care services and systems; physical therapy practitioners, too, are becoming valuable contributors to the interprofessional mental health care team.

The goal of the care team is to address the mental health needs of our clients in a coordinated, collaborative, and comprehensive way using evidence-based evaluation and intervention approaches that address the need of the whole client, not just the physical or mental health needs. This approach requires intentionality and understanding of the client's mental and physical health. It requires an understanding of the healthcare team and the healthcare system. It requires that occupational and physical therapy practitioners promote positive mental health across the spectrum of service delivery by helping clients take care of their physical and mental health care needs, engage in physical activity, and interact and build connections with people in their lives.

Activities

After examining the roles and responsibilities of occupational and physical therapy practitioners in mental health, consider the following:

- Occupational therapy has long been a central component of mental health care; physical therapy has not. Explain why this might be and describe how occupational and physical therapy practitioners can contribute to the mental health care team across the continuum of care.
- How can you integrate the Empowerment and Recovery Models of Care components into your evaluation and treatment?
- How can you design treatment for a client who has experienced trauma?
- What factors would you consider when a client is not making adequate progress in treatment?
- You are treating a client with a mental health disorder unfamiliar to you. What can you do to prepare for the visit?
- What strategies can you implement to reduce stress and burnout in your own life?

References

Abraham, S. (2016). Factors contributing to psychiatric patient falls. *Journal of Community Medical Health, 6*(410). doi:10.4172/2161-0711.1000410.

Adams, T., & Nguyen, T. (February 2022). *Mind the workplace 2022 report: Employer responsibility to employer mental health*. Alexandria VA: Mental Health America. https://mhanational.org/sites/default/files/MTW_Report_2022.pdf.

Allen, C., & Katz, N. (2006). *Routine task inventory - Expanded manual*. http://www.allen-cognitive-network.org/index.php/allen-model/ routine-task-inventory-expanded-rti-e.

Alonso, C., & Coe, C. L. (2001). Disruptions of social relationships accentuate the association between emotional distress and menstrual pain in young women. *Health Psychology: Official Journal of the Division of Health Psychology, American Psychological Association, 20*(6), 411–416.

Altman, B. M. (2016). Conceptual issues in disability: Saad Nagi's contribution to the disability knowledge base. Sociology looking at disability: What did we know and when did we know it. *Research in Social Science and Disability, 9*, 57–95. https://doi.org/10.1108/S1479-354720160000009006.

American Chronic Pain Association. (2021). *ACPA – Stanford Resource Guide To Chronic Pain Management An Integrated Guide to Comprehensive Pain Therapies*. https://med.stanford.edu/content/dam/sm/pain/documents/ACPA-Stanford-Resource-Guide-to-Chronic-Pain-Management-2021-Edition-4-18-21-.pdf

American Occupational Therapy Association. (2010). Specialized knowledge and skills in mental health promotion, prevention, and intervention in occupational therapy practice. *American Journal of Occupational Therapy, 64*(Suppl), S30–S43. doi:10.5014/ajot.2010.64u4.

American Occupational Therapy Association. (2017). Occupational therapy's role in medication management. *American Journal of Occupational Therapy, 71*(Suppl. 2), 7112410025p1–7112410025p20. doi:10.5014/ajot.2017.716S02.

American Occupational Therapy Association. (2020). Occupational therapy practice framework: Domain and process (4th ed.). *American Journal of Occupational Therapy, 74*(Suppl. 2), 7412410010. https://doi.org/10.5014/ajot.2020.74S2001.

American Physical Therapy Association. (2014). *Guide to physical therapy practice 3.0*. http://guidetoptpractice.apta.org.

American Physical Therapy Association. (2018). *Physical therapy can play a part in addiction treatment*. https://www.apta.org/news/2018/07/02/2018-next-physical-therapy-can-play-a-part-in-addiction-treatment.

American Physical Therapy Association. (2020). *The role of the physical therapist and the American physical therapy association in behavioral and mental health HOD P06-20-40-10 [Position]*. https://www.apta.org/apta-and-you/leadership-and-governance/policies/role-pt-apta-behavioral-mental-health.

American Psychiatric Association. (2013). *Diagnostic and statistical manual of mental disorders* (5th ed.). https://doi.org/10.1176/appi.books.9780890425596.

American Psychiatric Association. (2022). *Learn about the collaborative care model*. https://www.psychiatry.org/psychiatrists/practice/professional-interests/integrated-care/learn.

Anda, R. F., Felitti, V. J., Bremner, J. D., Walker, J. D., Whitfield, C., Perry, B. D., Dube, S. R., & Giles, W. H. (2006). The enduring effects of abuse and related adverse experiences in childhood. A convergence of evidence from neurobiology and epidemiology. *European Archives of Psychiatry and Clinical Neuroscience, 256*(3), 174–186. https://doi.org/10.1007/s00406-005-0624-4.

Anderson, P., Jané-Llopis, E., & Hosman, C. (2011). Reducing the silent burden of impaired mental health. *Health Promotion International, 26 Suppl 1*, i4–i9. https://doi.org/10.1093/heapro/dar051.

Andrasik, F., Flor, H., & Turk, D. C. (2005). An expanded view of psychological aspects in head pain: the biopsychosocial model. *Neurological Sciences: Official Journal of the Italian Neurological Society and of the Italian Society of Clinical Neurophysiology, 26 Suppl 2*, s87–s91. https://doi.org/10.1007/s10072-005-0416-7.

Arnd-Caddigan, M., & Pozzuto, R. (2008). Use of self in relational clinical social work. *Clinical Social Work Journal, 36*(3), 235–243.

Balagué, F., Mannion, A. F., Pellisé, F., & Cedraschi, C. (2012). Nonspecific low back pain. *The Lancet, 379*(9814), 482–491. https://doi.org/10.1016/S0140-6736(11)60610-7.

Ballantyne, J. C., Murinova, N., & Krashin, D. L. (2018). Opioid Guidelines Are a Necessary Response to the Opioid Crisis. *Clinical Pharmacology and Therapeutics, 103*(6), 946–949. https://doi.org/10.1002/cpt.1063

Bar-On, R. (2010). Emotional intelligence: an integral part of positive psychology. *South Africa Journal of Psychology, 40*(1), 54–62.

Baum, C., Christiansen, C., & Bass, J. (2015). Person-environment-occupational performance (PEOP) model. In C. Christiansen, C. Baum, & J. Bass (Eds.), *Occupational therapy: Performance, participation, well-being* (4th ed.). Thorofare, NJ: Slack.

Berrettini, W. (2016). Opioid neuroscience for addiction medicine: From animal models to FDA approval for alcohol addiction. *Progress in Brain Research, 223*, 253–267. https://doi.org/10.1016/bs.pbr.2015.07.030.

Brooks, R., & Bannigan, K. (2021). Occupational therapy interventions in child and adolescent mental health to increase participation: A mixed methods systematic review. *British Journal of*

Occupational Therapy, 84(8), 474–487. https://doi.org/10.1177/03080226211008718.

Brooks, R., Lambert, C., Coulthard, L., Pennington, L., & Kolehmainen, N. (2021). Social participation to support good mental health in neurodisability. *Child: Care, Health And Development, 47*(5), 675–684. https://doi.org/10.1111/cch.12876.

Browne, A., Miller, B., & Maguin, E. (1999). Prevalence and severity of lifetime physical and sexual victimization among incarcerated women. *International Journal of Law and Psychiatry, 22*(3-4), 301–322. https://doi.org/10.1016/S0160-2527(99)00011-4.

Butler, M., McCreedy, E., Schwer, N., Burgess, D., Call, K., Przedworski, J., Rosser, S., Larson, S., Allen, M., Fu, S., & Kane, R. L. (2016). *Improving cultural competence to reduce health disparities.* Agency for Healthcare Research and Quality (US).

Butler, D., & Mosley, L. (2020). *Explain pain* (2nd ed.). Noigroup Publications.

Campbell, J. N. (2016). The fifth vital sign was revisited. *Pain, 157*(1), 3–4. https://doi.org/10.1097/j.pain.0000000000000413.

Carswell, A., McColl, M. A., Baptiste, S., Law, M., Polatajko, H., & Pollock, N. (2004). The Canadian occupational performance measure: A research and clinical literature review. *Canadian Journal of Occupational Therapy. [Revue Canadienne d'Ergotherapie], 71*(4), 210–222. https://doi.org/10.1177/000841740407100406.

Centers for Disease Control and Prevention. (2018). *Mental health in the workplace.* https://www.cdc.gov/workplacehealthpromotion/tools-resources/pdfs/WHRC-Mental-Health-and-Stress-in-the-Workplac-Issue-Brief-H.pdf.

Centers for Disease Control and Prevention. (2020). *6 Guiding principles to a trauma-informed approach.* https://www.cdc.gov/cpr/infographics/6_principles_trauma_info.htm.

Centers for Disease Control and Prevention. (2021). *Diabetes and mental health.* https://www.cdc.gov/diabetes/managing/mental-health.html.

Centers for Disease Control and Prevention. (2022). *Whole school, whole community, whole child.* https://www.cdc.gov/healthyschools/wscc/index.htm.

Cioppa-Mosca, J. (2019). Rehabilitation: Keeping pace with societal needs. *HSS Journal - The Musculoskeletal Journal of Hospital for Special Surgery, 15,* 212–213. https://doi.org/10.1007/s11420-019-09716-9.

Cockburn, L. (2016). Evolution in psychosocial practice. In K. Terry, B. Kirsh, D. Pitts, & E. Fossey (Eds.), *Bruce and Borg's psychosocial frames of reference: theories, models, and approaches for occupation-based practice* (4th ed., pp. 17–29). Slack Incorporated.

Cocker, F., & Joss, N. (2016). Compassion fatigue among healthcare, emergency and community service workers: A systematic review. *International Journal of Environmental Research and Public Health, 13*(6), 618. https://doi.org/10.3390/ijerph13060618.

Compton-Phillips, A., & Mohta, N. (2018). *It's time to treat physical and mental health with equal intent: Care redesign survey.* New England Journal of Medicine Catalyst Report. https://cdn2.hubspot.net/hubfs/558940/It%E2%80%99s%20Time%20to%20Treat%20Physical%20and%20Mental%20Health%20With%20Equal%20Intent.pdf.

Cooper, M. (2007). Humanizing psychotherapy. *Journal of Contemporary Psychotherapy, 37*(1), 11–16.

Cooper, K., & Fink, M. (2014). The chemical induction of seizures in psychiatric therapy: were flurothyl (indoklon) and pentylenetetrazol (metrazol) abandoned prematurely? *Journal of Clinical Psychopharmacology, 34*(5), 602–607. https://doi.org/10.1097/JCP.0000000000000173.

Crombez, G., Eccleston, C., Van Damme, S., Vlaeyen, J., & Karoly, P. (2012). Fear-avoidance model of chronic pain: The next generation. *The Clinical Journal of Pain, 28*(6), 475–483.

Currid, T., & Pennington, J. (2010). Continuing education: Therapeutic use of self. *British Journal of Wellbeing, 1*(3), 35–41. doi:10.12968/bjow.2010.1.3.48645.

Curtiss, C. P. (2001). JCAHO: meeting the standards for pain management. *Orthopedic Nursing, 20*(2), 27–41. https://doi.org/10.1097/00006416-200103000-00008.

D'Amico, M. L., Jaffe, L. E., & Gardner, J. A. (2018). Evidence for interventions to improve and maintain occupational performance and participation for people with serious mental illness: A systematic review. *American Journal of Occupational Therapy, 72,* 7205190020. https://doi.org/10.5014/ajot.2018.033332.

Danielsen, K. K., Øydna, M. H., Strömmer, S., & Haugjord, K. (2021). "It's more than just exercise": Tailored exercise at a community-based activity center as a liminal space along the road to mental health recovery and citizenship. *International Journal of Environmental Research and Public Health, 18*(19), 10516. https://doi.org/10.3390/ijerph181910516.

Davidson, L., Rakfeldt, J., & Strauss, J. (2010). *Review of the roots of the recovery movement in psychiatry: Lessons learned.* Wiley-Blackwell.

Deighton, S., Neville, A., Pusch, D., & Dobson, K. (2018). Biomarkers of adverse childhood experiences: A scoping review. *Psychiatry Research, 269,* 719–732. https://doi.org/10.1016/j.psychres.2018.08.097.

Dewane, C. J. (2006). Use of self: a primer revisited. *Clinical Social Work Journal, 34*(4), 543–558.

Dickinson, H. O., Parkinson, K. N., Ravens-Sieberer, U., Schirripa, G., Thyen, U., Arnaud, C., Beckung, E., Fauconnier, J., McManus, V., Michelsen, S. I., Parkes, J., & Colver, A. F. (2007). Self-reported quality of life of 8-12-year-old children with cerebral palsy: a cross-sectional European study. *The Lancet, 369*(9580), 2171–2178. https://doi.org/10.1016/S0140-6736(07)61013-7.

Disability Data Briefing. (2002). *History of the international classification of functioning, disability and health (ICF).* Australian Institute of Health and Welfare, 21. https://www.aihw.gov.au/getmedia/5121aa5a-3df0-470b-8339-1969f75ef8da/ddb21.pdf.aspx?inline=true.

Dorn, L. D., Negriff, S., Huang, B., Pabst, S., Hillman, J., Braverman, P., & Susman, E. J. (2009). Menstrual symptoms in adolescent girls: association with smoking, depressive symptoms, and anxiety. *The Journal of Adolescent Health: Official Publication of the Society for Adolescent Medicine, 44*(3), 237–243. https://doi.org/10.1016/j.jadohealth.2008.07.018.

Doroshow, D. (2007). Performing a cure for schizophrenia: Insulin coma therapy on the wards. *Journal of the History of Medicine and Allied Sciences, 62*(2), 213–243.

Ernst, W. (2018). The role of work in psychiatry: Historical reflections. *Indian Journal of Psychiatry, 60*(Suppl. 2), S248–S252. https://doi.org/10.4103/psychiatry.IndianJPsychiatry_450_17.

Erskine, H. E., Baxter, A. J., Patton, G., Moffitt, T. E., Patel, V., Whiteford, H. A., & Scott, J. G. (2017). The global coverage of prevalence data for mental disorders in children and adolescents. *Epidemiology and Psychiatric Sciences, 26*(4), 395–402. https://doi.org/10.1017/S2045796015001158.

Evans, A. C., & Bufka, L. F. (2020). The critical need for a population health approach: Addressing the nation's behavioral health during the COVID-19 Pandemic and beyond. *Preventable Chronic Disease, 17,* 200261. http://dx.doi.org/10.5888/pcd17.200261.

Faria M. A., Jr. (2013). Violence, mental illness, and the brain - A brief history of psychosurgery: Part 1 - From trephination to lobotomy. *Surgical Neurology International, 4,* 49. https://doi.org/10.4103/2152-7806.110146.

Fazel, S., Hayes, A. J., Bartellas, K., Clerici, M., & Trestman, R. (2016). Mental health of prisoners: prevalence, adverse outcomes, and interventions. *The Lancet Psychiatry, 3*(9), 871–881. https://doi.org/10.1016/S2215-0366(16)30142-0.

Felitti, V. J., Anda, R. F., Nordenberg, D., Williamson, D. F., Spitz, A. M., Edwards, V., Koss, M. P., & Marks, J. S. (1998). Relationship of childhood abuse and household dysfunction to many of the leading causes of death in adults. The adverse childhood experiences (ace) study. *American Journal of Preventive Medicine, 14*(4), 245–258. https://doi.org/10.1016/s0749-3797(98)00017-8.

Fernandes, A., Jaeger, M., & Chudow, M. (2019). Post–intensive care syndrome: A review of preventive strategies and follow-up care. *American Journal of Health-system Pharmacy, 76*(2), 119–122.

Fisher, D. B. (1994). Health care reform based on an empowerment model of recovery by people with psychiatric disabilities. *Hospital & Community Psychiatry, 45*(9), 913–915. https://doi.org/10.1176/ps.45.9.913.

Fordyce, W. E. (1982). A behavioural perspective on chronic pain. *The British Journal of Clinical Psychology, 21*(Pt 4), 313–320. https://doi.org/10.1111/j.2044-8260.1982.tb00569.x.

Foronda, C., Baptiste, D. L., Reinholdt, M. M., & Ousman, K. (2015). Cultural humility: A concept analysis. *Journal of Transcultural Nursing, 27*(3), 210–217.

Gatchel, R. J., Peng, Y. B., Peters, M. L., Fuchs, P. N., & Turk, D. C. (2007). The biopsychosocial approach to chronic pain: scientific advances and future directions. *Psychological Bulletin, 133*(4), 581–624. https://doi.org/10.1037/0033-2909.133.4.581.

Gillen, G. (2014). Occupational therapy interventions for individuals. In B. A. B. Schell, G. Gillen, M. E. Scaffa, & E. S. Cohn (Eds.), *Willard and Spackman's occupational therapy* (12th ed., pp. 322–341). Philadelphia: Lippincott Williams & Wilkins.

Global Burden of Disease Pediatrics Collaboration, Kyu, H. H., Pinho, C., Wagner, J. A., Brown, J. C., Bertozzi-Villa, A., Charlson, F. J., Coffeng, L. E., Dandona, L., Erskine, H. E., Ferrari, A. J., Fitzmaurice, C., Fleming, T. D., Forouzanfar, M. H., Graetz, N., Guinovart, C., Haagsma, J., Higashi, H., Kassebaum, N. J., Larson, H. J., ... Vos, T. (2016). Global and national burden of diseases and injuries among children and adolescents between 1990 and 2013: Findings from the global burden of disease 2013 study. *JAMA Pediatrics, 170*(3), 267–287. https://doi.org/10.1001/jamapediatrics.2015.4276.

Gollaher, D. (1995). *Voice for the Mad*. The Free Press.

Grajo, L. C., Gutman, S. A., Gelb, H., Langan, K., Marx, K., Paciello, D., Santana, C., Sgandurra, A., & Teng, K. (2020). Effectiveness of a functional literacy program for sheltered homeless adults. *OTJR: Occupation Participation and Health, 40*(1), 17–26. https://doi.org/10.1177/1539449219850126.

Gu, J., Strauss, C., Bond, R., & Cavanagh, K. (2015). How do mindfulness-based cognitive therapy and mindfulness-based stress reduction improve mental health and wellbeing? A systematic review and meta-analysis of mediation studies. *Clinical Psychology Review, 37*, 1–12. https://doi.org/10.1016/j.cpr.2015.01.006.

Guimarães, J., Santos, B., Aperibense, P., Martins, G., Peres, M., & Santos, T. (2018). Electroconvulsive therapy: historical construction of nursing care (1989-2002). *Revista Brasileira de Enfermagem, 71*(Suppl. 6), 2743–2750. https://doi.org/10.1590/0034-7167-2018-0168.

Gutman, S. A. (2021). Eleanor Clarke Slagle lecture—Working with marginalized populations. *American Journal of Occupational Therapy, 75*, 7506150010. https://doi.org/10.5014/ajot.2021.756001.

Herrera-Escobar, J. P., Seshadri, A. J., Stanek, E., Lu, K., Han, K., Sanchez, S., Kaafarani, H., Salim, A., Levy-Carrick, N. C., & Nehra, D. (2021). Mental health burden after injury: It's about more than

just posttraumatic stress disorder. *Annals of Surgery, 274*(6), e1162–e1169. https://doi.org/10.1097/SLA.0000000000003780.

Huppert, F. A. (2005). Positive mental health in individuals and populations. In F. A. Huppert, N. Baylis, & B. Keverne (Eds.), *The science of well-being* (pp. 307–340). Oxford University Press. https://doi.org/10.1093/acprof:oso/9780198567523.003.0012.

Iacovides, S., Avidon, I., & Baker, F. C. (2015). What we know about primary dysmenorrhea today: a critical review. *Human Reproduction Update, 21*(6), 762–778. https://doi.org/10.1093/humupd/dmv039.

Ikiugu, M. N., Lucas-Molitor, W., Feldhacker, D., Gephart, C., Spier, M., Kapels, L., Arnold, R., & Gaikowski, R. (2019). Guidelines for occupational therapy interventions based on meaningful and psychologically rewarding occupations. *Journal of Happiness Studies, 20*, 2027–2053. https://doi.org/10.1007/s10902-018-0030-z.

Institute of Medicine. (2006). Committee on crossing the quality chasm: Adaptation to mental health and addictive disorders. In *Institute of Medicine, improving the quality of health care for mental and substance-use conditions: Quality chasm series*. Washington (DC): National Academies Press. https://www.ncbi.nlm.nih.gov/books/NBK19833/#.

Jacob, K. S. (2015). Recovery model of mental illness: A complementary approach to psychiatric care. *Indian Journal of Psychological Medicine, 37*(2), 117–119. https://doi.org/10.4103/0253-7176.155605.

Janssen, M., Heerkens, Y., Kuijer, W., van der Heijden, B., & Engels, J. (2018). Effects of mindfulness-based stress reduction on employees' mental health: A systematic review. *PLoS One, 13*(1), e0191332. https://doi.org/10.1371/journal.pone.0191332.

Jensen, M. P., Moore, M. R., Bockow, T. B., Ehde, D. M., & Engel, J. M. (2011). Psychosocial factors and adjustment to chronic pain in persons with physical disabilities: a systematic review. *Archives of Physical Medicine and Rehabilitation, 92*(1), 146–160. https://doi.org/10.1016/j.apmr.2010.09.021.

Jette, A. M. (2006). Toward a common language for function, disability, and health. *Physical Therapy, 86*(5), 726–734. https://doi.org/10.1093/ptj/86.5.726.

Joint Commission. (2015, September, 28). *Sentinel event alert: Preventing falls and fall-related injuries in health care facilities*. https://www.jointcommission.org/-/media/tjc/documents/resources/patient-safety-topics/sentinel-event/sea_55_falls_4_26_16.pdf.

Jordan, B. K., Schlenger, W. E., Fairbank, J. A., & Caddell, J. M. (1996). Prevalence of psychiatric disorders among incarcerated women. II. Convicted felons entering prison. *Archives of General Psychiatry, 53*(6), 513–519. https://doi.org/10.1001/archpsyc.1996.01830060057008.

Kabat-Zinn, J. (2015). Mindfulness. *Mindfulness, 6*(6), 1481–1483. doi:10.1007/s12671-015-0456-x.

Kellezi, B., Coupland, C., Morriss, R., Beckett, K., Joseph, S., Barnes, J., Christie, N., Sleney, J., & Kendrick, D. (2017). The impact of psychological factors on recovery from injury: a multicentre cohort study. *Social Psychiatry and Psychiatric Epidemiology, 52*(7), 855–866. https://doi.org/10.1007/s00127-016-1299-z.

Kelly, T. M., & Daley, D. C. (2013). Integrated treatment of substance use and psychiatric disorders. *Social Work in Public Health, 28*(3-4), 388–406. https://doi.org/10.1080/19371918.2013.774673.

Kilbourne, A. M., Beck, K., Spaeth-Rublee, B., Ramanuj, P., O'Brien, R. W., Tomoyasu, N., & Pincus, H. A. (2018). Measuring and improving the quality of mental health care: a global perspective. *World Psychiatry: Official Journal of the World Psychiatric Association (WPA), 17*(1), 30–38. https://doi.org/10.1002/wps.20482.

King, M. (2015). Attitudes of therapists and other health professionals towards their LGB patients. *International Review of Psychiatry, 27*(5), 396–404.

Koran, L. M., Thienemann, M. L., & Davenport, R. (1996). Quality of life for patients with obsessive-compulsive disorder. *The American Journal of Psychiatry, 153*(6), 783–788. https://doi.org/10.1176/ajp.153.6.783.

Lake, J., & Turner, M. S. (2017). Urgent need for improved mental health care and a more collaborative model of care. *The Permanente Journal, 21,* 17-024. https://doi.org/10.7812/TPP/17-024.

Leahy, R. (2008). The therapeutic relationship in CBT. *Behavioral Cognitive Psychotherapy, 36*(6), 685–693.

Lee, C., Chippendale, T., & McLeaming, L. (2020). Postoperative delirium prevention as standard practice in occupational therapy in acute care. *Physical & Occupational Therapy in Geriatrics, 38*(3), 264–270.

Leeuw, M., Goossens, M. E., Linton, S. J., Crombez, G., Boersma, K., & Vlaeyen, J. W. (2007). The fear-avoidance model of musculoskeletal pain: current state of scientific evidence. *Journal of Behavioral Medicine, 30*(1), 77–94. https://doi.org/10.1007/s10865-006-9085-0.

Leonardelli, C. A. (1988). *Milwaukee evaluation of daily living skills.* Thorofare, NJ: SLACK.

Levin, L. & Gildea. R. (2013). Bibliotherapy: tracing the roots of a moral therapy movement in the United States from the early nineteenth century to the present. *Journal of the Medical Library Association. 101,* 89–91. doi:10.3163/1536-5050.101.2.003.

Liberman, R. P., & Kopelowicz, A. (2005). Recovery from schizophrenia: a concept in search of research. *Psychiatric Services (Washington, D.C.), 56*(6), 735–742. https://doi.org/10.1176/appi.ps.56.6.735.

Livneh, H. (2001). Psychosocial adaptation to chronic illness and disability: A conceptual framework. *Rehabilitation Counseling Bulletin, 44,* 151–160. doi:10.1177/003435520104400305.

Livneh, H., & Martz, E. (2016). Psychosocial adaptation to disability within the context of positive psychology: Philosophical aspects and historical roots. *Journal of Occupational Rehabilitation, 26*(1), 13–19. https://doi.org/10.1007/s10926-015-9601-6.

Loden, M., & Rosener, J. B. (1991). *Workforce America! Managing employee diversity as a vital resource.* McGraw-Hill.

Louw, A., Diener, I., Butler, D. S., & Puentedura, E. J. (2011). The effect of neuroscience education on pain, disability, anxiety, and stress in chronic musculoskeletal pain. *Archives of Physical Medicine and Rehabilitation, 92*(12), 2041–2056. https://doi.org/10.1016/j.apmr.2011.07.198.

Lund, C., Breen, A., Flisher, A. J., Kakuma, R., Corrigall, J., Joska, J. A., Swartz, L., & Patel, V. (2010). Poverty and common mental disorders in low and middle income countries: A systematic review. *Social Science & Medicine, 71*(3), 517–528. https://doi.org/10.1016/j.socscimed.2010.04.027.

Marshall, C. A., Boland, L., Westover, L. A., Isard, R., & Gutman, S. A. (2021). A systematic review of occupational therapy interventions in the transition from homelessness. *Scandinavian Journal of Occupational Therapy, 28*(3), 171–187. https://doi.org/10.1080/11038128.2020.1764094.

Mazi, B., Kaddour, O., & Al-Badr, A. (2019). Depression symptoms in women with pelvic floor dysfunction: a case-control study. *International Journal of Women's Health, 11,* 143–148. https://doi.org/10.2147/IJWH.S187417.

Mental Health America (n.d.). *The federal and state role in mental health.* https://www.mhanational.org/issues/federal-and-state-role-mental-health.

Miaskowski, C., Blyth, F., Nicosia, F., Haan, M., Keefe, F., Smith, A., & Ritchie, C. (2020). A biopsychosocial model of chronic pain for older adults. *Pain Medicine (Malden, Mass.), 21*(9), 1793–1805. https://doi.org/10.1093/pm/pnz329.

Miles, J., Espiritu, R. C., Horen, N., Sebian, J., & Waetzig, E. (2010). *A public health approach to children's mental health: A conceptual framework.* Washington, DC: Georgetown University Center for Child and Human Development, National Technical Assistance Center for Children's Mental Health.

Milne, D. L., & James, I. A. (2002). The observed impact of training on competence in clinical supervision. *British Journal of Clinical Psychology, 41*(1), 55–72.

Mongelli, F., Georgakopoulos, P., & Pato, M. T. (2020). Challenges and opportunities to meet the mental health needs of underserved and disenfranchised populations in the United States. *Focus (American Psychiatric Publishing), 18*(1), 16. doi:10.1176/appi.focus.20190028.

Murison, R. (2016). The neurobiology of stress. *Neuroscience of Pain Stress and Emotion,* 29–49. doi:10.1016/b978-0-12-800538-5.00002-9.

Murphy, J. L., McKellar, J. D., Raffa, S. D, Clark, M. E., Kerns, R. D., & Karlin, B. E. (2014). *Cognitive behavioral therapy for chronic pain among veterans: Therapist manual.* Department of Veterans Affairs. https://www.va.gov/painmanagement/docs/cbt-cp_therapist_manual.pdf.

Nakao, M., Shirotsuki, K., & Sugaya, N. (2021). Cognitive-behavioral therapy for management of mental health and stress-related disorders: Recent advances in techniques and technologies. *BioPsychoSocial Medicine, 15*(1), 16. https://doi.org/10.1186/s13030-021-00219-w.

National Alliance on Mental Illness. (2020). *Mental health by the numbers.* https://www.nami.org/mhstats.

National Alliance on Mental Illness. (2022). *LGBTQI.* https://nami.org/Your-Journey/Identity-and-Cultural-Dimensions/LGBTQIhttps://www.nami.org/Your-Journey/Identity-and-Cultural-Dimensions/LGBTQI.

National Child Traumatic Stress Network. (2016). *Is it ADHD or child traumatic stress? Guide for clinicians.* http://www.nctsn.org/sites/default/files/assets/pdfs/adhd_and_child_traumatic_stress_final.pdf.

National Institute on Drug Abuse (NIDA). (2019). *Treatment approaches for drug addiction.* https://nida.nih.gov/publications/drugfacts/treatment-approaches-drug-addiction.

National Institute on Drug Abuse (NIDA). (2020). *Common comorbidities with substance use disorders research report - Part 1: The connection between substance use disorders and mental illness.* https://nida.nih.gov/publications/research-reports/common-comorbidities-substance-use-disorders/part-1-connection-between-substance-use-disorders-mental-illness.

National Institute of Mental Health (NIMH). (2022). *Research domain criteria initiative (RdoC).* https://www.nimh.nih.gov/research/research-funded-by-nimh/rdoc/about-rdoc.

National Institute of Mental Health (NIMH). (n.d.). *Substance use and co-occurring mental disorders.* https://www.nimh.nih.gov/health/topics/substance-use-and-mental-health#:,:text=Occurring%20Mental%20Disorders-,Overview,drugs%2C%20alcohol%2C%20or%20medications.

Nelson, G., Lord, J., & Ochocka, J. (2001). Empowerment and mental health in community: Narratives of psychiatric consumers/survivors. *Journal of Community & Applied Social Psychology, 11,* 125–142. doi:10.1002/casp.619.

Nguyen, T., & Davis, K. (2017). *The state of mental health in America 2017.* Alexandria, VA: Mental Health America. www.mentalhealthamerica.net/sites/default/files/2017%20MH%20in%20America%20Full.pdf.

Nijs, J., Meeus, M., Cagnie, B., Roussel, N. A., Dolphens, M., Van Oosterwijck, J., & Danneels, L. (2014). A modern neuroscience approach to chronic spinal pain: combining pain neuroscience education with cognition-targeted motor control training. *Physical Therapy, 94*(5), 730–738. https://doi.org/10.2522/ptj.20130258.

Oliver, M., Pearson, N., Coe, N., & Gunnell, D. (2005). Help-seeking behaviour in men and women with common mental health problems: Cross-sectional study. *British Journal of Psychiatry, 186*(4), 297–301. doi:10.1192/bjp.186.4.297.

Owen, B., & Bloom, B. (1997). *Profiling the needs of young female offenders: A protocol and pilot study.* US Department of Justice. https://www.ojp.gov/pdffiles1/nij/grants/179988.pdf.

Parker, R. M., Schaller, J., & Hansmann, S. (2003). Catastrophe, chaos, and complexity models and psychosocial adjustment to disability. *Rehabilitation Counseling Bulletin, 46,* 234–241.

Parcesepe, A. M., & Cabassa, L. J. (2013). Public stigma of mental illness in the United States: A systematic literature review. *Administration and Policy in Mental Health and Mental Health Services Research, 40*(5), 384–399.

Parry, M. (2006). Dorothea Dix (1802-1887). *American Journal of Public Health, 96*(4) 624–625. https://doi.org/10.2105/AJPH.2005.079152

Perry, B. D., & Szalavitz, M. (2017). *The boy who was raised as a dog: And other stories from a child psychiatrist's notebook — What traumatized children can teach us about loss, love, and healing.* Basic Books. https://doi.org/10.1111/j.1532-5415.2011.03788.x.

Peter, L. J., Schindler, S., Sander, C., Schmidt, S., Muehlan, H., McLaren, T., Tomczyk, S., Speerforck, S., & Schomerus, G. (2021). Continuum beliefs and mental illness stigma: a systematic review and meta-analysis of correlation and intervention studies. *Psychological Medicine, 51*(5), 716–726. doi:10.1017/S0033291721000854.

Phuphanich, M. E., Droessler, J., Altman, L., & Eapen, B. C. (2020). Movement-based therapies in rehabilitation. *Physical Medicine and Rehabilitation Clinics of North America, 31*(4), 577–591. https://doi.org/10.1016/j.pmr.2020.07.002.

Pietrzak, R. H., Goldstein, R. B., Southwick, S. M., & Grant, B. F. (2012). Physical health conditions associated with posttraumatic stress disorder in U.S. older adults: Results from wave 2 of the national epidemiologic survey on alcohol and related conditions. *Journal of the American Geriatrics Society, 60*(2), 296–303.

Pizzi, M. A., & Richards, L. G. (2017). Promoting health, well-being, and quality of life in occupational therapy: a commitment to a paradigm shift for the next 100 years. *The American Journal of Occupational Therapy, 71*(4), 7104170010p1–7104170010p5. https://doi.org/10.5014/ajot.2017.028456.

Ranjbar, N., & Erb, M. (2019). Adverse childhood experiences and trauma-informed care in rehabilitation clinical practice. *Archives of Rehabilitation Research and Clinical Translation, 1*(1-2), 100003.

Roberts, R., MacCann, C., Matthews, G., & Zeidner, M. (2010). Emotional intelligence: Towards a consensus of models and measures. *Social and Personality Psychology Compass, 4*(10), 821–840. doi:10.1111/j.1751-9004.2010.00277.x.

Robertson, I., & Flint-Taylor, J. (2010). Wellbeing in healthcare organizations: Key issues. *British Journal of Healthcare Management, 16*(1), 18–25.

Rodenbush, K. (2015). *The effects of trauma on behavior in the classroom [Presentation materials].* http://www.montereycoe.org/Assets/selpa/Files/Presentation-Materials/The%20Effects%20of%20Trauma%20on%20Behavior%20in%20the%20Classroom.pdf.

Rogers, J. C., & Holm, M. B. (1989). *Performance assessment of self-care skills.* http://pass@shrs.pitt.edu.

Rogers, J. C., & Holm, M. B. (2016). Functional assessment in mental health: lessons from occupational therapy. *Dialogues in Clinical Neuroscience, 18*(2), 145–154. https://doi.org/10.31887/DCNS.2016.18.2/jrogers.

Ross, S., & Peselow, E. (2012). Co-occurring psychotic and addictive disorders: Neurobiology and diagnosis. *Clinical Neuropharmacology, 35*(5), 235–243. https://doi.org/10.1097/WNF.0b013e318261e193.

Rueness, J., Augusti, E., Strøm, I., Wentzel-Larsen, T., & Myhre, M. (2020). Adolescent abuse victims displayed physical health complaints and trauma symptoms during post disclosure interviews. *Acta Paediatrica, 109*(11), 2409–2415.

Ryan, D. A., & Boland, P. (2021). A scoping review of occupational therapy interventions in the treatment of people with substance use disorders. *The Irish Journal of Occupational Therapy, 49*(2), 104–114. http://dx.doi.org/10.1108/IJOT-11-2020-0017.

Salime, S., Clesse, C., Jeffredo, A., & Batt, M. (2022). Process of deinstitutionalization of aging individuals with severe and disabling mental disorders: A review. *Frontiers in Psychiatry, 13,* 813338. https://doi.org/10.3389/fpsyt.2022.813338.

Savage, S. (2005). *Psychological adaptation to disability: Perspectives from chaos and complexity theory.* Science. https://www.redorbit.com/news/science/267083/psychological_adaptation_to_disability_perspectives_from_chaos_and_complexity_theory/.

Schnurr, P., Spiro, A., Aldwin, C., & Stukel, T. (1998). Physical symptom trajectories following trauma exposure: Longitudinal findings from the normative aging study. *The Journal of Nervous and Mental Disease, 186*(9), 522–528.

Shortell, S. M., Gillies, R. R., Anderson, D. A., Erickson, K. M., & Mitchell, J. B. (2000). *Remaking health care in America: The evolution of organized delivery systems* (2nd ed.). Jossey-Bass.

Smith, D. T., Mouzon, D. M., & Elliott, M. (2018). Reviewing the assumptions about men's mental health: An exploration of the gender binary. *American Journal of Men's Health, 12*(1), 78–89. https://doi.org/10.1177/1557988316630953.

Steadman, H. J., Osher, F. C., Robbins, P. C., Case, B., & Samuels, S. (2009). Prevalence of serious mental illness among jail inmates. *Psychiatric Services (Washington, D.C.), 60*(6), 761–765. https://doi.org/10.1176/ps.2009.60.6.761.

Stringer, H. (2019). Improving mental health for inmates. *Monitor on Psychology, 50*(3). https://www.apa.org/monitor/2019/03/mental-heath-inmates.

Substance Abuse and Mental Health Services Administration. (2022a). *Laws and regulations.* https://www.samhsa.gov/about-us/who-we-are/laws-regulations.

Substance Abuse and Mental Health Services Administration. (2022b). *Trauma and violence.* https://www.samhsa.gov/trauma-violence.

Taylor, R. R., Lee, S., Kielhofner, G., & Ketkar, M. (2009). Therapeutic use of self: A national survey of practitioners' attitudes and experience. *American Journal of Occupational Therapy, 63*(2), 198–206.

Thompson, L. K. (1992). *The Kohlman evaluation of living skills.* American Occupational Therapy Association.

Tohen, M., Hennen, J., Zarate, C. M., Jr., Baldessarini, R. J., Strakowski, S. M., Stoll, A. L., Faedda, G. L., Suppes, T., Gebre-Medhin, P., & Cohen, B. M. (2000). Two-year syndromal and functional recovery in 219 cases of first-episode major affective disorder with psychotic features. *The American Journal of Psychiatry, 157*(2), 220–228. https://doi.org/10.1176/appi.ajp.157.2.220.

Tordoff, D. M., Wanta, J. W., Collin, A., Stepney, C., Inwards-Breland, D. J., & Ahrens, K. (2022). Mental health outcomes in transgender and nonbinary youths receiving gender-affirming care. *JAMA Network Open, 5*(2), e220978. https://doi.org/10.1001/jamanetworkopen.2022.0978.

United States Department of Health and Human Services. (2022). *Opioid crisis statistics*. https://www.hhs.gov/opioids/about-the-epidemic/opioid-crisis-statistics/index.html#:,:text=In%20 2019%2C%20an%20estimated%2010.1,and%20745%2C000% 20people%20used%20heroin.&text=Appropriate%20prescribing %20of%20opioids%20is,and%20safety%20of%20Medicare%20 beneficiaries.

VanPuymbrouck, L., Carey, J., Draper, A., & Follansbee, L. (2021). Recognizing inequity: A critical step of health literacy for people with disability. *American Journal of Occupational Therapy, 75*, 7504180100. https://doi.org/10.5014/ajot.2021.045492.

Vlaeyen, J., & Linton, S. (2012). Fear-avoidance model of chronic musculoskeletal pain: 12 years on. *Pain (Amsterdam), 153*(6), 1144–1147.

Vyas, S., Rodrigues, A., Silva, J., Tronche, F., Almeida, O., Sousa, N., & Sotiropoulos, I. (2016). Chronic stress and glucocorticoids: From neuronal plasticity to neurodegeneration. *Journal of Neural Transplantation & Plasticity, 2016*, 6391686.

Waddell, C., Schwartz, C., Barican, J., Andres, C., & Gray-Grant, D. (2015). *Improving children's mental health: Six highly effective psychosocial interventions*. Vancouver, BC: Children's Health Policy Centre, Simon Fraser University. https://childhealthpolicy.ca/wp-content/uploads/2015/06/15-05-29-Waddell-Report.pdf.

Wheeler, S., & Richards, K. (2007). The impact of clinical supervision on counselors and therapists, their practice and their clients: A systematic review of the literature. *Counseling and Psychotherapy Research, 7*(1), 54–65.

Whitney, D. G., & Peterson, M. D. (2019). US national and state-level prevalence of mental health disorders and disparities of mental health care use in children. *JAMA Pediatrics, 173*(4), 389–391. https://doi.org/10.1001/jamapediatrics.2018.5399.

Wilburn, V. G., Hoss, A., Pudeler, M., Beukema, E., Rothenbuhler, C., & Stoll, H. B. (2021). Receiving recognition: A case for occupational therapy practitioners as mental and behavioral health providers. *The American Journal of Occupational Therapy: Official Publication of the American Occupational Therapy Association, 75*(5), 7505090010. https://doi.org/10.5014/ajot.2021. 044727.

Wirth, J. H., & Bodenhausen, G. V. (2009). The role of gender in mental-illness stigma: A national experiment. *Psychological Science, 20*(2), 169–173. https://doi.org/10.1111/j.1467-9280.2009.02282.x.

World Health Organization. (1980). *International classification of impairments, disabilities, and handicaps: A manual of classification relating to the consequences of disease, published in accordance with resolution WHA29.35 of the Twenty-ninth World Health Assembly, May 1976*. World Health Organization. https://apps.who.int/iris/handle/10665/41003.

World Health Organization. (1986). The 1st International Conference on Health Promotion, Ottawa, 1986. Ottawa Charter for Health Promotion. https://www.who.int/teams/health-promotion/enhanced-wellbeing/first-global-conference.

World Health Organization. (2022a). *International classification of functioning, disability and health (ICF)*. https://www.who.int/standards/classifications/international-classification-of-functioning-disability-and-health.

World Health Organization. (2022b). *Mental health: Strengthening our response*. https://www.who.int/news-room/fact-sheets/detail/mental-health-strengthening-our-response.

Wu, A., Roemer, E. C., Kent, K. B., Ballard, D. W., & Goetzel, R. Z. (2021). Organizational best practices supporting mental health in the workplace. *Journal of Occupational and Environmental Medicine, 63*(12), e925–e931. https://doi.org/10.1097/JOM.0000000000002407.

Zimney, K., Louw, A., & Puentedura, E. J. (2014). Use of therapeutic neuroscience education to address psychosocial factors associated with acute low back pain: a case report. *Physiotherapy Theory and Practice, 30*(3), 202–209. https://doi.org/10.3109/09593985.2013. 856508.

Zur, O. (2004). To cross or not to cross: Do boundaries in therapy protect or harm? *Psychology Bulletin, 39*(3), 27–32.

20

Integration of Health and Wellness Into Physical and Occupational Therapy Practice

DEBORAH ELGIN BUDASH, PhD, OTR/L; and KAREN MUELLER, PT, DPT, PhD, NBC-HWC

LEARNING OBJECTIVES

By the end of this chapter, the reader will be able to:

- Relate the principles of social determinants of health to the health and well-being of individuals and their communities.
- Describe the motivational requirements for sustained, autonomous health behavior change.
- Discuss the importance of autonomy, relatedness, and confidence as facilitators of health behavior change.

- Describe the process of behavior change as described in the transtheoretical model of change.
- Discuss the purpose and value of motivational interviewing as a relational approach that physical and occupational therapists can use to facilitate motivation for health behavior change.

CHAPTER OUTLINE

Background

As any student of an allied health profession has no doubt learned, the costs associated with healthcare are continually escalating. There are many reasons for the persistent increase in the cost of care. Due to these many and varied issues, recent healthcare reforms have focused on improving outcomes while controlling costs (American Occupational Therapy Association [AOTA], 2015, 2020; Scaffa & Reitz, 2020). Also, there has been an understanding that care is more cost-effective when administered in the community and proactively. These trends intersect as a population health approach to physical and occupational therapy providers from within the community.

An important recognition is that each individual can control some of these factors, which can then provide a level of management of these costs (Rosenfeld et al., 2022). By utilizing our knowledge of disease, exercise, and occupation, physical and occupational therapists can educate clients to limit disease progression and encourage healthier lifestyle choices to prevent disease and associated secondary effects. Viewing healthcare in this way provides occupational and physical therapists opportunities to educate and support clients in modifying their behaviors, ultimately leading to better health outcomes.

Escalating healthcare costs are attributed mainly to three factors: our aging population, a higher incidence of chronic disease that requires ongoing management, and the impact of the social determinants of health on health outcomes (Dexter et al., 2010; Skybova et al., 2021). Regarding the aging populace, the National Center for Chronic Disease Prevention and Health Promotion (NCCDPHP) (2022) estimates that 16% of the United States population is over 65 years old. Advanced age increases the risk of chronic disease. Dexter et al. (2010) estimated that 80% of older adults must cope with one or more chronic conditions.

Chronic diseases are more prevalent, and people now survive and live with chronic conditions (Dexter et al., 2010; United States Department of Health and Human Services (HHS), 2021c; Skybova et al., 2021). About 6 in every 10 Americans have a chronic condition that they must manage, and over 40% of those manage more than one condition (Buttorff et al., 2017). The NCCDPHP, part of the Centers for Disease Control and Prevention (CDC), reports that 90% of annual healthcare expenditures (which are estimated to be about $4.1 trillion annually) are directed to the care of chronic and mental health conditions (NCCDPHP, 2022). Many chronic conditions can be attributed to past lifestyle choices (Skybova et al., 2021). By extension, more health-focused lifestyle choices can prevent disease and limit disease progression (AOTA, 2015; American Physical Therapy Association [APTA] 2019a; Skybova et al., 2021). Healthcare professionals, such as occupational and physical therapists, can play an essential role in educating populations and providing resources and opportunities to support healthful decision-making (AOTA, 2015; APTA, 2019b).

Finally, there has been a recognition that specific characteristics of an individual's life can impact health outcomes, referred to as health disparities (CDC, 2017). These characteristics are classified as the social determinants of health (SDOH) (HHS, 2021c). Specifically, the social determinants of health are the circumstances connected to how individuals live and function, influencing health, risks, and outcomes. Some are changeable, and some are not (Fig. 20.1). The SDOH are divided into five categories, including economic stability, education access and quality, healthcare access and quality, neighborhood and built environment, and the social and community context (HHS, 2021c). These include concerns of poverty, access to affordable and quality education and healthcare, the nature of communities related to violence, personal safety, accessibility, and the support of healthy choices. The extent to which SDOH can be affected presents occupational and physical therapists with opportunities to support our clients' health and well-being. The SDOH will be explored in greater detail later in this chapter.

Healthy People 2030

Healthy People (HP) 2030 (US Department of Health and Human Services, 2020a) represents the current 10-year plan in the United States to improve the health of

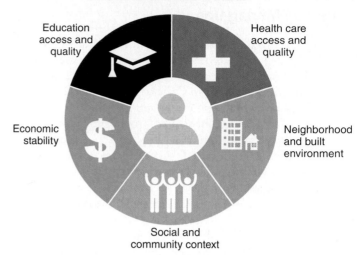

Social determinants of health

• **Fig. 20.1** Social Determinants of Health. (From United States Department of Health and Human Services, 2020a. *Healthy People 2030*, Office of Disease Prevention and Health Promotion. https://health.gov/healthypeople/objectives-and-data/social-determinants-health)

its population. Developed by the United States Department of Health and Human Services (HHS, 2021a), this plan identifies opportunities to improve health and well-being for all and identifies goals, offers resources, and collects data related to these efforts. HP 2030 aspires to five main goals, one directly addressing the SDOH: "Create social, physical, and economic environments that promote attaining the full potential for health and well-being for all" (HHS, 2020b, para 3). Overall, HP 2030 acknowledges the tremendous impact of health disparities, chronic conditions, and an aging population and focuses on more preventative and proactive care.

Prevention of disease and proactive disease management offer great potential in meeting the objectives of HP 2030 and the triple aim of healthcare reforms, specifically improved outcomes, reduction in healthcare costs, and enhanced healthcare experience (AOTA, 2015, 2020; Scaffa & Reitz, 2020). Occupational and physical therapy, as professions concerned with optimal health through occupation and physical activity, are poised to contribute greatly to the support of health for all individuals, groups, and populations (AOTA, 2020; Bezner, 2015). Occupational therapy's core belief is that health is impacted by engagement in occupations (AOTA, 2020). A key belief of physical therapy is that society can be changed and the human experience be optimized by movement (APTA, 2019b). In order to facilitate health through occupation and movement, prevention efforts can be provided from several levels, as described later in the chapter (AOTA, 2015). These varied approaches to prevention can provide comprehensive health management regardless of where the individual, group, or population exists on the spectrum of health.

The Role of Lifestyle Medicine in Chronic Disease Management

As noted, chronic disease can be considered an epidemic in the United States. Although these statistics are sobering, the potential for positive change is tremendous. According to the American College of Lifestyle Medicine, lifestyle factors such as poor diet and lack of exercise contribute to the development and progression of the top chronic disease conditions (Collings, 2021). These behaviors contribute to 80% of the total costs of treating chronic illnesses worldwide. However, with consistent lifestyle changes, particularly in nutrition, persons with chronic conditions, such as diabetes, can achieve remission (Rosenfeld et al., 2022).

In the realm of health protection, a study of 23,000 adults (Ford et al., 2009) demonstrated that adherence to a healthy lifestyle (defined as not smoking, healthy eating practices, optimal body mass, and regular physical activity) significantly impacted risk reduction for several chronic conditions. Specifically, this cohort demonstrated a 93% risk reduction for type 2 diabetes, an 81% reduction in myocardial infarction, and a 50% reduction in stroke. Moreover, even if not all four lifestyle behaviors were present, the risk of developing one or more chronic lifestyle-related diseases decreased commensurate with the number of positive lifestyle factors adopted. As a physical therapy or occupational therapy student, you will be better positioned to serve your patients (while enhancing your well-being and career engagement) by reflecting on your health behaviors and considering any beneficial changes. You can utilize evidence-based health behavior change interventions in the following sections to develop achievable wellness goals.

Primary prevention seeks to provide education to prevent disease onset and reduce the frequency of unhealthy behaviors (AOTA, 2015). As previously stated, the adoption of four lifestyle practices has a significant impact on reducing or eliminating the risk of chronic disease. Secondary prevention efforts involve screening and evaluation, the early identification of disease, and limiting the development of related secondary issues. For example, patients with stroke often have comorbidities such as hypertension and heart disease, which, if unmanaged, can lead to stroke recurrence and significant additional disability. Tertiary prevention services are designed to limit the progression of a condition, as in the initiation of a targeted exercise program for persons with Parkinson's disease (Crotty & Schwarzschild, 2020). These three approaches to prevention can provide comprehensive health management regardless of where the individual, group, or population exists on the spectrum of health (Fig. 20.2). Physical and occupational therapists are highly skilled in managing conditions across these levels of prevention. However, as evidence mounts for the value of primary prevention, OTs and PTs have a tremendous opportunity

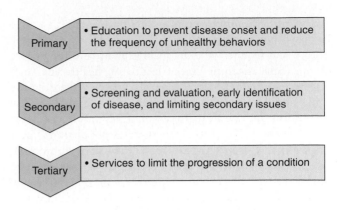

• **Fig. 20.2** Levels of Preventative Care

to engage their patients in health behavior change through lifestyle-focused intervention.

The concept of "lifestyle medicine" evolved from recognizing that most of our current diseases are decreasingly comprised of communicable microbial illnesses such as tuberculosis or influenza (Yeh & Kong, 2013). Rather, the current chronic disease burden is largely comprised of noncommunicable diseases resulting from the daily lifestyles of individuals and populations. The term "lifestyle medicine" first appeared in scientific literature in 1990. As recognition of the importance of personal health behaviors grew, the American College of Lifestyle Medicine (ACLM) was established in 2004, uniting physicians, healthcare professionals, and healthcare students in a shared commitment to developing evidence, education, and intervention supporting health behavior change (Benigas, 2019).

Today, lifestyle medicine is defined as "the use of a whole food, plant-predominant dietary lifestyle, regular physical activity, restorative sleep, stress management, avoidance of risky substances and positive social connection as a primary therapeutic modality for treatment and reversal of chronic disease" (American College of Lifestyle Medicine, 2022). In physical and occupational therapist practice, each of these six factors can be assessed in the context of the patient encounter. The Physical Therapy Healthy Lifestyle Appraisal (PTHLA) is a self-report measure that PTs and OTs can use to engage patients in conversations around health behavior change (Ingman et al., 2022).

The health behavior change process is multifaceted, incorporating the patient's health beliefs, resources, barriers, readiness, and confidence for change. Several health behavior theories have evolved in recent years, providing practitioners with a useful framework for intervention. Integrating these theories in clinical practice requires a different approach to patient intervention, specifically from a "top-down" directive approach to a collaborative, supportive one driven by the patient's needs, desires, and goals. The following sections will introduce these concepts and you are encouraged to consider their use in your patient interactions.

Factors Influencing Health Behavior Change

Social Determinants of Health

The ability to sustain personal health depends largely on our resources, many of which are beyond our realm of influence. For example, each of us needs access to food, clothing, and housing, and most live in communities that provide varying levels of access to these services. The CDC defines SDOH as "the conditions in the places where people live, learn, work, play, play, worship and age" (HHS, 2021c, para 1). The major components of these conditions can be grouped into five categories: economic stability, education access and quality, healthcare access and quality, neighborhood and built environment, and social and community context. Collectively, differences in SDOH have been declared by the World Health Organization to account for 30–55% of all health outcomes. Accordingly, evidence suggests that one of the strongest predictors of a person's health is their zip code. The SDOH model and the contributions of each level toward overall health are illustrated in Fig. 20.3.

Socioecologic Model

Health-related lifestyle choices are also governed by individual, environmental, and sociocultural factors, each of which must be addressed to optimize health outcomes. These factors are illustrated through the socioecological model, an integration of the socioeconomic model introduced by Urie Bronfenbrenner in 1977, and the biopsychosocial model developed by George Engel the same year (Engel, 1980). Together, these models integrate the biological, psychological, and environmental influences on health, providing a comprehensive framework for assessing and intervening in specific levels of health influence (Lehman et al., 2017). Accordingly, the socioecological model aligns with SDOH and can be used to identify focused strategies for health promotion and disease prevention. The following discussion provides examples of interventions at each level, and Fig. 20.4 illustrates the socioecological model.

At the intrapersonal (individual) level, health behavior change is influenced by the patient's knowledge, perceptions, and motivation. For example, a patient might know that increased vegetable intake is associated with better health but is unaware that fried potatoes are not included. When confronted with such patients, health providers often deliver directives and intimidating information such as "Didn't you know that shouldn't eat fried potatoes? They are bad for you! You shouldn't be eating them!" These directives leave patients confused and frustrated but lacking the necessary information and support for actual behavior change. To further illustrate this top-down approach's pitfalls, consider your response to such a directive. Most of us recoil at being told what to do. Thus interventions at the intrapersonal level must include support for one's motivation to change,

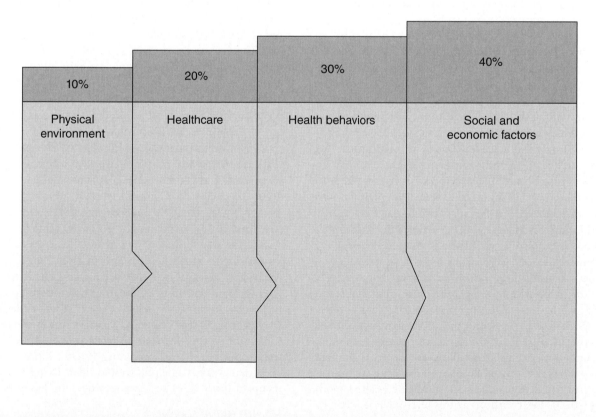

• **Fig. 20.3. Social Determinants of Health and Its Impact on Health Outcomes.** (Data from https://www.countyhealthrankings.org/explore-health-rankings/county-health-rankings-model)

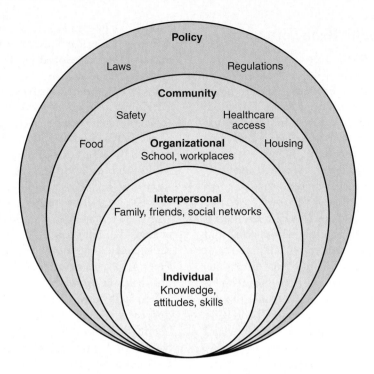

• **Fig. 20.4 The Socioecological Model of Health**

readiness and confidence to change, the barriers and resources that impair or support change, and any education needed to enhance these elements. The next section of this chapter will explore the behavioral approaches we can use to enhance these intrapersonal factors.

At the interpersonal level, health behaviors are deeply influenced by the patterns of our family and friends. For example, evidence suggests that adolescents whose friends and family smoke are significantly more likely to adopt this behavior (Joung et al., 2016). Thus health behavior interventions must include strategies to address these interpersonal influences. Interventions at this level include linking the patient's desire for health behavior change to their capacity for social interaction and family engagement. For example, an older person may be willing to exercise if it enables them to hike with their grandchildren. Thus identifying barriers and resources in your patients' social network can significantly impact their success in achieving desired health outcomes.

At the community level, it is important to consider the environmental features that either support or detract from the successful pursuit of health behaviors. For example, patients might be willing to include more fresh fruits and vegetables in their diet but have no access to such food in their neighborhood. Accordingly, a 2021 report from the Association of American Medical Colleges found that 23.5 million Americans, particularly persons of color and those in poverty, live in "food deserts," meaning communities without convenient access to affordable healthy foods (Haines, 2020). Interventions at this level include identifying community resources that can be accessed for support. For example, an elderly patient living alone but unable to cook safely might be connected with community agencies such as Meals on Wheels (Meals on Wheels America, 2022), an organization dedicated to reducing isolation and malnutrition among senior citizens.

Finally, to address the complex causes of many socioecologic health disparities, support is needed at the public policy level. For example, the Centers for Disease Control and Prevention's list of "Ten Great Public Health Achievements," including motor vehicle safety, tobacco control, and maternal and infant health—involve public policy change (Pollack-Porter et al., 2018). While these improvements helped to increase United States life expectancy to a peak of 78.9 years in 2019, this declined to 76.6 years in 2021 due to emerging public health challenges of the COVID pandemic and opioid epidemic (Centers for Disease Control and Prevention, National Center for Health Statistics, 2020). Further efforts are needed to address the underlying problems of income inequality and racial disparities that have contributed to this decrease.

As a future physical or occupational therapist, it will be important to engage your patients in discussions identifying the impact of social determinant/ecologic elements in their lives. These discussions will be essential to developing effective interventions at the relevant levels. You are likely familiar with these "environmental factors" in the International Classification of Functioning, Disability and Health (ICF) framework for clinical reasoning (CDC, 2020). Thus the ICF framework is a helpful tool for identifying relevant elements of the SDOH and socioecologic models of health.

Health Belief Model

What are the factors that lead people to make a health behavior change? The Health Belief Model (HBM) was

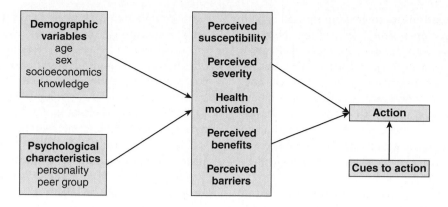

• **Fig. 20.5** The Health Belief Model

developed by psychologists Irwin Rosenstock, Godfrey Hochbaum, Stephen Kegeles, and Howard Leventhal during the 1950s for the United States Public Health Service to understand this process better (Cummings et al., 1978). This HBM model describes the impact of health beliefs and demographic and psychological factors on health motivation and action. Fig. 20.5 illustrates the components of the Health Belief Model.

The Health Belief Model states that a patient's perceived *susceptibility* and *severity* are important factors regulating health behavior (Rosenstock, 1974). For example, you might be willing to kiss your partner when they have a cold but not if they have COVID-19. Susceptibility and severity were two likely drivers of a 67% United States COVID-19 vaccination rate as of July 2022.

Most people are unwilling to invest the energy into making a health behavior change unless there is a considerable return on that investment; in other words, the health change must be *beneficial* and greater than any *barriers* to change. Thus thoroughly exploring the patient's perceived "cost/benefit ratio" around a health behavior change is critical. Motivation toward behavior change can be greatly enhanced when barriers are addressed or minimized and benefits are magnified. Many barriers and resources are related to the individual's SDOH and socioecologic status. Exploring these elements is an often neglected but critical factor for supporting desirable health outcomes. The Centers for Medicare and Medicaid have developed the Accountable Health Communities Health-Related Social needs screening tool for such exploration (Centers for Medicare and Medicaid, 2022). Typically, the decision to change a behavior evolves from a *cue to action*, an experience leading to the conviction that change is needed to live in a manner consistent with personal values. For example, after years of alcohol addiction and futile attempts at recovery, one patient decided to become sober after almost hitting a young child while driving under the influence. Until a person experiences a compelling cue to action, they may deny or minimize the need for change, despite warnings from their providers or public health entities. Accordingly, evidence suggests that graphic images of organs destroyed by smoking increase awareness of

smoking's health risks but do not affect smoking behavior. The health belief model emphasizes the importance of perceived benefits and self-efficacy and a person's confidence in their capacity to achieve their desired goal. Skillful practitioner communication can provide the needed support for strengthening needed abilities.

The next step in the behavior change process occurs when the patient commits to an action plan. Finally, the patient must take the actions needed to make and sustain the change. As you will discover in the following sections, the communication strategies emanating from Self-Determination Theory, the Transtheoretical Model of Change, and Motivational Interviewing are useful tools to move a patient toward the initiation and maintenance of health behavior change.

Self-Determination Theory

Self-determination is the freedom to live as one chooses, particularly the ability to make decisions of one's own volition. Self-Determination Theory (SDT) was developed by psychologists Richard Ryan and Edward Deci in 1985 to describe the necessary attributes and processes by which individuals arrive at such an internally motivated free choice, a state known as Intrinsic Motivation, the highest level of engagement (Deci & Ryan, 1985). Self-Determination Theory is grounded in the premise that each of us has innate tendencies toward personal growth, a process that begins with a physiologic or psychological need that activates a behavior. In SDT, the process of behavioral action is driven by three primary elements: autonomy, competence, and relatedness.

Autonomy pertains to freely chosen voluntary engagement in behavior because of its *personal value and fulfillment*. These are the primary features of intrinsic motivation. For example, consider the activities you do in your life because of their inherent satisfaction and value. Many of us engage in regular exercise for such reasons. Moreover, if we were forced to stop because of an injury or illness, our sense of well-being and self-esteem would likely suffer. Autonomy is vital to our well-being and a central principle of bioethics. Evidence suggests autonomy is best supported by offering choices, providing opportunities to give input into the plan of care, and shared decision-making. Thus in the context of health behavior change, our patients are most likely to be successful if provided with options and when they can contribute to and agree upon decisions related to their care. Competence arises from confidence, a faith in one's ability to complete the necessary actions to reach a goal. Confidence (and competence) are enhanced by sufficient knowledge and skills, ideally to the point where the challenges of a given task are within reach of the person's capacity for successful completion.

In our therapeutic interventions, meaningful patient outcomes rely on the appropriate balance between task difficulty and patient competence. When tasks are too easy, there is no challenge to competence and boredom ensues. In contrast, when tasks are too difficult, the challenge to competence is beyond the person's capacity, resulting in frustration and anxiety. Appropriate knowledge and skills and thoughtful task selection result in energizing, enjoyable, and growth-producing activity. Participation in such tasks often leads to a state of "flow," described as

> *a gratifying state of deep involvement and absorption that individuals report when facing a challenging activity and they perceive adequate abilities to cope with these challenges. (European Flow Research Network, 2014)*

Competence sufficient to reach the flow state is associated with many positive benefits, including increased attentional capacity, self-regulation, greater creativity, and higher levels of well-being. These attributes are essential elements of intrinsic motivation, making them important benchmarks for educational achievement (Heutte et al., 2021). One of the most satisfying clinical practice experiences is participating in a flow experience with our patients. In such cases, both parties benefit: The therapist gains a renewed sense of purpose and satisfaction, and the patient gains new learning, insights, and skills.

As PTs and OTs, we can enhance patient competence through various methods, including verbal instruction, demonstrations, and feedback (tactile or verbal). We can support autonomy and competence by seeking patient input about their strengths and resources. We can assist patients in identifying barriers and investigating their ideas for addressing these. We can collaborate in developing specific achievable goals within our patients' capacity and, most importantly, encourage their progress to build further strengths.

Relatedness is the sense of belonging, acceptance, feeling connected to others, and having a sense of personal value. As social creatures, we need interpersonal connections for optimal well-being. One recent study found that low social interaction was as deleterious to health as smoking 15 cigarettes a day and being an alcoholic (Holt-Lundstad et al., 2010). In contrast, evidence also suggests that strong social connections protect longevity by as much as 50% (Martino et al., 2015). OTs and PTs can engage patients toward desirable health behavior change by inviting them to explore their social networks and identifying sources of support for their desired goals. For example, some patients may prefer group exercise and others might benefit from joining a support group. We can also assist them in identifying barriers within their support system: for example, a patient is trying to lose weight but has a partner who continues to cook unhealthy food.

Another essential element of SDT theory is how a person moves toward intrinsic motivation. As mentioned, persons at this level perform certain behaviors because they are interesting, deeply satisfying, and affirm one's values and self-esteem. The term "wantivation" has been used to describe intrinsic motivation, highlighting the underlying full autonomy, competence, and social support required to "want" to act.

In contrast is extrinsic motivation, where an activity is performed for a reward, to avoid punishment, or because there are no other alternatives. For example, consider the structure of weight loss camps or residential substance abuse recovery programs. In both instances, the environment controls behavior. In these settings, there is no access to unhealthy food or addictive substance, and people will often experience considerable success if the environmental controls remain in place. Fig. 20.6 illustrates the SDT motivation continuum.

A compelling challenge in health behavior change is supporting our patients to move toward autonomously motivated wellness practices. This involves harnessing the patient's health belief system to embrace the target behavior's utility, value, and relevance. PTs and OTs can use thoughtful, open-ended questions to support autonomy by inviting our patients to express their values, interests, and reasons for change. We can provide information as needed to support competence. We can collaborate with our patients to explore personally enjoyable and meaningful activities, providing interventions that are just within reach of their competence. We can assist them in exploring resources in their social network and identifying ways to capitalize on these for success. Most importantly, we can use empathy and unconditional regard to support our patients, regardless of their place in the motivational continuum.

Transtheoretical Model of Change

Transitioning from extrinsic to intrinsic motivation is a stepwise process involving a series of identifiable stages. These stages are described in the Transtheoretical Model of Change (TTM). This model was developed by psychologists James Prochaska and Carlo DiClemente (Prochaska & DiClemente, 1983) and is one of the most commonly applied frameworks in behavior change. The stages of TTM and related intervention strategies are illustrated in Fig. 20.7 and discussed in the next section.

Precontemplation: (I can't or won't change)

In the precontemplation stage, there is no interest or sense of need to change behavior. Persons in this stage deny that the problem exists and lack insight into the severity and consequences of their behavior. They may also have failed at previous attempts to change and are too discouraged to try

The self-determination continuum					
Nonself-determined ....**Self-determined**					
Motivation	None	Extrinsic	Extrinsic	Extrinsic	Extrinsic	Intrinsic
Regulation style	None	External	Introjected	Identified	Integrate	Intrinsic
Motivation source	Impersonal	External	Somewhat external	Somewhat internal	Internal	Internal
Motivation regulator	Lack of control	Compliance, external rewards and punishment	Self-control, internal rewards and punishments	Personal importance, conscious valuing	Congruence, awareness, synthesis with self	Interest, enjoyment, inherent satisfaction

• **Fig. 20.6** Self-Determination Theory

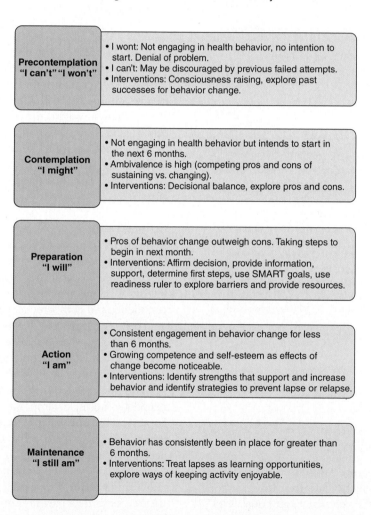

Precontemplation "I can't" "I won't"
- I wont: Not engaging in health behavior, no intention to start. Denial of problem.
- I can't: May be discouraged by previous failed attempts.
- Interventions: Consciousness raising, explore past successes for behavior change.

Contemplation "I might"
- Not engaging in health behavior but intends to start in the next 6 months.
- Ambivalence is high (competing pros and cons of sustaining vs. changing).
- Interventions: Decisional balance, explore pros and cons.

Preparation "I will"
- Pros of behavior change outweigh cons. Taking steps to begin in next month.
- Interventions: Affirm decision, provide information, support, determine first steps, use SMART goals, use readiness ruler to explore barriers and provide resources.

Action "I am"
- Consistent engagement in behavior change for less than 6 months.
- Growing competence and self-esteem as effects of change become noticeable.
- Interventions: Identify strengths that support and increase behavior and identify strategies to prevent lapse or relapse.

Maintenance "I still am"
- Behavior has consistently been in place for greater than 6 months.
- Interventions: Treat lapses as learning opportunities, explore ways of keeping activity enjoyable.

• **Fig. 20.7 The Stages and Strategies of the Transtheoretical Model of Change.**

new ones. As a result of prior failures, they may fixate on the negative side of change. Persons in the precontemplation stage may also attend healthcare appointments because of external pressure and may appear defiant. Although it can be challenging to address persons in the precontemplation stage, this is a time to engage the patient without judgment, focusing on self-exploration rather than action. Refer to Box 20.1 for precontemplation strategies.

Contemplation: (I might)
Individuals in the contemplation stage have a degree of awareness and acknowledgment of their problematic health

---

• BOX 20.1 Precontemplation Stage Strategies

1. Validate the patient's feelings about not being ready for change.
2. Assure the patient that the decision to change is theirs to make.
3. Encourage reevaluation of the current behavior:
   - What would need to happen for you to know that this is a problem?
   - What might be some warning signs that would tell you this is a problem?
4. Leverage existing strengths:
   - What things have you been successful at changing in the past?
   - What led you to make that change?
5. Explore their knowledge and raise consciousness: Use "Ask, Provide, Elicit"
   Ask, "May I provide you with some information on hypertension?
   Provide: "Untreated hypertension can lead to a heart attack or stroke":
   "Fortunately, hypertension can be treated to prevent these problems"
   Elicit: "What do you think about this information?"
6. Keep your door open to circle back on the initial discussion.
   - Can I contact you in a month to see how you are doing?

• BOX 20.2 Contemplation Stage Strategies: Decisional Balance

1. Pros of staying the same: What are the good things about smoking?
   - This question conveys positive regard.
2. Cons of staying the same: What could happen if you keep smoking?
   - This question raises awareness of the consequences.
3. Cons of changing: What are your concerns about quitting?
   - This question identifies barriers that can be addressed later
4. Pros of staying the same: What might be the benefits of quitting?
   - This question allows the patient to identify and personalize reasons for change.

Adapted from Velicer, W.F., DiClemente, C.C., Prochaska, J.O. & Brandenburg, N. (1985). Decisional balance measure for assessing and predicting smoking status. *Journal of Personality and Social Psychology*, 48(5), 1279–1289. doi:10.1037/0022-3514.48.5.1279

• BOX 20.3 Preparation Stage Strategies: Identifying the Initial Steps to Change

1. Where might be a good place to start?
2. Where do you think is the most important place to start?
3. What is one thing you could try?
4. Who can help?
5. What might you do to make this easier (addressing barriers)?

• BOX 20.4 Action Stage Strategies: Sustain Motivation

1. What are you doing to keep this change going?
2. What helps you be successful in making this change?
3. What is the best thing about making this change thus far?
4. What are you doing to prevent a return to your old behavior?

---

and are now ready to address it in the next 30 days. This stage is marked by information gathering, an important activity for later planning. Persons in this stage acquire the needed resources for change; they may purchase running shoes or join a weight loss support group. They might even experiment with different approaches to their problem (walking versus aerobic dance).

The preparation stage is the time for exploring resources and barriers and identifying the initial steps to change (Box 20.3).

Action: (I am)

A person in action has been engaging in health behavior for less than 6 months. They may be encouraged by improvements in their well-being and obvious physical improvements. A major benefit of this stage is a growing sense of confidence and competence. Persons at this stage are willing to receive support and may still benefit from rewards to sustain their motivation (Box 20.4).

Asking someone to contemplate what they are doing to prevent a return to their old behavior helps identify setback prevention strategies as the action stage is sometimes punctuated by lapses, a temporary return to the old behavior. Lapses differ from a relapse: Relapse is a longer or permanent return. It is helpful to acknowledge lapses as soon as they occur, inviting the patient to explore the antecedents and consequences as an opportunity for learning. Patients may also feel shame for their lapses, and it is empowering to realize that these are a part of human behavior and an opportunity to identify new strategies to prevent future setbacks.

Maintenance: (I still am)

At this point, the patient has sustained the health behavior change for more than 6 months. They are more confident in their ability to address challenges and less concerned about setbacks. At this point, the benefits of the behavior are likely to be self-reinforcing, an indication of intrinsic motivation. The patient's competence and autonomy are at

behavior. However, they are uncertain if they want to make an effort to change in the next 6 months. Thus the main feature of contemplation is ambivalence, an equal level of conflict between the pros and cons of change. A strategy known as decisional balance can be helpful at this stage. Decisional balance involves four questions that can lead to greater readiness for change (Velicer et al., 1985). Box 20.2 highlights decisional balance, using smoking as an example.

Preparation: (I will)

Persons in the preparation stage have resolved their ambivalence to the point where they acknowledge their problem

• BOX 20.5   Change Ruler Follow-up Questions

1. Why didn't you rate yourself lower?
   - This question engages patients in exploring underlying motivation, strengths, resources, or barriers that must be addressed for success.
   - For example, a person rating themselves as seven on the readiness ruler may answer, "I didn't rate myself lower because I know this is important" or "I want to get started but am not sure how."
2. What would need to happen for you to rate yourself higher?
   - This question opens the door for an exploration of additional requirements for success.
   - In many cases, these involve the resolution of barriers or the need for further information.

a level where support may be less needed. Nevertheless, lapses and relapses can still occur at this stage but may now be related to unexpected life events. Should this occur, an exploration of the patient's challenges, resources, and personal strengths can help the patient return to their desired behavior.

It is possible to determine your patient's stage of change using a "change ruler" (Clifford, 2019), a visual analog scale between 0–10. This scale can be used by asking your patient, "On a scale of 0–10, how *ready* are you to make this change?"

Typically, a person whose readiness rating is between 0 and 3 is not ready, placing them in the precontemplation stage. Ratings of 4–5 correspond to the contemplation stage, ratings of 6–7 to the preparation stage, and ratings of 8 or higher to the action and maintenance stages. This objective measure of the patient's readiness is an invaluable tool for enhancing motivation through two follow-up questions (Box 20.5).

In addition to readiness, the 0–10 scale can be used to assess two other domains, importance and confidence. These additional ratings can also provide opportunities to strengthen the patient's motivation by affirming their values (importance) and providing additional resources for success (confidence). Overall, the TTM is a powerful tool for understanding the process by which a person achieves intrinsic motivation. Armed with an understanding of SDT, physical and occupational therapists can facilitate this process by supporting the patient's autonomy, competence, and relatedness. In the next section, we will explore the conversational approach through which TTM and SDT can be used to support health behavior change.

Motivational Interviewing

Motivational interviewing (MI) was developed in the early 1980s by psychologists William Miller and Stephen Rollnick based on their experiences with problem drinkers (Miller, 1983). Since then, MI has gained widespread use as a tool for a wide spectrum of behavior change and has many uses in the context of physical and occupational therapy intervention. This section provides a brief overview of this powerful approach. You are encouraged to explore further resources (Clifford & Curtis, 2016) for integrating the related skills into your future practice.

MI is *"a collaborative, goal-oriented style of communication with particular attention to the language of change. It is designed to strengthen personal motivation for and commitment to a specific goal by eliciting and exploring the person's own reasons for change within an atmosphere of acceptance and compassion"* (Miller & Rollnick, 2013, p. 29). A central premise of MI is avoidance of the "righting reflex," a reference to the common health practitioner approach of "fixing" patients through top-down directives. Rather, MI is described more as a patient-practitioner "dance," in which the practitioner guides the patient through exploring their innate capacities and desire for change.

The resolution of ambivalence is another key concept of MI. In the early stages of readiness, ambivalence is a common and important feature of health behavior change. Strategies such as the previously described decisional balance questions are one approach to addressing ambivalence. Ambivalence can also be addressed by another MI tool known as "developing discrepancy." The discrepancy is developed through careful listening, which enables the practitioner to juxtapose patient statements supporting their capacities for change against those related to their concerns and justifications for sustaining negative health behaviors. An example of such a statement might be: *"on one hand, you aren't sure if you can stop drinking, but on the other hand, you were able to stay sober when you were pregnant. What made it easy then?"* Such conversations help the patient uncover and affirm existing strengths that enhance motivation. Regardless of whether decisional balance and developing discrepancy increase the patient's motivation, it is important to listen without judgment, avoid arguing, and express empathy.

MI can best be described as a way of being with patients. This way of being is described as "the spirit of MI" and involves collaboration between practitioner and patient, evoking the patient's ideas about change while emphasizing their autonomy and engaging with compassion. The spirit of MI can be applied through open-ended questions, affirmations, reflections, and summaries. Collectively, these approaches can be remembered through the acronym OARS.

Use o*pen-ended questions* (such as who, when, what, how, tell me about, what do you think about?). In contrast to closed-ended questions (typically involving a yes/no response), open-ended questions invite patients to express their ideas, values, and perspectives. When patients express these in their own words, their autonomy is supported. Careful listening to our patients' unique reasons and desires for change (known in MI as "change talk") provides opportunities for building motivation through patient-centered intervention.

Affirmations are practitioner statements that acknowledge and support patients' strengths, past successes, and efforts toward change. As opposed to practitioners' common use of generalized "cheerleading" statements (such as "you did great" or "I'm proud of you"), affirmations put a direct focus on a patient's change-enhancing attributes.

For example, "you showed great initiative by walking every day as you had planned" is empowering and motivation enhancing. Affirmations support competence and autonomy by enabling patients to honor and capitalize on their existing strengths.

Reflections are used by practitioners to express empathy and to demonstrate generous listening. They assure the patient that they have been heard. Reflections can be direct paraphrases, such as "you value your health." They can also be practitioner interpretations of what has been said. Either approach is helpful, and even if a reflection is inaccurate, it provides the patient with an opportunity for clarification.

Summaries can be described as a bouquet of patient reflections, highlighting change talk and other elements that will move the client toward further motivation and action. An example could be, "*You mentioned several reasons for working on healthy eating and meal planning, including being able to reduce your diabetes medications. You want to manage your diabetes to avoid the complications your mother had. You have not had success with meal planning in the past and would like some ideas.*"

MI conversations involve four steps: Engage, Focus, Evoke, and Plan. These can be described as follows:

The first step is to *engage* your patient by establishing rapport. Empathy, generous listening, and approaching your patient with genuine curiosity are essential tools in this process. In this step, you learn about your patient's life context, values, and goals, enabling you to collaborate towards meaningful outcomes.

The second step is *focus*. Here, you identify the patient's area of interest for behavior change. In many cases, the patient knows their behavior of interest. In other instances, they may not be certain, and it can sometimes be helpful to present the patient with a simple list of wellness elements: physical activity, nutrition, sleep and stress management.

The third step is to *evoke* the client's reasons for change and their readiness, confidence, and importance. The use of a change ruler can assist in clarifying these elements. It is also important to evoke the patient's

barriers and resources, exploring ways of minimizing the former and optimizing the latter.

Finally, the patient and practitioner develop a specific plan for addressing the change. The use of specific, measurable, achievable, relevant, and time-bound (SMART) goals provides a clear structure for the desired behavior (Table 20.1) (White et al., 2020).

Well-written SMART goals provide the framework for identifying and quantifying the elements of behavior change. SMART goals support patient autonomy by providing clear guidelines for performance. SMART goals enhance competence by assuring achievability and relevance. The aspect of relatedness can be specifically included in the various elements of the SMART goal structure; for example, a goal may be more achievable if it consists of another person, for example, "I will walk with my partner," or it may be more relevant when tied to social interaction: "I will be able to hike with my grandchildren." In many ways, SMART goals are not unlike the functional goals that OTs and PTs develop for their patients.

As a future healthcare provider, you will be better able to serve your patients if your health is optimal. You are encouraged to develop your own health-related SMART goals during your education. In this author's experience with physical therapy students, sufficient sleep, purposeful physical activity, and healthy nutrition are common areas to address.

Health and Wellness Coaching in PT and OT Practice

While any health professional can use the principles of health behavior change described in this section, skilled use of these strategies can be enhanced through training as a health and wellness coach. According to a recent systematic review (Wolever et al., 2013), the role of the health and wellness coach is defined as follows:

The coach is a healthcare professional trained in behavior change theory, motivational strategies, and communication

TABLE 20.1	SMART Goal Examples		
Specific	What is the single behavior?	I will walk...
Measurable	What is the observable evidence of behavior performance?	...three times a week for 30 minutes...
Achievable	What are the resources to achieve your goal?	...in my neighborhood on Monday, Wednesday, and Friday after breakfast. I will use my smartphone to time my walk. I will keep a log of my walking.
Relevant	Why is this goal vital for your overall well-being?	Walking will help me improve my endurance and will help me to sleep better.
Time-bound	How long will you do this action?	I will do this for the summer months of June and September.

techniques, which are used to assist patients to develop intrinsic motivation and obtain skills to create sustainable change for improved health and well-being. (Wolvever et al., 2013, p. 52)

The National Board for Health and Wellness Coaches (NBHWC) is the regulatory body to approve high-quality health and wellness coach training and educational programs. Successful completion of one of an NBHWC-approved training and the credentialing program (National Board for Health and Wellness Coaches, 2022) is a prerequisite to taking the national board certification exam, successful completion of which confers the credential of national board-certified health and wellness coach (NBC-HWC). Most health coach training programs take several months to a year for completion and involve both practical and written exams. Most of these training programs offer a stand-alone certification separate from the National Board for Health and Wellness Coaches. As of this writing, As of 2023, there are over 6700 national board-certified health and wellness coaches in the United States. As evidence supporting the success of health and wellness coaching grows, so does the demand for this practice area. As of 2020, health coaching was a $7.1-billion service market expected to reach $8.87 billion by 2025. According to a recent market analysis (LaRosa, 2021), the top three consumers of health coaching services include patients, physician offices, healthcare organizations, and corporate wellness programs. PTs and OTs are increasingly integrating health coaching into their clinical practices, and an increasing number are pursuing national board certification.

Moreover, the American Physical Therapy Association (APTA) approved the formation of the Health Promotion and Wellness Council in 2017, which is open to all members. In addition, many APTA academies (e.g., the Academy of Geriatrics and the Academy of Neurology) have practice-specific health and wellness and special interest groups. All these groups provide education and support for members.

The American Occupational Therapy Association (AOTA) also provides support, resources, and education on health and wellness as part of occupational therapy practice. Reitz and Scaffa (2020) penned AOTA's official statement on the role of occupational therapy in promoting health and well-being, describing the importance of occupational therapist intervention, specifically the role of occupational engagement. The AOTA (2022) is historically and currently a leading advocate for mental health promotion, prevention, and intervention across the lifespan.

Population Health PT and OT Skillset

In addition to understanding the theory of behavioral change to impact health, a community-based population health clinical practice requires a different and innovative pragmatic skill set for success (Scaffa & Reitz, 2020). Beyond the possession of broad clinical knowledge, population health practitioners must be knowledgeable in business as well as program-planning principles. These include a client-centered orientation to needs assessment, program planning, outcomes assessment, and a knowledge of the community and its inherent resources. Additional principles involve proficiency in working with diverse others or stakeholders who can contribute to or be involved in service delivery to ensure relevant and meaningful programming. Community practice further involves applying core professional knowledge in new and different contexts. It requires a thorough understanding of the community and the resources available and the ability to connect key stakeholders to available resources in order for them to build coalitions within communities. Understanding health education and behavior decision-making processes helps foster and understand behavioral change. Finally, community practice requires fundraising awareness and skills, as few structures currently exist to support this practice. Fundraising awareness and skills involve routinely surveying resources for grant funding, identifying and seeking corporate sponsorship, advocacy for legislation to support efforts, and more traditional fundraising approaches, all of which are a more active approach to service provision as opposed to providing services based on what third-party payers will cover (Scaffa & Reitz, 2020).

For occupational therapists, opportunities exist for supporting occupational engagement with many populations. Some exciting innovative community-based programming identified in the literature include reducing recidivism with individuals following incarceration (Jaegers et al., 2020); support of youth with disabilities in managing transitions within and as they exit secondary schools (Podvey & Myers, 2018); early identification of at-risk families to help develop enriched environments to foster the achievement of developmental milestones (Coffin & Gropack, 2015); facilitating preparation for support of youth in the foster care system in their transition into the community through various life skills and career preparation initiatives (Paul-Ward & Lambdin-Pattavina, 2016); the development of inclusive programming to support individuals with disabilities within the community (Scaffa & Reitz, 2020); wellness coaching for individuals with substance use disorder (Armstrong, 2020); occupation engagement, exploration, and environmental modification for homeless children, youth, and families (Benoit, 2019; O'Donnell & McKinnon, 2022); programs supporting survivors of intimate partner violence to develop life skills and self-sufficiency (Javaherian-Dysinger et al., 2021); and programs that support the maintenance of health and well-being of well elderly in the community (Stancanelli, 2020).

For physical therapists, Benzer (2015) discusses areas that may involve identifying opportunities for sleep, smoking cessation, stress management, and nutrition. APTA (2019) further outlines physical therapy roles in active living, workplace and community-based injury prevention programs, and reproductive and sexual health. In 2017, the APTA launched the Health Promotion and Wellness Council, free to all members and devoted to providing education, recent evidence, and research opportunities related to lifestyle intervention. Current initiatives include the development of the

Physical Therapy Healthy Lifestyle Appraisal (Ingman et al., 2022), the development of a website for nutrition and physical therapy, and the formation of a task force exploring the inclusion of mental and behavioral health as consideration for physical therapist practice. Each of these opportunities represents potential growth for our professions in new and exciting ways and the ability for physical and occupational therapists to impact the nation's health more broadly. Perhaps most importantly, this population-based perspective positions our professions to be leaders in our respective areas related to the health and well-being of populations.

Barriers and Considerations

There are currently obstacles to practice in these areas, many of which originate from our respective professions. A population-based perspective is distinct from yet complementary to the medical model of care (Scaffa & Reitz, 2020). Many occupational and physical therapists are most comfortable functioning within the medical model, and exploring our scopes of practice in different areas can be challenging. If our practitioners cannot perceive the opportunities, then a limited number of practitioners will be open or willing to explore these areas, hindering growth (Benzer, 2015). Realities of the medical model (e.g., high productivity standards) limit the time to explore new practice areas.

Community-based population health services require a certain comfort with ambiguity as practitioners address new goals and perspectives (Scaffa & Reitz, 2020). This approach is more entrepreneurial than a medical model approach and requires a certain level of risk tolerance that not all practitioners possess. Finally, there is a lack of funding for population-based services (Armstrong, 2020; Bezner, 2015; Scaffa & Reitz, 2020). Progress has been made (e.g., for lifestyle redesign programming for weight loss). Still, funding and reimbursement are not universal, requiring proactive actions on the part of practitioners to secure funding through fundraising, grantsmanship, active participation in legislative efforts related to policy, and fee-for-service paradigms (Scaffa & Reitz, 2020).

Future Directions for Health and Wellness Practice

Because of the substantial burden of chronic-related disease, health and wellness interventions are becoming a key element of physical and occupational therapy practice. To prepare for best practices in this area, physical and occupational therapy education programs must prepare their graduates for emerging competencies. The final portion of this section will outline the opportunities that lie ahead.

Health and Wellness Coaching Reimbursement

In January 2021, the American Medical Association, in collaboration with the National Board of Health and Wellness Coaching, approved the creation of three new current procedural technology (CPT) category codes for health coaching. These include:

- 0591T: Health and Well-Being Coaching face-to-face; individual, initial assessment
- 0592T: Individual, follow-up session, at least 30 minutes
- 0593T: Group (two or more individuals), at least 30 minutes

These codes were approved as category III, a temporary code applied to interventions considered "emerging technology." For these codes to be used, any non-physician provider must hold certification from the National Board for Health and Wellness Coaching or The National Commission for Health Education Credentialing.

These temporary codes provide sufficient evidence that health coaching services are being used in the United States adequately and that these services have clinical efficacy. While reimbursement for category III codes is optional, the goal is for these to become fully reimbursable (category I) in the next few years. Thus using these codes by qualified PTs and OTs represents a tremendous opportunity for establishing the value of health and wellness coaching and will hopefully lead to a larger body of evidence supporting the value of this intervention.

MI Training in PT and OT Education Programs

As evidence of the value of MI training in managing chronic pain, physical activity, and older adult frailty accrue (Physiopedia, 2022), physical and occupational therapy educational programs can support using this approach in their educational programs. Currently, it is unknown how many educational programs include MI training, but anecdotal evidence suggests that many programs have begun to include this. As a relational approach to patient-centered care, MI training can be easily integrated into communication, health and wellness courses, and professionalism. By integrating MI throughout the curriculum, our future practitioners can become better prepared to develop lifestyle-focused interventions for patients of all ages and conditions.

Increased Education on Nutrition

Although health benefits can accrue from regular exercise alone, recent evidence suggests that a high-quality diet is also needed to reduce mortality from cardiovascular disease and cancer (Ding et al., 2022). Similar evidence has also emerged around other health conditions such as hypertension and diabetes (Jurik & Stasny, 2019; Rosenfeld et al., 2022). Lack of adequate nutrition education has been documented in United States medical schools. In 2019, the Liaison Committee on Medical Education, the accrediting organization for United States medical schools, recommended no less than 25 hours of nutrition education across the 4-year medical school curriculum. Despite this recommendation, more training may be needed to address the nutritional complexities of many chronic illnesses.

PTs and OTs are highly skilled in exercise-related interventions but probably receive inadequate nutritional education. Concerns about practice act violations have likely contributed to this deficiency, but this has changed in recent years. Accordingly, a 2019 position statement of the American Physical Therapy Association states:

> "It is within the professional scope of physical therapist practice to screen for and provide information on diet and nutritional issues" (APTA, 2019b).

The occupational therapy practice framework (AOTA, 2020) has long asserted that eating, feeding, and the specific instrumental activities of daily living of meal preparation and grocery shopping are part of the occupational therapist's domain of practice. These occupations present a natural opportunity to address nutritional concerns as part of occupational engagement.

While there is no standardized nutrition education for United States physical therapy schools, educational programs must include nutritional content as part of the accreditation process. Further exploration is needed to determine appropriate levels of education. In the meantime, guidelines for clinical practice have been identified, providing a useful starting place for continued discussion (Berner et al., 2021).

Conclusion

There are many health concerns that a population health practice can address. Daily, needs are identified that are particularly amenable to this approach. For example, Houtrow et al. (2020) described how children with disabilities and their families were disproportionately impacted by the COVID-19 pandemic and the recent associated lockdown policies. Occupational and physical therapists can address many of the needs of these children and families. By adopting a service perspective to population health needs, therapists can help their respective professions flourish and situate themselves for leadership roles as these needs evolve and change over time.

References

American College of Lifestyle Medicine. (2022). *About us.* https://lifestylemedicine.org/about-us/. Accessed August 15, 2023.

American Occupational Therapy Association (AOTA). (2015). *Occupational therapy's role in health promotion.* https://www.aota.org/~/media/Corporate/Files/AboutOT/Professionals/WhatIsOT/HW/Facts/FactSheet_HealthPromotion.pdf.

American Occupational Therapy Association (AOTA). (2020). Occupational therapy in the promotion of health and well-being. *American Journal of Occupational Therapy, 74,* 7403420010. https://doi.org/10.5014/ajot.2020.743003.

American Occupational Therapy Association. (2022). *Mental health promotion, prevention and intervention across the lifespan.* https://www.aota.org/-/media/Corporate/Files/Practice/MentalHealth/Distinct-Value-Mental-Health.pdfAmerican.

Physical Therapy Association (APTA). (2019a). *Physical therapists' role in prevention wellness, fitness, health promotion, and management of disease and disability.* https://www.apta.org/apta-and-you/leadership-and-governance/policies/pt-role-advocacy.

American Physical Therapy Association. (2019b). *House of delegates policy P06-19-08-44; Role of the physical therapist and APTA in diet and nutrition.* https://www.apta.org/apta-and-you/leadership-and-governance/policies/role-of-pt-diet-nutrition.

Armstrong, M. (2020). *Occupational therapy practice in community mental health: Four case examples.* https://www.aota.org/publications/student-articles/career-advice/community-mental-health.

Benigas, S. (2019). American College of Lifestyle Medicine: Vision, tenacity, transformation. *American Journal of Lifestyle Medicine, 14*(1), 57–60.

Benoit, E. (2019). *Rediscovering humanity to redefine homelessness: An occupational therapy perspective.* https://www.aota.org/publications/ot-practice/ot-practice-issues/2019/fieldwork-issues-homelessness

Berner, P., Bezner, J. R., Morris, F., & Lein, D. H. (2021). Nutrition in physical therapist practice: Setting the stage for taking action, *Physical Therapy, 101*(5), pzab062.

Bezner, J. R. (2015). Promoting health and wellbeing: Implications for physical therapist practice. *Physical Therapy, 95*(10), 1433–1444.

Buttorff, C., Ruder, T., & Bauman, M. (2017). *Multiple chronic conditions in the United States.* Rand Corporation. https://www.rand.org/content/dam/rand/pubs/tools/TL200/TL221/RAND_TL221.pdf.

Centers for Disease Control and Prevention. (2017). *Health disparities.* https://www.cdc.gov/aging/disparities/index.htm.

Centers for Disease Control and Prevention. (2020). *The ICF: An overview.* https://www.cdc.gov/nchs/data/icd/icfoverview_finalforwho10sept.pdf. Accessed August 15, 2023.

Centers for Disease Control and Prevention, National Center for Health Statistics. (2020). *Changes in life expectancy at birth, 2010-2018.* https://www.cdc.gov/nchs/data/hestat/life-expectancy/life-expectancy-2018.htm#Table1.

Centers for Medicare and Medicaid Services. (2022). *The Accountable Health-Related Social Needs Screening Tool.* https://innovation.cms.gov/files/worksheets/ahcm-screeningtool.pdf. Accessed August 15, 2023.

Clifford, D., & Curtis, L. (2016). *Motivational interviewing in nutrition and fitness.* New York: Guilford Press.

Clifford, D. (2019). Dawn Clifford's MI tips. *MI tip of the day: The change ruler.* (Video) YouTube. https://youtu.be/bm3sAwmBetg.

Coffin, D. A., & Gropack, S. J. (2015). *The effect of a community-based program on the development of at-risk preschoolers.* https://ajot.aota.org/article.aspx?articleid=2490955.

Collings, C. (2021). *The power of lifestyle medicine to treat disease.* Presentation for American College of Lifestyle Medicine. https://www.lifestylemedicine.org/ACLM/Education/Webinar_Archive_Open_Source/The_Power_of_Lifestyle_Medicine.aspx.

Crotty, G. F., & Schwarzschild, M. A. (2020). Chasing protection in Parkinson's disease: Does exercise reduce risk and progression? *Frontiers in Aging Neuroscience, 12,* 186.

Cummings, K. M., Jette, A. M., & Rosenstock, I. M. (1978). Construct validation of the health belief model. *Health Education & Behavior, 6*(4), 394–405.

Deci, E. L., & Ryan, R. M. (1985). *Intrinsic motivation and self-determination in human behavior.* Plenum New York: Plenum Press.

Dexter, P. R., Miller, D. K., Clark, D. O., Weiner, M., Harris, L. E., Livin, L., Myers, I., Shaw, D., Blue, L. A., Kunzer, J., & Overhage, J. M. (2010). Preparing for an aging population and improving chronic disease management. *AMIA 2010 Symposium Proceedings, 2010,* 162–166.

Ding, D., Van Buskirk, J., Nguyen, B., Stamatakis, E., Elbarbary, M., Veronese, N., Clare, P. J., Lee, I., Ekelund, U., & Fontana, L. (2022). Physical activity, diet quality and all-cause cardiovascular disease and cancer mortality: A prospective study of 346 627 UK Biobank participants. *British Journal of Sports Medicine,* bjsports-2021-105195. doi:10.1136/bjsports-2021-105195.

European Flow Research Network. (2014). *What is flow - Current definition.* https://efrn.eu.

Engel, G. L. (1980). The clinical application of the biopsychosocial model. *American Journal of Psychiatry, 137,* 535–544.

Ford, E. S., Bergmann, M. M., Kröger, J., Schienkiewitz, A., Weikert, C., & Boeing, H. (2009). Healthy living is the best revenge: Findings from the European prospective investigation into cancer and nutrition—Potsdam study. *Archives of Internal Medicine, 169*, 1355–1362.

Haines, M. (2020). Pandemic worsens food deserts for 23.5 million Americans. *Voice of America.* https://www.voanews.com/a/usa_pandemic-worsens-food-deserts-235-million-americans/6189526.html.

Heutte, J., Fenouillet, F., Martin-Krumm, C., Gute, G., Raes, A., Gute, D., Bachelet, R., & Csikszentmihalyi, M. (2021). Optimal experience in adult learning: Conception and validation of the flow in education scale (EduFlow-2). *Frontiers in Psychology, 12*, 828027.

Holt-Lunstad, J., Smith, T. B., & Layton, J. B. (2010) Social relationships and mortality risk: A meta-analytic review. *PLoS Medicine, 7*(7), e1000316.

Houtrow, A., Harris, D., Molinero, A., Levin-Decanini, T., & Robichaud, C. (2020). COVID-19's impact on the practice of pediatric medicine: Insights and recommendations. *Journal of Pediatric Rehabilitation Medicine, 13*(3), 415–424.

Ingman, M. S., Bezner, J. B., & Black, B. B. (2022). Development and reliability of the physical therapy healthy lifestyle appraisal: A new assessment tool to guide behavior change. *Cardiopulmonary Physical Therapy Journal, 33*, 77–86.

Jaegers, L. A., Skinner, E., Conners, B., Hayes, C., West-Bruce, S., Vaughn, M. G., Smith, D. L., & Barney, K. F. (2020). Evaluation of the jail-based occupational therapy transition and integration services program for community reentry. *American Journal of Occupational Therapy, 74*(3), 7403205030.

Javaherian-Dysinger, H., Dalida, E., Maclang, C., Cho, E., Simbolon, H., & Santiago, M. (2021). Intimate partner violence and OT: A systematic review. *American Journal of Occupational Therapy, 75*(2). doi:10.5014/ajot.2021.75S2-PO380

Joung, M. J., Han, M. A., Park, J., & Ryu, S. Y. (2016). Association between family and friend smoking status and adolescent smoking behavior and e-cigarette use in Korea. *International Journal of Environmental Research and Public Health, 13*(12), 1183.

Jurik, R., & Stastny, P. (2019). Role of nutrition and exercise programs in reducing blood pressure: A systematic review. *Journal of Clinical Medicine, 8*(9), 1393.

LaRosa, J. (2021). *$7 billion US health coaching market gains favor among consumers, insurers and employers.* https://blog.marketresearch.com/7-billion-u.s.-health-coaching-market-gains-favor-among-consumers-insurers-employers.

Lehman, B. J., David, D. M., & Gruber, J. A. (2017). Rethinking the biopsychosocial model of health: Understanding health as a dynamic system. *Social and Personality Psychology Compass, 11*, e12328.

Martino, J., Pegg, J., & Frates, E. P. (2015). The connection prescription: Using the power of social interactions and the deep desire for connectedness to empower health and wellness. *American Journal of Lifestyle Medicine, 11*(6), 466–475.

Meals on Wheels America. (2022). *Meals on wheels America.* https://www.mealsonwheelsamerica.org/learn-more/national.

Miller, W. (1983). Motivational interviewing with problem drinkers. *Behavioural Psychotherapy, 11*(2), 147–172.

Miller, W. R., & Rollnick, S. (2013). *Motivational interviewing: Helping people to change* (3rd ed.). New York: Guilford Press.

National Board for Health and Wellness Coaches. (2022) *Approved training programs.* https://nbhwc.org/find-an-approved-training-program/#!directory/ord=rnd.

National Center for Chronic Disease Prevention and Health Promotion (NCCDPHP). (2022). *Promoting health in older adults.* https://www.cdc.gov/chronicdisease/resources/publications/factsheets/promoting-health-for-older-adults.htm.

O'Donnell, M. & McKinnon, S. (2022). Health policy perspectives - Advocating for change to meet the developmental needs of young children experiencing homelessness. *American Journal of Occupational Therapy, 76*, 7605090010. https://doi.org/10.5014/ajot.2022.050114

Paul-Ward, A., & Lambdin-Pattavina, A. (2016). New roles for occupational therapy to promote independence among youth aging out of foster care. *American Journal of Occupational Therapy, 70*, 7003360010.

Physiopedia. (2022). *Motivational interviewing.* https://www.physiopedia.com/Motivational_Interviewing.

Pollack Porter, K. M., Rutkow, L., & McGinty, E. E. (2018). The importance of policy change for addressing public health problems. *Public Health Reports, 133*(Suppl. 1), 9S–14S.

Podvey, M. C., & Myers, C. T. (2018). *Transitions for children and youth: How occupational therapy can help.* https://www.aota.org/-/media/Corporate/Files/AboutOT/Professionals/WhatIsOT/CY/Fact-Sheets/Transitions.pdf.

Prochaska, J. O., & DiClemente, C. C. (1983). Stages and processes of self-change of smoking: Toward an integrative model of change. *Journal of Consulting and Clinical Psychology, 51*(3), 390–395.

Reitz, S. M., & Scaffa, M. E. (2020). Occupational therapy in the promotion of health and well-being. *American Journal of Occupational Therapy, 74*(3), 7403420010p1–7403420010p14.

Rosenfeld, R. M., Kelly, J. H., & Agarwal, M. (2022). Dietary interventions to treat type 2 diabetes in adults with a goal of remission: An expert consensus statement from the American College of Lifestyle Medicine. *American Journal of Lifestyle Medicine, 16*(3), 342–362.

Rosenstock, I. M. (1974). Historical origins of the health belief model. *Health Education Monographs, 2*(4), 328–335. doi:10.1177/109019817400200403.

Scaffa, M. E., & Reitz, S. M. (2020). *Occupational therapy in community and population health practice* (3rd ed.). F. A. Davis.

Skybova, D., Slachtova, H., Tomaskova, H., Dalecka, A., & Madar, R. (2021). Risk of chronic diseases limiting longevity and healthy aging by lifestyle and social-economic factors during the life course - A narrative review. *Medycna Pracy, 72*(5), 535–548.

Stancanelli, J. (2020). Teaching occupational therapy's role on health and wellness for community-based older adults. *SIS Quarterly Practice Connection, 5*(4), 9–12.

US Department of Health and Human Services. (2020a). *Healthy people 2030.* https://health.gov/healthypeople.

US Department of Health and Human Services. (2020b). *Healthy people 2030 framework.* https://health.gov/healthypeople/about/healthy-people-2030-framework.

US Department of Health and Human Services. (2021c). *Social determinants of health.* https://health.gov/healthypeople/priority-areas/social-determinants-health.

Velicer, W. F., DiClemente, C. C., Prochaska, J. O., & Brandenburg, N. (1985). Decisional balance measure for assessing and predicting smoking status. *Journal of Personality and Social Psychology, 48*(5), 1279–1289.

White, N. D., Bautista, V., Lenz, T., & Cosimano, A. (2020). Using the SMART-EST goals in lifestyle medicine prescription. *American Journal of Lifestyle Medicine, 14*(3), 271–273. https://www.ncbi.nlm.nih.gov/pmc/articles/PMC7232896/pdf/10.1177_1559827620905775.pdf.

Wolever, R. Q., Simmons, L. A., Sforzo, G. A., Dill, D., Kaye, M., Bechard, E. M., Southard, M. E., Kennedy, M., Vosloo, J., & Yang, N. (2013). A systematic review of the literature on health and wellness coaching: Defining a key behavioral intervention in healthcare. *Global Advances in Health and Medicine, 2*(4), 38–57.

Yeh, B. I., & Kong, I. D. (2013). The advent of lifestyle medicine. *American Journal of Lifestyle Medicine, 3*(1), 1–8.

21

Care Coordination and Case Management

MELISSA K. TRAVELSTED, DNP, APRN, FNP-C, PTA, AANP

LEARNING OBJECTIVES

By the end of this chapter, the reader will be able to:

1. Define relevant terminology regarding care coordination and case management.
2. Discuss the components of care coordination across the lifespan.
3. Describe the role of quality and safety in healthcare.
4. Discuss how care coordination can prevent burnout and facilitate the achievement of the Quadruple Aim.
5. Describe the role of rehabilitative services in care coordination.

CHAPTER OUTLINE

The United States healthcare system is transitioning from fee-for-service to a value-based payment program to control costs and improve quality care (Beck da Silva Etges et al., 2020). *Mirror, Mirror 2021: Reflecting Poorly* is the latest in a series of reports released by the Commonwealth Fund, a private foundation that supports healthcare research to improve quality and policy in healthcare (Schneider et al.,

2021). The goal of the *Mirror, Mirror* report is to compare the healthcare systems of 11 high-income countries (Australia, Canada, France, Germany, the Netherlands, New Zealand, Norway, Sweden, Switzerland, the United Kingdom, and the United States) using data from the Organization for Economic Co-operation and Development (OECD) and the World Health Organization (WHO). Despite spending

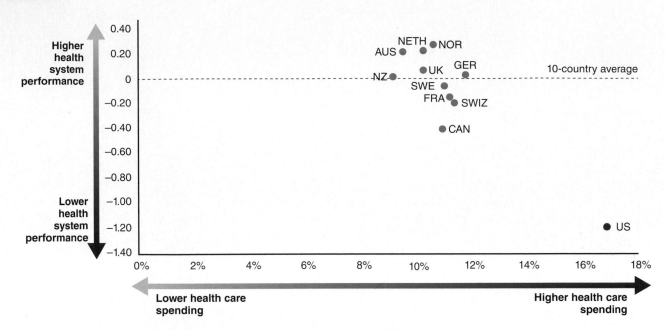

• **Fig. 21.1** Healthcare in the United States Compared With Other High-Income Countries. (Eric C. Schneider et al., Mirror, Mirror 2021 — Reflecting Poorly: Health Care in the U.S. Compared to Other High-Income Countries (Commonwealth Fund, Aug. 2021). https://www.commonwealthfund.org/publications/fund-reports/2021/aug/mirror-mirror-2021-reflecting-poorly)

more on healthcare, the US healthcare system ranks last compared with these other high-income countries (Schneider et al., 2021). Americans spent 16.8% of the gross domestic product on healthcare in 2019, yet the United States healthcare system ranks last overall in performance (Fig. 21.1). The United States also has the lowest life expectancy at 78.6 years, compared with the OECD's 26 high-income member countries (Tikkanen & Abrams, 2020). The average life expectancy of OECD countries is 80.7 years.

In 2020, healthcare spending in the United States reached $4.1 trillion (Centers for Medicare & Medicaid Services [CMS], 2021). According to the National Quality Forum (NQF), inefficiencies in communication and patient care fragmentation increase errors, cost, and unnecessary pain (NQF, 2012). Care coordination has been identified as a tool to reduce fragmentation of care, minimize inefficiencies, and reduce the cost of care (Doty et al., 2020).

Care Coordination and Case Management Defined

The distinction between care coordination and case management is unclear, as the terms have been used interchangeably and inconsistently throughout the literature. Overall, care coordination and case management are similar in that they are collaborative efforts to ensure patients receive the most appropriate care. However, they are both defined based on the perspective of the individual or organization. Thus the next two sections will define case management and care coordination.

Case Management

Case management is defined in this chapter as overseeing a specific disease or condition, focusing on the allocation of funds and occurring within a facility, care setting, or health system (Kuo et al., 2018). Case managers are often registered nurses (RNs) or social workers with specific skills and knowledge of the populations they serve. The case manager's responsibility is to coordinate care to include transitions through the continuum of care (Cesta, 2018). The continuum of care spans over time from setting to setting and from illness to wellness. The case manager is the gatekeeper for the patient through the continuum of care to ensure that the patient receives the necessary care in a timely and efficient manner. Necessary care includes patient education, discharge planning, and facilitating the patient's interdisciplinary healthcare team.

Care Coordination

Care coordination occurs primarily outside the acute care setting to facilitate the appropriate healthcare services, in the right order, at the right time, and in the right setting (McDonald et al., 2007). Care coordination in the outpatient or community setting is the responsibility of the primary care provider (Doty et al., 2020). A commonly accepted definition of care coordination was adopted by the Agency for Healthcare Research & Quality (AHRQ) in 2006. The AHRQ is a subdepartment of the United States Department of Health and Human Services (HHS) and is the leading federal agency focused on quality and safety improvement in the healthcare of the United States (AHRQ,

2016a). The AHRQ-funded study developed a broad definition of care coordination following a systematic review of more than 40 definitions in the literature. AHRQ describes care coordination as:

> *the deliberate organization of patient care activities between two or more participants (including the patient) involved in a patient's care to facilitate the appropriate delivery of health care services. Organizing care involves the marshaling of personnel and other resources needed to carry out all required patient care activities and is often managed by the exchange of information among participants responsible for different aspects of care.* (McDonald et al., 2007, p. 41)

Several organizations accept this definition of care coordination, but no universal definition has been identified due to the variations of the stakeholders and activities involved in care coordination (NQF, 2021). The AHQ also developed a visual definition of care coordination due to the vast variety of definitions (Fig. 21.2) (McDonald et al., 2014, Chapter 2). The central goal of care coordination ("meet patient needs and preferences in delivery of high quality, high-value care") appears inside the triangle of perspectives (McDonald et al., 2014, Chapter 2). The triangle represents the three perspectives of care: patient/family, healthcare professionals, and system representatives, while the surrounding circles represent the possible participants, settings, and information

along the care path. The blue circle represents care coordination and the linkages to all aspects of patient care.

Care Coordination Across the Lifespan

All patients require care coordination; however, coordination varies with patient populations (Antonelli et al., 2009). Care should be person-centered, focusing on the patient's individual needs and values (American Geriatrics Society Expert Panel on Person-Centered Care, 2016). Our most vulnerable populations (frail, elderly persons with cognitive deficiencies, children with special healthcare needs, and those with multiple chronic diseases) are at the greatest risk of fragmented care (McDonald et al., 2014).

Pediatric Care Coordination

Pediatric care coordination is provided in a health care team integrated with a community-based, primary care medical home (PCMH) setting. The PCMH is a care model for children and adults and has five functions and attributes: comprehensive care, patient-centered, coordinated care, accessible services, and quality and safety (AHRQ, 2021). Under the direction of the primary care provider (PCP), the pediatric medical home is the central point of care and is family-centered (Cady et al., 2020). The team provides opportunities for families to express their needs and concerns and connects the patient and family with appropriate

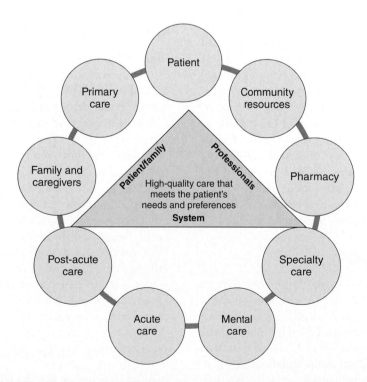

• **Fig. 21.2** The Care Coordination Ring. (McDonald KM, Schultz E, Albin L, Pineda N, Lonhart J, Sundaram V, Smith-Spangler C, Brustrom J, Malcolm E, Rohn, L. and Davies, S. Care Coordination Atlas Version 4 (Prepared by Stanford University under subcontract to American Institutes for Research on Contract No. HHSA290-2010-00005I). AHRQ Publication No. 14-0037- EF. Rockville, MD: Agency for Healthcare Research and Quality. June 2014.)

services and resources, minimizing care fragmentation and improving health outcomes. Antonelli et al.'s (2009, p. 8) definition of pediatric care coordination is:

> *Pediatric care coordination is a patient-and family-centered, assessment-driven, team-based activities designed to meet the needs of children and youth. Care coordination addresses interrelated medical, social, developmental, behavioral, educational, and financial needs in order to achieve optimal health and wellness outcomes, and efficient delivery of health-related services and resources within and across systems.*

This definition is supported by the American Academy of Pediatrics (AAP), emphasizing that care coordination is a core element of the PCMH (AAP, 2014). Care coordination is the preeminent factor for developing and nurturing relationships across the care continuum (patients/families, healthcare providers, community resources, and care settings). These relationships are the basis of the PCMH.

Children with special healthcare needs require additional layers of care coordination (Cady et al., 2020). Approximately 18% of children in the United States have special healthcare needs (National Academy for State Health Policy [NASHP], 2020). Children and Youth with Special Health Care Needs (CYSHCN) are at increased risk for chronic illness due to physical, developmental, behavioral, or emotional conditions (Maternal and Child Health Bureau [MCHB], 2021). CYSHCN requires special consideration due to the increased need for services, additional specialists, and changes in care related to growth and maturity, which is especially significant in children with medical complexities (CMC) (NASHP, 2020). CMC are medically fragile and comprise less than 1% of children in the United States. With increased medical care comes an increase in care providers (Cady et al., 2020). CMC families and caregivers require a single point of contact with the care team. This point of contact is usually an RN or social worker functioning as the care coordinator. Effective care coordination involves consideration of all aspects of care that will address the child's healthcare needs and quality of care, including the continuum of health, education, early childcare, early intervention, nutrition, mental/behavioral/emotional health, community partnerships, and social services (AAP, 2014)

Geriatric Care Coordination

The United States population is aging (Administration on Aging [AOA], 2021). In 2019, the United States population aged 65 years and older was 54.1 million, comprising 16% of the population, an increase of 14.4 million over the last 10 years. By 2040, the percentage of adults 65 years and older is estimated to be 21.6% of the population.

Care of older adults can be complicated by multiple chronic diseases and functional limitations (AGS, 2016). The goals for the care of older adults are healthcare safety, quality, and coordination. The IOM report *Crossing the*

Quality Chasm: A New Health System for the 21st Century identified patient-centered care as one of the six aims for quality improvement in healthcare (IOM, 2001). Patient-centered care is the gold standard for healthcare in the United States and abroad and facilitates effective care coordination for older adults. There are eight essentials to realizing patient-centered care:

- An individualized, goal-oriented care plan based on a person's preferences
- Ongoing review of the person's goals and care plan
- Care supported by an interprofessional team in which the person is an integral team member
- One primary or lead point of contact on the healthcare team
- Active coordination among all healthcare and supportive service providers
- Continual information sharing and integrated communication
- Education and training for providers and, when appropriate, the person and those important to the person
- Performance measurement and quality improvement using feedback from the person and caregivers (AGS, 2016, p. 16)

History of Care Coordination

Care coordination occurs with all patient care, whether formal or informal. Formal care coordination is increasingly emphasized due to the focus on quality improvement and cost containment (NQF, 2012).

National Quality Forum (NQF)

In the 1960s, quality improvement in healthcare became a distinct field of study (Namburi & Lee, 2021). The Institute of Medicine's (IOM) 1999 report, *To Err Is Human*, highlighting the positive relationship between quality healthcare and patient safety, spurred the establishment of the NQF (Kohn et al., 2000). The NQF is a public, nonprofit organization designated to develop a national quality improvement and reporting strategy. The NQF has determined that care coordination in combination with effective communication is essential to improved outcomes, decreased medication errors, decreased ER visits, and hospital readmissions resulting in an overall reduction in healthcare cost (NQF, 2021). NQF defines care coordination as "the deliberate synchronization of activities and information to improve health outcomes to ensure patients' and families' needs and preferences for healthcare and community services are met throughout their treatment and care" (NQF, 2021, p. 12).

National Transitions of Care Coalition (NTOCC)

It is not uncommon for an elderly patient or a patient with chronic disease to have multiple healthcare providers and receive care in various healthcare settings (NTOCC, 2010). Transitions from one healthcare provider to another, from unit to unit in a facility, or from one facility to another along the care continuum are vulnerable times for patients. Poor transitions between healthcare providers and settings can result in:

- Compromised safety and quality of care
- Increased burden on patients and their families
- Increased cost of care (NTOCC, 2008)

The NTOCC is a team of interdisciplinary healthcare leaders focusing on effective transfers of care to improve healthcare quality. The NTOCC developed the Care Transition Bundle with seven essential intervention categories: medication management, transition planning, patient and family engagement/education, information transfer, follow-up care, healthcare provider engagement, and shared accountability across providers and organizations. Clear and timely communication, efficient care coordination, and patient-centered care are three primary components of safe transitions of care (NTOCC, 2008).

NTOCC defines care coordination as the transition between two particular care settings involving coordinated communication among providers and health plan administrators across various settings to ensure optimal patient care (NTOCC, 2010). Communication should include providers, patients, and family caregivers. A survey by the Commonwealth Fund of primary care providers in 11 countries found that in the United States, less than half of the primary care providers received notification of a change by a specialist in a patient's plan of care or medications (Doty et al., 2019).

Role in Quality and Safety

Safety and quality have been issues in healthcare for centuries; in fact, Florence Nightingale voiced her concerns in the 1800s (Wakefield, 2008). The IOM's *To Err Is Human* in 2000 noted that errors in healthcare ranked as one of the leading causes of death and injury (Kohn et al., 2000). This revelation brought quality and safety to the attention of the public as well as legislators (Wakefield, 2008). The IOM report agreed that humans make mistakes and identified the need for improved design of healthcare processes to limit errors and improve safety (Kohn et al., 2000). *Crossing the Quality Chasm: A New Health System for the 21st Century* was the IOM's follow-up report in 2001. The IOM committee identified four aspects of care responsible for inadequate quality of care: advances in complexity of healthcare due to advancing medical knowledge and technology, increased incidence of chronic disease, poorly organized healthcare processes and systems, and limits on utilization of information technology. This report established six healthcare system improvement aims (IOM, 2001). These aims suggest that healthcare should be:

- **Safe:** Care should be safe with the avoidance of injury.
- **Effective:** Care should be evidence-based and provided to those who would benefit from treatment (avoid underuse and overuse).
- **Patient-centered:** Care should be based on the preferences and values of the patient.

- **Timely:** Care should be provided in a timely fashion.
- **Efficient:** Care should avoid the waste of resources (equipment, supplies, ideas, and energy).
- **Equitable:** Care quality should be equal to all and not based on gender, ethnicity, geographic location, and socioeconomic status.

The third IOM report published in 2003, *Priority Areas for National Action: Transforming Health Care Quality,* initiates safety and quality measures to develop priority conditions as recommended in *Crossing the Quality Chasm* (IOM, 2003). Care coordination was one of the 20 priority areas identified. The committee determined that improvements in care coordination would positively impact healthcare processes across the continuum of care, especially in patients with serious illnesses and those with chronic diseases. Chronic disease is on the rise and the 2018 National Health Interview Survey (NHIS) reveals that 51.8% of United States adults suffer from at least one chronic condition and 27.02% from multiple chronic conditions (Boersma et al., 2020). Compared with adults without chronic conditions, adults with multiple chronic conditions have decreased quality of life, increased healthcare costs, and increased mortality. The IOM (2003) committee determined that care coordination over time between multiple health care providers and different settings is crucial for patients with chronic illness.

The IOM embarked on a quest in 1996 to assess and improve healthcare in the United States (National Academies Press, 2022). Since then, the IOM has released a series of 12 reports on safety and quality (Box 21.1), each with a different focus.

Legislation

The Patient Protection and Affordable Care Act (ACA) of 2010 (also known as Obamacare) required the establishment

---

• BOX 21.1 IOM's Quality Chasm Collection

- To Err Is Human: Building a Safer Health System (2000)
- Crossing the Quality Chasm: A New Health System for the 21st Century (2001)
- Priority Areas for National Action: Transforming Health Care Quality (2003)
- Health Professions Education: A Bridge to Quality (2003)
- Fostering Rapid Advances in Health Care: Learning from System Demonstrations (2003)
- Leadership by Example: Coordinating Government Roles in Improving Health Care Quality (2003)
- Keeping Patients Safe: Transforming the Work Environment of Nurses (2004)
- Patient Safety: Achieving a New Standard for Care (2004)
- Quality Through Collaboration: The Future of Rural Health (2005)
- Improving the Quality of Health Care for Mental and Substance-Use Conditions (2006)
- Preventing Medication Errors (2007)
- Improving Diagnosis in Health Care (2015)

Note. The individual reports at the National Academies Press website https://www.nap.edu/collection/62/quality-chasm

of the National Quality Strategy (NQS) by the United States Department of Health and Human Services to guide local, state, and national quality improvement efforts (Tikkanen et al., 2020). The NQS was first published in 2011 as the National Strategy for Quality Improvement in Healthcare with the three main objectives of better care, healthy people and communities, and affordable care (AHRQ, 2016b).

Triple Aim to Quadruple Aim

The healthcare objectives of the NQS reflect the Institute for Healthcare Improvement's (IHI) Triple Aim (Bodenheimer & Sinsky, 2014). The IHI developed a framework to optimize the healthcare system referred to as the Triple Aim, composed of the three foundational goals of "improving the individual experience of care; improving the health of populations; and reducing the per capita costs of care for populations" (Berwick et al., 2008, p. 759).

Primary care providers report adoption of the Triple Aim; however, they report an inability to succeed due to stress and burnout of clinicians and staff (Bodenheimer & Sinsky, 2014). The extent of physician and healthcare worker burnout stimulated Bodenheimer and Sinsky to expand the Triple Aim to the Quadruple Aim in 2014 to include "care of the patient requires care of the provider" (Bodenheimer & Sinsky, 2014, p. 573). Each aim depends on and influences the other aims (Fig. 21.3).

The three dimensions of burnout are emotional exhaustion, cynicism with job detachment, and a sense of professional ineffectiveness (National Academies of Sciences, Engineering, and Medicine [NASEM], 2019). Burnout is associated with many adverse outcomes in healthcare workers, such as increased rates of anxiety, depression, and substance abuse (Prasad et al., 2021). Healthcare worker burnout is also associated with poorer-quality care, reduced patient satisfaction, and increased costs (NASEM, 2019). The COVID-19 pandemic has worsened stress and burnout in healthcare providers (Prasad et al., 2021).

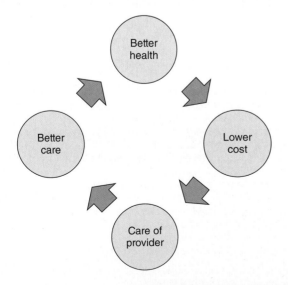

• **Fig. 21.3** The Institute for Healthcare Improvement Quadruple Aim: Each aim builds and influences the others.

Achieving an improved healthcare delivery system depends on a healthy workforce (NASEM, 2019). If well structured with support staff, care coordination may be associated with decreased burnout; however, burnout may occur if implemented with an increased task burden (Apaydin et al., 2021). Increased burnout can threaten the achievement of the Quadruple Aim of better care, better health, lower healthcare costs, and care of the provider.

Accountable Care Organization (ACOs)

An ACO is a group of providers (physicians, hospitals, and other healthcare providers) accountable for the costs of care for a population based on pre-designated performance standards (Bartels et al., 2015). ACOs receive prospective payments for the covered patients and clinical outcomes–based incentive payments. The program began in 2012 with an emphasis on preventive care and decreased hospital readmissions through care coordination programs that link reimbursement with quality measures.

The ACA authorized ACOs for patients with Medicare to decrease costs and improve care (CMS, 2021; Kuo et al., 2018). ACOs are patient-centered and utilize care coordination to facilitate safe care at the right time and place (CMS, 2021). ACOs are especially advantageous for patients with medical complexities such as CMC and the elderly with multiple chronic conditions (Kuo et al., 2018; Bartels, 2015).

Health Information Technology

The Health Insurance Portability and Accountability Act (HIPAA) was passed in 1996 (Office of the National Coordinator for Health Information Technology [ONC], 2021). HIPAA requires establishing standards for electronic health care transactions, and the HIPAA Privacy Rule defines what protected information is and how information can be used. The American Recovery and Reinvestment Act (ARRA), passed in 2009, established the Health Information Technology for Economic and Clinical Health Act (HITECH Act) to promote the adoption of health information technology (HHS, 2017). Meaningful Use in the HITECH Act incentivized provider use of electronic health records (EHR) (ONC, 2019). Meaningful Use has now transitioned into the Medicare EHR Incentive Program (MU) under the Merit-Based Incentive Payment System (MIPS). The four aims of MIPS are:
- Improving quality, safety, efficiency, and a reduction in health disparities
- Engaging patients and families
- Improving care coordination and population/public health
- Maintaining health information privacy and safety

Electronic medical records (EMR) and EHR are used interchangeably; however, their meanings differ. An EMR is a digital medical record (replacing the paper chart) and is contained in a single practice, while an EHR is a complete health record from multiple providers and can be shared electronically between providers (Fig. 21.4) (O'Connor, 2020). The EHR is a tool healthcare providers utilize for

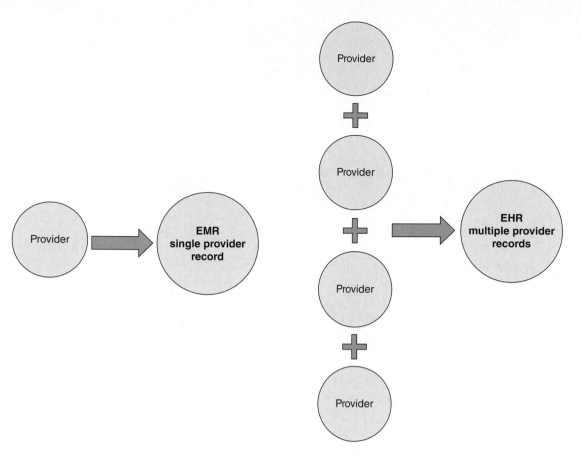

• **Fig. 21.4** Electronic Medical Record (EMR) Versus Electronic Health Record (EHR)

documentation, billing, and care coordination activities such as ordering tests, prescribing medications, and making referrals to other providers (NQF, 2021). The overreaching goal of EHR compliance is to improve clinical outcomes and population health, increase transparency and efficiency, empower individuals, and develop more robust research related to health systems.

Communication and Standardized Documentation

The IOM report, *To Err Is Human*, found that poor communication contributes to medical errors and impaired patient safety (Kohn et al., 2000). Whether verbal or written, communication in healthcare is considered inadequate if the information is inaccurate, incomplete, ill-timed, confusing, or unnecessary (The Joint Commission [TJC], 2017). Standardized terminology is paramount to patient safety and healthcare documentation (Fennelly et al., 2021). In 2004, TJC issued its "do not use" list of abbreviations to avoid dangerous misinterpretation of written documentation (TJC, 2018).

Communication and Safety With Hand-offs

Appropriate communication is the key to safety, especially at patient hand-offs between healthcare providers. A hand-off

occurs when the responsibility of a patient's care transfers from one healthcare provider and is accepted by another. The Joint Commission is a nonprofit organization that aims to ensure patient safety, quality healthcare, and patient advocacy through the accreditation of healthcare facilities and practices (Wadhwa & Huynh, 2021). TJC published National Patient Safety Goals (NPSG) and in 2006 released National Patient Safety Goal 2E (NPSG 2E), which called for standardized hand-off communication (AHRQ, 2019). NPSG 2E established specific guidelines for the standard of care for hand-off communication (Fig. 21.5). Hand-off communications should be done face-to-face or by phone with limited interruptions and should be interactive with the opportunity to ask questions (AHRQ, 2019; TJC, 2017). The information provided should be up-to-date and accurate (TJC, 2017). The standard also encourages using a standardized communication tool, EHR, to supplement communication and include patient or family input with hand-offs.

Situation-Background-Assessment-Recommendation

A standardized communication tool benefits a safe transition (TJC, 2017). The Situation-Background-Assessment-Recommendation (SBAR) tool is a standardized communication tool used by healthcare providers when discussing a patient's condition or used at hand-off (Leonard et al.,

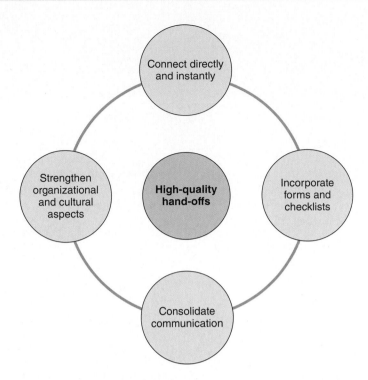

• **Fig. 21.5** Consolidated Joint Commission Hand-Off Commination Tips. (Adapted from https://www.vocera.com/blog/4-steps-address-joint-commissions-sentinel-event-alert-hand-communication; https://www.jointcommission.org/-/media/tjc/documents/resources/patient-safety-topics/sentinel-event/sea_8_steps_hand_off_infographic_2018pdf.pdf?db=web&hash=F4BCE57E34ED03DF76411EB9E302038E&hash=F4BCE57E34ED03DF76411EB9E302038E)

2017; TJC, 2017). The S or situation section of the tool should answer the question *why*. If a provider calls a physician, the information provided should answer why they called. The B or background section provides all pertinent information about the patient's background (e.g., diagnosis, current medications, allergies, labs, vitals, code status). The A is your assessment of the situation and the R is your recommendation or what you want from the communication. The strength of the SBAR is communicating critical information necessary for immediate attention due to a change in a patient's condition (AHRQ, 2020). Starmer et al. (2012) expressed the concern that a limitation of the SBAR is that it would not apply to the complex patient at the time of hand-off. See Table 21.1 for an example of the SBAR tool.

I PASS the BATON

Team Strategies & Tools to Enhance Performance and Patient Safety (TeamSTEPPS) curriculum is a set of teamwork tools resulting from a collaboration between the Department of Defense (DOD) and AHRQ to facilitate teamwork in healthcare (King et al., 2008). The TeamSTEPPS program strives to optimize communication and teamwork skills between healthcare providers. In response to the JCT NPSG 2-E requiring all healthcare organizations to implement standardized hand-offs with the opportunity for the receiving provider to ask questions, the I PASS the BATON communication tool was developed (DOD, 2005).

The I PASS the BATON mnemonic for hand-off communication can be utilized during nearly all simple and complex healthcare hand-offs (AHRQ, 2020; DOD, 2005). Accurate and complete transition communication must convey the patient plan of care to include treatment and services, current condition, and changes in patient condition or care, both recent and anticipated (DOD, 2005). During I PASS the BATON communication, the healthcare provider should (I) introduce themselves to the oncoming provider, (P) patient identification, (A) assessment; the history of the current illness, (S) situation; the patient's status/current condition, (S) safety concerns, (B) background; patient's past medical history, (A) action; provide a list with rationale, (T) timing; action list urgency and prioritization, (O) ownership; identify who is responsible for including healthcare team and patient/family, and (N) next; what is the plan. See Table 21.1 for an example of the I PASS the BATON tool.

I-PASS

I-PASS is another standardized communication tool to optimize hand-offs (Starmer et al., 2012). Starmer et al. developed the I-PASS acronym based on the I PASS the BATON mnemonic from TeamSTEPPS. Feedback from providers identified a need to shorten and simplify the mnemonic. The I-PASS acronym is I (illness severity), P (patient summary), A (action list), S (situation awareness and contingency planning), and S (synthesis by the receiver). See Table 21.1 for an example of the I-PASS tool.

TABLE 21.1   **Examples of Hand-off Tools With Scenarios**

SBAR

S	**Situation** • Provide information to answer *why* the therapist is calling	• Dr. Jones, this is Sharon Smith, PT • I am seeing Mr. Thomas in CCU Room 3A16 for physical therapy • He is a 60-year-old man who looks pale and diaphoretic • He is confused, weak, and complaining of chest pressure after sitting on the edge of the bed
B	**Background** • Provide pertinent information about the patient's background (e.g., diagnosis, current medications, allergies, labs, vitals, code status)	• He has a history of hypertension • He was admitted for chest pain two days ago • His BP is 90/50, his pulse is 120 BPM, and O_2 sat 94%
A	**Assessment** • Provide an assessment of the situation	• He is presenting with an altered cardiovascular response to activity
R	**Recommendation** • Provide a recommendation or what is wanted from the communication	• I will be holding physical therapy at this time and will require resumption of care orders • I have discussed the situation with Jill Brown, RN in CCU

IPASS the BATON

I	**Introduction** • Introduce yourself and your role/job (including the patient)	• Dr. Jones, this is Sharon Smith, PT • I am seeing Bob Thomas for physical therapy
P	**Patient** • Name, identifiers, age, sex, location	• Mr. Thomas is a 60-year-old male in CCU Room 3A16
A	**Assessment** • Presenting chief complaint, vital signs and symptoms, and diagnosis	• He was admitted with chest pain two days ago • He is confused, weak, and complaining of chest pain sitting edge of the bed • He is also pale and diaphoretic • His BP is 90/60, pulse 120 BPM, and O_2 sat 94%
S	**Situation** • Current status/circumstances, including code status, level of (un)certainty, recent changes, response to treatment	• Mr. Thomas is a full code • He had been performing well with PT until today
S	**Safety Concerns** • Critical lab values/reports, socioeconomic factors, allergies, alerts (e.g., falls, isolation)	• Labs have not been drawn today. His last HGB was 13.6 and HCT 39 at noon yesterday. • NKDA • No falls since in the hospital, but he is at risk of falling due to weakness and confusion

The

B	**Background** • Co-morbidities, previous episodes, current medications, family history	• He has a history of hypertension • He is currently taking amlodipine 10 mg daily, simvastatin 10 mg at bedtime, and citalopram 20 mg daily
A	**Actions** • What actions were taken or are required AND provide a brief rationale	• I have reported concerns to the RN, Jill Brown • I am holding PT
T	**Timing** • Level of urgency and explicit timing, prioritization of actions	• This is an urgent situation
O	**Ownership** • Who is responsible (nurse/doctor/team) including patient/family responsibilities?	• Jill Brown, RN is in the room with him now
N	**Next** • What will happen next? Anticipated changes? What is the PLAN? Contingency plans?	• Holding PT • I will await resumption orders for PT from you

Continued

TABLE 21.1	**Examples of Hand-off Tools With Scenarios—cont'd**	
IPASS		
I	**Illness Severity** • Stable, "watcher," unstable	• Unstable
P	**Patient Summary** • Summary statement • Events leading up to the admission • Hospital course • Ongoing assessment • Plan	• Mr. Bob Thomas was admitted two days ago with chest pain • He is now complaining of chest pain when sitting on the edge of the bed. He is confused, pale, diaphoretic, and weak • I will hold PT at this time and will await the resumption of care orders
A	**Action List** • To-do list • Timeline and ownership	• I have returned him to the bed, and the nurse (Jill Brown) is in the room with him now
S	**Situation Awareness & Contingency Planning** • Know what is going on • Plan for what might happen	• He has an altered cardiovascular response to activity that is a change from yesterday
S	**Synthesis by Receiver** • The receiver summarizes what was heard • Asks questions • Restates key action/to-do items	• Dr. Jones's questions and response: • How was he feeling lying in bed before sitting up? • Has he had a bowel movement/passed any blood in his stool? • Does he have any nausea or vomiting? • Yes, please hold PT at this time, and I will order STAT labs and speak with the RN, Jill Brown

Adapted from Leonard, M., Bonacum, D., & Graham, S. (2017). *SBAR: Situation-background-assessment-recommendation*, example 1. https://www.mhanet.com/mhaimages/SQI/3_IHI%20SBAR%20tool.pdf; Department of Defense (2005).
Department of Defense Patient Safety Program: Healthcare communications toolkit to improve transitions in care, p. 3. https://login.ssmhealth.com/MyHR/Shared%20Documents/Nurse%20Residency%20Program%20Material/Class%206/I%20Pass%20The%20Baton%20REFERENCE.pdf; and Starmer, A. J., Spector, N. D., Srivastova, R., Allen, A. D., Landrigan, C. P., SEctish, T. C., & the I-PASS Study Group. (2012). *I-PASS, a mnemonic to standardize verbal hand-offs*, p. 203. https://www.ipassinstitute.com/hubfs/I-PASS-mnemonic.pdf

Rehabilitation Services and Teamwork for Effective Care Coordination

Teamwork facilitates effective care coordination with clear communication and smooth transitions (Lamb & Newhouse, 2018). The IOM report *To Err Is Human* proposed promoting effective team functioning to positively impact continuity of care and prevent errors in care such as an incomplete or incorrect plan of care (POC) (Kohn et al., 2000). Teams in healthcare function through interprofessional collaboration (IPC) to successfully attain the goal of efficient, coordinated, high-quality care (Wong et al., 2016).

Healthcare teams are members from various disciplines and professions, such as physicians, nurse practitioners, registered nurses (RN), physical therapists (PT), occupational therapists (OT), speech-language pathologists, and medical social workers. Each discipline or profession has a distinct educational and practice background with a unique focus and patient care goals. Lancaster et al. (2015) compared the dynamics of interdisciplinary communication and collaboration to an orchestra, with each member experiencing care from a different perspective. The individual's perspective is underpinned by their unique knowledge, expertise, and experience. Collaboration is paramount to producing a symphony of efficient patient care as with an orchestra.

TeamSTEPPS

Healthcare teams' effective and safe patient care requires planning, cultivation, training, and practice (Clancy & Tornberg, 2019). TeamSTEPPS is an evidence-based curriculum developed by the DOD in collaboration with AHRQ to promote quality and safety in healthcare (Clancy & Tornberg, 2019; King et al., 2008; Wong et al., 2016). The curriculum fosters mutual respect of the team members and is focused on four areas: team leadership, situation monitoring, mutual support, and communication (Clancy & Tornberg, 2019).

Interprofessional Education Competencies Collaborative

In 2010, the WHO released a *Framework for Action on Interprofessional Education and Collaborative Practice* to alleviate the global shortage of healthcare workers and improve individual and population health outcomes through collaborative care (WHO, 2010). The framework is based on more than 50 years of research indicating that effective collaborative care results from effective interprofessional education (WHO, 2010). Fig. 21.6 demonstrates the positive effects of IPE, resulting in a collaborative-practice ready workforce that strengthens health systems and improves health outcomes.

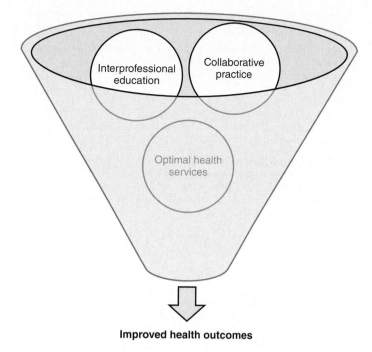

Improved health outcomes

• **Fig. 21.6** WHO Framework for Action on Interprofessional Education and Collaborative Practice. (From https://www.who.int/publications/i/item/framework-for-action-on-interprofessional-education-collaborative-practice)

Interprofessional education (IPE) is defined as "when students from two or more professions learn about, from, and with each other to enable effective collaboration and improve health outcomes" (WHO, 2010, p.10). IPE participants benefit by improving team communication skills, developing respect for other health professions, eliminating harmful stereotypes, and establishing patient-centered practice (WHO, 2010). IPE is the foundation for effective care coordination and improved quality and safety in healthcare.

Interprofessional Education Collaborative (IPEC)

IPEC was established in 2009 to prepare future healthcare workers for team-based practice for improved health outcomes (IPEC, 2016). In 2011, the collaboration of professionals from six founding disciplines (i.e., dentistry, nursing, medicine, osteopathic medicine, pharmacy, and public health) published core competencies for interprofessional practice. The *IPEC Core Competencies for Interprofessional Collaborative Practice* was updated in 2016 to reaffirm, organize and broaden the competencies originally released in 2011. Due to the extensive dissemination of the 2011 and 2016 competencies, interest in interprofessional education has surged, and the IPEC expanded to include 21 national associations (Table 21.2) (IPEC, 2022b).

The 2016 IPEC core competencies are values/ethics for interprofessional practice, roles/responsibilities, interprofessional communication, and teams and teamwork, as outlined in Fig. 21.7 (IPEC, 2016). In 2021, IPEC launched a working group to revise the core competencies to utilize

TABLE 21.2	**IPEC Members: National Associations**

- Accreditation Council for Education in Nutrition and Dietetics (ACEND)
- American Association of Colleges of Nursing (AACN)
- American Association of Colleges of Osteopathic Medicine (AACOM)
- American Association of Colleges of Pharmacy (AACP)
- American Association of Colleges of Podiatric Medicine (AACPM)
- American Association for Respiratory Care (AARC)
- American Council of Academic Physical Therapy (ACAPT)
- American Dental Education Association (ADEA)
- American Occupational Therapy Association (AOTA)
- American Psychological Association (APA)
- American Speech-Language Hearing Association (ASHA)
- Association of Academic Health Sciences Libraries (AAHSL)
- Association of American Medical Colleges (AAMC)
- Association of American Veterinary Medical Colleges (AAVMC)
- Association of Chiropractic Colleges (ACC)
- Association of Schools and Colleges of Optometry (ASCO)
- Association of Schools and Programs of Public Health (ASAHP)
- Council on Social Work Education (CSWE)
- National League for Nursing (NLN)
- Physician Assistant Education Association (PAEA)

Note: List of national association members can be found at https://www.ipecollaborative.org/membership

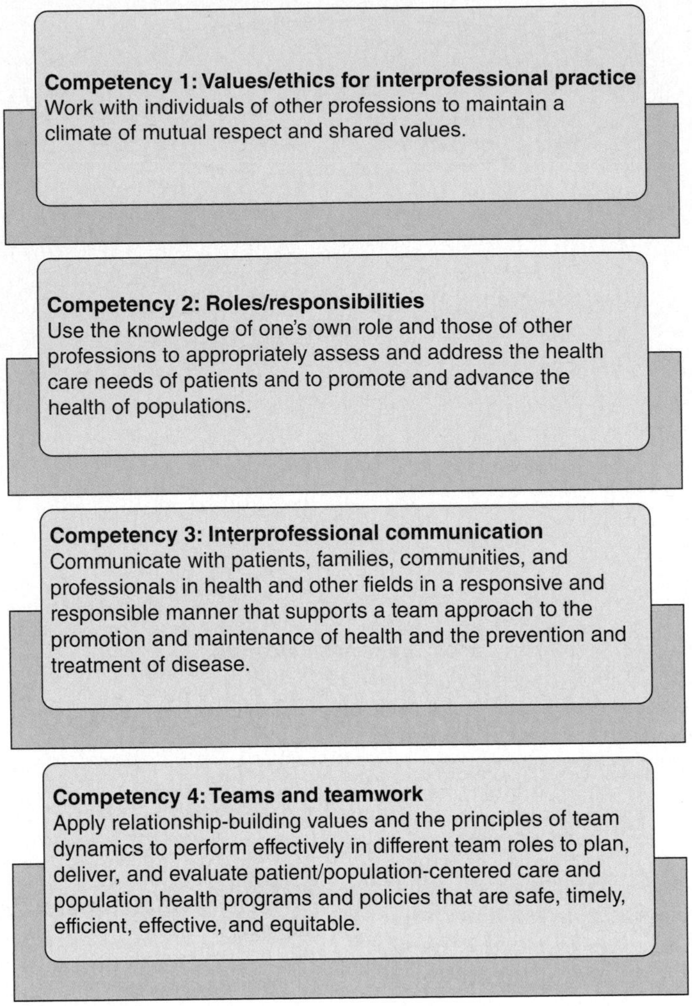

• **Fig. 21.7** Core Competencies for Interprofessional Collaborative Practice. (Adapted from Interprofessional Education Collaborative (2016). *Core competencies for interprofessional collaborative practice: 2016 update*, p. 10. https://www.ipecollaborative.org/ipec-core-competencies)

updated research related to IPE and collaborative practice (CP) (IPEC, 2022a). The tentative release date of the updated competencies is 2023.

Physical Therapy Interprofessional Education and Practice

The American Physical Therapy Association (APTA) is a supporting organization of IPEC and recommends the incorporation of the IPEC core competencies for interprofessional collaborative practice into education and practice initiatives through position statement HOD P06-19-69-33 (APTA, 2019). The APTA *Standards of Practice for Physical Therapy* identifies coordination as one of the 10 standards for administering physical therapy services (APTA, 2020). "Physical therapy personnel collaborate with all health services providers and with patients, clients, caregivers, and others as appropriate; and use a team and person-centered approach in coordinating and providing physical therapist services" (APTA, 2020, p. 3).

The PT collaborates with the patient and those pertinent to the patient's care in developing a plan of care and management

plan (APTA, 2020). The PT's patient management responsibilities include communication, coordination, and documentation of all aspects of care. Communication is the sharing of information regarding patient care and includes the patient, physical therapy staff, and other disciplines involved in the patient's course of care (APTA, 2018). Patient management documentation is a critical professional and legal responsibility in quality patient outcomes (APTA, 2018). Documentation consists of any entry in the patient's medical record and should demonstrate evidence-based practice, patient-centered care, cultural competence, and a record of the patient's clinical course of care. Documentation should be clear and function as a communication tool between physical therapy personnel and other disciplines.

Physical Therapy Core Competencies for Entry-Level Practice in Acute Care

The acute care PT requires the ability to efficiently analyze and implement specialized knowledge and skills in an evolving environment to communicate the appropriate needs

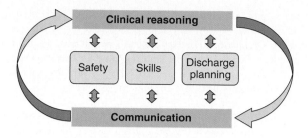

• **Fig. 21.8** The Five Areas of Core Competencies for Entry-Level Practice in Acute Care Physical Therapy. (From Greenwood, K., Stewart, E., Milton, E., Hake, Mitchell, L, & Sanders, B. (2015). *Core competencies for entry-level practice in acute care physical therapy*, p. 4. https://www.aptaacutecare.org/page/corecompetencies)

regarding physical therapy with the patient, family/caregiver, and interprofessional healthcare team (Greenwood et al., 2015). The APTA outlined five core competencies for entry-level PTs in acute care: clinical decision-making, communication, safety, patient management, and discharge planning. Collaboration with the interprofessional team, patient, and family is a consistent entry-level activity in all five core competencies. Fig. 21.8 represents the continuous relationship between the five core competencies.

Occupational Therapy Interprofessional Education and Practice

Occupational therapy began as an interprofessional discipline (Robinson et al., 2016). In 1917, the National Society for the Promotion of Occupation Therapy, now known as The American Occupational Therapy Association (AOTA), was created to promote the profession of occupational therapy. The six founders were from diverse professions, such as OTs, RNs, art educators, architects, and physicians (Hattjar, 2018). The origin of occupational therapy evolved from a need to care for individuals with physical or psychiatric illnesses holistically and compassionately. The founders impressed the importance of a therapeutic relationship with the patient and developing a patient-centered treatment plan focused on the patient's environment, values, goals, and desires (AOTA, 2020).

AOTA is a supporting member of IPEC and has developed interprofessional education standards through the Accreditation Council for Occupational Therapy Education (ACOTE) (IPEC, 2016). ACOTE is the accrediting agency for AOTA establishing, enforcing, and maintaining educational standards for occupational therapy and occupational therapy assistant programs (ACOTE, 2022a). The 2018 ACOTE standards address care coordination, case management, and interprofessional team dynamics (ACOTE, 2022b). Standard B.4.20 Care Coordination, Case Management, and Transition Services state that OT providers (OTs and Occupational Therapy Assistants) should participate to the extent of their education in traditional and emerging practice environments. Standard B.4.25 Principles of

Interprofessional Team Dynamics states that all levels of OT providers should:

> *Demonstrate knowledge of the principles of interprofessional team dynamics to perform effectively in different team roles to plan, deliver, and evaluate patient- and population-centered care as well as population health programs and policies that are safe, timely, efficient, effective, and equitable.* (ACOTE, 2022b, p. 33)

The AOTA *Occupational Therapy Scope of Practice* identifies care coordination, case management, and transition services as a component of the practice of OT in the definition for use in state regulations (AOTA, 2021a). The AOTA *Standards of Practice for Occupational Therapy* include in Standard I, the responsibilities of the OTs to function as effective advocates for the client, providing client-centered services, and practicing as an integral member of the interprofessional collaborative (AOTA, 2021b).

OT practitioners are well equipped to participate in care coordination and case management, as the educational curriculum includes functional assessments, task analysis, environmental assessments, adaptation, compensation, and remediation (Robinson et al., 2016). OT students learn how psychosocial, physical, cognitive, cultural, and environmental supports affect the patient's functional status, communicate with the patient and family effectively, and collaborate with other providers (Moyers & Metzler, 2014).

Physical Therapy, Occupational Therapy, and Primary Care

The Commonwealth Fund's *Mirror, Mirror 2021* report highlights the deficits of the United States healthcare system (Schneider et al., 2021). Fragmented care, the increasing prevalence of chronic disease, and diminishing access to primary care in the United States have worsened care outcomes and increased costs. A significant distinguishing feature of countries that outperform the United States is an investment in primary care. Primary care utilization is associated with improved medical outcomes; however, utilization of primary care in the United States is decreasing (Primary Care Collaborative [PCC], 2020).

Care coordination primarily occurs in the primary care setting (McDonald et al., 2007). Practitioners in PT and OT are well positioned to practice in primary care (Garber, 2020; Halle et al., 2018; Moyers & Metzler, 2014). Integrating PT and OT practitioners in a primary care setting can decrease the burden on the primary care provider (PCP), increase the capacity of care of the practice, and improve patient outcomes (Bodenheimer et al., 2021; Halle et al., 2018).

Musculoskeletal conditions are the leading cause of morbidity in the United States, account for a significant cost in care, and are a frequent cause of primary care visits (Carvalho et al., 2018). The PT embedded in a primary care practice can primarily manage the patient with a musculoskeletal complaint, thus potentially improving access to care, decreasing cost, improving patient satisfaction, and cost savings (Garber, 2020).

OT practitioners are well equipped to improve patient outcomes as interprofessional team members in the primary care setting (Halle et al., 2018). The OT practitioner is uniquely situated to function as a case manager in primary care (Robinson, 2016). By focusing on a holistic approach to care through health promotion, patient-centered goals, social support evaluation, environmental situation evaluation, and physical evaluation, the OT can assist the patient in achieving mental and physical outcomes (Robinson, 2016).

Achieving the quadruple aim and improving patient care with care coordination is possible through interprofessional teamwork (Bodenheimer & Sinsky, 2014). Primary care is the basis for quality patient care while decreasing costs (PCC, 2020). Better health outcomes are associated with a larger supply of primary care providers. As the United States population outgrows the primary care workforce (PCC, 2020), PT and OT practitioners are poised to fill the gaps (Bodenheimer et al., 2021; Halle et al., 2018).

References

Accreditation Council of Occupational Therapy Education. (2022a). *About.* https://acoteonline.org/about/.

Accreditation Council for Occupational Therapy Education. (2022b, January). *2018 Accreditation Council for Occupational Therapy Education (ACOTE) standards and interpretive guide.* https://acoteonline.org/accreditation-explained/standards/.

Administration on Aging. (2021). *2020 profile of older Americans.* Administration for Community Living. https://acl.gov/sites/default/files/Aging%20and%20Disability%20in%20America/2020ProfileOlderAmericans.Final_.pdf.

Agency for Healthcare Research and Quality. (2016a). *Agency for healthcare research and quality: A profile.* https://www.ahrq.gov/cpi/about/profile/index.html.

Agency for Healthcare Research and Quality. (2016b). *The national quality strategy: Fact sheet.* https://www.ahrq.gov/workingforquality/about/nqs-fact-sheets/fact-sheet.html.

Agency for Healthcare Research and Quality. (2019, September). *Patient safety 101: Hand-offs and signouts.* Patient Safety Network. https://psnet.ahrq.gov/primer/handoffs-and-signouts.

Agency for Healthcare Research and Quality. (2020). *Pocket guide: Team STEPPS.* https://www.ahrq.gov/teamstepps/instructor/essentials/pocketguide.html.

Agency for Healthcare Research and Quality. (2021). *Defining the PCMH.* https://www.ahrq.gov/ncepcr/tools/pcmh/defining/index.html.

American Academy of Pediatrics. (2014). Patient-and family-centered care coordination: A framework for integrating care for children and youth across multiple systems. *Pediatrics, 133*(5), e1451–e1460.

American Geriatrics Society Expert Panel on Person-Centered Care. (2016). Person-centered care: A definition and essential elements. *Journal of the American Geriatrics Society, 64*(1), 15–18.

American Occupational Therapy Association. (2020). Occupational therapy practice framework: Domain and process fourth edition. *The American Journal of Occupational Therapy, 74*(2), 7412410010p1–7412410010p87.

American Occupational Therapy Association. (2021a). Occupational therapy scope of practice. *The American Journal of Occupational Therapy, 75*(Suppl. 3), 7513410020. http://research.aota.org/ajot/

article_pdf/75/Supplement_3/7513410020/73923/7513410020.pdf.

American Occupational Therapy Association. (2021b). Standards of practice for occupational therapy. *The American Journal of Occupational Therapy, 75*(Suppl. 3), 7513410030. http://research.aota.org/ajot/article-pdf/75/Supplement_3/7513410030/73808/7513410030.pdf.

American Physical Therapy Association. (2018, May 18). *Documentation overview.* https://www.apta.org/your-practice/documentation/overview.

American Physical Therapy Association. (2019). *Commitment to interprofessional education and practice.* https://www.apta.org/apta-and-you/leadership-and-governance/policies/commitment-to-interprofessional-education-and-practice.

American Physical Therapy Association. (2020). *Standards of practice for physical therapy.* https://www.apta.org/siteassets/pdfs/policies/standards-of-practice-pt.pdf.

Antonelli, R. C., McAllister, J. W., & Popp, J. (2009). *Making care coordination a critical component of the pediatric health system: A multidisciplinary framework.* Commonwealth Fund. https://www.commonwealthfund.org/publications/fund-reports/2009/may/making-care-coordination-critical-component-pediatric-health.

Apaydin, E. A., Rose, D. E., McClean, M. R., Yano, E. M., Shekelli, P. G., Nelson, K. M., & Stockdale, S. E. (2021). Association between care coordination tasks on non-VA community care and VA PCP burnout: An analysis of a national cross-sectional survey. *BMC Health Services Research, 21,* 809.

Bartels, S. J., Gill, L., & Naslund, J. A. (2015). The Affordable Care Act, accountable care organizations, and mental health care for older adults: Implications and opportunities. *Harvard Review of Psychiatry, 23*(5), 304–319.

Beck da Silva Etges, A. P., Ruschel, K. B., Polanczyk, C. A., & Urman, R. D. (2020). Advances in value-based healthcare by application of time-driven activity-based costing for inpatient management: A systematic review. *Value in Health, 23*(6), 812–823.

Berwick, D. M., Nolan, T. W., & Whittington, J. (2008). The triple aim: Care, health, and cost. *Health Affairs, 27*(3), 759–769.

Bodenheimer, T., Kucksdorf, J., Torn, Al., & Jerzak, J. (2021). Integrating physical therapists into primary care within a large health care system. *Journal of the American Board of Family Medicine, 34*(4), 866–870. https://www.jabfm.org/content/34/4/866.

Bodenheimer, T., & Sinsky, C. (2014). From triple to quadruple aim: Care of the patient requires care of the provider. *Annals of Family Medicine, 12*(6), 573–576.

Boersma, P., Black, L. I., & Ward, B. W. (2020). Prevalence of multiple chronic conditions among US adults, 2018. *Preventing Chronic Disease, 17,* E106. https://www.cdc.gov/pcd/issues/2020/pdf/20_0130.pdf.

Cady, R., Bushaw, A., Davis, H., Mills, J., & Thomasson, D. (2020). Care coordination for children with medical complexity. *The Nurse Practitioner, 45*(6), 11–17. doi:10.1097/01.NPR.0000666172.10978.4f.

Carvalho, E., Bettger, J. P., Bowlby, L., Carvalho, M., Dore, D., Corcoran, M. W., Harris, A. A., Bond, J., & Gooded, A. P. (2018). Integration of musculoskeletal physical therapy care in the patient-centered medical home (IMPaC): Protocol for a single site randomized clinical trial. *BMJ Open, 8,* e022953.

Centers for Medicare & Medicaid Services. (2021). *Accountable Care Organizations (ACOs).* https://www.cms.gov/Medicare/Medicare-Fee-for-Service-Payment/ACO.

Cesta, T. (2018). *Coordination of care and the role of the case manager.* Relias Media. https://www.reliasmedia.com/articles/142793-coordination-of-care-and-the-role-of-the-case-manager.

Clancy, C. M., & Tornberg, D. N. (2019). TeamSTEPPS: Assuring Optimal teamwork in clinical settings. *American Journal of Medical Quality, 34*(5), 436–438. https://journals.sagepub.com/doi/10.1177/1062860607300616.

Department of Defense. (2005). *Department of Defense Patient Safety Program: Healthcare communications toolkit to improve transitions in care.* https://login.ssmhealth.com/MyHR/Shared%20Documents/Nurse%20Residency%20Program%20Material/Class%206/I%20Pass%20The%20Baton%20REFERENCE.pdf.

Doty, M. M., Tikkanen, R., Shah, A., & Schneider, E. C. (2019). *International survey: Primary care physicians in US struggle more to coordinate care and communicate with other providers but offer patients more health IT tools.* The Commonwealth Fund. https://www.commonwealthfund.org/publications/journal-article/2019/dec/international-survey-primary-care-physicians-eleven-countries

Doty, M. M., Tikkanen, R., Shah, A., & Schneider, E. C. (2020). Primary care physicians' role in coordinating medical and health-related social needs in eleven countries. *Health Affairs, 39*(1), 115–123.

Fennelly, O., Grogan, L., Reed, A., & Hardiker, N. R. (2021). Use of standardized terminologies in clinical practice: A scoping review. *International Journal of Medical Informatics, 149,* 1–11.

Garber, M. B. (2020). Physical therapists in the patient centered medical home: Improving cost, quality, and access. *Orthopaedic Practice, 32*(3), 127–129. https://www.orthopt.org/uploads/content_files/files/127%20Physical%20Therapists%20in%20the%20Patient.pdf.

Greenwood, K., Stewart, E., Milton, E., Hake, M. L., & Sanders, B. (2015). *Core competencies for entry-level practice in acute care physical therapy.* APTA Acute Care. https://www.aptaacutecare.org/page/corecompetencies.

Halle, A. D., Mroz, T. M., Fogelberg, D. J., & Leland, N. E. (2018). Occupational therapy and primary care: Updates and trends. *The American Journal of Occupational Therapy, 72*(3), 7203090010p1–7203090010p6.

Hattjar, B. (Ed.). (2018). *Fundamentals of occupational therapy: An introduction to the profession.* Thorofare, NJ: SLACK.

Institute of Medicine. (2001). *Crossing the quality chasm: A new health system for the 21st Century.* Washington, D.C.: The National Academies Press.

Institute of Medicine. (2003). *Priority areas for national action: Transforming health care quality.* http://nap.edu/10593.

Interprofessional Education Collaborative. (2016). *Core competencies for interprofessional collaborative practice.* https://www.ipecollaborative.org/ipec-core-competencies.

Interprofessional Education Collaborative. (2022a). *IPEC core competencies revision, 2021-2023.* https://www.ipecollaborative.org/index.php?option=com_content&view=article&id=70:2021-2023-core-competencies-revision&catid=20:site-content&Itemid=158.

Interprofessional Education Collaborative. (2022b). *Membership.* https://www.ipecollaborative.org/membership.

King, H. B., Battles, J., Baker, D. P., Alonso, A., Salas, E., Webster, J., Toomey, L., & Salisbury, M. (2008). TeamSTEPPS: Team Strategies and Tools to Enhance Performance and Patient Safety. In Henriksen, K., et al. (Eds.), *Advances in patient safety: New directions and alternative approaches (Vol. 3: Performance and Tools).* Agency for Healthcare Research and Quality. https://www.ncbi.nlm.nih.gov/books/NBK43686/.

Kohn, L. T., Corrigan, J. M., & Donaldson, M. S. (Eds.). (2000). *To err is human: Building a safer health system.* The National Academies Press.

Kuo, D. Z., McAllister, J. W., Rossignol, L., Turchi, R. M., & Stille, C. J. (2018). Care coordination for children with medical complexity: Whose care is it, anyway? *Pediatrics, 141*(Suppl. 3), s223–s232.

Lamb, G., & Newhouse, R. (2018). *Care coordination: A blueprint for action for RNs.* American Nurses Association.

Lancaster, G., Kalakowsky-Hayner, S., Kovacich, J., & Greer-Williams, N. (2015). Interdisciplinary communication and collaboration among physicians, nurses, and unlicensed assistive personnel. *Journal of Nursing Scholarship, 47*(3), 275–284.

Leonard, M., Bonacum, D., & Graham, S. (2017). *SBAR: Situation-background-assessment-recommendation.* Institute for Healthcare Improvement. https://www.mhanet.com/mhaimages/SQI/3_IHI%20SBAR%20tool.pdf.

Maternal and Child Health Bureau. (2021). *Children and youth with special health care needs (CYSHCN).* Health Resources & Services Administration. https://mchb.hrsa.gov/programs-impact/focus-areas/children-youth-special-health-care-needs-cyshcn#:,:text=CYSHCN%20are%20children%20who%20have,that%20required%20by%20children%20generally.

McDonald, K. M., Sundaram, V., Bravata, D. M., Lewis, R., Lin, N., Kraft, S. A., McKinnon, M., Paguntalan, H., & Owens, D. K. (2007). *Closing the quality gap: A critical analysis of quality improvement strategies volume 7—care coordination [Technical Review Number 9].* Agency for Healthcare Research and Quality. https://www.ncbi.nlm.nih.gov/books/NBK44015/pdf/Bookself_NBK44015.pdf.

McDonald, K. M., Schultz, E., Albin, L., Pineda, N., Lonhart, J., Sundaram, V., Smith-Spangler, C., Brustrom, J., Malcolm, E., Rohn, L., & Davies, S. (2014). *Care coordination atlas: version 4.* Agency for Healthcare Research and Quality. https://www.ahrq.gov/ncepcr/care/coordination/atlas.html.

Moyers, P. A., & Metzler, C. A. (2014). Interprofessional collaborative practice in care coordination. *The American Journal of Occupational Therapy, 68*(5), 500–505.

Namburi, N., & Lee, L. S. (2021). *National quality forum.* StatPearls. https://www.ncbi.nlm.nih.gov/books/NBK549854/.

National Academy for State Health Policy. (2020). *National care coordination standards for children and youth with special health care needs.* https://www.nashp.org/national-care-coordination-standards-for-children-and-youth-with-special-health-care-needs/#toggle-id-1.

National Academies of Sciences, Engineering, and Medicine. (2019). *Taking action against clinician burnout: A systems approach to professional well-being.* The national Academies Press.

National Academies Press. (2022). *Quality chasm collection.* https://www.nap.edu/collection/62/quality-chasm.

National Quality Forum. (2012) *Care coordination endorsement maintenance2012: Phases 1 and 2 [Technical Report].* https://www.qualityforum.org/Projects/c-d/Care_Coordination_Endorsement_Maintenance/Care_Coordination_Endorsement_Maintenance.aspx.

National Quality Forum. (2021). *Leveraging electronic health record (EHR)-Sourced measures to improve care communication and coordination [Literature Review Draft #4].* https://www.qualityforum.org/EHR_Care-Coordination.aspx.

National Transitions of Care Coalition. (2008). *Improving on transitions of care: How to implement and evaluate a plan.* https://pdf4pro.com/amp/view/the-national-transitions-of-care-coalition-ntocc-1e4edb.html.

National Transitions of Care Coalition. (2010). *Improving transitions of care: Findings and considerations of the vision of the national transitions of care coalition.* https://pdf4pro.com/amp/view/improving-transitions-of-care-ntocc-org-1d4d7f.html.

O'Connor, S. (2020). *EHR vs EMR: What are the key differences.* Advanced Data Systems Corporation. https://www.adsc.com/blog/ehr-vs-emr-what-are-the-key-differences.

Office of the National Coordinator for Health Information Technology. (2019). *Meaningful use.* HealthIT.gov. https://www.healthit.gov/topic/meaningful-use-and-macra/meaningful-use.

Office of the National Coordinator for Health Information Technology. (2021). *21st Century cures act.* HealthIT.gov. https://www.healthit.gov/topic/laws-regulation-and-policy/health-it-legislation.

Prasad, K., McLoughlin, C., Stillman, M., Poplau, S., Goelz, E., Taylor, S., Nankivil, N., Brown, R., Linzer, M., Cappelucci, K., Barouche, M., & Sinsky, C. A. (2021). Prevalence and correlates of stress and burnout among US healthcare workers during the COVID-19 pandemic: A national cross-sectional survey study. *EClinical Medicine, 35,* 100879.

Primary Care Collaborative. (2020). *Primary care spending: High stakes, low investment.* https://www.pcpcc.org/sites/default/files/resources/PCC_Primary_Care_Spending_2020.pdf.

Robinson, M., Fisher, T. F., & Broussard, K. (2016). Role of occupational therapy in case management and care coordination for clients with complex conditions. *The American Journal of Occupational Therapy, 70*(2), 7002090010p1–7002090010p6.

Schneider, E. C., Shah, A., Doty, M. M., Tikkanen, R., Fields, K., & Williams, R. D. (2021). *Mirror, mirror 2021: Reflecting poorly healthcare in the US compared to other high-income countries.* Commonwealth Fund. https://www.commonwealthfund.org/publications/fund-reports/2021/aug/mirror-mirror-2021-reflecting-poorly.

Starmer, A. J., Spector, N. D., Srivastova, R., Allen, A. D., Landrigan, C. P., Sectish, T. C., & the I-PASS Study Group. (2012). I-Pass, a mnemonic to standardize verbal hand-offs. *Pediatrics, 129*(2), 201–204.

The Joint Commission. (2017). *Sentinel event alert 58: Inadequate hand-off communication.* https://www.jointcommission.org/resources/patient-safety-topics/sentinel-event/sentinel-event-alert-newsletters/sentinel-event-alert-58-inadequate-hand-off-communication/#.YkSGbChKiUl.

The Joint Commission. (2018). *The Joint Commission fact sheet: Official "do not use" list.* https://www.jointcommission.org/-/media/tjc/documents/resources/patient-safety-topics/patient-safety/do_not_use_list_9_14_18.pdf.

Tikkanen, R., & Abrams, M. K. (2020). *US health care from a global perspective, 2019: Higher spending, worse outcomes?* Commonwealth Fund.

Tikkanen, R., Osborn, R., Mossialos, E., Djordjevic, A., & Wharton, G. A. (2020). *International health care system profiles: United States.* Commonwealth Fund. https://www.commonwealthfund.org/international-health-policy-center/countries/united-states#ensuring-quality-of-care.

US Department of Health and Human Services. (2017). *HITECH Act enforcement interim final rule.* Health Information Privacy. https://www.hhs.gov/hipaa/for-professionals/special-topics/hitech-act-enforcement-interim-final-rule/index.html.

Wadhwa, R., & Boehning, A. P. (2021, March). The Joint Commission. In *StatPearls.* StatPearls Publishing. https://www.ncbi.nlm.nih.gov/books/NBK557846/?report=printable.

Wakefield, M. K. (2008). *Patient safety and quality: An evidence-based handbook for nurses.* Agency for Healthcare Research and Quality. https://www.ncbi.nlm.nih.gov/books/NBK2677/.

Wong, A. H. W., Gang, M., Szyld, D., & Mahoney, H. (2016). Making an "attitude adjustment" using a simulation-enhanced interprofessional education strategy to improve attitudes toward teamwork and communication. *Simulation in Healthcare, 11*(2), 117–125.

World Health Organization. (2010). *Framework for action on interprofessional education & collaborative practice.* https://www.who.int/publications/i/item/framework-for-action-on-interprofessional-education-collaborative-practice.

Index

Note: page numbers followed by "b" indicate boxes, "f" indicate figures, and "t" indicate tables.

TTM. *see* Transtheoretical model
Turf war, interprofessional collaboration and, 66–67

U
UHC. *see* Universal Health Care
Underinsured, 208–209t
Uninsured, 208–209t
Unit limits, of insurance, 208–209t
Units per visit, for physical therapy practices, 243
Universal Health Care (UHC), 2, 3b
Unstructured opportunities, for professional development, 101–103
  continuing education courses, 101–102
  other certification, 103, 104t
  specialist or advanced certification, 102–103, 103t, 104t
US Central Intelligence Agency World Fact Book, 20
US Department of Health and Human Services (USDHHS), 19, 62
US Department of Housing and Urban Development (HUD), 22
US Department of Veterans Affairs, 33
US healthcare systems, 1–17
  contemporary health reform era, 14
  contemporary public and population health in, 14
  corporate era, 14
  development and reform of, 9–10
  factors impacting, 2t
  health disparity in, 12–13, 12f
    paradigm shift, 13, 13f
    substance abuse, 12–13
  historical overview of, 2–6
  national health insurance programs in, 10–12
    Medicare and Medicaid, 10–11, 11f
    State Children's Health Insurance Program, 11–12
  origins of, 3–6, 4f
  social influences on, 6–9
    of disease, 8–9, 8f, 9f
    war, 6–7, 6f, 7t

V
Validity, of data-informed care, 200
Value, of data-informed care, 200
Value proposition, 238–239
Variety, of data-informed care, 200
Velocity, of data-informed care, 199
Veracity
  of data-informed care, 200
  in healthcare, 81
  principles of, 84t

Verbal communication, 145–146
Verification, of insurance, 208–209t
Veterans affairs (VA) coverage, 215–216t
Veterans Healthcare Administration (VHA), 33
Vietnam War, physical therapy during, 93, 93f
Virtual reality (VR), 56, 56f
Virtue ethics, 80
Vision, 73–77
  of American Medical Association, 74, 74f
  of American Occupational Therapy Association, 75–77, 77f, 77t, 78f
  of American Physical Therapy Association, 75, 76f, 76t
  for business ideas, 234–236, 236t
  of organization, 179, 179f
  of World Health Organization, 74, 75f
Visit limits, of insurance, 208–209t
Visualization, of data-informed care, 200
Volatility, of data-informed care, 200
Volume, of data-informed care, 199
VR. *see* Virtual reality
Vulnerability, of data-informed care, 200

W
Wantivation, 340
Waste, 209–210
  monitoring of, 210
  steps to avoid, 210
Wheelchair seating and mobility, 59
WHO. *see* World Health Organization
Whole School, Whole Community, Whole Child Model (WSCC), 316
Workers' compensation, 215–216t
Workers' compensation, reimbursement and, 262
World Health Organization (WHO), core values, mission, and vision, 74, 75f
World War I
  occupational therapy during, 90
  physical therapy during, 93
World War II
  occupational therapy during, 90, 91f
  physical therapy during, 93
Written communication, 148–149
  HIPAA, 148–149, 149b

Z
Zero reject policy, 299